SEPSIS – AN ONGOING AND SIGNIFICANT CHALLENGE

Edited by **Luciano Azevedo**

Sepsis – An Ongoing and Significant Challenge
http://dx.doi.org/10.5772/2958
Edited by Luciano Azevedo

Contributors

Johan Sebastián Hernández Botero, María Cristina Florián Pérez, Safiah Mai, Momina Khan, Patricia Liaw, Alison Fox-Robichaud, Neville Azzopardi, Manuel Fenech, Tonio Piscopo, Ayse Belin Ozer, Mustafa Bayar, Peixin Huang, Ding You Li, Daniel P. Heruth, Li Qin Zhang, Dmitry N. Grigoryev, Shui Qing Ye, Ricardo Fernandez, Claudio Acuña-Castillo, Zeljko Lausevic, Mirjana Lausevic, Lixin Xie, Aristotelis Perrakis, Volker Müller, Werner Hohenberger, Roland S. Croner, Radha Swathe Priya M., Emma P. Córcoles, Bernhard Resch, Nora Hofer, Wilhelm Müller, C. Savagner, B. Leboucher, G. Gascoin-Lachambre, C. Gras-Leguen, Efraín Riveros Pérez, Marilynn R. Fairfax, Hossein Salimnia, Andries William Dreyer, Renato Finkelstein, Ilana Oren, Rekha Chandran, Morgan Hakki, Stephen Spurgeon, F.J. García-Miguel, Marie Mullen

Published by InTech
Janeza Trdine 9, 51000 Rijeka, Croatia

Publishing Process Manager Mirna Cvijic
Technical Editor InTech Prepress, Novi Sad
Cover InTech Design team

Additional hard copies can be obtained from orders@intechopen.com

Hydrogen Storage, Edited by Lianjun Liu
p. cm.
ISBN 978-953-51-0731-6

For EU product safety concerns:
IN TECH d.o.o., Prolaz Marije Krucifikse Kozulić 3, 51000 Rijeka, Croatia,
info@intechopen.com or visit our website at intechopen.com.

Meet the editor

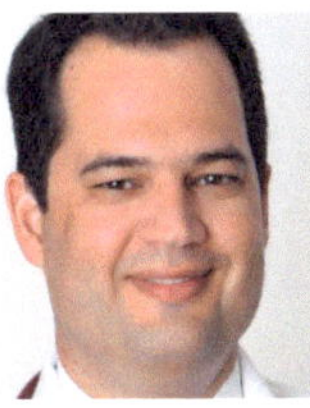

Dr. Luciano Azevedo obtained his medical degree from Federal University of Paraíba, Brazil, in 1996. After deciding to study critical care, he moved to São Paulo where he finished medical residencies in Internal Medicine and Critical Care Medicine at the University of São Paulo in 1998 and 1999, respectively. By this time, he was completely absorbed by the study of sepsis and this led him to complete his PhD in this area at the University of São Paulo in 2004. Nowadays, he is a professor at the Emergency Medicine Department at the University of São Paulo and the coordinator of the Intensive Care and Anesthesiology Experimental Laboratory at the Instituto Sirio-Libanes de Ensino e Pesquisa in São Paulo. He is author of 50 peer-review articles and 32 book chapters, has edited three books and served as a reviewer for 15 journals in the fields of intensive care, anesthesiology and translational science.

Contents

Preface

Sepsis, the inflammatory response after an infection, comprises a spectrum of conditions ranging from systemic inflammatory response syndrome to septic shock and multisystem organ failure, the deadly forms of the disease. Sepsis is the major cause of death in non-cardiologic intensive care units around the world. Every year, billions of dollars are consumed in the treatment of patients with this condition as well as in research in order to understand its complex pathophysiology and therefore obtain future therapeutic opportunities. Despite the efforts of the scientists and medical practitioners, the mortality rates are still very high, mainly for underdeveloped and developing countries. In addition, the annual incidence of the disease is increasing, probably due to progressive aging of the population, improvements in critical care support and in immunosuppressive therapies so that individuals with immunosuppression now have increased life expectancy.

In this book we intend to provide an update on several fields of this disease. Starting from the history of sepsis and finishing with treatment of sepsis-associated organ dysfunctions, this book offers a wide scope of well-written and complete reviews concerning several pathophysiological and therapeutic aspects of sepsis. We hope that the laborious work of the authors will provide an important forum of discussion on the topic, and increase the awareness of the healthcare team regarding the important aspects of early recognition and treatment of this severe condition.

I would also like to acknowledge the assistance of the publishing team and the invitation of the publisher to edit such an interesting and important book.

Finally, I would like to thank all of the authors for their excellent contributions.

Luciano CP Azevedo
State University of São Paulo School of Medicine
Federal University of São Paulo
Instituto Sirio-Libanes de Ensino e Pesquisa, São Paulo
Brazil

Section 1

History of Sepsis

Chapter 1

The History of Sepsis from Ancient Egypt to the XIX Century

Johan Sebastián Hernández Botero and María Cristina Florián Pérez

Additional information is available at the end of the chapter

http://dx.doi.org/10.5772/51484

1. Introduction

Throughout history, mankind has succumbed to endless infectious diseases which have been responsible of great historical changes; classic examples like "The Black Death" during the late Medieval period, a disease being the cause of profound demographical and social changes that prelude The Renaissance; we can also mention the smallpox epidemic during the New World conquest in the XVI century, a disease which was a direct cause of the pre-Columbian Mesoamerican cultures' holocaust. These are mere examples of well characterized infectious diseases which have had a definite contribution, among other factors, to the development of great scientific and historical changes. As oppose to these notoriously famous infectious diseases, sepsis cannot be categorized as a unique nosological entity studied by medical historians through the history of western medicine. This is the reason why we feel obliged to go beyond a simple description of sepsis throughout history from ancient Egypt to pre-modern times. Therefore, this text also intends to demonstrate how the study and clinical approach of the phenomena in the past, that we've come to know as sepsis, gave way to the development of many important medical revolutions in the XVI and XIX century, especially in the fields of surgery and microbiology respectively.

To make a historical detailed description of sepsis referred to a variety of nosologic entities such as pulmonary, intestinal and/or urinary tract infections is yet a very difficult task, perhaps an impossible one, the latter due to the heterogeneous character of its etiology, also the diverse clinical manifestations, its wide range of complications, these summoned to a whole array of concepts, theories and conjectures applied within many determined cultural contexts in their attempt to describe and understand the meaning of sepsis. Nevertheless, the phenomena we've come to know as sepsis, considered as a potential consequence of any type of wound, was a clinical phenomena well identify since the Ancient Egypt and can be traced as a defined clinical entity through western civilization history. The time relation between a wound and the appearance of fever was well recognized, as were also the signs of local inflammation and the secondary systemic involvement. This is the reason why we have chosen to approach the history of sepsis through the study of traumatic lesions, and its importance in the development of the germ theory and the rise of modern surgery. Having this approach, we're allow to understand the direct relation between trauma and infection and also the evolution in the concept of sepsis: from the birth of the word itself and its introduction as a medical concept, its etiology and pathophysiology as a disease, to the diverse forms of treatments proposed previous to contemporary medicine; all this in a fascinating journey from the ancient Egypt to the XIX century.

2. Historical evolution of the word sepsis and its introduction as a medical concept

The word sepsis has an unequivocal Greek origin derived mainly from the word [σηψις], which is the original Greek word for "decomposition of animal or vegetable organic matter". We come across the word for the first time in Homer's poems, where Sepsis is a derivative of the verb form sepo [σηπω] which means "I rot" (Geroulanos and Douka 2006). Homer used the word in the 24th song of the Iliad where Priam was led by Hermes, into the Greek camps to beg Achilles for the return of Hector`s body. In vers 414, when Priam is asked for his son`s body, a slave answers: "Neither hounds nor vultures have yet devoured him; he is still just lying at the tents by the ship of Achilles, and though it is now twelve days that he has lain there, his flesh is not wasted nor have the worms eaten him although they feed on warriors." At the end, the Greek hero Achilles is convinced by Priam to return the body and Hector's funerals are carried out (Lattimore 1961). The term is immersed in Greek classic literature and was used by authors like Aristotle among others. Its use and its concept in the ancient Greek world could be the object for a complete revision (Majno 1991). Later on, when we talk about Greece, we will expand this concept along with its antithesis: Pepsis and its importance in the Greek ars medica (see ahead in this chapter: "Ancient Greece: Giving birth to the word Sepsis.") In the context of medical literature we can find the word sepsis in the Hippocratic corpus (Hippocrates 1849; Geroulanos and Douka 2006), cited in the Epidemics book (B. 2,2, Prorret. I.99). Its use was related to an Egyptian concept that will be mentioned later and which explains the origin of some diseases as a consequence of self-intoxication with harmful products derived from the colon. Undoubtedly, the use of this word in Hippocratic literature gave cause to its persistence in some ancient books for more than 2500 years. However, its use as a medical term declined and, on the other hand, a big portion of the classic medical literature was unknown until the Renaissance, because of several philosophical and historical reasons implicit in the Middle Ages, so that the word sepsis, even though persisted in the dusty shelves of ancient collections, undoubtedly was of little use in the Medieval medical context. One of the first bibliographic references in a medical context appears thanks to Matthaeus Silvaticus (circa 1280- circa 1342) a physician from the famous Salerno School who wrote one of the most famous medical encyclopedias in the late Middle Ages. His Text Pandactae Medicinae was printed in at least eleven editions in various countries between the invention of the printing press and 1500 (López Piñeros 2002). In this text a description of the terms "sepsis" and "virtus" or "septic property" ("Sepsis: Putredo"; "Séptica Virtus: Putredine inducens") is provided, undoubtedly offering a clear reference to the classic Greek concept of sepsis (Silvaticus 1541). This is not surprising. The Salerno Medical School was influenced by Greek classic work translations from Arabic, something very common in the late Middle Ages and the period preceding the Renaissance (Crombie 1987). With this gradual recovery of the most faithful translations of the classic Greek works through the Arab physicians and translators, European physicians could appropriate many concepts that had partially disappeared as it happened with the word sepsis. It is important to remember, however, that Greek medicine gave a lot of importance to the environment and its influence on health, so it is not surprising that the putrefactive phenomena were associated to the disease, reason why we cannot find the first medical uses of the term sepsis in literature related to public health, without a doubt in clear relation to the concept miasma (see ahead in this chapter ""Why then and not before: Germs before the microbiologic era"). Because of this, in 1750 Sir John Pringle, the father of military healthiness, uses for the first time in history the word in his work Experiments upon septic and antiseptic substances (Pringle 1750), a text that made him deserving of the Copley Medal because of his contributions to the birth of Military Healthiness. Pringle was among the first persons to see the importance of these principles in hospitals and camps (Thurston 2000). Some of the first references about the use of the term in several European languages can be found. In English they date from 1858 with the inclusion of the word sepsis in the Oxford English Dictionary. However, we can find the use of the term in previous specialized works. The word sepsis is introduced for the first time in a French medical dictionary in 1834, long before the microbiological revolution, and it is defined simply as putrefaction (Béclard 1834). Similarly, a German medical dictionary from 1845 uses the term in the context of the disease (Busch 1845). By the end of the XIX century the concept sepsis was already well assimilated by the medical community, using it indistinctively with the word septicaemia (Van Arsdale 1886), reason why its use had already been related with the works of microbiology founding fathers (see ahead in this chapter: "Sepsis and the birth of the germ theory"). At the end of the XIX century sepsis and septicaemia were not the only words related; also, words like pyemia (a disease produced by the absorption of pyogenic bacteria and the pressence of pus in the blood) or sapremia (a constitucional disorder due to chemical poisoning by products of bacteria that occurs as a result of putrefactive processes set up by certain forms of bacteria in a wound), (Van Arsdale 1886) had been introduced.

3. Sepsis in the Ancient Egypt

From prehistory, human beings have tried to take care of their wounds in a practice that has evolved from the shamans´ magical approach to the therapies and methods used presently (Broughton 2006). However, some of the practices that remained for centuries and that we would consider modern, have their origins in the ancient Egypt (Mejía Rivera 2002; Broughton 2006).

The oldest report we have about sepsis associated with wounds goes back to Edwin Smith's discovery of a papyrus in 1862 in the Luxor, Egypt outskirts (Breasted 1980). Written arounnd 1600 BC, this papyrus seems to be the copy of another much older manuscript dated in 3000 BC, reason why it is considered the oldest known surgery treatise (Bishoy 2004; Stiefel 2006). Reference to 48 cases of traumatic lesions between wounds, fractures and dislocations in different parts of the body are mentioned in this masuscript explaining their symptoms, signs and their follow up, prognosis and treatment (Breasted 1980). This treatise demonstrates the clinical richness or the Egiptian physician who founded his diagnostic appreciations in a rigorous semiological and systematic method based on the clinical pehnomenon observation through the senses, including the inspection and palpation of the lesions such as a contermporary physician would do it (Mejía Rivera 2002). This empirism allowed the Egyptian general practitioner the construction of the prognosis with a minimum of magic or divinatory elements, supported in the assessment of the primary lesion as well as its subsequent evolution, thus allowing the search for emerging secondary complications, as it would be for us, sepsis evidenced semiologically by a systemic inflammatory response.

In five out of the forty-eight cases there are clear references to fever as a secondary phenomenon in the wound,1 making special emphasis in its detection during subsequent clinical assessment monitoring the patients' evolution. In some cases fever modifies both treatment and prognosis. Even explanatory notes are made in which concern related with the severity and persistence of the fever profile is shown (Breasted 1980). Nonetheless, fever is not the only sign of infectious complication. In several of the described cases the presence of pus (ryt) as a secondary and late phenomenon is described and associated with a bad prognosis. This is how the Egyptian physicians limited their efforts when performing surgical explorations because of the possibility to promote the lesion suppuration (Blum 2002). Egyptian physicians, without knowing the concept of infection or inflammation, identified some clear signs of what today we know as local suppuration and systemic infection.

In the forty-seventh case, an open wound of shoulder with its flesh turning black is described, and clarifications and therapeutic suggestions in case fever persists are made (Breasted 1980). The identification of a wound with necrotic appearance in the context of a secondary feverish profile demonstrates the capacity of the Egyptian physicians to diagnose what today we know as a gangrenous necrosis phenomenon , accompanied by a systemic inflammatory response. However, the case that surprises the most, because of its semiological accuracy when finding septic and suppurative complications, is the seventh case in whcih the care of a penetrating cranial wound which perforated the sutures is exposed (Breasted 1980; Seara Valero 1995). A clinical case whose diagnostic evaluation is carried out in two moments: a first moment in which the severity of the trauma and

---

[1] We found fever in the following cases: Case 7: head wound; Case 28: throat wound; Case 23: jaw wound; Case 41: thoracic lesion; Case 47: shoulder with gangrene (Breasted 1980) . All of them are explanations of fever as far as prognosis and treatment.

associated neurological consequences are corroborated, considering it still a treatable wound; it only is considered incurable when, after a second clinical assessment, fever accompanied by flush, perspiration, neck stiffness, convulsions and ram urine odor in the wound are detected (Breasted 1980; Seara Valero 1995). This description evidences the expertise of the ancient Egyptian physicians in the detection of a secondary infecious complication. As we know, presently such profile is compatible with a intracranial suppurative complication accompanied by meningism in the context of a systemic inflamatrory response (Adams 1999). The Egyptian physicians were pioneer in the making of the diagnostic approach of a feverish profile originated in an infected wound, establishing the bases for the Western semiological method to deal with septic patients.

It is well known that before the XIX century a theory about germs did not exist and even less in the ancient Egypt. Nevertheless, even though the Egyptians could not see microorganisms in the intestinal flora, they knew that the intestine contained some type of dangerous material. Egyptians postulated that a dangerous principle spelled WHDW (that tentatively can be pronounced as "ukhedu") could be found there. This dangerous substance could find a way though the blood vessels and intoxicate the complete body (Majno 1991). With the "ryt" and the "ukhedu" concepts it is not surprising that the Egyptians searched for materials that did not decompose and that, consequently, prevented suppuration and bad odors form the lesions. About the therapeutic Egyptian methods one can find disagreements. Some authors propose that Egyptian medicine practiced a therapeutic practice similar to the prehistoric rituals and pharmacopoeia in accordance with pre-technical medicine and, as a consequence, it did not generate greater advances in the wounds infection control (Robinson 1947; Forrest 1982). Nontheless, other authors rehabilitate the therapeutic richness of Egyptian medicine through experiments with different substances used in antiquity (Majno 1975). Other works also support this hypothesis by means of the most rigorous study of the last archeological and historical evidences (Mejía Rivera 2002). Even though some of the first references about wounds cleaning and dressing date from the Sumerians about 2100 BC, we know that the most conservative and apyogenic techniques for wounds care were developed in Egypt. Even though it is difficult to establish whether the Egyptian physician found any association between suppuration and the subsequent development of sepsis, something in their therapeutic practices was oriented to avoid pus formation. In Eber's papyrus (dated in 1400 BC) also found by Smith in the Luxor outskirts in 1862, the use of honey and grease on open wounds as well as pus removal to promote wounds healing are established (Broughton 2006). Some of these principles came to Greek medicine during the IV century BC through physicians trained in Egypt such as Crisipo de Gnido who discovered the use of hemostatic dressing as well as other blodless methods in the management of traumatic lesions. These methods were adopted by some of Crisipo's eminent students like Herófilo (c. 335 BC - 280 BC) and Erasistrato (c. 304 – 250 BC) (Robinson 1947). Diverse ancient texts commonly suggest wound wash with beer, hot water and honey, to cover them subsequently with grease impregnated with herbs and grease dressings (Majno 1975; Forrest 1982). Presently it has been proved that the ancient Egyptians' ointments based on honey and grease have bactericide action: a mixture with one third of honey and two thirds of butter diminish the S. Aureus y E. Coli count from 105 to 102 in only 24 hours (Broughton 2006). The use of compresses impregnated with wine were also used in former times with an approximate 10% alcohol content as well as the presence of malvoside and enoside pigments (Majno 1975), winw can kill E. Coli colonies in only 60 minutes (Broughton 2006). Botanic studies show that nearly 2,500 plants possess microbiological activities and it is possible that many of them had been used in former times for wounds treatment without having any knowledge about it (Forrest 1982). The reason why these peoples promoted the use of such substances was maybe because of their good aroma and their slow decomposition. Within this framework the Egyptian physician is the pioneer in the observation of nature to try to find tools for apyogen care of wounds (Forrest 1982). As it will be seen in the paragraphs below, through Western history the cleaning of wounds was more the exception to the rule, and it is only natural that all possible means to promote supuration were looked for, an objective which was outstandingly achieved by the Middle Age physicians.

4. Ancient Greece: Giving birth to the word sepsis

In the ancient Greece, medicine suffers deep transformations and the seeds of the care and treatment of wounds paradigm were planted for the centuries to come. Although the Hippocratic body writers were not aware of the concept of microorganism, they identified the suppurative infections clinical manifestations, excelling in their correct description (Siegel 1960). Greeks were perfectly aware of the inherent dangers of the continuous loss of skin, to which respect Hippocratic literature describes: "When a cut becomes inflamed, the neighboring tissues become intumiscent, and the lesion flush and heat spreads through the vessels. If the lesion is located in the leg, the tumors will develop in the groin; if it is in the arm they will prefer the armpit" (Grmek 1991). We can then see how the Hippocratic physicians, without any conceptual knowledge about infection or lymphatic system, accurately describe a skin primary lesion with subsequent local spread, evidenced by lymphangitis and secondary lymphadenitis. Likewise, Greek physicians were well aware of the dangers of a systemic compromise: "A local lesion, heated by humor afflux, makes the whole body become feverish. One can die because of this, especially on odd numbered days" (Joly 1970). This description demonstrates identification of the clinical phenomenon that we know today as sepsis with its deadly consequences, but supporting its pathogenesis through the classic humorism (Forrest 1982). These interactions between humors, tissues, and their implications in the origin of systemic inflammation, explain the therapeutic approach of purulent lesions in ancient Greece but, in order to understand this, first we must review what humorism was and how Greeks conceived disease. In the Hippocratic text Airs, Waters, and Places Hippocrates perfects the theory of elements proposed half a century before by the philosopher and physician Empedocles of Agrigentum (circa. 490–430 BC). In this theory Hippocrates proposed that human beings are composed by four fundamental humors (blood, phlegm, yellow bile, and black bile), representation of the four elements (air, water, fire, and earth). The health of a particular individual depended then from the adequate equilibrium of such humors (eucrasia), as well as the individual's harmony with the environment. Hippocrates believed that disequilibrium in the humors (dyscracia) was the essential cause for disease to occur (Francis 1985). This would be the support for the Hippocratic-Galen model of physiological-environmental style, a model which would become a dogma until far after the Middle Ages (the implications of this model in the infections approach will be discussed ahead). For the Hippocratic Corpus pus formation in external wounds can appear because of decomposition of mistreated tissues, because of extravasated blood, or because of humor afflux (Grmek 1991). The process was different for internal no traumatic lesions in which purulent collections formed such as abdominal abscesses or empyemas. This process happened because of accumulation and stagnation of blood in the area in addition to the secondary rupture of small vessels or the displacement of phlegm which drained in the area and generated the collection (Grmek 1991). Likewise, Greeks had a different conception about the role of humors in primary systemic infections. They observed the characteristics of these patients' extracted blood and, in the context of feverish-septic clinical manifestations they interpreted the blood physical changes as an increase in the black bile (Majno 1982; Francis 1985; Abbas 2002). These changes consisted of a precipitation of the form component and a darkening of the blood as a consequence of the increase in the globular sedimentation speed and the desaturation of the sample respectively (Shoemaker 1971; Pastrana 2006). As it is known nowadays, these processes are the result of a systemic inflammation which increases the acute phase reactants (Gabay 1999) and diminishes the saturation of venous blood (Shoemaker 1971). This last one is a consequence of the decrease in oxygen transportation, the increase of its tissular extraction or mitochondrial microcirculatory dysfunction (Trzeciak 2005; Cinel 2007). The etiopathogenic conceptions from the humoralism view point made the treatment change if the case was a medical profile originated from an "invisible" inflammation or if the case was a suppurative profile from a traumatic origin with secondary systemic compromise.

Although it seems paradoxical, for the Hippocratic physician suppuration could have a benign or a harmful character. To understand this it is necessary to review two very important Greek concepts: SEPSIS and PEPSIS. These two concepts, which could be understood as some sort of Ying-yang, are fundamental in order to understand suppuration and wounds care. It is difficult to translate accurately and literally the sepsis and pepsis concepts but essentially they represent the decomposition or disintegration processes which could be subject to live matter (Majno 1991). Sepsis is very close to the concept of putrefaction as we understand it nowadays, and it necessarily implies "bad odors" and "putrefaction" processes that occurred in the colon inside the body (maybe this concept was associated with the Egyptian term "ukhedu") and was also associated with the stinking swamps and rotten organic matter (see ahead miasmas). On the other hand, PEPSIS was closer to "firing", "maturation", and "fermentation". The digestive processes in the stomach, as well as tears of milk formation were maturation peptic processes of humors (Majno 1991).

This way we can understand that despite there was not a microorganisms theory, somehow in the ancient world the macroscopic consequences of three phenomena caused by the microbian world could be observed: Putrefaction (SEPSIS) to which all living matter was exposed when it died; fermentation (PEPSIS) which was used to produce wine, vinegar among other ferments and ripe food products; and infection, especially wounds, which somehow was similar to sepsis and that was first explained through the humoral theory, then through miasmas and finally through infection and the germs theory as it will be presented at the end of this chapter.

For the Greeks there existed transformation processes which were subject to humors during the course of the illness either to cause it or to solve it (Grmek 1991). These processes consisted of the body substances maturation and the formation of pus in a lesion did not escape from this principle. Depending on the type of process (benign pepsis, or harmful sepsis) the lesion suppuration essence itself would be explained (Grmek 1991). For this reason, there is a clear distinction from Greek semiology between desirable and undesirable pus. For the Hippocratic physician a darker, abundant, heterogeneous, fetid and bloody secretion was interpreted as part of a bad prognosis inflammatory profile (Grmek 1991), undoubtedly closer to the concept of sepsis. Different from this type of undesirable pus, suppuration could be part of healing only if it had benign semiological characteristics or closer to the humors pepsis. In this context, suppuration helped by means of destruction of already necrotic tissues. For this reason, it is not surprising that the total absence of pus production was interpreted as an ominous sign (Grmek 1991). Nowadays we know that an absence of pyogenic response may indicate an insufficiency of secondary local inflammatory response to the immune system, even more in the context of a malnourished, elderly or weakened patient (McFarlane 1976; Opal 2005). As a result, the Hippocratic physician focused part of his therapeutic efforts in allowing a rather conservative and limited suppuration of the lesions (Grmek 1991). Although there is no clarity about any specific procedure carried out to control excessive suppuration, Greeks are attributed the implementation of abscesses-drainage. In the year 280 BC, a Greek barber invented what we could call nowadays syringe (pyúlkos or pus extractor) which was commonly used to drain purulent foci (Majno 1975). With the disappearance of Greek civilization the surgical drainage practice was buried, to be rescued only a couple of centuries ago when it started to play the fundamental role in the management of sepsis it has today (Dellinger 2008).

It is important to highlight that in the classic Mediterranean world each wound suffered infection to a greater or a lesser extent which made improbable to distinguish between healing on first intention or as a part of the resolution of a secondary infectious process with superimposed suppuration (Majno 1975; Grmek 1991). These physiopathological precisions explain the apparent ambiguity of Greek therapeutics as far as the desire to promote or restrict pus formation. In the first part of the book About Ulcers this therapeutic dilemma is illustrated and referring to the care of a recent ulcer, the Hippocratic Corpus says:

"Recent ulcers, both the ulcers themselves and the surrounding parts, will be least exposed to inflammation if one shall bring them to a suppuration as expeditiously as possible, and if the matter is

not prevented from escaping by the mouth of the sore; or, if one should restrain the suppuration, so that only a small and necessary quantity of pus may be formed, and the sore may be kept dry by a medicine which does not create irritation." [Afterwards on the origin of suppuration] "A sore suppurates when the blood is changed and becomes heated; so that becoming putrid, it constitutes the pus of such ulcers." (Francis 1985)

Erroneously, authors suggest that for the Greek the appearance of pus was not necessary for the positions of defense of wounds healing (Forrest 1982). As it was stated before, for the Hippocratic corpus suppuration was a sign of the transformation process which allowed the wound healing through the maturation of humors (Grmek 1991). Interpreted as a clinical sign, pus could be interpreted as an adequate evolution or a compilation of the wound, a distinction which limited the Greek efforts when promoting pus formation in a conservative approach contrasting with Roman and Medieval medicine.

Hippocratic literature is prolific in the number of substances that can be applied on a wound (Majno 1975; Francis 1985). Postures defending cautery with boiling oil can be found in the texts (Blum 2002), as well as other more conservative postures such as the use of ointments, bandages and baths with wine, water and vinegar (Forrest 1982; Francis 1985; Broughton 2006). Even some references indicated keeping the wounds dry (Francis 1985; Francis 1985). Bandages as a bloodless haemosthasis and healing method were fundamental in the Greek therapeutics. Greeks made of this technique an art reaching great mastery in their production using them for diverse purposes (Majno 1975; Francis 1985; Francis 1985). Its use was accompanied by different substances that impregnated them, favoring the use of wine (Francis 1985), verdigris, green copper ore (Forrest 1982 escences and ointments (Majno 1975). It was also common that venesection was promoted to evacuate blood contanied in the lesion, perhaps with the intention to reduce the blood afflux and the excessive pus formation (Forrest 1982). All these procedures would be adopted by the Medieval Roman medicine, with some qualitative changes as it will be shown below.

5. From Rome to the Medieval Age. *Pus bonum et laudabile*[2] and the downfall of surgery

"Those diseases which medicines do not cure iron cure; those which iron cannot cure, fire cures; and those which fire cannot cure, are to be reckoned wholly incurable." Hippocrates from Cos. V - IV Centuries BC.

The Roman Empire received many of their knowledge from Greek science (Haggard 1947). In general, during the Roman period of Greek medicine the same antiseptic components were used, adding a few ones such as silver nitrate (Broughton 2006). Galen and Dioscorides

[2] "Pus bonum et laudabile" In Spanish: "Pus buena y digna de alabanza". (from Latin: Bonus: Useful and on purpose for something and Laudabilis: praiseworthy). Concept proposed by Galen from Pergamo (129 – 200 d. C.) who made public that wounds healed on second intention and that pus formation was fundamental for healing. This concept stimulated the indiscriminate use of cautery during the Middle Ages, as well as ointment composed by rotten or caustic substances to facilitate suppuration of a lesion.

were authors who standed out in the Medieval Ages as a mandatory reference, being their texts followed as dogmas until the Renaissance. Galen (129 – 200 AD), who would become the undisputed medical authority for the next fifteen centuries, did not contribute too much to the a-pyogen wound care strengthening the previous ideas about the importance of suppurative healing, introducing the concept of Pus bonum et laudabile (Pollak 1970; Forrest 1982; Thurston 2000; Blum 2002). This concept stated that wounds were cured on second intention and that pus formation was fundamental for their healing. This approach stimulated the indiscriminate use of cautery during the Middle Ages period, as well as the use of ointments composed by rotten or caustic substances to facilitate suppuration in the lesion (Blum 2002). Celsus (45 BC- AD 25) was the first Western physician in characterizing the four cardinal signs of inflammation: "Notae vera inflammationis sunt quattuor; rubor et tumor cum calore et dolore". (Forrest 1982; Blum 2002). Regarding wounds, Celsus proposed different treatments from those proposed by Hyppocrates and Galen, applying some of the Alexandrian school3 developing the first acceptable approximation to haemosthasis (Robinson 1947). However, his work was lost during the Medieval period; his text De Medicina rescued from a church in Milan in 1443 (Paget 2005) was one of the first medicine books printed after Gütemberg's dead (Forrest 1982). In this text Celsus proposed a first line bloodless haemostatic method which consisted in packing the wound with linen moistened with water, vinegar or wine (Celsus 1961). After having the hemorrhage controlled, the edges of skin were moistened with rose oil and butter, and the use of bandages with water continued along with a light diet and rest (Davies 1970). Cautery with caustics was considered the third line and was only used when the vessel ligature had failed in containing the hemorrhage (Forrest 1982). Some of the principles promulgated in his work are the foundation of today's haemosthasis which tried to stop bleeding without destroying tissues or promoting infection (Hontanilla Calatayud 1999). The objective of the classic Greek and Greek-Roman therapeutics in the treatment of wounds qualitatively was the same. Their difference lied on the gradual importance suppuration gained as a fundamental element in wounds' healing. This evolution was evident from the relatively a-pyogenic healing of the Alexandrians (Robinson 1947) to the pus bonum et laudabile concept adopted in the Middle Ages (Forrest 1982; Thurston 2000; Blum 2002).

After the peak of Roman medicine, Arabians became the receivers of medical science by accumulating, translating and commenting many of the classic texts that would serve as a reference for the physicians during the Middle Ages (Haggard 1947). Medical texts survived thanks to the efforts of great translators and commentators such as Hunayn, Avicenna, Rhazes and Averroes who compiled knowledge in important Greek-Arabic summaries allowing discrete advances in clinic (Robinson 1947). Nonetheless, surgery did not share the same luck; as the Middle Ages progressed, the sacred character of nature became preponderant, the human body as a divine creation at God's image and

[3] As mentioned before, it is possible that Celsus had as sources some texts or sources from Alexandrian physicians such as Erasistratus and Herophilus whose master, Crisipo of Gnido was educated in the apyogen surgical techniques in Egypt.

likeness, became an inexplorable taboo which made inacceptable any diagnostic or therapeutic technique that could outrage its sacred character (Mejía Rivera 1990; Mejía Rivera 2005). This giving up of the human being corporal reality exploration added up to the academic and social tendency to see surgery as a "second category" discipline, causing its gradual transformation into an empirical and despicable task separated from the distinguished academic environment of that period. These reasons explain why surgical treatises fell into the ostracism (Haggard 1947). Regarding this, Albucasis, one of the greatest Arabian surgeons, would comment: "The surgical art has disappeared between us almost without leaving any mark. Only in the writings of some ancients we find references: but these, wrongly translated, erroneous and altered have become unintelligible and useless" (Robinson 1947). Undoubtedly Arab literature is influenced mainly by Galen texts whose treatments supported the value of suppuration in the healing of wounds: consequently, during the Middle Ages the use of sutures, wounds exploration and vessels ligature were pushed into the background, making of the painful cautery the appropriate procedure for all kinds of lesions (Robinson 1947; Forrest 1982; Forrest 1982). As it has been discussed so far, the most conservative approaches practiced by Alexandrian and Greek physicians got lost in time and would only be taken up again in the Renaissance thanks to the recovery of lost texts and to the new scientific spirit of that period which allowed the development of an empirical mental attitude that would confront the old preestablished dogmas.

The practice of surgery in Europe remained unaltered during the late Middle Ages because of the use of cautery, a consequence of the unanimous acceptance of pus bonum et laudabile, and it was only in the XIII century that some authors dared to contradict Galen. The first of them was the surgeon from Bologna Teodorico de Borgognoni (1205-1298) who proposed in his work Chirurgia (a compilation of his father's Hugh of Lucca, who was the founder of the Bologna Surgery School teachings) the use of clean dressings to try to keep the wounds dry thus avoiding caustic substances which promoted pus appearance (Forrest 1982). At the same time, in Montpellier, Henri de Mondeville (1260-1320) criticized Galen work, particularly wound healing, and in his work Cyrurgia from 1320 he proposed the use of spring water or boiled water to clean wounds (Blum 2002). In line with this, William of Saliceto (1210-1280) maintained ardently that pus formation was deleterious for both, the patient and the wound, suggesting that healing must be given on first intention (Thurston 2000). However, these works did not have a lot of impact in this period: most of these authors were attacked by their contemporary authors who defended passionately the status quo and the continuity of the Galen paradigm as a dogma. We could summarize the causes of the failure of these new proposals as follows: 1) the lack of a change in the philosophical corpus of each period which epistemologically supported the change of a model; 2) the absence of some anomaly which systematically challenged the paradigm in each period; 3) authors, times, and places cohesion which coincided and supported a growing corpus of evidence that challenged the old paradigm. These obstacles would be surmounted thanks to the Renaissance and the introduction of gunpowder in the war, as well as the great men such as Ambroise Paré, Paracelsus and subsequently the fathers of microbiology.

6. Firearms, the end of the Medieval Ages and the Renaissance. The role of sepsis in the birth modern surgery

As it can be inferred from the previously described, sepsis became a silent partner for barber surgeons in hospices and battle fields taking innumerable lives in olden days. This tragedy was a consequence of the Galen dogma bomun et laudabile, a concept that defined the wounds treatment for many centuries. What made such somnolence of medicine possible? In the first place, many of the surgical procedures in the olden days, particularly the Greek and Alexandrian -less iatrogenic and perhaps more effective- were abandoned or simply lost the medical corpus allowing cautery to become the surgical tool of choice during the last half of the Middle Ages (Hernández Botero 2009). Secondly, within the scientific framework of the period, there existed neither a philosophical nor a scientific corpus which allowed the development of new paradigms in medicine. In this way, the Galen postulates were the guideline, wounds continued to be treated with fire, the injured burned in fever and the pus stench was the norm, and, even though there were isolated and fruitless efforts to fight sepsis, the scientific spirit of that period simply was not ready for a change in paradigm (Kuhn 2004; Hernandez Botero 2009).

In the period of arrows and swords, wounds in the torso or the head ended up being lethal; as a consequence, most of the ancient texts focused on the management of wounds in the limbs which could have a relatively benign prognosis if hemorrhagic shock was not present (Helling 2000). The war surgeon's arsenal in olden days was limited and the efforts were focused in the search for homeostasis through a diversity of techniques from poultice, dressings, and packaging to ligature and cautery (Castiglioni 1941; Singer 1962; Laín Entralgo 1979). Amputation was very-little practiced and the necessary surgical techniques to perform this procedure had not been developed (Majno 1975; Forrest 1982; Helling 2000; Broughton 2006; Hernandez Botero 2009). As we can see, medicine could not offer much for the development of an appropriate surgical management of infected wounds.

Firearms checkmated the Western surgical knowledge because they hastened a dramatic change in the wounds pattern during armed confrontations from their gradual introduction by the second half of the XIV century (Singer 1962; Blum 2002; Chase 2003; Broughton 2006). The primary lesion was now accompanied by the bullet contaminant material, external debris and gunpowder residues (Chase 2003). Serious burns, open fractures, avulsions and extensive lacerations, undoubtedly associated with a significant increase in mortality (Blum 2002; Broughton 2006). This new lesion pattern, as well as an unquestionable increase in mortality produced by non-hemorrhagic shock, started to generate the wrong perception that wounds were being poisoned by harquebus gunpowder. Although the specific author who suggested this hypothesis is unknown, some pioneer surgeons who defended this posture stand out: German surgeon Hieronymus Brunschwig (1450 – 1533), one of the first war surgery text authors, proposed that the increase in mortality was due to a "blood poisoning" caused by gunpowder, and he even proposed in his book Chirurgia in 1497, that the treatment must have been focused in extracting this dangerous substance: *"In case a man has been shot with a gun and the bullet is still in place, he is poisoned by the powder, or part of the powder is still in the body, in the arm or leg or wherever the wound may be. Take a seton, push it through the wound, and pull it back and forth to force the powder out... You may then insert a lint plug moistened with bacon or lubricated with ox grease."* (Brunschwig 1497). Giovanni de Vigo (1460 – 1520), Italian author introduces the most copied and translated surgical text in his time, Practica in arte chirurgica copiosa (Roma 1514). He makes popular, because of his Galen Midievalist essence, the use of boiling oil on the wounds as an efficient way to counteract the poisoning with gunpowder, and, without any doubt, something equally efficient in producing abundant pus quantity (Robinson 1947). On the other hand, the Italian physician Alfonso Ferri (1515 – 1595) aptly proposed in 1552 that portions of the armor and clothes that remained deep in the wounds were responsible for suppuration and even he encouraged their removal (Thurston 2000). When interpreting these innovative works in war surgery, one can conclude that the increase in mortality was due to an accentuation of sepsis as a secondary phenomenon to the initial wound. This was an awaited situation because of the appearance of more extensive, exposed and contaminated wounds, factors which increased their susceptibility to infection. The so called "blood poisoning" would rather have corresponded to an increase in the sepsis and septic shock cases behind the battle front due, not only to the wounds pattern and contamination, but also to the different treatment promoting their suppuration.

Once the Middle Ages period finished, the Renaissance started and more than two hundred years went by since the harquebus in the European battle fields started to sound in order to have real advances in the war wounds treatment (Singer 1962; Pollak 1970; Forrest 1982; Broughton 2006). The first one happened thanks to the great Swiss physician and surgeon Paracelsus (1493-1541), an angry critic of Hippocratic and Galen medicine who furiously claimed against what was called *"the reprehensible precept that teaches that it is necessary to make wounds suppurate"* (Robinson 1947). His declarations were undoubtedly revolutionary: *"The true physician of wounds is nature. All treatment must be reduced to infection prevention. Complexion, humors, diet and time, and the stars don't have any influence. The results will be determined by a treatment which allows nature to act in peace"* (Robinson 1947). If Paracelsus was the great innovator theorist in the XVI century, it was a French barber who, through empirical evidence, was able throw one more shovelful of soil on the pus bonum et laudabile. This happened in Italy in 1536 when out of serendipity (Mejía Rivera 2004) the French surgeon and father of modern surgery, Ambroise Paré (1509 -1590) decided to put to an end the indiscriminate production of pus. It was during the siege of Turin that the young surgeon found himself in the obligation to use dressings and poultice instead of the standard treatment with boiling oils because of the scarcity of supplies. The anecdote of this finding published in his text *The Method of Curing Wounds Made by Arquebus and Other Firearms* (1545), is well-known:

"The soldiers within the castle, seeing our men come on them with great fury, did all they could to defend themselves, and killed and wounded many of our soldiers with pikes, harquebus, and stones, whereby the surgeons had all their work cut out for them. Now I was at this time a fresh water soldier; I had not yet seen wounds made by gunshot at the first dressing. It is true I had read in Giovanni de Vigo's first book, "Of wounds in general", eighth chapter [Practica in arte chirurgica

copiosa (Roma 1514)], that wounds made by firearms partake venenosity, by reason of the powder; and for their cure he bids you cauterize them with oil of elders scalding hot, mixed with a little treacle. And to make no mistake, before I would use the said oil, knowing this was to bring great pain to the patient, I asked first before I applied it, what other surgeons did for the first dressing; which was to put the said oil, boiling well, into the wounds, with tents and setons; wherefore I took courage to do as they did. At last my oil ran short, and I was forced instead thereof to apply a digestive made of the yolk of eggs, oil of roses and turpentine. In the night I could not sleep in quiet, fearing some default in not cauterizing, that I should find the wounded to whom I had not used the said oils dead from the poison of their wounds; which made my rise very early to visit them, where beyond my expectation I found that those to whom I had applied my digestive medicament had but little pain, and their wounds without inflammation or swelling, having rested fairly well that night; the others, to whom the boiling oil was used, I found feverish, with great pain and swelling about the edges of the wounds. Then I resolved never more to burn thus cruelly poor wounded men. [...] See how I learned to treat gunshot wounds; not by books." (Paget 2005)

These observations have deep epistemological implications. First of all, it is a prototype of what we know today as clinical test with control; in the second place, this discovery through the mixture of the scientific method and out of serendipity actions, in the context of therapeutic difficulties posed by the use of firearms, achieves the beginning of an experimental evidence corpus that would serve to bury Galen dogma that had prevailed for centuries (Kuhn 2004; Mejía Rivera 2004). It is then that young Paré, with only twenty-six years of age, abandons boiling oil, recovering from ostracism, among other things, ligature as a more asceptic hemostasia technique (Robinson 1947), thus reducing significantly the occurrence of infection and setting the bases for new and revoluationary surgical developments (Baskett 2004; Drucker 2008). Even though Paré himself continued being reluctant to surgical exploration of wounds and only performed it when he was going to pull out foreign bodies and fragments of bone (Helling 2000), in few years great advances in exploration of surgical techniques would be achieved. This happened with the publication of his fellow countryman Pierre Joseph Desault (1744-1759) who managed to introduce the modern debridement concept (Broughton 2006). Desault observed that tissue inflammation produces constriction inside the fascias or aponeurosis and attributed to it the cause of gangrene (Broughton 2006). Similarly John Hunter (1728 -1793) identified the deleterious effect devitalized and necrotic tissues have for wounds healing and he proposed their surgical removal (Hunter 1985; Ellis 2001). Subsequently, the Russian military surgeon Carl Reyher (1846 – 1899) combined antiseptic techniques along with the careful mechanical cleaning through surgical techniques, thus giving shape to debridement as we know it today (Helling 2000). Before Desault, Hunter and Reyher, the lesions surgical approach consisted basically in removing the bullet from the wound, inflicting more damage and introducing more contaminants (Ellis 2001). Debridement could generate a preventive approach by allowing the removal of desvitalized tissues thus preventing infection and, similarly, it allowed the surgical approach of the already established sepsis.

In this context, it is necessary to ask: How was the clinical course of the injured person after the introduction of gunpowder in combat? When a soldier receives an extensive damage in a limb because of a cannonball or an explosion, the wound process suffered a characteristic natural history (Helling 2000):

1. The patient could die during the first hours because of hemorrhagic shock because of extensive vascular damage.
2. If the patient survived the initial hemorrhage, a period of thirty days called "the first inflammation" started, period in which the following might happen in the exact order it appears below:
- Dead produced by non-hemorrhagic posttraumatic shock, this struck within the first 48 hours and was independent from the hemorrhage or gangrene.
- If the patient survived the shock, gangrene started within the five or seven days following the lesion, surely accompanied by fatal septic shock.
3. If the patient still continued alive, he was at the mercy of chronic infections stressed by malnutrition as well as any other preexistent or new disease.

During the primary inflammation period we can differentiate between post-trauma shock and septic shock because of the starting time and their clinical characteristics. Following, Nocholas Senn describes a shock pot-trauma case during the war between The United States and Spain:

"A young soldier has been struck down by a fragment of a bursting shell, which has almost completely severed both legs just below the knee-joint. The patient lies on the ground, motionless. He has lost little blood, but his lips are pale ...the hands are cold, and the pulse at the wrist cannot be felt. The respirations are irregular ...it takes repeated questions to elicit the simplest answer."(Senn 1900)

In those first post-trauma hours many surgeons were aware that the patient's dead might strike from the shock in spite of an adequate control of the bleeding (Helling 2000). This shock of difficult explanation was attributed to neurological causes because of the deceitful characteristics of its appearance and to the patient's inability (Larrey 1812). Nontheless, the specific physiopathology of this shock resides in the molecular response the seriously injured tissues develop; a powerful inflammatory response with systemic consequences which can cause multiple organic dysfunction even if there is not infection (Lenz 2007). The mechanisms responsible of this response have been philogenetically preserved to react energically before diverse inflammatory stimulus (O'Neill 1998; Opal 2000; Beutler 2001). This inflammatory post-traumatic response continues to be a problem nowadays, not only because of the organic damage it generates, but also because it increases the possibilities of systemic superimpossed infection. This association has been called the two impact theory which suggests that the initial inflammatory response is the bridge to develop sepsis through the apoptosis of immune cells or splachnic perfusion with bacterial translocation from the intestinal light (Border 1987; Keel 2005)

Up to this point we have seen the gradual development of some surgical techniques. However we have not tackled amputation, a procedure that, even though bloody and horrible, would be the only hope for seriously injured soldiers during the pre-antibiotic period. Amputation was not a very popular practice through history and there is a variety of cultural and scientific reasons for that. In the primitive societies this practice was only performed for religious or punishment reasons, never as a medical intervention; primitive human beings were terrified to go to the supernatural world with incomplete bodies (Pollak 1970). Centuries later, Hippocratic physicians did not know how to amputate, but they witnessed how gangrenous limbs of some patients which, without evidence of infection self-mummyfied and fell, process that was called melasmas (Majno 1975). During the rest of the Greek-Roman period amputation continued out of the medical practice and even thouhg some Greek schools improved fundamental techniques to perform this procedure such as the vessel ligature (Robinson 1947), they were never used in the context of such surgery (Helling 2000). Later, during the Middle Ages, these techniques were buried with the rest of the ancient surgical knowledge at the expense of the use of cautery, making it impossible to develop an appropriate amputation technique (Robinson 1947; Helling 2000; Hernandez Botero 2009). Ever since the new and harmful war artefacts were introduced, the need came up to reconsider the approach of a patient with a smashed limb and whose final destination in most cases would be death. Amputation would be the answer to approach these types of patients not only for the bleeding control, but also for the traumatic shock and, of course, the infection. However, it was a hard way.

At the beginning of the XVI century, amputation was seen as a second line therapy and it was reserved as the treatment for established gangrene being treated only when other procedures such as poultice, dressings and cautery had already been used (Helling 2000). Vessels ligature, a fundamental technique when amputating, had not been rescued yet and did not make a part of the surgical knowledge. As a consequence, when amputation was considered, it was performed on the established necrotic tissue in order to avoid hemorraghe, which did not allow to avoid a subsequent systemic infection (Helling 2000). After the advances of surgery in the XVI and XVII centuries, amputation started to earn the place it deserved in the sepsis surgical control.

XIX century: two nations at war, France and England; two conflicting strategists, Napoleon Bonaparte and Field Marshal Arthur Wellesley, Duke of Wellington. Amidst this bloody conflict, their respective surgeons would demonstrate that science goes beyond flags and conflicts. Napoleon's surgeon at that time, Dominic Jean Larrey (1766 - 1842), proposed the use of early amputation as a way to reduce mortality. In his memories he adds: "amputation must be performed instantly. Otherwise, the damaged areas will soon become gangrene" (Larrey 1812). Larrey creates the concept of early amputation, changing an affected limb into a small wound, less contaminated, with more possibilities to control hemorraghe and where infeccion would be inevitable. With great expertise in this procedure, Larrey performed more tha two hundred amputations per day in the Borodino Campaign (Ellis 2001), and could report an approximate of 75% survival rates (Larrey 1812). This concept of early amputation was of paramount importance to avoid both sepsis and the feared post-trauma shock.

On his side, the British surgeon, George James Guthrie (1785-1856), who was Wellington chief surgeon (called "the British Larrey"), describes in his Treatise on Gunshot Wounds the typical clinical profile of a septic shock which could be observed after the Battle of Waterloo (1815). A clear difference compared with the post-trauma shock description can be seen: *"Pain, heat, redness, tumefaction of neighbouring parts constituting inflammation comes on, which speedily runs into suppuration or gangrene... fever becomes more violent and frequently ends in death in the course of a few day."* (Guthrie 1827). As it can be seen, a temporal distinction between local inflammation and sepsis development in the following days is made, evidenced by the continuous in character feverish profile with a fast physiological decline which ends up in death. In the context of the pre-antibiotic period, early amputation proposed by Larrey was the only option to give hope to a seriously injured soldier because it limited the systemic response to the lesion thus diminishing the damaged tissues to be susceptible of patogen colonization.

However, only a few agreed with Larrey about tissue damaged by itself as the stimulus for "shock and prostration of strength" and about removal using early amputation being an effective way to avoid gangrene. In fact, this point provoked a great debate between the XVII and the XIX centuries; to amputate or not to amputate, that was the question (Helling 2000). Several medical figures added to this controversy, even John Hunter himself, who was inclined towards a more conservative and late use of amputation, arguing that the battle field was the least suitable to perform a surgery of these characteristics (Hunter 1985; Ellis 2001). Even so, history and multiple wars would give Larrey the reason. Guthrie himself collected the Battle of Waterloo data about the total population of 596 soldiers and he found that in the 371 group of patients who were performed amputation in the battle field, mortality was only 22% while in the 225 soldiers group who were performed late amputations (possibly after 30 days), mortality was 37% (Helling 2000). Similar results were observed during the American Civil War (Otis 1883). These data show us that during the pre-intibiotic period the early performance of such procedure had an impact in mortality reducing the incidence of complications such as post-trauma shock and sepsis.

With the disappearance of the pus bonum et laudabile concept it is evident so far how important the advances in the field of surgery were for the sepsis control. However, in spite of the expertise gained with the scalpel, very few has been attained in the identification of the real enemy of the septic patient: microorganisms. Towards the XIX century it was a heroic deed to come out alive from an operating room, and it is no surprise that before the asepsis and antisepsis techniques appeared, surgeries could draw mortality rates higher than 90% (Robinson 1947; Pollak 1970; Ledermann 2008). It was well put by the Scottish physician James Young Simpson in 1847: *"The man laid on the operating table in one of our hospitals, is exposed to more chances of death than the English soldier on the field of Waterloo.*"(Pollak 1970).

7. Why then and not before: Germs before the microbiologic period

Let's analyze some approximations to the theory of contagion and infection before the XIX century in which the emphasis will be placed on the reasons why these postulates did not have a greater incidence in the medical corpus in their respective period, and we will stop in a case that perfectly can summarize the epistemological framework of the rest. Let's begin in Greece again. It was not difficult for the Greek to identify that some of the signs of intoxication such as vomit, diarrhea and, in some cases, fever were similar to the clinical profiles caused by infections. For them, the fact that some diseases, especially feverish ones, affected groups of people closely related or even complete populations did not go unnoticed. What was this poison that could intoxicate, alter humors and also affect a great number of people at the same time and in the same place? Greek physicians did not take long in finding the similarity stinking exhalations had in those sick with the plague and the foul vapors emanating from marshes. These stinking exhalations, called miasmas, were nothing different from the odors rising from putrefaction (in the Greek sense of the word sepsis) of undesirable substances. The putrid swamp areas filled with mosquitoes were clearly related with the appearance of malaria (mal'aria, Roman word for "bad air"),so that Greeks, Romans, and everyone from them on, associated the appearance of feverish diseases with the bad environmental odors that intoxicated the body and caused humorous disorder. This explained for them the appearance of disease like that, in a great number of people in the same place and at the same time (Castiglioni 1941). Another approximation consisted of contagion (from latin 'contigere' meaning 'to touch') which argued that a venous, non volatile material caused the disease while intoxicating the part of the body it contacted permitting humor sepsis to happen. These two theories, both miasmas and contagion, were not something different from a part of the Galen postulates from physiological-environmental essence: according to Galen, disease was the expression of a disorder in proportion to humors or their quality which occurred because of the conjunction of three factors:

- Initial causes: external factors such as heat, cold, miasmas that might produce damaging changes in the humors.
- Precedent Cause: It is the personal predisposition to a disorder which explains why some individuals are more susceptible than others to a determined disease.
- Cohesive Cause: It is the alteration in composition, proportion or quality of humors (dyscrasia) and that could be triggered by the union of precedent and initial causes. The disease was a manifestation of the cohesive cause in which the other factors (initial or precedent) had already acted as a whole or separately.

Which was the fundamental detail here? All therapeutics was directed to this cohesive cause or humorous disorder in order to achieve eucrasia (the adequate humor proportion). In this sense, the initial cause, whichever it was, was an "associated factor" and it was not seen as a neither necessary nor sufficient cause for the maintenance of a disease (Nutton 1983). This indicates that any postulate that intended to pose the existence of invisible living forms able to cause a disease could only be seen as one of the many factors which caused the disease, and different from what is stated in the germs theory in the XIX century, it would hardly be seen as a determinant factor to be attacked with the therapeutics to solve the disease.

Were there in olden days similar approximations to what we know today as germs or different approaches to the humoralism-environmental theory? The truth is that there were.

Years after Hippocrates times, in his book about the generation of animals (Generation of animals. III.xi), Aristotle explains that new animals are born from putrid material4, and he added that sepsis produce small creatures, especially in the putrid mud and in stinking swamps (Majno 1991). These ideas were not forgotten and the Roman writer Marcus Terentius Varro (116 a. C. - 27 a. C.) wrote a text known as Agricultural Topics in three books devoted to his wife Fundania in which he mentions: "In swampy places a multitude of small animals develop which can not be perceived by the eye, but the penetrate the body through the mouth and thenose, and cause terrible diseases."5 These postulates were inside the Humoralism framework because they identified putrefaction in the swamps as the origin of small and dangerous animals, and these would not be something different from an initial cause, another element that would contribute to humorous disorder. Other authors, on the other hand, certainly opposed Hippocratic conceptions. The origins of some of these theories date centuries back reaching Pre-Socratic philosophers from the atomic mechanism such as Leucippus and Democritus (IV and V centuries BC) who suggested the existence of infinite, in varied forms, indivisible and always moving particles which conformed all reality. These atomists postulates would be adopted by Greek physicians such as Caelius Aurelianus, Philo and Asclepiades, representatives of the Methodist medical school from the I and II Centuries AD, who posed an atomic-ontological approach. This approach stated the origin of disease is in the greater or lower particles cohesion which breeds the ground so that, under the concept of atomic entities, diseases can be appropriated to singularities dynamic in character, imperceptible to the eye, and that can affect its environment. The Methodist postulates were treated apathetically because of the medical status quo between the III and the XVI centuries; this is not surprising since they proposed an ontological concept of the disease which was irreconcilable with the Galen doctrines of physiological-environmental type. Later, Arabians who were great receivers of Greco-Roman science increased quantitatively the knowledge about infectious diseases but assumed the physiological-environmental model as a dogma. Authors like Avicenna preferred Galen explanations of air corruption with miasmas, atmospheric changes and astrologic influences instead of any approximation coming from microscopic life as the cause of disease. So, it is not surprising that the seeds of disease, a concept closer to the germs theory stayed asleep in the shelves of the medieval knowledgeable without any practical approximation.

The search for sepsis seeds continues until the mid XVI century. Paré had just published in France his experiences in the Villaine Castle and Paracelsus lied in his grave in Salzburg leaving behind an immense legacy. It was in 1546, in Padua, and emblematic Renaissance city where only three years back Copernicus and Vesalius had published their great works, when a great poet and physician's text saw the light: Girolamo Fracastoro (1478 – 1553). Native form Verona, this author proposed in his text De Contagione et Contagiosis Morbis

---

[4] This principle, known as the spontaneous generation of life, remained unaltered as a dogma until Luis Pasteur, in the XIX century demonstrated that it was false, thanks to his experiments with microorganisms (see next section).

[5] Rerum Rusticarum – De agricultura Libri Tres: *"...siqua loca palusteria, et quod [arescunt] crescunt animalia quaedam minuta, quae non possunt pculi consequi, et per aera intus in corpus per os ac nares perueniunt atque efficiunt difficilis morbos."* (Terrencio Varrón 1992)

et Eorum Curatione (Wright 1930) what seemed to be an approximation to the modern concept of contagion6. Because of Fracastoro's presence in the historical framework of great medical revolutions during the Renaissance, a favorable reaction from the different contemporary authors did not take long to come and they considered his text as the first scientific declaration about the true nature of contagion which, suposedly, would anticipate what would become the current germs theory. They also compared the importance of their achievement with that achieved by Puré, Vesalius, and Paracelsus (Singer 1917; Castiglioni 1941; Robinson 1947; Pollak 1970; Howard-Jones 1977). Nevertheless, based in the originality of his conception, the practical application of his context and the scope of his influence, it can be stated that Fracastoro did not have the historical-scientific relevance confered on him. Three reasons can be given for this: 1) Were his postulates original? No. It is well-known that during Fracastoro's times the disease seeds lied, maybe as their bibliographic sources, in three Galen texts; some Plutarch's passages referring to the Methodists; passages from the teologist Isidore making reference to Lucretious7 and some Roman and Medieval agricultural sciences ancient texts (Nutton 1983.; Terrencio Varrón 1992); 2) Did they have some practical application? No. Fracastoro's seeds made part of the multiple initial causes that could have contributed to unchain illness. If the seeds were or were not present was irrelevant because they were not understood as a necessary cause for the disease appearance. In this sense, theorizing about the seeds was a philosophical luxury without immediate medical applications because the therapeutics in that period was focused in correting the humoral disorder as such, and it was not focused on the hypotetical entities that had already acted to unchain it. Within the framework of the old paradigma, it was impossible to accept, until it had not been observed in the microscope and after studies that demonstrated its role in the disease, that a particular entity (semina morbi) was the necessary cause for the appearance of an infection. This ontological approach would only be possible thanks to the disappearance of humoralism and the appearance of the cellular theory and, obviously, the development of microbiology (Howard-Jones 1977; Nutton 1983.; Grissom 2004); 3) Did he have any immediate or subsequent influence? Fracastoro was not an influential professor in a big European university and he was only known locally. His writings, very little disseminated, were hardly rescued the century before last when their first translations appeared in the XIX century which will conclude with the first translation into English in 1930 (Wright 1930). Which was then the real value of Fracastoro? He was a

[6] In 1930 Wilber C. Wright was the first one to translate and publish G. Fracastoro's text in English. A version brilliantly translated into Spanish is available in the collection Clásicos *de la Medicina, Medicina Renacentista III. Gerolamo Fracastoro: De Contagione Et Contagiosis Morbus. Revista MD En Español, Octubre, 1970. p: X1-X8.* In his text, Fracastoro argues that infection is not produced because of unknown causes but because of seeds of the disease: *semina morbi* o *seminaria,* which are imperceptible particles composed by different elements and propagate (*propagare*) and breed (*gignere*) other seeds, and cause corruption at the level of the constituent particles of things. However, at no time Fracastoro specifies that those are living organisms or makes clear precisions about the difference between contagion and infection, or about any of the conceptual meanings.

[7] Lucrecio, great poet in the century I BC, would say in his book *De Rerum Nature*: "I have already shown that there are many seeds useful for our life, but also there are many others that fly around bringing diseases and death" (Nutton 1983). This poet, contemporary author from Asclepiades, probably had access to Methodist texts, or he knew Aristotelian explanations on the animals' formation, or he had access to the hidden but devastating critics that Galen used to do of the Methodists and their texts.

poet and writer who, as a good Renancentist dominated a variety of fields such as geology, physics and geography (Nutton 1983). As a medical author, he took the liberty of leaving behind physiological and environmental-humoralist explanations, and described contagious diseases in purely ontologic terms (Nutton 1983). Even though his vision of disease could not be empirically confirmed and its seeds could not be demonstrated as etiological agents until the introduction of the microscope, Fracastoro is one of the signs of the epistemological rupture with the Galen humoralism which finishes in the XIX century. Fracastoro, in his historical-scientific context, is a clear example of the changes that, as a whole, science, philosophy, and even human beings themselves who practice them, must go through in order to accept a new paradigm. Seen from modern historiography, the reading made of Fracastoro's work is, in essence, a clear example of an anachronistic interpretation of medical historiography because of a clear overvaluation on the side of historian-physicians by the end of the XIX century and beginnings of the XX century that saw in their semina morbi a singular likeness with the microbial pathogen theories which were in their zenith in those years.

During the XVI and XVII centuries there were some theoreticians and scientists who started to question the Galen concept on physiology of the disease and consequently, preestablished conceptions about infection. These men would plant the seeds that later would be harvested during the XIX century. The first of them was the Jesuit Athanasiuus Kircher (1602-1680). This great German scientist whose contributions extend from Biology to Philosophy, transcended Fracastoro and suggested that contagion was due to living organisms (contagia animata), an approach derived from his investigations in the plague patients' blood and pus. Kircher was the first one to infer that the recently discovered animalcules must have been the cause of the disease. However, his microscopic techniques did not allow him to see some free living protozoa without any relation with the disease (Bustíos Romaní 2004).

8. Sepsis and the birth of the germ theory

Until the end of the XVIII century the breaking with Galen humoralism had started consolidating with the anatomopathologic approach inaugurated by Morgagni which allowed locating the disease in a specific place (organ) and with a demonstrable cause, and later, with the works of the German doctor Rudolph Virchow (1821 - 1902) who, after many hours of study with the microscope started to postulate the cellular theory (Omnis cellula e cellula), which invited to find the causes of the disease in the tissular and cellular structures (Pollak 1970). However, and still within this context, humoralists' ideas from the Greco-Roman era about pus were still sounding and the origin of that secretion continued to be a mystery (Grmek 1991; Hernandez Botero 2009). With the development of cellular theory proposed it was already known that cells could only originate from preexistent cells and not from amorphous material which allowed elucidating the cellular character of suppuration. One of his most outstanding students, Julius Cohnheim (1839-1884), published a controversial work in 1873: Neue Untersuchungen ubre die Entzündung (New Studies on Inflammation) in which, based on previous studies about the local origin of white cells present in pus, could verify diapedesis and the importance of blood vessels in its production through the ingenious studies in frogs mesentery (Malkin 1984). These first advances allowed future advances in the understanding of chemotaxis, diapedesis, and locall inflammation, and they, laid down the foundations for the beginning of immunological and physical chemical studies that opened new ways to understand the phenomenon off inflammation (López Piñeros 1974).

This way we arrive to the XIX century. By this time microbiology was a branch of Botanic, and it will be within some few decades that microbiology not only will change medicine forever, but also the human beings' destiny. Everything begins with a martyr prophet of science: the Hungarian obstetrician Ignaz Semmelweis (1818 – 1865). His story is well known. Semmelweis was able to associate the physicians and medicine students' contaminated hands during autopsies with the increase of puerperal sepsis and theorized that it was cadaverous particles and not "cosmic, hygromatic or telluric" influences the responsible ones for the significant increase in mortality in a maternity ward at the general hospital in Vienna, and through simple hygienic measurements, he could diminish dramatically puerperal sepsis mortality (Charles 1994; Henao 1999; De Costa 2002). Nevertheless, his observations are not accepted by the medical community and after a long struggle for disseminating his theory, he is accused of having lost his mind and he is hospitalized against his will in a psychiatric hospital in Vienna where he dies alone. Through his clinical observations, Semmelweis makes the first attempt to consolidate the ontological character of sepsis, based on the evident etiological specificity of its theory. However, the necessary biological concepts to give a scientific sense to his observations did not exist. It is sad to know that only some years would go by after his dead when Pasteur, without knowing Semmelweis' work (Debré 2000), would isolate streptococcus from purulent lochia of women to whom Semmelweis could have saved (Charles 1994; Henao 1999; Magner 2009).

During the XIX century a good corpus of evidence had already been collected which demonstrated how bacteria appeared to be responsible for sepsis. Vichow's famous helper, the German student Edwin Klebs (1834–1913), reviewed under the microscope multiple samples of autopsies that he collected while serving as military physician during the Franco-Prussian war in 1879. In his revision of more than one-hundred specimens, Klebs found bacteria in almost every case and, even though he supposed erroneously that all of them were all the same type of organism which he called *Microsporon Septicum*, he was one of the first scientist in seeing and relating what no one had seen before: the agents causing sepsis and their role in the clinical phenomena itself (Magner 2009). This revolutionary finding would not have been important if the works of other great researchers who developed the microbiological theory and demonstrated the importance that converting the invisible and theoretical in something practical and visible had not been combined. The concepts about what bacteria are and how they are related to the disease still needed to be matured, answers that would come from both sides of the war in which Klebs had served: France and Germany.

The first lights came from France where a rather mediocre student who desired to be a painting teacher, would revolutionize all the fields of knowledge he dealt with. Louis Pasteur (1822 – 1895), after his prolific career in Chemistry, started to study in depth the world of microorganisms and, after several years of work, he summarized and published in 1865 the results of a fermentation in which he refutes spontaneous generation of life and demonstrated in an irrefutable way the existence of microorganisms.

His works gave cause for important conclusions: He demonstrated that the air is filled with microbes ready to develop and that the putrid liquids can be sterilized by heating. About half way through his career, his studies about fermentation gave him the possibility to state that contagious diseases might be caused by microscopic organisms (Aguirre 1996; Restrepo 1996). After these studies, Pasteur would carry a prolific academic career that would not only allow him great developments in the newborn infectology, but also his works would be the scientific bases , among others, for the practical development that later on would be known as asepsis and antisepsis.

If Pasteur opened the way for bacteriology, a German doctor, Robert Koch (1843 – 1910) consolidated its development as a discipline. After multiple achievements harvested in the study of bacterial etiology of diverse diseases, Koch started to worry since 1887 about the growth of bacteria in wounds and in surgical incisions. From his observations he published that same year the book Untersuchungen über die Aetiologie der Wundinfektionskrankheiten (About Etiology of Traumatic Infective Diseases) in which he exposes his experiments infecting wounded animals with putrid substances. In his work he would explain: "*I conclude that bacteria are not present in the blood or tissues of healthy animals,*" however, "bacteria are present in all sick animals [in blood and tissues], and their number and distribution is in such a way that they perfectly explain the symptoms of the disease" (Brock 1999). These observations are a rough draft of what would become Koch's postulates. Without any doubt these postulates could causally relate microbes and sepsis and thus constituted a first look at the disease pathogenesis. Nontheless, Koch's works had a problem: they were completely carried out with animals. But he didi not take too long in establishing a relation in humans thanks to the Scotish physician Alexander Ogston (1844 - 1929),who used the same methods Koch used and could establish in an unequivocal way the relation between bacteria and sepsis and even detailed two different types of coccus: staphylococcus and streptococcus which were present in blood and pus of many septic patients. His publications were pioneer without any doubt and constituted a cornerstone for the study of sepsis in the areas of pathology, surgery and bacteriology (Van Arsdale 1886; Brock 1999; Magner 2009).

The English surgeon Joseph Lister (1827 – 1912) took his observation to the practice even when he did not know his enemy: the microbe. His works were already well advanced when he had access to the first pioneer works in bacteriology and he could start collating his practical results with the experimental and theoretical evidence of the microbiology colossus (Ledermann 2008). In his work what stands out is his particular worry for diminishing infections in open fractures, traumatic lesions and the surgical act in general. Lister observed that fractures where the skin was intact healed without infection while in the open fractures sepsis and pus drainage were common (Thurston 2000). His observations on amputation wounds and infected wounds took him to conclude that dust of disease was responsible for these complications (Lister 1867; Walker 1956; Ledermann 2008). When Pasterur's work came into his hands, he could finally see the connection between his observations on wounds and the microscopic bacteria responsible for fermentation (Thurston 2000). That is how in 1867 he publishes his work about the antiseptic management of open fractures with carbolic acid (Lister 1867; Lister 1870) which changed forever the treatment of this type of lesions (Schwartz 1932). Lister started to become active in the microbiology studies and he attended the Seventh International Medical Congress in London in the summer of 1881 where he could exchange opinions with Koch and Pasteur. Later he continued updated with these two researchers' work and even he received a copy of the first germs microphotographs in septic rabbits' tissues taken by Koch during his investigations about etiology of infective traumatic diseases (Robinson 1947; Brock 1999).

With the bacterial etiology of sepsis established by the end of the XIX century, many concepts about bacteria already made part of the surgery and pathology texts: Terms like pyaemia, sapremia, purulent infection, putrid infection, septicemia, surgical sepsis and traumatic fever were used indistinctively for the systemic condition that we know today derives from the invasion of bacteria after the colonization of a wound (Van Arsdale 1886). Through their conclusive scientific evidences Koch and Pasteur change animalcules, semina morbi, contagia animata, cadaveric particles, disease powder, in the microbiological revolution, while Lister can take all these concepts into practice saving innumerable lives thus changing medicine practice forever.

9. Conclusions

"...when a man has been wounded who can be saved, there are in the first place two things to be kept in mind: that he should not die from hemorrhage or inflammation" Aurelius Cornelius Celsus. I Siglo d.C.

The identification of the phenomenon we know as sepsis today, secondary to any type of wound, was a constant from olden times to the Middle Ages. The temporal association between lesion and subsequent appearance of fever was well known, as well as the different inflammation signs in the primary lesion and the secondary systemic compromise. The interpretation of these phenomena changed from magical-religious conceptions to the classic humoralism which dominated western medicine for more than a thousand years. The governing paradigm in each period supported the medical and surgical management of wounds, beginning with the relatively a-pyogen healing from the Ancient Egypt and Alexandria, going through the surgical and non surgical management of the classic Greek and Greco- Roman medicine whose therapeutic objective, though qualitatively was the same, varied in the gradual importance suppuration as fundamental healing process gained. Finally, during the Middle Ages, an imminently Galen approach, Arab medicine performed a determined defense of suppuration as a comprehensive part of the treatment and favored non surgical procedures as cautery in order to facilitate it. This historical evolution was sprinkled by multiple facts of epistemological relevance, In the first place, during the Middle Ages there was a split between the medical knowledge and surgery allowing the gradual loss of surgical knowledge from the classic texts, which explains why during this period the use of sutures, wound exploration and vessels ligatures were pushed into the background turning the painful cautery in the suitable conduct for all types of lesions. Secondly, none of the intents to defeat the Galen dogma "pus bonum et laudabile" succeeded: without a philosophical corpus that supported the paradigm changes, without experimental coincident evidences in time-place which could force such change, and without any anomaly that placed a doubt on the established conceptions, this task would continue to be a chimera. These factors of a strictly epistemological order, explain why the Galen dogma continued taking lives through the Middle Ages until after the Renaissance. Sepsis, understood as an anomaly in Khunian terns, put in crisis the Galen paradigm allowing important developments in medicine; change would finally come with the transformation in the philosophical conception of the disease in which it was accepted that it could be caused by entities and not by simple deviations of normality. This turn from the physiological to the ontological provided the support that would allow the acceptance that those gracious animalcules seen through the microscope lenses, microorganisms, are the real enemies of the injured and infected patient.

Many of the quantitative novelties achieved by medicine during the XX century are nothing but reforms, subtractions and contributions to those models which pioneers from past centuries conceived. As we could observe, these deep ruptures needed a fertile soil in the scientific spirit and in the minds of men of science in order to assume the doctrinal and practical changes which allowed facing up to the scientific challenges. Historiographic misunderstandings like the ones raised by Fracastolo's work, or scientific tragedies such as Semmelweis' life, are irrefutable proof that the development of a discipline is neither an isolated fact from the rest of the sciences and human activities since that discipline nurtures with them, nor an isolated fact from society since it is immersed in it and serves its purposes. To conclude, we might ask a last question: Is sepsis nowadays an overcome challenge? Definitively, no. Sepsis constitutes, today, one of the main challenges in intensive care: it is the main cause of death in non coronary ICUs, up to 35% of patients in these units will suffer the disease. 18 million cases per year with a global mortality of 30% are reported each year. It is responsible for more deaths than AIDS and its incidence will increase in 8% annually. After 40 years of exhaustive research mortality has been reduced in only 10% (Martin 2003; Jaimes 2005). 17 billion dollars per year in costs and attention are spent yearly and, from the medicines researched, several dozen in three decades only two have marginally diminished mortality. It is not surprising then that sepsis has been called with sarcasm "the pharmaceutics cemetery". All these factors show a problem: Is sepsis becoming a systematic challenge for the present medical paradigm? It is very possible since many factors in our world are analogous in medical and social consequences to the challenges that allowed sepsis to take innumerable lives in olden days. Our immune system evolved in a context which demanded the most vigorous answers before the invading pathogen, a killing or dying fight; however, the game rules have changed. Present and unavoidable conditions in our modern world such as population aging, microbial endurance, immunosuppression, increasing intravenous and other types of invasions are related with an increase in the incidence and seriousness of the disease. These factors not only give advantages to microorganisms but also exert a tremendous evolutionary pressure on us. We have a permanent armed race in which our invaders will always have an advantage over us and we find ourselves unrelentingly urged to innovate from the biomedical sciences. In conclusion, maybe sepsis imposes new challenges of great magnitude in the following years that can allow us, and force us to open new ways to develop new paradigms in this century's medicine… at least that is what the costly lessons of the past teach us.

Author details

Johan Sebastián Hernández Botero
Departamento de Ciencias Básicas para la Salud, Universidad de Caldas, Colombia
Departamento de Ciencias Básicas Biológicas, Universidad Autónoma de Manizales, Colombia

María Cristina Florián Pérez
Departamento Clínico-Quirúrgico, Universidad de Caldas, Colombia
Unidad de Cuidados Intensivos, Hospital Departamental Santa Sofía ESE, Colombia

Acknowledgement

Orlando Mejía Rivera, Julián David Bohórquez Carvajal, Oscar Jaramillo Robledo, Eliana Andrea Castrillon Soto.

10. References

Abbas, A. (2002). Inmunidad Innata - Respuestas fisiológicas y patológicas al lipolisacárido bacteriano. *Inmunología celular y molecular*. A. Abbas, Lichtman, AH., Pober, JS. Madrid, McGraw Hill - Interamericana: 287.

Adams, R., Victor, M., Ropper, AH. (1999). Infecciones del Sistema Nervioso. *Principios de Neurología.* R. Adams, Victor, M., Ropper, AH. Mexico D.F, McGraw Hill - Interamericana: 604-643.

Aguirre, C. (1996). "El Legado de Louis Pasteur." *Iatreia* 9(1): 16-21.

Baskett, T. (2004). "Ambroise Paré and the arrest of haemorrhage." *Resucitation* 62: 133-135.

Béclard, R., Cloquet, H., Cloquet, J., Orfilia, M. (1834). *Nouveau Dictionnaire de Médecine, Chirurgie, Pharmacie, Chimie, Histoire Naturelle.* Paris, Deville Cavellin.

Beutler, B., Poltorak, A. (2001). "Sepsis and evolution of the innate immune response." *Crit Care Med* 29(7): (Suppl):2-6.

Bishoy, M. (2004). "Surgery on Papyrus." *Student BMJ* 12: 338-339.

Blum, Y., Esterhai, J. (2002). "The history of the treatment of musculoskeletal infection." *Oper Tech Orthop* 12(4): 226-231.

Border, J., Hasset, J., LaDuca, J., Seibel, R., Steinberg, S., Mills, B., Losi, P., et al. (1987). "The gut origin of septic states in blunt multiple trauma." *Ann Surg* 206: 427-448.
Breasted, J. H. (1980). *The Edwin Smith Surgical Papyrus*, Chicago University. Chicago Press.
Brock, T. D. (1999). *Robert Koch: a life in medicine and bacteriology*. Washington, American Society for Microbiology Press.
Broughton, G., Janis, JE., Attinger, CE. (2006). "A brief history of wound care." *Plast Reconstr Surg* 117(7): (suppl):6-11.
Brunschwig, H. (1497). *Das Buch Der Cirurgia*. Strassburgo, Johann Grüninger
Busch, D., Dieffenbach, JF., Hecker, JF., Horn, E., Jüngken, JC., Link, HF., Miller, J. (1845). *Encyclopädisches Wörterbuch der medicinischen Wissenschaften*. Berlin, Verlag von Veit - J.W. Boike.
Bustíos Romaní, C. (2004). Higiene y Sanidad en el Mundo occidental. *Cuatrocientos años de Salud Publica en Perú*. C. Bustios Romaní. Lima, UNMSM: 34-35.
Castiglioni, A. (1941). *A History of Medicine*. New York, A.A. Knopf.
Celsus, A. C. (1961). De Medicina. W. T. Spencer. Cambridge, Harvard University Press.
Cinel, I., Dellinger, P. (2007). "Advances in pathogenesis and management of sepsis." *Curr Opin Infect Dis* 20: 345-352.
Crombie, A. (1987). La recepción de la ciencia greco-arabe en el mundo occidental. *Historia de las Ciencias, De San Agustín a Galileo.* A. Crombie. Madrid, Alianza Universidad. 1: 44-67.
Charles, J., Charles, D. (1994). Infeccion posparto. *Infecciones Obstétricas y Perinatales*. D. Charles. Madrid, Mosby / Doyma: 61-67.
Chase, K. (2003). *Firearms: A Global History to 1700*. Cambridge, Cambridge University Press.
Davies, R. (1970). "Some Roman Medicine." *Med Hist* 14(1): 101-106.
De Costa, C. (2002). ""The contagiousness of childbed fever": a short history of puerperal sepsis and its treatment." *Med J Aust* 177(12): 668-671.
Debré, P., Forster, E. (2000). *Louis Pasteur*. Baltimore, Jonhs Hopkins University Press.
Dellinger, P., Levy, MM., Carlet, JM., Bion J., Parker, MM., Jaeschke, R., Reinhart, K, et al. (2008). "Surviving Sepsis Campaign: international guidelines for management of severe sepsis and septic shock." *Crit Care Med* 36(1): 296-327.
Drucker, C. (2008). "Ambroise Paré and the birth of the gentle art of surgery." *Yale J Biol Med* 81(4): 199-202.
Ellis, H. (2001). "John Hunter's teachings on gunshot wounds." *J R Soc Med* 94: 43-45.
Forrest, R. (1982). "Development of wound therapy from the Dark Ages to the present." *J R Soc Med.* 75: 268-273.
Forrest, R. (1982). "Early history of wound treatment." *J R Soc Med.* 75: 198-205.
Francis, A. (1985). *The Genuine Works Of Hippocrates*. New York, Classics of Medicine Library / Gryphon Editions Ltd.
Francis, A. (1985). Hippocrates: On Fractures. *The Genuine Works Of Hippocrates.* A. Francis. New York, Classics of Medicine Library / Gryphon Editions Ltd.: 157-166.
Francis, A. (1985). Hippocrates: On Regimen on Acute Disease. *The Genuine Works Of Hippocrates.* A. Francis. New York, Classics of Medicine Library / Gryphon Editions Ltd.: 59 - 97.
Francis, A. (1985). Hippocrates: On Surgery. *The Genuine Works Of Hippocrates.* A. Francis. New York., Classics of Medicine Library / Gryphon Editions Ltd.: 157-204.

Francis, A. (1985). Hippocrates: On Ulcers. *The Genuine Works Of Hippocrates*. A. Francis. New York, Classics of Medicine Library / Gryphon Editions Ltd: 325-336.
Gabay, C., Kushner, I. (1999). "Acute-phase proteins and other systemic responses to inflammation." *N Engl J Med* 340(6): 448-454.
Geroulanos, S. and E. T. Douka (2006). "Historical perspective of the word "sepsis"." *Intensive Care Med* 32(12): 2077.
Grissom, J. (2004). Explaining Plague in Early Modern Europe: The Role of Contagion in the Theories of Girolamo Fracastoro and Thomas Willis. *History of Science*. Norman, Oklahoma., University of Oklahoma. Master of Arts.: 91.
Grmek, M. (1991). *Diseases in the ancient greek world*. Baltimore and London, The John Hopkins University Press.
Guthrie, G. (1827). *A treatise on Gun-shot Wounds*. London, Burges and Hill.
Haggard, H. W. (1947). *El Médico en la Historia*. Buenos Aires, Editorial Sudamericana.
Helling, T., McNabney, WK. (2000). "The role of amputation in the management of Battlefield Casualities: A History of Two Millenia." *J Trauma* 49: 930-939.
Henao, G. (1999). "La lucha de I. F. Semmelweis en la génesis de un nuevo paradigma." *Iatreia* 12(3): 149-156.
Hernandez Botero, J. (2009). "Recuento histórico y análisis epistemológico de la sepsis secundaria a lesiones y su control quirúrgico: Desde el papiro de Edwin Smith hasta el "pus bonum et laudabile"." *Iatreia* 22(3): 292-300.
Hippocrates (1849). Of Epidemics. *The Genuine Works Of Hippocrates*. A. Francis. London, Sydenham Society: 339-381.
Hontanilla Calatayud, B. (1999). *Cirugía Menor*. Madrid, Marban.
Howard-Jones, N. (1977). "Fracastoro and Henle: A re-appraisal of their contribution to the concept of communicable diseases." *Med Hist* 21: 61-68.
Hunter, J. (1985). *A treatise on the blood, inflammation and Gun-Shot Wounds*. Birmingham, Classics of Surgery Library / Gryphon Editions.
Jaimes, F. (2005). "A literature review of the epidemiology of sepsis in Latin America." *Rev Panam Salud Publica* 18(3): 163-171.
Joly, R., Ed. (1970). *Hippocrates: Des maladies IV*. París, Société d'édition Les Belles Lettres.
Keel, M., Trentz, O. (2005). "Pathophysiology of polytrauma." *Injury* 36(6): 691-709.
Kuhn, T. S. (2004). *La estructura de las revoluciones científicas*. Buenos Aires, Fondo de Cultura Económica.
Laín Entralgo, P. (1979). *Historia Universal de la Medicina*. Barcelona, Salvat.
Larrey, J. (1812). *Memoires de Chirurgie Militaire et Campagnes*. Paris, Tallandier.
Lattimore, R. (1961). *The Iliad of Homer*. Chicago, University of Chicago Press.
Ledermann, W. (2008). "En memoria de Lister." *Rev Chil Infect* 25(5): 351-356.
Lenz, A., Franklin, GA., Cheadle, WG. (2007). "Systemic inflammation after trauma." *Injury* 38(12): 1336-1345.
Lister, J. (1867). "On a new method of treating compund fracture, abscess etc., with observations on the conditions of suppuration." *Lancet*: 326-329, 357-359, 387-389, 507-509.
Lister, J. (1870). "The antiseptic system of treatment in surgery." *Lancet* 2: 287.
López Piñeros, J. (1974). Patología y medicina interna en Alemania. *Historia Universal de la medicina*. P. Lain-Entralgo. Barcelona, Salvat. 6: 123-155. Volumen VI.
López Piñeros, J. (2002). *La Medicina en la Historia*. Madrid, La esfera de los libros.

Magner, L. (2009). *A History of Infectious Diseases and the Microbial World*. New York, Praeger Publishers.

Majno, G. (1975). *The Healing Hand: Man and Wound in the Ancient World*. Cambridge, Harvard University Press.

Majno, G. (1991). "The ancient riddle of sigma eta psi iota sigma (sepsis)." *J Infect Dis* 163(5): 937-945.

Majno, G., Cotran, RS., Kaufman N., Ed. (1982). *Current topics in inflamation and infection.* International Academy of Pathology Monograph. Baltimore., Wlliams & Wilkins.

Malkin, H. (1984). "Julius Cohnheim (1839-1884). His life and contributions to pathology." *Ann Clin Lab Sci* 14(5): 335-342.

Martin, G., Mannino, DM., Eaton, S., Moss, M. (2003). "The epidemiology of sepsis in the United States from 1979 through 2000." *N Engl J Med* 348: 1546-1554.

McFarlane, H. (1976). "Malnutrition and impaired immune response to infection." *Proc Nutr Soc.* 35(3): 263-272.

Mejía Rivera, O. (1990). *Humanismo y Antihumanismo*. Manizales., Fondo Editorial Universidad de Caldas.

Mejía Rivera, O. (2002). *De la prehistoria a la Medicina Egipcia*. Manizales, Centro Editorial Universidad de Caldas.

Mejía Rivera, O. (2004). *Los descubrimientos serendípicos. Aproximaciones epistemológicas al contexto del descubrimiento científico.* Manizales, Universidad de Caldas, Facultad de Ciencias para la Salud

Mejía Rivera, O. (2005). "El nuevo paradigma genético y la naturaleza humana." *Acta Med Colomb* 30: 68-72.

Nutton, V. (1983.). "The seeds of disease: An explanation of contagion and infection from the greeks to the renaissance." *Med Hist* 27: 1-34.

O'Neill, L., Greene, C. (1998). "Signal Transduction pathways activated by the IL-1 receptor family: Ancient Signaling machinery in mammals, insects and plants." *J Leukoc Biol* 63: 650-657.

Opal, S. (2000). "Phylogenetic and functional relationships between coagulation and the innate immune response." *Crit Care Med.* 28(9): suppl: 77-80.

Opal, S., Girard, TD., Ely, EW. (2005). "The immunopathogenesis of sepsis in elderly patients. ." *Clin Infect Dis.* 15(41): Suppl 7:S504-512.

Otis, G. (1883). *The Medical and Surgical History of the War of the Rebellion*. Washington, US Govermment Printing Office.

Paget, S. (2005). *Ambroise Pare and His Times 1510 to 1590*. Whitefish Montana, Kessinger Publishing.

Pastrana, J., García, JP., Civeira, J., Prieto, M. (2006). Bioquímica Hemática: Velocidad de sedimentación globular. *Balcells: La Clínica y el Laboratorio.* J. Valtueña Prieto. Barcelona, Elsevier-Masson: 111-115.

Pollak, K. (1970). *Los discípulos de Hipocrates, Una historia de la Medicina*. Barcelona, Círculo de Lectores.

Pollak, K. (1970). *Los discípulos de Hipocrates, Una historia de la Medicina.* Barcelona, Círculo de Lectores.

Pringle, J. (1750). Experiments upon septic and antiseptic substances. *Philosophical Transactions, of the Royal Society of London*. D. W. A. Millar, T. Durham T. Payne. London, Bulmer, W.

Restrepo, A. (1996). "Louis Pasteur: In memoriam." *Iatreia* 9(1): 22-27.

Robinson, V. (1947). La Medicina Árabe en la Edad Media. *La Medicina en la Historia*. V. Robinson. Buenos Aires, Ediciones del Tridente: 95-96.

Robinson, V. (1947). La Medicina en el Antiguo Egipto. *La Medicina en la Historia*. V. Robinson. Buenos Aires, Ediciones del Tridente: 19-32.

Robinson, V. (1947). La Medicina en la Edad Media. *La Medicina en la Historia*. V. Robinson. Buenos Aires, Ediciones del Tridente: 127-175.

Robinson, V. (1947). *La Medicina en la Historia*. Buenos Aires, Ediciones del Tridente.

Robinson, V. (1947). *La Medicina en la Historia*. Buenos Aires, Ediciones del Tridente.

Robinson, V. (1947). La Medicina Griega en Alejandría. *La Medicina en la Historia*. V. Robinson. Buenos Aires, Ediciones del Tridente: 34-80.

Schwartz, R. (1932). "The historical derivation of the physiological principles underlying the treatment of fractures." *J Bone Joint Surg Am* 14: 17-26.

Seara Valero, M. (1995). *Magia y Medicina*. Madrid, Ediciones Contrastes.

Senn, N. (1900). *Medico-Surgical Aspects of The Spanish American War*. Chicago, American Medical Association.

Shoemaker, W. (1971). "Cardiorespiratory patterns in complicated and uncomplicated septic shock." *Ann Surg.* 174: 119-125.

Siegel, R. (1960). "Epidemic and Infectious Diseases at the Time of Hippocrates: Their Relation to Modern Accounts." *Gesnerus* 17: 77-99.

Silvaticus, M. (1541). Pandectae medicinae. T. Paganum. Salerno: 14.

Singer, C., Singer D. (1917). "The scientific position of Girolamo Fracastoro." *Ann Med Hist*: 1-34.

Singer, C., Underwood, EA. (1962). *A Short History of Medicine*. New York, Clarendon Press.

Stiefel, M., Shaner, A., Schaefer, S. (2006). "The Edwin Smith papyrus: The birth of analytical thinking in medicine and otolaryngology." *The Laryngoscope* 116(2): 182-188.

Terrencio Varrón, M. (1992). *De las cosas del Campo. Traducido por Domingo Tirado Benedí*. México DF, Universidad Autonoma de México.

Thurston, A. (2000). "Of Blood, Inflamation And Gunshot Wounds: The history of the control of Sepsis." *Aust N Z J Surg* 70: 855-861.

Trzeciak, S., Rivers, EP. (2005). "Clinical manifestations of disordered microcirculatory perfusion in severe sepsis. ." *Critical Care* 9(suppl 4): S20-S26.

Van Arsdale, W. (1886). "Sepsis. On the present state of knowledge in bacterial science in its surgical relations." *Ann Surg.* 3(4): 321-333.

Walker, K. (1956). *Joseph Lister*. London, Hutchinson.

Wright, W. (1930). *Gerolamo Fracastoro: De contagione et Contagiosis Morbis Et Eorum Curatione*. New York, GP Putman's Sons - Library of New York Academy of Medicine.

Section 2

Sepsis Pathophysiology and Animal Studies

Chapter 2

Experimental Sepsis Models

Safiah Mai, Momina Khan, Patricia Liaw and Alison Fox-Robichaud, on behalf of the Canadian Critical Care Translational Biology Group (CCCTBG)

Additional information is available at the end of the chapter

http://dx.doi.org/10.5772/52876

1. Introduction

Sepsis is a devastating condition characterized by the systemic activation of inflammatory and coagulation pathways in response to microbial infection of normally sterile parts of the body. Severe sepsis, defined as sepsis with at least one dysfunctional organ, is the leading cause of death in non-coronary intensive care units and is associated with mortality rates of 30-50%. The development of experimental sepsis models to elucidate the progression and pathophysiology of clinical sepsis spans the past eight decades. Studies utilizing models of intra-abdominal sepsis began in the 1930's with the isolation of endotoxin and the intravenous or peritoneal infusion of live organisms, a model which dominated sepsis research for over 30 years. In the 1960's, a transition was made from endotoxemia models to a focus on bacteremia. Such models include the injection of live bacteria (Pseudomonas aeruginosa, Escherichia coli, and Staphylococcus aureus), inoculation of feces, and intramuscular, intraperitoneal and subdermal implantation of feces-containing capsules and sponges. Following the use of endotoxemia and bacteremia models, various models involving ischemia and bowel perforation were developed. These models led to the development of the most frequently used sepsis model today, cecal ligation puncture (CLP) and more recently, the colon ascendens stent peritonitis (CASP) model. Over the years several large animal models of sepsis have also been developed, of which canine, ovine, bovine, rabbit, and non-human primates have proven to be most useful. However, the translation of findings and inferences from animal sepsis models to human sepsis remains a challenge. In this chapter, we will provide an overview of experimental models of sepsis, with focus on the merits and limitations of each model. We will also focus on strategies that may improve the translation of results from animal studies to human sepsis. This requires consideration of the limitations of current sepsis models including supportive therapies, considering age, gender, obesity, and exposure to pathogens in animals used, and addressing the risk of bias in experimental sepsis models.

2. History of experimental sepsis models

Sepsis is a serious, complicated, heterogeneous condition involving a dysregulated host response to an initial infection and subsequent hemodynamic, cardiovascular, respiratory, metabolic, hormonal, inflammatory, innate and adaptive immune changes (1;2). Experimental sepsis models have been utilized extensively and developed over the last eight decades to study the progression and pathophysiology of clinical sepsis (3-5). Intra-abdominal sepsis models were introduced in the 1930s with the isolation of endotoxins and the intravenous or peritoneal infusion of live organisms, models which dominated sepsis research for thirty years. Upon the discovery of new antimicrobial compounds, treatment of intra-abdominal abscesses became a clinical focus in the 1960s and a transition was made from the endotoxin model to the bacterial model of infection (4). These models used fecal pellets and the addition of an adjuvant to induce infection with the goal of studying peritonitis rather than isolated abscess formation (3). However, these models fell short as mortality rates relied heavily on bacterial counts and bacterial composition which varied widely between both species and individual subjects. Additionally, the bacterial overload at non-physiologically relevant levels and lack of a sterile environment contributed to a much greater mortality rate in experimental sepsis compared to what was observed clinically (4).

To overcome these limitations, the introduction of defined bacterial inoculum models in the 1970s improved sepsis modeling immensely. These models were also used in landmark studies which uncovered the two-stage nature of intra-abdominal sepsis with gram-negative enteric bacteria inducing the peritonitis phase and anaerobic bacteria responsible for subsequent abscess formation (3). Antibiotic agents tested using defined bacterial models were successful in either improving survival or reducing abscess formation but were not successful in improving both criteria. This led to the development of models which more closely resembled the progression clinical sepsis.

In the '60s and '70s, the Clowes group and Wright group were able to create septic conditions in dogs by ligating the cecum at the ileocecal valve, successfully demonstrating both the initial hyperdynamic phase and later hypodynamic phase of sepsis, but neither groups documented bacterial cultures to validate dissemination of pathogens in the peritoneum or circulation (6-9). A small animal model was later introduced by Ryan *et al* whereby the rat cecum is ligated distal to the ileocecal valve, devascularizing the cecum and introducing a necrotic component to experimental sepsis (10). It is this latter model which lead to the most frequently used animal model of sepsis, cecal ligation and puncture.

3. Common models of polymicrobial sepsis

3.1. Cecal Ligation and Puncture (CLP)

The CLP model of intra-abdominal sepsis was introduced by Wichterman, Baue, and Chaudry in 1980. The group published an insightful review of previous models and introduced a novel sepsis model still widely regarded as the gold standard for modelling polymicrobial sepsis today—the cecal ligation and puncture (CLP) model. Rats were fasted, their cecum was ligated distal to the ileocecal valve, the antimesenteric cecal surface was punctured twice with an 18G ½ needle, and received subcutaneous saline post-operatively. This model induced polymicrobial infection (blood cultures positive for *Escherichia coli, Streptococcus bovis, Proteus mirabilis, Enterococcus,* and *Bacteroides fragilis)* and bacteremia (peritoneal cavity fluid positive for the above microbes as well as *Streptococcus viridians* and *Clostridium sporogenes)* and a 70% mortality rate. Mildly ill rats sacrificed 10 hours following CLP demonstrated the early hyperdynamic phase of sepsis (increased blood flow to organs, hyperinsulinemia, and hyperglycemia) while rats sacrificed 16-24 hours post-operative represented a hypodynamic late septic state (decreased blood flow to organs, hypoinsulinemia, hypoglycemia, and high serum lactate levels) (3). The results of this model correlate with clinical sepsis conditions as patients who are initially normotensive, show an increase in cardiac output, have low peripheral resistance, and increased total oxygen consumption, conditions which reverse in late septic shock (3).

Multiple aspects of the CLP procedure address the complex, of the clinical course of sepsis. CLP induces polymicrobial infection of the peritoneum with a localized infectious focus, release of bacteria and endotoxic molecular components of pathogens (pathogen-associated molecular patterns or PAMPs) into normally sterile areas in the host, and subsequent translocation of enteric bacteria into the bloodstream, modelling the stages of intra-abdominal clinical sepsis (3). Under anaesthesia, the cecum is exposed and trauma is induced via a midline skin laparotomy and blunt dissection of the peritoneum to exteriorize the cecum. Avoiding damage to the mesenteric vessels, the cecum is ligated with suture distal to the ileocecal valve, punctured once or twice (through-and-though) from the mesenteric to anti-mesenteric direction halfway between the ligation and cecal end, and aspirated for trapped gasses (3). A small amount of fecal content is extruded to allow for patency of the puncture(s) and continuous flow of feces post-operatively. The cecum is returned into the peritoneal cavity taking care not to spread fecal content on the incision and the peritoneum and abdomen are closed separately with sutures (11).

3.1.1. Host response to CLP

Significant elements of the host response to CLP-induced polymicrobial sepsis are present in clinical sepsis. The hemodynamic profiles, cardiovascular response, metabolic phases, systemic involvement of cytokine responses (ex. profiles of interleukins), changes in the innate and adaptive immune response, and abnormalities in mediators of coagulation which occur following CLP are also observed in the clinical course of sepsis (12). Moreover, CLP involves multiple, complicated elements which are unaccounted for by models of endotoxemia and bacterial inoculum. These include a laparotomy which mimics surgery-induced trauma in the septic patient, the presence of inflamed tissue (peritonitis), necrosis via ligation of the cecal end, apoptosis of specific leukocytes, bacteremia induced by pathogens from a host-derived flora (fecal spillage), and translocation of enteric, living, multiplying bacteria into the bloodstream (12). The inclusion of these elements as part of the CLP model improves the clinical relevance of outcomes from these preclinical studies.

As observed in clinical sepsis, the hyperinflammatory state which occurs during the systemic inflammatory response syndrome (SIRS) transitions to an immunosuppressed state characterized by a compensatory acute response (CARS) (12;13). However, the point at which this transition occurs in both clinical and experimental sepsis is unclear. The early hyperdynamic stage of sepsis and the later hypodynamic state following the CLP procedure is indicated by changes in response to immune challenge and changes in peripheral blood cells, plasma levels of cytokines, and chemokines. Neutropenia and lymphopenia are characterized by significant peripheral blood alterations rapidly following CLP parallel to leukocytosis or leukocytopenia observed in the clinical SIRS condition (1;12-14). Following CLP, total white blood cells, polymorphonuclear cells, and lymphocytes increase rapidly within the first 2 hours, decrease from 2-4 hours, and plateau until endpoint at 8 hours following CLP (15). The pro-inflammatory response is also characterized by significant increases in cytokines TNFα and IL-6 and chemokines KC, MIP-2, and MCP-1 from non-detectable plasma levels that increase and remain elevated over an 8 hour period (12;15). Several studies have demonstrated the importance of an early pro-inflammatory response in the progression of sepsis. Antibody-mediated blockade of IL-6 (16;17), complement factor C5a or C5a receptor (18-20), and depletion of neutrophils offered protective effects and increased survival of animals subjected to CLP.

While anti-inflammatory proteins like IL-10 and glucocorticoids are crucial for dampening and terminating the inflammatory response (21-23), the hypoinflammatory phase of experimental sepsis characterized by neutrophil paralysis (shutting down of signaling pathways), apoptosis of lymphocytes and dendritic cells, and elevations in anti-inflammatory mediators significantly increase the susceptibility of the septic host to nosocomial infection. It is during this hypoinflammatory, immunosuppressed state when most mortality is observed in clinical sepsis (21) however it is unknown if this holds true in animal sepsis.

3.1.2. Modifying severity in CLP

Multiple elements of the CLP procedure can be modified to model the wide spectrum of conditions observed in clinical sepsis. These factors include the number of cecal punctures, gauge of needle used to puncture the cecum, and the length of cecum ligated in the animal (3). However, there are conflicting findings as to whether the number of cecal punctures affects disease severity. One group reported that two cecal punctures does not result in a significant increase in mortality but is associated with a decrease time to endpoint (24). Variations in the CLP protocol can be used to produce different disease severities and mimic various stages of the sepsis spectrum from the rapid onset of a robust, hyperinflammatory state to a gradual progression of severe sepsis to an immunosuppression in septic shock. For instance, modifications such as using a smaller gauge/thicker needle (18G ½ rather than a 26G½) or ligating a larger amount of cecum (by placing the suture proximal to the ileocecal valve) can increase the severity and produce a mortality rate that may be more clinically relevant (25).

The flexibility in modeling various severities of disease, ability to recreate hemodynamic, metabolic, and immune changes, the inclusion of surgical trauma, necrosis, and apoptosis of specific cell types which more closely correlate with clinical sepsis contribute to the acceptance of CLP as the gold standard for modeling polymicrobial, intra-abdominal sepsis.

3.2. Colon Ascendens Stent Peritonitis (CASP)

Almost two decades following the introduction of the CLP model by Chaudry et al., Zantl et al. introduced a polymicrobial, peritonitis sepsis model termed colon ascendens stent peritonitis or CASP (26). The CASP model is a reproducible model suitable for studying the pathophysiology of abdominal sepsis and can be successfully varied by using stents of different diameters ranging from 14G to 22G (26;27). It can also be used to study surgical interventions which involve the elimination of the infectious focus by stent removal (27). The prevalence of the CASP model in sepsis studies has only recently increased. Currently, the number of studies utilizing the CLP sepsis model far exceed those using CASP (25).

In the CASP procedure, a laparotomy is performed to exteriorize the cecum, terminal ileum, and ascending colon. The ascending colon wall is pierced and the suture is fixed on the colon wall 15 mm distal from the ileocecal valve. A prepared stent or cannula is used to puncture the ascending colon around 1-2 mm proximal from the suture and the cannula is inserted into the colon and sutured securely. Fecal content is milked through the stent which provides a pathway between the intestinal lumen and the peritoneum, allowing unobstructed influx of enteric bacteria into the peritoneal cavity (26;28). Disease severity of this model, can be modified by adjusting the size of the cannula used for stenting from 14 G to 20 G (100% lethality and less than 50% mortality at 48 hours following surgery, respectively) (24;28). Within 3 hours of stent implantation, levels of circulating and systemic cytokines and chemokines including TNFα, IFN-γ, IL-1, IL-12, IL-18, KC/GRO-α, MCP-1, and anti-inflammatory IL-10 increase (26;29;30). Unlike CLP however, progression of sepsis in the CASP model appears less dependent on the initial immune response elicited by TNFα and more heavily focused on innate immune activation via toll-like receptors (TLRs) and TLR signalling. In several studies, progression of sepsis required the TLR adaptor molecule MyD88 and antibody mediated inhibition of TLR4/MD2 prevented lethality induced by CASP (31;32). IL-12 and inducible nitric oxide synthase (iNOS) offer some antibacterial and immunoprotective effects since mice genetically deficient of IL-12 and iNOS are more susceptible to CASP-induced sepsis (33). Additionally, exogenous addition of complement factor C3 (34) and activated protein C (35) offered cytoprotective and anti-inflammatory effects against CASP-induced lethality.

The CASP model of polymicrobial sepsis and peritonitis appears to have substantial utility, however our understanding of signalling pathways and the pathobiology which results in disease in this model are lacking. Animals subjected to CASP appear to mount a rapid, stronger immune response than animals subjected to CLP but further experimentation is required to determine the efficacy of using CASP as a sepsis model. Undoubtedly, the use of CASP will increase in prevalence as the pathophysiology and underlying mechanisms of disease which produce the septic conditions are uncovered.

3.3. CLP vs. CASP

Notable differences in the host response to CLP versus CASP-induced sepsis have been documented. The progression of sepsis in the CLP model involves TNFα-mediated activation of the immune response while the CASP model is less dependent on the initial immune response elicited by TNFα and more so dependent on TLR activation and signalling (12;25;29). One study comparing the two distinct models found that bacterial counts of peritoneal lavage, liver, lung, and serum levels of TNFα, IL-1β, and IL-10 increase steadily over a 24 hour period in the CASP model and were significantly higher than that of mice subjected to CLP (24). In this study, the authors observed continuously low bacterial counts and cytokine levels at all time-points as well as abscess formation around the cecum in mice subjected CLP. In light of these observations, it has been suggested that CASP is a true model of peritonitis with early SIRS, while CLP more closely mimics abscess formation (24;25). Alternatively, others interpret the rapid elevations in systemic cytokines, bacterial counts and strong immune response following CASP to be comparable to that observed in endotoxemia models and the inflammatory reactions characterized by protracted cytokine profiles following CLP to more closely reflect clinical sepsis (12).

Discrepancies between the host response to CLP versus CASP have been observed in studies using genetically-modified animals, although consensus on the interpretation of these results is lacking. While TNFα-deficient mice were protected in a CLP model, TNFRp55/TNFR1-deficient mice did not appear to have an altered resistance to CASP-induced sepsis (26;36). However, the differences observed may be due to the incomplete abolishment of TNFα activity as these mice may be deficient in only one of two TNF receptors, abolishing the cytotoxic TNFR1 and leaving the protective TNFR2 intact (37). Additionally, IFNγ exhibited protective effects in a CASP model and not in CLP-induced sepsis (26;36). Abolishing cytokine IL12p40 rendered the host more susceptible to CASP-induced sepsis while the same deficiency was found to either have no significant effect in some CLP studies (36) or increase susceptibility to sepsis in others CLP studies (38). The discrepancies in experimental outcomes of studies using CLP and CASP may be results of differences in the host response between these sepsis models, and an incomplete understanding of the pathophysiology of each model. Careful consideration should be taken to choose an appropriate model to address the primary research question to be investigated.

3.4. Limitations of current models

Earlier models of endotoxemia and bacterial inoculum fall short in modelling the complex changes which occur in clinical sepsis. Many cardiovascular, respiratory, metabolic, hormonal, inflammatory, innate and adaptive immune changes associated with the spectrum of septic conditions cannot be sufficiently reproduced by a single injection of endotoxin or bacteria (12). Injection of isolated microorganisms fails to mimic the host response to the diversity of causative agents in clinical sepsis. A specific instance is the injection of an endotoxin like lipopolysaccharide (LPS, a component of the cell wall of gram-negative bacteria) (4). LPS endotoxemia is dependent on TLR4 signalling and represents one specific aspect of the immune response, not the complex interactions of multiple signalling pathways during the progression of sepsis. Endotoxin injection and bacterial inoculum are followed by rapid elevations in cytokines which are much higher than what is observed in human sepsis (4). These models are more reflective of endotoxic shock rather than sepsis due to the overload of endotoxins in murine animals which exhibit a much higher endotoxin resistance than humans, further decreasing the clinical relevance of these studies (12). Moreover, these increases are transient, occurring in a short time span, and fail to reflect the complex physiological response in clinical sepsis.

Although surgical polymicrobial sepsis models show a greater clinical relevance than earlier models of endotoxemia and bacterial or fecal injections, both CLP and CASP are not without limitations. While the severity of experimental sepsis can be controlled by modifying certain elements of a CLP protocol (e.g. length of ligated cecum) these factors may also decrease the consistency between animals and reproducibility of the study, as the amount of cecum ligated may vary between subjects (3). More contributing factors to inter-animal variability include differences in the amount of fecal content in the cecum at the time of surgery, the size of cecum of each animal, and bacterial flora in different animals. Moreover, conflicting findings over the effect of the number of punctures on disease severity further highlight differences that may result due to surgical manipulation at the hands of different experiments (24). Another limitation of CLP and CASP……..

Another limitation of CLP and CASP is the inter-study variations due to differences in protocols used between investigators. The number of cecal punctures and sizes of needles used to perforate the bowels vary between studies using the CLP model. Likewise, differences in the diameter of catheter used, location of stent insertion and suturing in the CASP model also influence disease severity (24;25). While some of these limitations will inevitably affect the consistency and reproducibility of sepsis studies in animals, standard protocols can be enforced to reduce potential discrepancies.

4. Sepsis in large animal models

Small size, shorter reproductive cycles as well as less housing and maintenance costs are some advantages of utilizing small animals for scientific research. However certain physiological features of small animals vary considerably from its human counterparts (39). In addition, serial tissue and blood samples cannot be extracted from small animals, increasing the number of animals required to study whether an affect exists. Large animals, on the other hand not only allow serial sampling but also have very similar immunological and physiological functions to humans, rendering them better subjects to model clinical sepsis and drug testing. The Food and Drug Association (FDA) also recognizes the value of large animals requiring all new drug applications to include data from at least one non-rodent animal. In this section the rabbit, canine, porcine, ovine and non human primate models of sepsis and their limitations will be discussed.

4.1. Rabbit models of sepsis

A rabbit model of pneumococcal sepsis was developed in 1970. It encompasses several aspects of clinical sepsis including increased cardiac output and body temperature (40;41). This model involves the use of *Diplococcus pneumoniae* to induce sepsis and an inoculum of 1 ml of medium containing rabbit blood and tryptase soy broth with 10^8 to10^9 colony forming units is administered intraperitoneally (40) Several other rabbit models of sepsis were developed to study lung injury. Matute Bello et al. observed that a dose of 10^9 cfu/clot induced a more persistent infection compared to 10^8 cfu/clot, while inoculation of 10^{10} cfu/clot had lethal effects in a rabbit model of peritonitis (42). In this model, polymorphonuclear leukocyte (PMNs) function in the peritoneal cavity was perturbed suggesting potential contribution in the development of septic shock (42). Overall, the rabbit model of sepsis has been used to investigate physiological and immunological responses during sepsis and septic shock (43).

4.2. Canine models of sepsis

The canine models of endotoxemia and bacteremia have been used extensively to study cardiovascular function during sepsis. Dogs subjected to septic shock, show responses that parallel human sepsis. For example, there is a severe but reversible decrease in systolic ventricular function (44), a 32-108% increase in cardiac output, decrease in mean arterial pressure, and leukocytosis as well as increase in plasma epinephrine and norepinephrine levels during septic shock (45). Cytokine profiles in the canine model of endotoxemia also mirror those reported in human sepsis patients with a 62 fold increase in IL-6 mRNA in peripheral blood mononuclear cells (PBMC) and 4.5 fold increase in TNFα within the first hours compared to controls (46).

Despite the analogous physiological responses, there are several limitations of this model pertaining to clinical relevance. Canines have an adrenergic sensitive sphincter around the hepatic vein which constricts during sepsis increasing intestinal venous pressure and damaging the mucosal barrier, increasing its relevance to a gut injury model (47;48). Another important limitation is the resistance of canines to endotoxins and the requirement of high LPS dosage to induce sepsis (39;49). This requirement for increased endotoxemia results in a severe hypodynamic response in canines (50) which does not mimic hyperdynamic human sepsis.

4.3. Porcine models of sepsis

Pigs are popular animals for since they are readily available and relatively easy to handle. Continuous infusion of live bacteria, endotoxins as well as CLP are some of the methods used to induce sepsis in pigs. Porcine models of sepsis have been used extensively to investigate therapeutic agents focusing on improving renal, hepatic, intestinal and cardiovascular function (51-53). For instance, using a porcine model of LPS induced shock, Cohen et al. observed that increasing levels of nitric oxide (NO) improves renal blood flow and glomerular filtration rate (51). In addition, the porcine model of fecal peritonitis has been previously used to investigate the impact of adding low dose arginine vasopressin (AVP) to norepinephrine infusion for improving organ function (52). In the AVP treatment group, renal function was significantly improved, and significantly less hepatic apoptosis compared to the group treated with norepinephrine alone, suggesting that the addition of AVP to norepinephrine improves renal function (52).

The porcine model of fecal peritonitis has also been used to study acute lung injury associated with sepsis. Septic pigs have decreased left ventricular function, respiratory dysfunction as well as hemorrhage, pulmonary congestion associated with neutrophil infiltration characteristic of acute lung injury (53). This model has been further used to study effects of certain therapeutic agents such as N-acetylamrinone and L-arginine (54;55).

Due to the close similarity between pig and human anatomies, these animals have also been utilized to develop techniques commonly performed on sepsis patients such as laparoscopy (56). Porcine models of neonatal sepsis also closely mimic the clinical course of neonatal sepsis with a significant decrease in systemic blood pressure (71 ± 3 mmHg in sepsis and 64 ± 3 mmHg in control at 3 h) and increases in serum levels of endotoxins, TNFα, and IL-6 (57). Anatomical and physiological similarities between porcine and human anatomy have allowed for the successful testing of techniques and study of therapeutic agents which translate to human sepsis.

4.4. Ovine models of sepsis

In sheep, infusion of endotoxins (58), live bacteria as well as administration of fecal content into the abdominal cavity are some methods used to induce sepsis. The ovine model of sepsis has distinct similarities to human sepsis and several advantages over other animal models specifically regarding cardiopulmonary responses. One similarity between sheep and human sepsis is the biphasic cardiovascular profile. In endotoxemia models of ovine sepsis, two phases of cardiopulmonary function are observed (59). Within the first hour, the animal is in a hypodynamic state with a low cardiac index, myocardial contractility, high mean pulmonary arterial pressure, and pulmonary vascular resistance (59). The first phase is followed by a hyperdynamic state with significant increase in cardiac output (59).

The ovine is also a popular specie to study sepsis associated with lung injury. Daniel Traber is a pioneer in developing the ovine model of 'smoke injury' which involves insufflating sheep with smoke from burning cotton cloth (60) and the 'ovine burn model' which involves third degree burns and smoke injury (61). Smoke inhalation is induced using a modified bee smoker filled with 40 g of burning cotton cloth attached to a tracheostomy tube through a modified endotracheal tube (61). Based on similar principles, the ovine model of 'smoke inhalation and septic shock' was developed to study sepsis associated with pneumonia that develops due to acute lung injury (ALI) and acute respiratory distress syndrome (ARDS) after smoke inhalation (62). In this model, the aforementioned technique of 'smoke inhalation' is used to induce lung injury (63), followed by instilling bacteria such as *Pseudomonas aeruginosa* into the lungs (63;64).

Using the 'ovine smoke inhalation and septic shock' model several therapeutic agents have been investigated for sepsis management. Necrosis and apoptosis in this model were improved by administration of WW-85, a peroxynitrite decomposition catalyst. Other notable changes include improved gas exchange, decreased levels of myeloperoxidase (MPO) and lung 3-nitrotyrosine (65). There was also an overall improvement in pulmonary function suggesting that blocking nitric oxide-peroxynitrite pathway may ameliorate some effects of septic shock (65).The ovine model of sepsis and septic shock has made important contributions in the areas of cardiovascular (66) and pulmonary research as well as in determining the efficacy of fluids (58) and therapeutic agents (67), such as anticoagulants (68) and recombinant human protein C (69) to improve sepsis outcomes.

4.5. Non-human primate models of sepsis

Due to genetic similarities to humans, non-human primates are an ideal model for testing species-specific therapies (70). The method of inducing sepsis and septic shock in baboons utilizes an intravenous infusion of live *E.coli* (70). Using the baboon model of sepsis, several therapeutic discoveries have been made, the most prominent one being Activated Protein C (APC) (71;72). Taylor et al. reported that co-administration of APC with E. coli at lethal doses reduces coagulopathic and hepatotoxic effects induced by E. coli. This blocking of lethal effects of *E.coli* disappeared when protein C activation was blocked *in vivo* (73). More recently Xu et al. also reported that histone levels increase following *E.coli* administration in baboons. Extracellular histones released in response to inflammatory stimuli and during sepsis contributes to endothelial dysfunction, organ failure and death (71). Xu et al. discovered that baboons co-administered with both APC and *E.coli*, were rescued from mortality (71). The success of APC in baboon model of sepsis, allowed for its use in the clinical setting, until its recent withdrawal from the market following a further phase III trial. Despite the advantages associated with baboon models of sepsis, risk of infectious disease transmission, high housing and maintenance costs, as well as the ethical concerns deter many investigators from utilizing these animals for sepsis research (49).

4.6. Limitations of large animal models of sepsis

Large animal models have provided tremendous insight into the pathophysiology of sepsis, however there are certain limitations to the use of these animals. Due to their large size, they are also more difficult to handle, house, and anaesthetize and in the case of primates, pose risks of cross transmissible diseases (47).

5. Co-morbidities and sepsis

There have been several therapeutic agents with positive outcomes in animal models however majority failed to show efficacy in clinical settings. This disconnect is partially due to discrepancies in translating findings from animal models to clinical sepsis. Defined human target populations and established severities of sepsis would allow for more realistic and applicable animal modelling.

Clinical studies report that individuals with co-morbidities such as diabetes are at a higher risk of mortality and morbidity from infectious diseases (74-77). It has also been estimated that greater than 50% of septic patients have at least one additional co-morbid condition (78). Therefore, incorporating co-morbid conditions into animal models is one method by which modeling clinical sepsis in animal models could be improved.

5.1. Sepsis and diabetes

Several animal studies and clinical trials have demonstrated that diabetes increases the risk of infections and mortality (74-77). A retrospective cohort study from Ontario, Canada by Shah et al. reported that almost half of the diabetic patients in their study (n=513,749) had a minimum of one case of infectious disease for which they were either hospitalized or received a physician claim (74). It was also found that bacterial infections and infections in general were also more commonly found in diabetics (74). From animal models of type II diabetes it is known that sepsis induced inflammation is more severe in diabetic animals (79). Septic diabetic animals also have increased bacteria load (80;81), altered levels of cytokine expression (81;82) and dysfunctional immune cells such as PMNs contributing to poor outcomes.

Studies in animal models of obesity parallel the findings in diabetic animals. Strandberg et al. reported that mice fed a high fat diet (HFD) with saturated fats, had higher mortality rates when challenged with *Staphylococcus aureus* compared to mice fed a low fat diet (LFD) (83). The HFD fed group had increased bacterial load, decreased immune cell-mediated clearance of bacteria, and significantly elevated pro and anti-inflammatory cytokine levels compared to mice on a LFD (83). Therefore obesity can influence the response of immune cells to infections such as sepsis and thus have direct impact on sepsis outcomes.

5.2. Urinary tract infection and sepsis

The urogenital tract is the focus of infection in approximately 25% of all sepsis cases (84). Urinary tract infection (UTI) associated sepsis is predominantly found in elderly individuals, diabetics and immuno-suppressed patients (85). Several animal models have been developed to study different aspects of these co-morbid conditions. Harberg et al. developed a model of *E.coli* induced UTI by infecting urinary bladders of female mice by administrating bacteria via a urethral catheter (86). Pyelonephritis isolates (HU734) and normal fecal (414) *E. coli* were used to induce infection, where the pyelonephritis strains were discovered to remain in the system longer (86). UTI associated sepsis animal models have also been used to test potential therapeutic strategies. Reid et al. investigated whether competitive exclusion of uropathogenic bacteria would occur when animals were treated with indigenous bacteria (87). In female rats with chronic UTI induced by periurethral injections of agar beads with bacteria, rats exposed to indigenous bacteria , *Lactobacillus casei*, 21 days before the uropathogen challenge, had no pathogenic bacteria or immune responses in the bladder and kidney for up to 60 days (87). Given the prevalence of UTi-associated sepsis in the clinical setting, using animal models which involve co-morbidities and common clinical infections will increase the relevance of these animal studies.

5.3. Genetics and sepsis

Several studies have identified the implications of genetic variance, for immune responses to sepsis. Even while comparing across different strains of septic mice, mortality rates, liver MPO activity, metallothione mRNA, leptin as well as IL-10 levels are significantly higher in C57BL/6J compared to A/J mice (88). Thus, genetic differences in mice and possibly humans are associated with differences in the inflammatory processes initiated in response to infection that ultimately affects sepsis outcomes (88).

Transgenic animal models have also been utilized extensively in sepsis research (89). Transgenic apolipoprotein (ApoE) polymorphs, ApoE3TR and ApoE4TR, generated by replacing mouse ApoE allele with its human counterpart coding sequences were used to investigate if ApoE genotype affects sepsis outcomes (89). ApoE is a ligand for low density lipoprotein (LDL) receptor, responsible for clearance of VLDLs and chylomicrons residues. ApoE plays key role in lipid metabolism (90) and mediates removal of inflammatory apoptotic substances (91). Mice with the human APOE4 allele have greater inflammatory response (with two to four fold increase in synthesis of cytokine) as well increased time to mortality (89).

ApoE knockout mice (apoE -/-) generated by gene targeting are more susceptible to endotoxemia and K. *pneumoniae* compared to LDLr-/- mice implicating the role of apoE in modulating LPS induced inflammatory responses (92). Haraguchi et al. have reported using the ApoE-/- strain that administration of pioglitazone suppresses inflammation and improves survival in these mice, providing support for the use of peroxisome proliferator-activated receptor gamma (PPAR-γ) agonist as potential treatment option for severe sepsis (93).

Other strains of transgenic mice have also been utilized for sepsis research such as mice with inactivated beta$_2$ integrin CD11b. These transgenic mice are partially protected against micro-vessel permeability and edema formation, suggesting key role of Cd11b in lung PMN sequestration and vascular injury during the early phase of gram-negative sepsis (94). Lectin-like oxidized low density lipoprotein receptor 1 knockout (LOX-1-/-) mice have been used to investigate the role of LOX-1 in sepsis induced mortality. Wu et al. reported that LOX-1-/- mice with CLP-induced sepsis had decreased systemic inflammation, neutrophil migration to sites of infection, levels of pro-inflammatory cytokines, and lung edema as well as increased bacterial clearance implicating the key role of LOX-1 in systemic inflammation (95). Important findings have also been discovered in toll like receptor knockout mice (TLR-/-) . Toll like receptors (TLRs) recognize different components of bacteria cell wall and mediate immune responses to infection. TLR-4 for instance interacts with LPS, activating the expression of target genes. TLR-/- knockout mice have been utilized to study dendrititc cell maturation and cytokine production (96), infections of the urogenital organs (97) and defense against infections such as murine tuberculosis (98) among several others aspects of adaptive and immune responses.

Transgenic mice such as ob/ob have also been used to examine the effects of leptin deficiency on sepsis outcomes (99). Leptin deficiency, in ob/ob mice, is associated with greater organ dysfunction and increased mortality rates during sepsis (99). Leptin signaling appears to improve survival and may be required for immune responses, implicating therapeutic potential for leptin analogues for sepsis. Thus transgenic mice have made important contributions to Improve our understanding of sepsis at physiological, immunological and cellular levels.

6. Emerging preclinical research in sepsis: Neutrophil Extracellular Trap (NET) formation

An emerging area of sepsis research involves the formation of neutrophil extracellular traps. In 2004, Brinkmann et al. characterized a novel mechanism of innate immunity exhibited by neutrophils. Upon stimulation by endotoxins or pro-inflammatory mediators, activated neutrophils released chromatin material composed of a DNA backbone and antimicrobial granular proteins in the form of neutrophil extracellular traps (NETs) (100). NETs ensnare circulating microorganisms, preventing further dissemination of pathogens in the vasculature while providing a scaffold for neutrophil granular proteins. This creates a high, local concentration of proteins with antimicrobial properties (100) and allows for microbicidal synergy, concentrating their ability to disarm and kill microorganisms (101).

6.1. NETosis

The formation of NETs, recently coined NETosis (100;102) is an active process. Cleavage of histones by neutrophil elastase is sufficient to cause decondensation of nuclear material (103) which can be observed before disintegration of nuclear and granule membranes. Chromatin material mixes with nuclear and granular proteins with potent antimicrobial properties and is released extracellularly (102;104) forming stretches of DNA and globular proteins with diameters of 15-17 nm and 25 nm respectively which can aggregate to form thicker threads around 50 nm in diameter (100). The process of NETosis is distinct from that of necrosis (the plasma membrane remains intact while nuclear and cytoplasmic granular components mix) and that of apoptosis (no phosphatidylserine exposure signaling phagocytosis, or nucleosomal cleavage) (102;105).

NETosis can be experimentally induced by exposure to endotoxins (e.g. LPS), gram-negative and gram-positive bacteria, fungi, pro-inflammatory mediators (e.g. IL-8, phorbol myristate acetate or PMA a protein kinase activator), and activated platelets (103;106-111). NET formation in experimental conditions results in the release of proteins which degrade virulence factors expressed on the pathogen surface and create a toxic environment for invading microorganisms (102;107;112-115). NET-associated azurophilic granule proteins which have antimicrobial or immunomodulating effects include histones with specific post-translational modifications (and histone cleavage products like buforin), cathepsin G, elastase, MPO, pentraxin, gelatinase (matrix metalloproteinase-9), catalase, lactoferrin, peptidoglycan recognition proteins (PGRPs), and bactericidal permeability-increasing protein (BPI) (100;107;116). NETs have also been shown to kill infectious organisms and impair pathogenic invasion of gram-negative bacteria (e.g. *Shigella flexneri), gram-positive bacteria (e.g. Staphylococcus aureus, Group A streptococcus),* fungi (e.g. *Candida albicans),* and even viruses (e.g. influenza A virus) (100;102;106;107;107-110;112;114-117).

6.2. NETosis in infection and sepsis

In 2007, a landmark paper published by the Kubes group characterized the mechanism by which platelet-neutrophil interactions contribute to pathogenesis of severe sepsis. It was observed that LPS-induced endotoxemia in mice as well as plasma from severe sepsis patients were able to trigger NET formation but at a cost to the host. Upon detection of TLR4 ligands (e.g. LPS), platelets bind to neutrophils adhered to the endothelium (118). Within minutes, TLR4-dependent platelet-neutrophil interactions resulted in the robust release of granules and DNA in the form of NETs the integrity of which was maintained under flow conditions reflective of physiologic shear forces in the microvasculature (0.5 dyne/cm^2). NET-mediated bacterial clearance through trapping and ensnaring of bacteria was primarily observed in liver sinusoids and lung capillaries, areas with the greatest capacity for immobilizing bacteria due to the decreased lumen size of vessels (118). However, formation of NETs is not without a cost as it was also found to cause cellular and tissue damage to the host. *In vitro,* NET formation resulted in endothelial cell damage marked by increased staining of propidium iodide, a nucleic acid stain impermeable to viable cells (118). *In vivo,* NET formation was also found to cause hepatotoxicity in LPS-challenged mice indicated by the decreased perfusion of liver sinusoids and increase in levels of alanine aminotransferase, associated with platelet-mediated neutrophil activation. Given these findings, the authors propose that platelets act as a sensor or barometer (partially via TLR4 receptors) for pathogens in the blood, inducing a last resort immune response mediated by neutrophils to ensnare and kill bacteria at the expense of the host's tissues (118). In the already immune-deregulated state of the septic host, NETs can exacerbate sepsis by releasing high concentrations of potent proteases, inducing further endothelial damage, and forming a chromatin meshwork, trapping host cells (erythrocytes, leukocytes, and platelets) which can potentiate inflammation, coagulation, ischemia, and hypoxia in downstream tissues.

6.3. NET pathogenicity

NETs induce pathogenic effects via multiple mechanisms. Platelet-mediated NET formation trapped platelets, leukocytes, and red blood cells causing microvascular plugging and areas of ischemia in downstream tissues (118;119). Ischemic conditions increase the production of IL-8 (120) and reactive oxygen species (121) both of which can induce further NET formation (122). Several lines of evidence also suggest that NETs exert pro-coagulant effects in sepsis and other conditions of deregulated coagulation and inflammation. In studies of thrombosis, NETs were found to interact closely with fibrin and platelets via von Willebrand factor, fibronectin, and fibrinogen, effectively stabilizing platelet-rich clots (119;123). NETs perfused with blood or platelet-rich plasma stimulated platelet aggregation and promoted thrombus formation (124). Another *in vivo* study observed that both DNA and RNA provide a surface template on which activation of the contact pathway via XIIa/XIa promoting fibrin-rich thrombus formation and decreased plasma clotting times (125). Antimicrobial proteins associated with NETs also exert pro-coagulant effects which are pathogenic to the host. Positively-charged histones promote red blood cell accumulation and platelet aggregation by electrostatic interactions with the negatively-charged cells (126). NET-associated histones also impair the natural anticoagulant protein C, activate platelets, and induce thrombin generation via platelet TLR2 and TLR4-mediated mechanisms (124;127-129). Additionally, histones induce prothrombinase activity, increased P-selectin expression, phosphatidylserine exposure, and FV activation (127).

NETs and NET-associated proteins have also been found to exert pro-inflammatory effects. MPO released during NET formation binds the negatively-charged, proteoglycan-rich endothelium, inducing endothelial cell damage and vascular permeability (130;131). Incubation of NETs with human platelets and THP-1 cells resulted in the release of pro-inflammatory cytokines including IL-1β, IL-8, and TNFα (132).

The pathogenic nature of NETs is also supported by studies showing improved outcome associated with NET destruction via DNase administration (133). Furthermore, DNaseI-deficient mice develop lupus-like symptoms induced by NET formation, indicating that NET removal is likely a crucial process in the proper immune response (123). The formation of NETs and release of NET-associated proteins (e.g. histones) potentiate the pro-inflammatory and pro-coagulant response, both of which contribute to end organ morphology in sepsis. These changes include neutrophil adherence to microvascular endothelium, inflammatory infiltration, vacuolization of epithelial and endothelial cells, fibrin deposition, microvascular ruptures with intra-alveolar hemorrhaging, and the formation of platelet-rich micro- and macrovascular thrombi (118;127;129;134;135). While clinical isolates have been shown to have the ability to generate NETs *in vitro,* there is to date no clear evidence to show whether this phenomena occurs in septic patients, or whether this is associated with organ dysfunction or mortality.

7. Translation of preclinical studies to clinical outcomes

Despite the success of many therapeutic agents in improving outcome in preclinical studies of sepsis, many have failed to demonstrate efficacy in the clinical setting. To illustrate, studies investigating the efficacy of anti-TNF therapies (5;5;136;137) and activated protein C (APC) were promising in animal studies, but this success failed to translate to clinical outcomes (35;73;138). Neutralization of TNF was beneficial in some models of endotoxemia challenge with viable gram-negative bacteria (e.g. group B streptococci) (139-145) but in other preclinical studies where microorganisms such as Candida, S. pneumoniae, Listeria, or mycobacteria were used, neutralizing TNF exacerbated outcome in animals subjected to the pathogenic challenge (36;70;136;137;146-149). In complex models of sepsis, no consistent harm or benefit was validated and some clinical studies found an increased mortality associated with anti-TNF therapy (150;151). Similar to anti-TNF therapy, some preclinical studies demonstrated the protective or therapeutic effect of APC (35;73;138) but these results failed to translate in some clinical studies (72). The therapeutic efficacy of anti-TNF therapy and APC in preclinical studies is largely influenced by the animal model used. Thus the appropriate translation of findings and inferences from preclinical studies to clinical outcomes in sepsis remains a heavily debated area.

7.1. Critical appraisal of preclinical sepsis studies

Limitations in both the use of animal models and design of experimental studies contribute to the poor translation of preclinical animal studies to clinical sepsis. Some limitations are inherent to the use of animals to model any clinical condition. It is commonly the case that young animals of a specific gender, species, genetic background, and nutritional status housed in a pathogen-free, sterile facility unexposed to the natural environment are used (5). Many of these elements are tightly controlled to maintain consistency at the expense of clinical relevance. However, an attempt at balancing both consistency and clinical relevance can be made if the investigator designs treatment groups for different animals (e.g. separate treatment groups for females and males, groups for young and aged mice, etc.) given the heterogeneity of the sepsis patient population.

Other limitations may be appropriately addressed by establishing clear research questions and implementing an experimental protocol which would adequately investigate these questions. For instance, if the objective of an animal study is to test the clinical applicability of a therapeutic agent, it would be more clinically relevant if therapies currently used for the management of sepsis including the adequate administration of resuscitation fluids, antibiotics, and supportive therapies (14) were incorporated into the experimental protocol of the animal study. Additionally, the experimental protocol of animal studies can be modified to include clinically relevant management procedures such as constant monitoring and assessment for hemodynamic parameters, tissue perfusion, or dehydration as would occur in clinical sepsis. Other factors which may contribute to the gap between findings in experimental and clinical studies include the time at which therapeutic agents are administered, the lack of staging of sepsis to reflect disease progression at different severities on the sepsis continuum or different patient populations, and the risk of experimenter bias in animal studies (5;12)

7.2. Limitations to the clinical relevance of animal studies

7.2.1. Age

It is commonly the case that murine studies of sepsis utilize 8 week-old mice, the physiological equivalent of a young adulthood in humans. However, the sepsis patient population consists largely of patients over 60 years of age which is not adequately represented in sepsis literature using animal models (152). There are limitations to examining the true pathophysiology and clinical treatment of a condition which occurs most commonly in the aging population when findings are extrapolated from preclinical studies using young, healthy mice exclusively. For example, aging is associated with increased apoptosis of rapidly dividing epithelial cells of the gut and spleen in animal sepsis (153).

This may contribute to the increased mortality in aged septic mice, a factor which would not accounted for when using young animals to model sepsis occurring in an aging population. The effect of age in sepsis in a clinical setting can be appreciated in the PROWESS trials. Substantial difference in absolute risk reduction of mortality were found to be associated with age in clinical sepsis (154). Age should be considered in animal studies of sepsis to increase the clinical relevance to human sepsis.

7.2.2. *Gender*

In addition to limitations produced by using young animals exclusively, male animals are almost exclusively chosen in intra-abdominal sepsis studies which poorly reflects the incidence of clinical sepsis in both genders around 40% of which is female (155). Male mice are often chosen over females to avoid confounding effects and variables posed by varied expression of biomarkers and circulating cells associated with different phases of the estrous cycle. For instance, steroid hormones are implicated in the expression of adhesion molecules resulting in different peripheral blood leukocyte concentrations and an altered coagulant response (156;157). Neutrophil concentrations and response to stimulation also vary considerably during different phases of the estrous cycle (158). For consistency, male mice are often chosen of sepsis studies, despite the similar occurrence of sepsis in males and females however, an investigator should consider, if feasible, treatments with one group for each gender of animal used.

7.2.3. *Fluid resuscitation*

The importance of early goal-directed treatment including adequate fluid resuscitation and treatment with antibiotics has been thoroughly demonstrated in severe sepsis and septic shock (159). Correction of hemodynamic abnormalities and hypovolemia associated with sepsis is integral to reducing mortality rates and improving sepsis outcomes. Hypovolemia compromises tissue oxygenation due to inadequate blood flow within the microvasculature and is the prime cause of organ dysfunction and failure (159). In order to differentiate pathology due to sepsis from pathology resulting solely from circulatory decline and lack of hemodynamic support, the administration of balanced fluids is crucial. This is supported by findings showing significant differences between the hemodynamic profiles of under-resuscitated animals versus those with adequate supportive fluids, and aggressive fluid resuscitation was required to replicate hemodynamic profiles observed in patients with severe sepsis (47). In canines with septic shock, animals that received combination therapy of antibiotics and cardiovascular support (via fluid resuscitation and dopamine) had a 43% improvement in survival rates compared to septic animals treated with either therapy alone (160;160). Furthermore, experiments elucidating the effects of various fluid regimes on resuscitation in sepsis have demonstrated that lactated Ringer's crystalloid solution but not saline-based solutions reduced sepsis-induced leukocyte recruitment in the liver of mice subjected to CLP (161). Based on these studies, an appropriate fluid regime which would account for surgical losses and provide adequate hemodynamic support to maintain circulatory and cardiovascular function, as would occur in the management of clinical sepsis, should be considered in preclinical studies of sepsis (12).

7.2.4. Patient heterogeneity

The human septic population is diverse and highly heterogeneous. Clinical cases of sepsis are often much more complex than sepsis induced in animal studies. The diversity of infectious agents as well as sites of infection in clinical sepsis are not always reflected in animal studies, factors which should be considered in the translation of preclinical to clinical studies. For instance, clinical sepsis may result from trauma and subsequent fecal spillage into a sterile peritoneum or staphylococcal bacteremia in an elderly patient with congestive heart failure. Evidently, animal models like those inducing sepsis via injections of endotoxic bacterial components or even live bacteria fail to induce the range of conditions observed in a septic patient (5). To decrease this gap, one may choose to consider introducing cormorbidities as previously described or other trauma or infectious injuries to animal sepsis models.

Animal	Species, genetic background, gender, age, nutritional status following insult, comorbidities incorporated in model
Source of Infection	Single versus multiple organisms, local versus systemic challenge, addition of adjuvants, presence and extent of tissue damage from challenge
Intervention	Dose and timing of intervention compared to septic insult (administered before, concurrent with, or following insult)
Co-interventions	Fluid resuscitation, antibiotics, analgesics, source removal
Experimental Design	Risk bias (blinding or randomization methods are used), assay methodology
Markers of Outcome	Parameters used as markers of outcome (choice of biomarker and quantification methods, physiological response, inflammatory parameters, survival)

Table 1. Limitations to the Clinical Relevance of Preclinical Studies

7.3. Summary of limitations

Factors which limit the translation of preclinical studies to clinical outcomes include the following (5): the animal used for experimental studies (species, genetic background, gender, age, nutritional status following insult, comorbidities incorporated in model), the source of infection (organism, local vs. systemic challenge, adjuvants, tissue damage from challenge), dose and timing of intervention (administered before, concurrent with, or following insult), co-interventions (fluid resuscitation, antibiotics, analgesics, source removal), experimental design (risk bias, blinding, randomization, assay methodology), and parameters used as markers of outcome (quantification and choice of biomarker, physiological response, inflammatory parameters, survival) which can significantly alter response to treatment. These potential limitations are summarized in Table 1 adapted from Marshall et al, 2005.

7.4. Considerations to improve the translation of preclinical studies to clinical outcomes

It is evident that experimental design greatly influences the findings of both experimental and clinical studies in sepsis. One method to increase the transparency, reproducibility, consistency, and efficacy of sepsis research is to increase standards for reporting of animal sepsis studies. The Consolidated Standards of Reporting Trials (CONSORT 1996, 2001, and 2010) statement is a rigorous and highly standardized approach to conducting clinical research which addresses variability of results due to the study design and reporting of clinical trials (162-164). In an attempt to limit the variability in both the use of animal studies and reporting of results, Marshall et al. propose that a similar checklist should be required for preclinical studies (5). The checklist includes the following variables which should be explicitly described and recorded in detailed manner to ease pooling of results from various preclinical studies, define a framework from which to understand divergent results, improve the consistency of reporting of results, and enhance the reliability of reported results. The standards for reporting animal research in bioscience were raised further in 2010 with the publication of the ARRIVE guidelines, Animals in Research: Reporting *In Vivo* Experiments (165). Below is an adaptation of the Consolidated Standards of Reporting Trials Checklist for Preclinical Studies proposed by Marshall et al. in 2005 with descriptions of methods by which these reporting standards could be maintained as suggested by Kilkenny et al. (Table 2).

7.4.1. Sepsis definition

In the design and reporting of a preclinical sepsis study, a basic but crucial aspect that one should consider is the very definition of sepsis, the conditions and presentation of which differ from one animal model to another. Clinical sepsis is defined by meeting specific criteria which involve inflammatory, hemodynamic, organ dysfunction, and tissue perfusion variables. Sepsis is no longer defined solely by changes in physiological parameters (e.g. body temperature, heart rate, respiratory rate, and white blood cell count) which are common to many other conditions. Likewise, defining sepsis based on levels of several biomarkers of inflammation, for instance fails to capture the complexity of cardiovascular, hormonal, metabolic, innate and adaptive immune changes which occur in this heterogeneous condition. Although it would be helpful to document changes in biomarkers and physiological parameters (e.g. heart rate, etc.), current preclinical studies are limited as the criteria which define sepsis (and the severity) in various animals have not been clearly elucidated. There is currently no consensus over the physiological parameters, levels of biomarkers, or variables of end organ health which would indicate sepsis in an animal although these parameters are much more clearly outlined by clinical sepsis definition guidelines (1). This limitation will need to be addressed in future preclinical sepsis studies. Other parameters which may be informative of the septic condition in animals include appearance (perfusion of mucous membranes), urine production, and bacterial cultures from the blood, peritoneal fluid, and local site of infection, which may be considered in the design of animal studies. Successful animal studies should establish a clear definition of the conditions which would indicate a septic animal, explicitly defining the severity of disease induced as part of the study protocol (167).

Sepsis Definition	Clear sepsis definition as indicators of sepsis, severe sepsis, or septic shock in the animal used (166)
Animal	Species, strain, genetic background, gender, age, weight, handling, housing, feeding conditions
Experimental Design	Method of sepsis induction (details which indicate severity), intervention (timing and dose), experimental methodology, controls included, randomization methods, blinding of experimenter
Analytic Plan	Primary and secondary endpoints, power calculations for sample size determination, intention-to-treat analysis, criteria for animals excluded from studies (substitute endpoints)
Co-Interventions	Resuscitation fluids, antibiotics, source removal, feeding
Results	Flowchart of included and excluded animals, establish mortality rates in studies conducted

Table 2. Checklist for the Reporting of Animal Studies

7.4.2. Experimental design

In the interests of reproducibility and reliability, the method of sepsis induction, intervention (timing and dose), experimental protocol, inclusion of proper controls, randomization methods, and methods of experimenter blinding should be documented in detail. Although experimental methodologies are commonly recorded, there is a significant lack of attention to reduce experimenter bias by randomization and blinding, despite the confounding effects recently addressed in a systematic review of literature of studies using animal sepsis models. It was observed that only 2% of systematic reviews and meta-analyses appraised the risk of bias or clinical relevance of the underlying animal research despite a significant proportion of the literature extrapolating results from animal studies to clinical sepsis (168). In one review of studies using animal models, more than 80% of research papers surveyed did not report the use of methods to minimize the risk of bias by the investigator (165;169). To improve the translation of inferences and findings from experimental sepsis to clinical sepsis in future studies, one should consider reducing the effects of experimenter bias by randomizing animals in the treatment groups of the study and blinding the experimenter to the intervention provided given that implementation of these elements would not compromise the protocol or results of the study (5;166;167).

7.4.3. Randomization

In the absence of randomization, the results of clinical and animal studies may be unintentionally biased by factors which may influence study outcomes. Nonrandomized clinical studies have frequently shown a larger treatment effect than randomized control trials, an effect which should be studied and addressed in animal studies (168;170-173). Randomization involves taking proactive measures in assigning subjects to a treatment or control group in studies testing the efficacy of a potential treatment drug versus a placebo control or potential treatment drug versus a pre-existing treatment (167;173). The systematic randomization of subjects or animals minimizes allocation or selection bias by eliminating influences from unknown or known prognostic variables (like the hemodynamics in septic and nonseptic animals) which may influence the response to treatment, mortality, or outcome, unduly producing biased results in a study (166;170-172). Randomization also ensures that protocols and procedures are conducted consistently and systematically in treatment and control groups. Elements of animal studies where randomization may offer an efficacious benefit include the procedure to induce sepsis (preventing unintentional bias by variations in sepsis severity), treatment (consistent timing, route, and method of administering treatments or controls), monitoring of subjects following sepsis induction and treatment, and resuscitation procedures of the study groups (169;173).

Although various methods of randomization have been established and recommended for different clinical trials, consensus and literature on randomization in pre-clinical and experimental studies are lacking. Simple randomization methods such as the "repeated fair coin-tossing" have been recommended for large clinical studies ($n > 200$), but are inadequate for studies with small samples sizes like experimental animal studies (167;173). Restricted randomization methods like permutated-block randomization where allocation ratios are used to specify the number of subjects in each group (or ratio of subjects in one treatment group to another) (170-172) successfully address this issue, but restricted randomization methods have not been validated in animal studies. Given that the risk of allocation and selection bias have been shown to unduly influence the results of clinical studies and that randomization and blinding have successfully minimized these risks, it is crucial that the same level of criticism and caution be applied in the experimental design and conducting of experimental studies by addressing these risks (167;170-173).

7.4.4. Blinding

In addition to randomization, blinding of investigators also minimizes the risk of bias at many levels of the preclinical study. Blinding decreases differential treatment of animals in the study groups (more intensive monitoring or closer supervision of one treatment group over another) to unintentional biases in analyzing data and adjudicating outcomes (5;166). For instance, markers of disease severity or mortality outcome such as organ histology may be interpreted in a biased manner in an untreated control group versus the treated group if the investigator is not blinded to the treatment received (169). Likewise, marginal findings may be analyzed in a biased manner when interpretation of the outcome marker is subjective. In studies where substitute endpoints are used (such is the case when mortality is not used as endpoints for ethical reasons), blinding reduces the chance of experimenters prolonging the time to endpoint (in an attempt to establish a therapeutic effect when one does not exist) or decreasing the time to a substitute endpoint or even excluding animals (if unexpected results are observed in either treatment or control groups) (165;167;170;172). Blinding of the investigator to the treatment or control substance received minimizes the risk of experimenter bias.

7.4.5. Analytic plan

The analytic plan should be described in detail such that the procedure is reproducible by others and variations in models used by other investigators can be appreciated (e.g. size and number of enterotomies and location of ligature in a CLP model) when comparing various preclinical studies (5). Primary and secondary endpoints of the study should be clearly outlined, whether they are to determine the efficacy of a potential therapy, improve prognosis, or diagnosis of sepsis. If the primary objective is to investigate a potential therapy, endpoints and markers of outcome of the animal study should also be clinically relevant (166;173;174). The measurement of outcome should also appropriately reflect markers relevant to the potential therapy being tested. For example, the coagulant state of the animals should be measured if the drug being tested acts via its anticoagulant effects. While mortality is the most informative marker of outcome in clinical sepsis, organ health and dysfunction are useful surrogate markers of outcome due to their relevance to clinical sepsis (173).

7.4.6. Power calculations

In studies elucidating the therapeutic potential of a compound, power calculations can be used to reliably determine the sample size required to show that an effect is associated with treatment as well as exclude an effect when none exists (5). The magnitude of a treatment effect is most commonly expressed as the relative risk reduction (RRR, RRR = [1-(X/Y)] x 100 where Y is the proportion of animals that expired in the treatment group and X is the proportion of animals that expired in the control group (175). Given that mortality (and therefore the power of the study) will be altered should any subjects be excluded, the exclusion of subjects should only occur if subjects meet pre-established criteria.

7.4.7. Exclusion criteria

As in clinical studies, conditions under which subjects will be excluded should be clearly outlined before the animal study (169). The study should account for all animals, including those that do not complete the experimental protocol and observations and reasons for excluded animals should be appropriately documented. This is important to determine whether prognosis independent of the treatment may in actuality be related to the exclusion of certain subjects (5;174). Data should also be recorded and kept for subjects excluded from the study for any post-hoc analyses, standards which are expected of clinical studies.

7.4.8. Animal welfare

Many animal ethics and welfare committees are preventing the use of mortality as an endpoint and encouraging the use of surrogate markers of death. However, investigators and funding agencies are critical of such studies which do not use changes in mortality as a measure of therapeutic efficacy. There is currently no consensus nor scientific validation of clinically relevant, reliable substitute markers of death in septic animals (5;174). Moreover, there is concern over the use of analgesics and anaesthetics which have been shown to interfere with components in the natural progression of sepsis and even exert protective, anti-inflammatory effects. For example, *in vivo* and *in vitro* studies have elucidated that pentobarbital significantly reduces the LPS-induced inflammatory response by suppressing TNF α mRNA and protein expression by NF-κB and p38 MAP kinase (176). The concern over analgesics and anaesthetics Interfering with disease progression and treatment response may cause some reluctance towards the appropriate use of analgesics and anaesthetics in preclinical studies. Although scientific concern is warranted, these findings highlight the importance of considering drug effects and incorporating them into the experimental design, as it should be noted that analgesics and anaesthetics are clinically relevant to treatment and management of the septic patient, and from the standpoint of relevance (not to mention from an ethical standpoint), should not be excluded in animal studies. To improve clinical relevance and translation of studies utilizing experimental models, the appropriate use of these drugs with further understanding of their effects should be integrated rather than avoided in preclinical studies of sepsis (5;165).

7.5. Recommendations for a thorough validation of therapeutic efficacy in preclinical studies

Given the potential limitations of preclinical studies when designing preclinical studies with potential clinical applications, one should take a critical approach when validating the therapeutic efficacy of a potential drug in preclinical studies. Recommendations for conducting preclinical studies with clinical applications will be provided with the intent to address the concerns raised previously. Literature by Marshall et al. suggest that early proof of concept studies should 1) delineate a potential pathological role for the target in question by quantifying its increases in a simple acute model like endotoxemia or bacteremia (LPS or E. coli challenge) and 2) demonstrate that attenuating such target may improve outcome or offer some therapeutic benefit by a measurable decrease in harmful effects of the initial challenge or insult (5;165;174). If a proof of concept can be established, time course studies should be conducted to determine if the potential treatment offers therapeutic effects if administered before, during the progression of, or after the insult in both simple acute and complex models (e.g. LPS challenge and CLP). Experimental methodology and design of further studies should consider the results of studies on targets with similar biological or pathophysiological effects. Any adverse effects of the intervention, like impairment of the host's natural anti-microbial immune function or further dysregulation of the coagulant state should be determined in a high-risk model using live organisms as the challenges. (5;174) Moreover, the systemic physiological and biological responses to the therapeutic intervention (e.g. cardiac output, oxygenation, glomerular filtration) should be determined in a large animal model, given the limitations of small rodent models of sepsis. Interventions used in the management of clinical sepsis such as fluid resuscitation, ventilatory support, and hemodynamic monitoring, can be incorporated into the study design of preclinical trials using large animal models (5).

8. Goals for the future of experimental sepsis research

Goals for the future use of experimental sepsis models ought to focus on improving the relevance, translation, and applicability of results and inferences from animal studies to what is observed clinically. This requires consideration of the limitations of current sepsis models described such as considering age, gender, genetic background, nutritional status, and the environment of the housing facility, incorporating cormorbidities and supportive therapies which may be clinically relevant, and finally addressing the risk of bias by randomization and blinding methods in preclinical studies of sepsis.

Author details

Safiah Mai, Momina Khan and Patricia Liaw*
McMaster University, Canada
David Braley Research Institute, Canada

Alison Fox-Robichaud*
McMaster University, Canada
David Braley Research Institute, Canada
Hamilton Health Sciences, Canada

---

* on behalf of the Canadian Critical Care Translational Biology Group (CCCTBG)

9. References

[1] Levy MM, Fink MP, Marshall JC, Abraham E, Angus D, Cook D, et al. 2001 SCCM/ESICM/ACCP/ATS/SIS International Sepsis Definitions Conference. Crit Care Med 2003, 31:1250-6.
[2] Namas R, Zamora R, Namas R, An G, Doyle J, Dick TE, et al. Sepsis: Something old, something new, and a systems view. J Crit Care 2012, 27:314-11.
[3] Wichterman KA, Baue AE, Chaudry IH. Sepsis and septic shock--a review of laboratory models and a proposal. J Surg Res 1980, 29:189-201.
[4] Deitch EA. Rodent models of intra-abdominal infection. Shock 2005, 24 Suppl 1:19-23.
[5] Marshall JC, Deitch E, Moldawer LL, Opal S, Redl H, Poll Tvd. Preclinical Models of Shock and Sepsis: What Can They Tell Us? Shock 2005, 24 Suppl 1:1-6.
[6] Clowes GH, Jr., Zuschneid W, Turner M, Blackburn G, Rubin J, Toala P, et al. Observations on the pathogenesis of the pneumonitis associated with severe infections in other parts of the body. Ann Surg 1968, 167:630-50.
[7] Sloane DR, Clowes GJ. Traumatic intramural haematoma of the duodenum. Med J Aust 1968, 2:1184-5.
[8] Wright NG, Cornwell HJ, Thompson H. Canine adenovirus nephritis. J Small Anim Pract 1971, 12:657-64.
[9] Wright NG, Thompson H, Cornwell HJ. Canine adenovirus pneumonia. Res Vet Sci 1971, 12:162-7.
[10] Ryan CJ, Benjamin IS, Blumgart LH. Portacaval transposition in the rat: a new technique and its effects on liver and body weight. Br J Surg 1974, 61:224-8.
[11] Rittirsch D, Huber-Lang MS, Flierl MA, Ward PA. Immunodesign of experimental sepsis by cecal ligation and puncture. Nat Protocols 2008, 4:31-6.
[12] Dejager L, Pinheiro I, Dejonckheere E, Libert C. Cecal ligation and puncture: the gold standard model for polymicrobial sepsis? Trends Microbiol 2011, 19:198-208.
[13] Bone RC. Sir Isaac Newton, sepsis, SIRS, and CARS. Crit Care Med 1996, 24:1125-8.
[14] Dellinger RP, Levy MM, Carlet JM, Bion J, Parker MM, Jaeschke R, Reinhart K, Angus DC, Brun-Buisson C, et al. Surviving Sepsis Campaign: International guidelines for management of severe sepsis and septic shock. Intensive Care Med 2008, 34:17-60.
[15] Remick DG, Newcomb DE, Bolgos GL, Call DR. Comparison of the mortality and inflammatory response of two models of sepsis: lipopolysaccharide vs. cecal ligation and puncture. Shock 2000, 13:110-6.
[16] Riedemann NC, Guo RF, Ward PA. Novel strategies for the treatment of sepsis. Nat Med 2003, 9:517-24.
[17] Riedemann NC, Guo RF, Hollmann TJ, Gao Hong, Neff TA, Reuben JS, et al. Regulatory role of C5a in LPS-induced IL-6 production by neutrophils during sepsis. The FASEB Journal 2004, 18:370-2.
[18] Huber-Lang M, Sarma VJ, Lu KT, McGuire SR, Padgaonkar VA, Guo RF, et al. Role of C5a in multiorgan failure during sepsis. J Immunol 2001, 166:1193-9.

[19] Huber-Lang MS, Riedeman NC, Sarma JV, Younkin EM, McGuire SR, Laudes IJ, et al. Protection of innate immunity by C5aR antagonist in septic mice. FASEB J 2002, 16:1567-74.
[20] Czermak BJ, Sarma V, Pierson CL, Warner RL, Huber-Lang M, Bless NM, et al. Protective effects of C5a blockade in sepsis. Nat Med 1999, 5:788-92.
[21] Hotchkiss RS, Coopersmith CM, McDunn JE, Ferguson TA. The sepsis seesaw: tilting toward immunosuppression. Nat Med 2009, 15:496-7.
[22] Muenzer JT, Davis CG, Chang K, Schmidt RE, Dunne WM, Coopersmith CM, et al. Characterization and modulation of the immunosuppressive phase of sepsis. Infect Immun 2010, 78:1582-92.
[23] Hotchkiss RS, Nicholson DW. Apoptosis and caspases regulate death and inflammation in sepsis. Nat Rev Immunol 2006, 6:813-22.
[24] Maier S, Traeger T, Entleutner M, Westerholt A, Kleist B, Huser N, et al. Cecal ligation and puncture versus colon ascendens stent peritonitis: two distinct animal models for polymicrobial sepsis. Shock 2004, 21:505-11.
[25] Schabbauer G. Polymicrobial sepsis models: CLP versus CASP. Drug Discovery Today: Disease Models 2012, 9:e17-e21.
[26] Zantl N, Uebe A, Neumann B, Wagner H, Siewert JR, Holzmann B, et al. Essential Role of Gamma Interferon in Survival of Colon Ascendens Stent Peritonitis, a Novel Murine Model of Abdominal Sepsis. Infection and Immunity 1998, 66:2300-9.
[27] Buras JA, Holzmann B, Sitkovsky M. Animal Models of sepsis: setting the stage. Nat Rev Drug Discov 2005, 4:854-65.
[28] Traeger T, Mikulcak M, Eipel C, Abshagen K, Diedrich S, Heidecke CD, et al. Kupffer cell depletion reduces hepatic inflammation and apoptosis but decreases survival in abdominal sepsis. Eur J Gastroenterol Hepatol 2010 Sep, 22:1039-49.
[29] Emmanuilidis K, Weighardt H, Maier S, Gerauer K, Fleischmann T, Zheng XX, et al. Critical role of Kupffer cell-derived IL-10 for host defense in septic peritonitis. J Immunol 2001, 167:3919-27.
[30] Hammer M, Echtenachter B, Weighardt H, Jozefowski K, Rose-John S, Mannel DN, et al. Increased inflammation and lethality of Dusp1-/- mice in polymicrobial peritonitis models. Immunology 2010, 131:395-404.
[31] Daubeuf B, Mathison J, Spiller S, Hugues S, Herren S, Ferlin W, et al. TLR4/MD-2 monoclonal antibody therapy affords protection in experimental models of septic shock. J Immunol 2007, 179:6107-14.
[32] Weighardt H, Kaiser-Moore S, Vabulas RM, Kirschning CJ, Wagner H, Holzmann B. Cutting edge: myeloid differentiation factor 88 deficiency improves resistance against sepsis caused by polymicrobial infection. J Immunol 2002, 169:2823-7.
[33] Markus E, Traeger T, Westerholt A, Holzmann B, Stier A, Pfeffer K, Maier S, Heidecke CD. Impact of interleukin-12, oxidative burst, and iNOS on the survival of murine fecal peritonitis. International Journal of Colorectal Disease 2006, 21:64-70.

[34] Yuan Y, Ren J, Wu X, Cao S, Li J. Exogenous C3 postpones complement exhaustion and confers organ protection in murine sepsis. J Surg Res 2011, 168:e87-e94.
[35] Kerschen EJ, Fernandez JA, Cooley BC, Yang XV, Sood R, Mosnier LO, et al. Endotoxemia and sepsis mortality reduction by non-anticoagulantΓÇôactivated protein C. The Journal of Experimental Medicine 2007, 204:2439-48.
[36] Echtenacher B, Falk W, M+ñnnel DN, Krammer PH. Requirement of endogenous tumor necrosis factor/cachectin for recovery from experimental peritonitis. The Journal of Immunology 1990, 145:3762-6.
[37] Ebach DR, Riehl TE, Stenson WF. Opposing effects of tumor necrosis factor receptor 1 and 2 in sepsis due to cecal ligation and puncture. Shock 2005, 23:311-8.
[38] Moreno SE, Alves-Filho JC, Alfaya TM, da Silva JS, Ferreira SH, Liew FY. IL-12, but not IL-18, is critical to neutrophil activation and resistance to polymicrobial sepsis induced by cecal ligation and puncture. J Immunol 2006, 177:3218-24.
[39] Michie HR. The value of animal models in the development of new drugs for the treatment of the sepsis syndrome. Journal of Antimicrobial Chemotherapy 1998, 41 Suppl 1:47-9.
[40] Guckian JC, Morrey BF, Kirby HB. Role of Lysosomes and Cathepsin Inhibitor in Plasma during Pneumococcal Infection. The Journal of Infectious Diseases 1970, 122:290-302.
[41] Chiavolini D, Pozzi G, Ricci S. Animal Models of Streptococcus pneumoniae Disease. Clinical Microbiology Reviews 2008, 21:666-85.
[42] Matute-Bello G, Frevert C, Kajikawa O, Skerrett S, Goodman R, Park D, et al. Septic Shock and Acute Lung Injury in Rabbits with Peritonitis. American Journal of Respiratory and Critical Care Medicine 2001, 163:234-43.
[43] Guckian JC. Coagulopathy in Experimental Sepsis with Streptococcus pneumoniae in Rabbits: Effect of Drug Therapy and Splenectomy. Journal of Infectious Diseases 1976, 134:150-7.
[44] Natanson C, Fink MP, Ballantyne HK, MacVittie TJ, Conklin JJ, Parrillo JE. Gram-negative bacteremia produces both severe systolic and diastolic cardiac dysfunction in a canine model that simulates human septic shock. J Clin Invest 1986, 78:259-70.
[45] Nagy S, Tárnoky K TLBMKG. A canine model of hyperdynamic sepsis induced by intestinal ischemia. Acta Physiol Hung 1990, 75:303-20.
[46] Song R, Kim J, Yu D, Park C, Park J. Kinetics of IL-6 and TNF-+¦ changes in a canine model of sepsis induced by endotoxin. Veterinary Immunology and Immunopathology 2012, 146:143-9.
[47] Zanotti-Cavazzoni SL, Goldfarb RD. Animal Models of-áSepsis. Crit Care Clin 2009, 25:703-19.
[48] Reilly PM, Wilkins KB, Fuh KC, Haglund U, Bulkley GB. The mesenteric hemodynamic response to circulatory shock: an overview. Shock 2001, 15:329-43.
[49] Fink MP, Heard SO. Laboratory models of sepsis and septic shock. Journal of Surgical Research 1990 Aug, 49:186-96.

[50] Spapen H, Zhang H, Wisse E, Baekeland M, Seynaeve C, Eddouks M, et al. The 21-Aminosteroid U74389G Enhances Hepatic Blood Flow and Preserves Sinusoidal Endothelial Cell Function and Structure in Endotoxin-Shocked Dogs. Journal of Surgical Research 1999, 86:183-91.
[51] Cohen R, Hassell A, Marzouk K, Marini C, Liush S, Scharf S. Renal Effects of Nitric Oxide in Endotoxemia. American Journal of Respiratory and Critical Care Medicine 2001, 164:1890-5.
[52] Ji MH, Yang JJ, Wu J, Li RQ, Li GM, Fan YX, et al. Experimental sepsis in pigs- effects of vasopressin on renal, hepatic, and intestinal dysfunction. Ups J Med Sci 2012, 117: 257-63.
[53] Azevedo LCP, Park M, Noritomi DT, Maciel AT, Brunialti MK, Salomúo R. Characterization of an animal model of severe sepsis associated with respiratory dysfunction. Clinics 2007, 62:491-8.
[54] Luiking YC, Poeze M, Ramsay G, Deutz NEP. The Role of Arginine in Infection and Sepsis. Journal of Parenteral and Enteral Nutrition 2005, 29:S70-S74.
[55] Allen EM, Rowin M, Pappas JB, Vernon DD, Dean JM. Hemodynamic effects of N-acetylamrinone in a porcine model of group B streptococcal sepsis. Drug Metabolism and Disposition 1996, 24:1028-31.
[56] Greif WM, Forse RA. Interventions to improve cardiopulmonary hemodynamics during laparoscopy in a porcine sepsis model. Journal of the American College of Surgeons 1999, 189:450-8.
[57] Kato T, Hussein MH, Sugiura T, Suzuki S, Fukuda S, Tanaka T, et al. Development and Characterization of A Novel Porcine Model of Neonatal Sepsis. Shock 2004, 21:329-35.
[58] Ertmer C, Kampmeier TG, Rehberg S, Morelli A, K+Âhler G, Lange M, et al. Effects of balanced crystalloid vs. 0.9% saline-based vs. balanced 6% tetrastarch infusion on renal function and tubular integrity in ovine endotoxemic shock*. Critical Care Medicine 2011, 39:783-92.
[59] Noda H, Noshima S, Nakazawa H, Meyer J, Herndon DN, Redl H, et al. Left ventricular dysfunction and acute lung injury induced by continuous administration of endotoxin in sheep. Shock 1994, 1:291-8.
[60] Traber DL, Herndon DN, Stein MD, Traber LD, Flynn JT, Niehaus GD. The pulmonary lesion of smoke inhalation in an ovine model. Circ Shock 1986, 18:311-23.
[61] Soejima K, Schmalstieg FC, Sakurai H, Traber LD, Traber DL. Pathophysiological analysis of combined burn and smoke inhalation injuries in sheep. American Journal of Physiology - Lung Cellular and Molecular Physiology 2001, 280:L1233-L1241.
[62] Shirani KZ, Pruitt B, Mason ADJ. The Influence of Inhalation Injury and Pneumonia on Burn Mortality. Annals of Surgery 1987, 205:82-7.
[63] Traber DL, Herndon DN, Stein MD, Traber LD, Flynn JT, Niehaus GD. The pulmonary lesion of smoke inhalation in an ovine model. Circ Shock 2012, 18:311-23.

[64] Maybauer MO, Maybauer DM, Traber LD, Westphal M, Enkhbaatar P, Morita N, et al. Gentamicin Improves Hemodynamics in Ovine Septic Shock After Smoke Inhalation Injury. Shock 2005, 24:226-31
[65] Maybauer DM, Maybauer MO, Szab+¦ C, Cox RA, Westphal M, Kiss L, et al. The Peroxynitrite Catalyst WW-85 Improves Pulmonary Function in Ovine Septic Shock. Shock 2011, 35:148-55.
[66] Calzavacca P, Ramchandra R, Booth L, Bellomo R, May CN. Cardiovascular effects of beta-blockade in a sheep model of severe sepsis. Critical Care 2011, 15 Suppl 3:P36.
[67] Lange M, Ertmer C, Rehberg S, Morelli A, K+Âhler G, Kampmeier T, et al. Effects of two different dosing regimens of terlipressin on organ functions in ovine endotoxemia. Inflammation Research 2011, 60:429-37.
[68] Su F, Huang H, He X, Simuen D, Xie J, Orbach A, et al. Effects of a Novel Anticoagulant Compound (TV7130) in an Ovine Model of Septic Shock. Shock 2010, 34:622-7.
[69] Waerhaug K, Kuklin V, Kirov M, Sovershaev M, Langbakk B, Ingebretsen O, et al. Recombinant human activated protein C attenuates endotoxin-induced lung injury in awake sheep. Critical Care 2008, 12:R104.
[70] Redl H, Bahrami S. Large Animal Models: Baboons for Trauma, Shock, and Sepsis Studies. Shock 2005, 24:88-93.
[71] Xu J, Zhang X, Pelayo R, Monestier M, Ammollo CT, Semeraro F, et al. Extracellular histones are major mediators of death in sepsis. Nat Med 2009, 15:1318-21.
[72] Ranieri VM, Thompson BT, Barie PS, Dhainaut JF, Douglas IS, Finfer S, et al. Drotrecogin alfa (activated) in adults with septic shock. N Engl J Med 2012, 366:2055-64.
[73] Taylor FB, Chang A, Esmon CT, D'Angelo A, Vigano-D'Angelo S, Blick KE. Protein C prevents the coagulopathic and lethal effects of Escherichia coli infusion in the baboon. J Clin Invest 1987, 79:918-25.
[74] Shah BR, Hux JE. Quantifying the Risk of Infectious Diseases for People With Diabetes. Diabetes Care 2003, 26:510-3.
[75] Jacober SJ, Sowers JR. An Update on Perioperative Management of Diabetes. Arch Intern Med 1999, 159:2405-11.
[76] Browne JA, Cook C, Pietrobon R, Bethel MA, Richardson WJ. Diabetes and Early Postoperative Outcomes Following Lumbar Fusion. Spine 2007, 32:2214-9.
[77] Kornum JB, Thomsen RW, Riis A, Lervang HH, Sch+©nheyder HC, S+©rensen HT. Diabetes, Glycemic Control, and Risk of Hospitalization With Pneumonia. Diabetes Care 2008, 31:1541-5.
[78] Moss M. Epidemiology of Sepsis: Race, Sex, and Chronic Alcohol Abuse. Clinical Infectious Diseases 2005, 41 Suppl 7:S490-S497.
[79] Jacob A, Steinberg ML, Yang J, Dong W, Ji Y, Wang P. Sepsis-induced inflammation in exacerated in an animal model of type II diabetes. Int J Cli Exp Med, 1:22-31.
[80] Edwards MS, Fuselier PA. Enhanced susceptibility of mice with streptozotocin-induced diabetes to type II group B streptococcal infection. Infection and Immunity 1983, 39:580-5.

[81] Yamashiro S, Kawakami K, Uezu K, Kinjo T, Miyagi K, Nakamura K, et al. Lower expression of Th1-related cytokines and inducible nitric oxide synthase in mice with streptozotocin-induced diabetes mellitus infected with Mycobacterium tuberculosis. Clinical & Experimental Immunology 2005, 139:57-64.

[82] Graves DT, Naguib G, Lu H, Leone C, Hsue H, Krall E. Inflammation is More Persistent in Type 1 Diabetic Mice. Journal of Dental Research 2005, 84:324-8.

[83] Strandberg L, Verdrengh M, Enge M, Andersson N, Amu S, +ûnnheim K, et al. Mice Chronically Fed High-Fat Diet Have Increased Mortality and Disturbed Immune Response in Sepsis. PLoS ONE 2009, 4:e7605.

[84] Brun-Buisson C. The epidemiology of the systemic inflammatory response. Intensive Care Medicine 2000, 26 Suppl 1:S64-S74.

[85] Wagenlehner FME, Pilatz A, Weidner W. UrosepsisΓÇöfrom the view of the urologist. International Journal of Antimicrobial Agents 2011, 38 Suppl 0:51-7.

[86] Hagberg L, Engberg I, Freter R, Lam J, Olling S, Svanborg Ed+®n C. Ascending, unobstructed urinary tract infection in mice caused by pyelonephritogenic Escherichia coli of human origin. Infection and Immunity 1983, 40:273-83.

[87] Reid G, Chan RC, Bruce AW, Costerton JW. Prevention of urinary tract infection in rats with an indigenous Lactobacillus casei strain. Infection and Immunity 1985, 49:320-4.

[88] Stewart D, Fulton WB, Wilson C, Monitto CL, Paidas CN, Reeves RH, et al. Genetic Contribution to the Septic Response in A Mouse Model. Shock 2002, 18:342-7.

[89] Wang H, Laskowitz DT, Sullivan PM, Christensen DJ. APOE genotype affects outcome in a murine model of sepsis: implications for a new treatment strategy. Anaesthesia and Intensive Care 2009, 37:38-45.

[90] Zhang SH, Reddick RL, Piedrahita JA, Maeda N. Spontaneous hypercholesterolemia and arterial lesions in mice lacking apolipoprotein E. Science 1992, 258:468-71.

[91] Grainger DJ, Reckless J, McKilligin E. Apolipoprotein E Modulates Clearance of Apoptotic Bodies In Vitro and In Vivo, Resulting in a Systemic Proinflammatory State in Apolipoprotein E-Deficient Mice. The Journal of Immunology 2004, 173:6366-75.

[92] de Bont N, Netea MG, Demacker PNM, Verschueren I, Kullberg BJ, van Dijk KW, et al. Apolipoprotein E knock-out mice are highly susceptible to endotoxemia and Klebsiella pneumoniae infection. Journal of Lipid Research 1999, 40:680-5.

[93] Haraguchi G, Kosuge H, Maejima Y, Suzuki JI, Imai T, Yoshida M, et al. Pioglitazone reduces systematic inflammation and improves mortality in apolipoprotein E knockout mice with sepsis. Intensive Care Medicine 2008, 34:1304-12.

[94] Gao XP, Liu Q, Broman M, Predescu D, Frey RS, Malik AB. Inactivation of CD11b in a mouse transgenic model protects against sepsis-induced lung PMN infiltration and vascular injury. Physiological Genomics 2005, 21:230-42.

[95] Wu Z, Sawamura T, Kurdowska AK, Ji HL, Idell S, Fu J. LOX-1 Deletion Improves Neutrophil Responses, Enhances Bacterial Clearance, and Reduces Lung Injury in a Murine Polymicrobial Sepsis Model. Infection and Immunity 2011, 79:2865-70.

[96] Kaisho T, Akira S. Dendritic-cell function in Toll-like receptor- and MyD88-knockout mice. Trends in immunology 2001, 22:78-83.

[97] Zhang D, Zhang G, Hayden MS, Greenblatt MB, Bussey C, Flavell RA, et al. A Toll-like Receptor That Prevents Infection by Uropathogenic Bacteria. Science 2004, 303:1522-6.

[98] Sugawara I, Yamada H, Li C, Mizuno S, Takeuchi O, Akira S. Mycobacterial infection in TLR2 and TLR6 knockout mice. Microbiol Immunol 2003, 47:327-36.

[99] Tschop J, Nogueiras R, Haas-Lockie S, Kasten KR, Castaneda TR, Huber N, et al. CNS Leptin Action Modulates Immune Response and Survival in Sepsis. The Journal of Neuroscience 2010, 30:6036-47.

[100] Brinkmann V, Reichard U, Goosmann C, Fauler B, Uhlemann Y, Weiss DS, et al. Neutrophil extracellular traps kill bacteria. Science 2004, 303:1532-5.

[101] Papayannopoulos V, Zychlinsky A. NETs: a new strategy for using old weapons. Trends Immunol 2009, 30:513-21.

[102] Fuchs TA, Abed U, Goosmann C, Hurwitz R, Schulze I, Wahn V, et al. Novel cell death program leads to neutrophil extracellular traps. J Cell Biol 2007, 176:231-41.

[103] Papayannopoulos V, Metzler KD, Hakkim A, Zychlinsky A. Neutrophil elastase and myeloperoxidase regulate the formation of neutrophil extracellular traps. J Cell Biol 2010, 191:677-91.

[104] Remijsen Q, Kuijpers TW, Wirawan E, Lippens S, Vandenabeele P, Vanden Berghe T. Dying for a cause: NETosis, mechanisms behind an antimicrobial cell death modality. Cell Death Differ 2011, 18:581-8.

[105] Vandenabeele P, Galluzzi L, Vanden Berghe T, Kroemer G. Molecular mechanisms of necroptosis: an ordered cellular explosion. Nat Rev Mol Cell Biol 2010, 11:700-14.

[106] Bruns S, Kniemeyer O, Hasenberg M, Aimanianda V, Nietzsche S, Thywissen A, et al. Production of extracellular traps against Aspergillus fumigatus in vitro and in infected lung tissue is dependent on invading neutrophils and influenced by hydrophobin RodA. PLoS Pathog 2010, 6:e1000873.

[107] Urban CF, Reichard U, Brinkmann V, Zychlinsky A. Neutrophil extracellular traps capture and kill Candida albicans yeast and hyphal forms. Cell Microbiol 2006, 8:668-76.

[108] Urban CF, Ermert D, Schmid M, Abu-Abed U, Goosmann C, Nacken W, et al. Neutrophil extracellular traps contain calprotectin, a cytosolic protein complex involved in host defense against Candida albicans. PLoS Pathog 2009, 5:e1000639.

[109] Bianchi M, Hakkim A, Brinkmann V, Siler U, Seger RA, Zychlinsky A, et al. Restoration of NET formation by gene therapy in CGD controls aspergillosis. Blood 2009, 114:2619-22.

[110] Springer DJ, Ren P, Raina R, Dong Y, Behr MJ, McEwen BF, et al. Extracellular fibrils of pathogenic yeast Cryptococcus gattii are important for ecological niche, murine virulence and human neutrophil interactions. PLoS One 2010, 5:e10978.

[111] Hakkim A, Furnrohr BG, Amann K, Laube B, Abed UA, Brinkmann V, et al. Impairment of neutrophil extracellular trap degradation is associated with lupus nephritis. Proc Natl Acad Sci U S A 2010, 107:9813-8.

[112] Buchanan JT, Simpson AJ, Aziz RK, Liu GY, Kristian SA, Kotb M, et al. DNase expression allows the pathogen group A Streptococcus to escape killing in neutrophil extracellular traps. Curr Biol 2006, 16:396-400.

[113] Brinkmann V, Reichard U, Goosmann C, Fauler B, Uhlemann Y, Weiss DS, et al. Neutrophil extracellular traps kill bacteria. Science 2004, 303:1532-5.

[114] Beiter K, Wartha F, Albiger B, Normark S, Zychlinsky A, Henriques-Normark B. An endonuclease allows Streptococcus pneumoniae to escape from neutrophil extracellular traps. Curr Biol 2006, 16:401-7.

[115] Guimaraes-Costa AB, Nascimento MT, Froment GS, Soares RP, Morgado FN, Conceicao-Silva F, et al. Leishmania amazonensis promastigotes induce and are killed by neutrophil extracellular traps. Proc Natl Acad Sci U S A 2009, 106:6748-53.

[116] Ramos-Kichik V, Mondragon-Flores R, Mondragon-Castelan M, Gonzalez-Pozos S, Muniz-Hernandez S, Rojas-Espinosa O, et al. Neutrophil extracellular traps are induced by Mycobacterium tuberculosis. Tuberculosis (Edinb) 2009, 89:29-37.

[117] McCormick A, Heesemann L, Wagener J, Marcos V, Hartl D, Loeffler J, et al. NETs formed by human neutrophils inhibit growth of the pathogenic mold Aspergillus fumigatus. Microbes Infect 2010, 12:928-36.

[118] Clark SR, Ma AC, Tavener SA, McDonald B, Goodarzi Z, Kelly MM, et al. Platelet TLR4 activates neutrophil extracellular traps to ensnare bacteria in septic blood. Nat Med 2007, 13:463-9.

[119] Martinez VF, Balada E, Ordi-Ros J, Vilardell-Tarres M. DNase 1 and systemic lupus erythematosus. Autoimmun Rev 2008, 7:359-63.

[120] Tew MB, Johnson RW, Reveille JD, Tan FK. A molecular analysis of the low serum deoxyribonuclease activity in lupus patients. Arthritis Rheum 2001, 44:2446-7.

[121] Balada E, Ordi-Ros J, Hernanz S, Villarreal J, Cortes F, Vilardell-Tarres M, et al. DNASE I mutation and systemic lupus erythematosus in a Spanish population: comment on the article by Tew et al. Arthritis Rheum 2002, 46:1974-6.

[122] Bodano A, Gonzalez A, Balada E, Ordi J, Carreira P, Gomez-Reino JJ, et al. Study of DNASE I gene polymorphisms in systemic lupus erythematosus susceptibility. Ann Rheum Dis 2007, 66:560-1.

[123] Napirei M, Wulf S, Mannherz HG. Chromatin breakdown during necrosis by serum Dnase1 and the plasminogen system. Arthritis Rheum 2004, 50:1873-83.

[124] Fuchs TA, Brill A, Duerschmied D, Schatzberg D, Monestier M, Myers DD, Jr., et al. Extracellular DNA traps promote thrombosis. Proc Natl Acad Sci U S A 2010, 107:15880-5.

[125] Kannemeier C, Shibamiya A, Nakazawa F, Trusheim H, Ruppert C, Markart P, et al. Extracellular RNA constitutes a natural procoagulant cofactor in blood coagulation. Proc Natl Acad Sci U S A 2007, 104:6388-93.

[126] Shak S, Capon DJ, Hellmiss R, Marsters SA, Baker CL. Recombinant human DNase I reduces the viscosity of cystic fibrosis sputum. Proc Natl Acad Sci U S A 1990, 87:9188-92.

[127] Semeraro F, Ammollo CT, Morrissey JH, Dale GL, Friese P, Esmon NL, et al. Extracellular histones promote thrombin generation through platelet-dependent mechanisms: involvement of platelet TLR2 and TLR4. Blood 2011, 118:1952-61.
[128] Semeraro N, Ammollo CT, Semeraro F, Colucci M. Sepsis, thrombosis and organ dysfunction. Thromb Res 2012, 129:290-5.
[129] Xu J, Zhang X, Pelayo R, Monestier M, Ammollo CT, Semeraro F, et al. Extracellular histones are major mediators of death in sepsis. Nat Med 2009, 15:1318-21.
[130] Marshall CJ, Nallaratnam M, Mocatta T, Smyth D, Richards M, Elliott JM, et al. Factors influencing local and systemic levels of plasma myeloperoxidase in ST-segment elevation acute myocardial infarction. Am J Cardiol 2010, 106:316-22.
[131] Baldus S, Eiserich JP, Mani A, Castro L, Figueroa M, Chumley P, et al. Endothelial transcytosis of myeloperoxidase confers specificity to vascular ECM proteins as targets of tyrosine nitration. J Clin Invest 2001, 108:1759-70.
[132] Keshari RS, Jyoti A, Kumar S, Dubey M, Verma A, Srinag BS, et al. Neutrophil extracellular traps contain mitochondrial as well as nuclear DNA and exhibit inflammatory potential. Cytometry A 2012, 81:238-47.
[133] Wartha F, Beiter K, Normark S, Henriques-Normark B. Neutrophil extracellular traps: casting the NET over pathogenesis. Curr Opin Microbiol 2007, 10:52-6.
[134] Esmon CT. Extracellular histones zap platelets. Blood 2011, 118:3456-7.
[135] Xu J, Zhang X, Monestier M, Esmon NL, Esmon CT. Extracellular histones are mediators of death through TLR2 and TLR4 in mouse fatal liver injury. J Immunol 2011, 187:2626-31.
[136] Lorente JA, Marshall JC. Neutralization of tumor necrosis factor in preclinical models of sepsis. Shock 2005, 24 Suppl 1:107-19.
[137] Hinshaw LB, Tekamp-Olson P, Chang AC, Lee PA, Taylor FB, Jr., Murray CK, et al. Survival of primates in LD100 septic shock following therapy with antibody to tumor necrosis factor (TNF alpha). Circ Shock 1990, 30:279-92.
[138] Lay AJ, Donahue D, Tsai MJ, Castellino FJ. Acute inflammation is exacerbated in mice genetically predisposed to a severe protein C deficiency. Blood 2007, 109:1984-91.
[139] Maderazo EG, Breaux S, Woronick CL, Krause PJ. Efficacy, toxicity, and pharmacokinetics of pentoxifylline and its analogs in experimental Staphylococcus aureus infections. Antimicrobial Agents and Chemotherapy 1990, 34:1100-6.
[140] Teti G, Mancuso G, Cusumano V, Blandino G, Fera MT, Carbone M. Effects of anti-cytokine treatments in neonatal sepsis models. J Chemother 1995, 7 Suppl 4:96-8.
[141] Mancuso G, Cusumano V, Cook JA, Smith E, Squadrito F, Blandino G, et al. Efficacy of tumor necrosis factor +¦ and eicosanoid inhibitors in experimental models of neonatal sepsis. FEMS Immunology & Medical Microbiology 1994, 9:49-54.
[142] Freudenberg MA, Galanos C. Tumor necrosis factor alpha mediates lethal activity of killed gram-negative and gram-positive bacteria in D-galactosamine-treated mice. Infect Immun 1991, 59:2110-5.

[143] Papasian CJ, Silverstein R, Gao JJ, Bamberger DM, Morrison DC. Anomalous Role of Tumor Necrosis Factor Alpha in Experimental Enterococcal Infection. Infection and Immunity 2002, 70:6628-37.

[144] Hinshaw LB, Emerson TE, Jr., Taylor FB, Jr., Chang AC, Duerr M, Peer GT, et al. Lethal Staphylococcus aureus-induced shock in primates: prevention of death with anti-TNF antibody. J Trauma 1992, 33:568-73.

[145] Stevens DL, Bryant AE, Hackett SP, Chang A, Peer G, Kosanke S, et al. Group A Streptococcal Bacteremia: The Role of Tumor Necrosis Factor in Shock and Organ Failure. Journal of Infectious Diseases 1996, 173:619-26.

[146] Beutler B, Milsark IW, Cerami AC. Passive immunization against cachectin/tumor necrosis factor protects mice from lethal effect of endotoxin. Science 1985, 229:869-71.

[147] Tracey KJ, Fong Y, Hesse DG, Manogue KR, Lee AT, Kuo GC, et al. Anti-cachectin/TNF monoclonal antibodies prevent septic shock during lethal bacteraemia. Nature 1987, 330:662-4.

[148] Eskandari MK, Bolgos G, Miller C, Nguyen DT, DeForge LE, Remick DG. Anti-tumor necrosis factor antibody therapy fails to prevent lethality after cecal ligation and puncture or endotoxemia. J Immunol 1992, 148:2724-30.

[149] Echtenacher B, Hultner L, Mannel DN. Cellular and molecular mechanisms of TNF protection in septic peritonitis. J Inflamm 1995, 47:85-9.

[150] Cohen J. Adjunctive therapy in sepsis: a critical analysis of the clinical trial programme. Br Med Bull 1990, 55:212-25.

[151] Fisher CJ, Agosti JM, Opal SM, Lowry SF, Balk RA, Sadoff JC, et al. Treatment of Septic Shock with the Tumor Necrosis Factor Receptor:Fc Fusion Protein. N Engl J Med 1996, 334:1697-702.

[152] Martin GS, Mannino DM, Eaton S, Moss M. The Epidemiology of Sepsis in the United States from 1979 through 2000. N Engl J Med 2003, 348:1546-54.

[153] Turnbull IR, Buchman TG, Javadi P, Woolsey CA, Hotchkiss RS, Karl IE, et al. Age disproportionately increases sepsis-induced apoptosis in the spleen and gut epithelium. Shock 2004, 22:364-8.

[154] Bernard GR, Vincent JL, Laterre PF, LaRosa SP, Dhainaut JF, Lopez-Rodriguez A, et al. Efficacy and Safety of Recombinant Human Activated Protein C for Severe Sepsis. N Engl J Med 2001, 344:699-709.

[155] Wichmann MW, Inthorn D, Andress HJ, Schildberg FW. Incidence and mortality of severe sepsis in surgical intensive care patients: the influence of patient gender on disease process and outcome. Intensive Care Med 2000, 26:167-72.

[156] Hrekova SP, Vodianyk MO, Chernyshov VP. [Effect of progesterone and 17beta-estradiol on proinflammatory cytokine costimulatory proliferative activity]. Fiziol Zh 2002, 48:63-9.

[157] England JM, Bain BJ. Total and differential leucocyte count. Br J Haematol 1976, 33:1-7.

[158] Northern AL, Rutter SM, Peterson CM. Cyclic changes in the concentrations of peripheral blood immune cells during the normal menstrual cycle. Proc Soc Exp Biol Med 1994, 207:81-8.
[159] Rivers E, Nguyen B, Havstad S, Ressler J, Muzzin A, Knoblich B, et al. Early Goal-Directed Therapy in the Treatment of Severe Sepsis and Septic Shock. N Engl J Med 2001, 345:1368-77.
[160] Natanson C, Danner RL, Reilly JM, Doerfler ML, Hoffman WD, Akin GL, et al. Antibiotics versus cardiovascular support in a canine model of human septic shock. American Journal of Physiology - Heart and Circulatory Physiology 1990, 259:H1440-H1447.
[161] Ondiveeran HK, Fox- Robichaud AE. Pentastarch in a Balanced Solution Reduces Hepatic Leukocyte Recruitment in Early Sepsis. Microcirculation 2004, 11:679-87.
[162] Schulz KF, Altman DG, Moher D. CONSORT 2010 statement: updated guidelines for reporting parallel group randomised trials. Int J Surg 2011, 9:672-7.
[163] Moher D, Schulz KF, Altman DG. The CONSORT statement: revised recommendations for improving the quality of reports of parallel-group randomized trials. Ann Intern Med 2001, 134:657-62.
[164] Begg C, Cho M, Eastwood S, Horton R, Moher D, Olkin I, et al. Improving the quality of reporting of randomized controlled trials. The CONSORT statement. JAMA 1996, 276:637-9.
[165] Kilkenny C, Browne WJ, Cuthill IC, Emerson M, Altman DG. Improving bioscience research reporting: the ARRIVE guidelines for reporting animal research. PLoS Biol 2010, 8:e1000412.
[166] Bebarta V, Luyten D, Heard K. Emergency medicine animal research: does use of randomization and blinding affect the results? Acad Emerg Med 2003, 10:684-7.
[167] Piper RD, Cook DJ, Bone RC, Sibbald WJ. Introducing Critical Appraisal to studies of animal models investigating novel therapies in sepsis. Crit Care Med 1996, 24:2059-70.
[168] Lamontagne F, Briel M, Duffett M, Fox-Robichaud A, Cook DJ, Guyatt G, et al. Systematic review of reviews including animal studies addressing therapeutic interventions for sepsis. Crit Care Med 2010, 38:2401-8.
[169] Kilkenny C, Parsons N, Kadyszewski E, Festing MF, Cuthill IC, Fry D, et al. Survey of the quality of experimental design, statistical analysis and reporting of research using animals. PLoS One 2009, 4:e7824.
[170] Chalmers TC, Celano P, Sacks HS, Smith H, Jr. Bias in treatment assignment in controlled clinical trials. N Engl J Med 1983, 309:1358-61.
[171] Sacks H, Chalmers TC, Smith H, Jr. Randomized versus historical controls for clinical trials. Am J Med 1982, 72:233-40.
[172] Colditz GA, Miller JN, Mosteller F. How study design affects outcomes in comparisons of therapy. I: Medical. Stat Med 1989, 8:441-54.

[173] Guyatt GH, Sackett DL, Cook DJ. Users' guides to the medical literature. II. How to use an article about therapy or prevention. A. Are the results of the study valid? Evidence-Based Medicine Working Group. JAMA 1993, 270:2598-601.
[174] Marshall JC, Creery D. Pre-clinical models of sepsis. Sepsis 1998, 2:187-97.
[175] Guyatt GH, Sackett DL, Cook DJ. Users' guides to the medical literature. II. How to use an article about therapy or prevention. B. What were the results and will they help me in caring for my patients? Evidence-Based Medicine Working Group. JAMA 1994 , 271:59-63.
[176] Contopoulos-Ioannidis DG, Ntzani E, Ioannidis JP. Translation of highly promising basic science research into clinical applications. Am J Med 2003 , 114:477-84.

Chapter 3

Sepsis, the Liver and the Gut

Neville Azzopardi, Manuel Fenech and Tonio Piscopo

Additional information is available at the end of the chapter

http://dx.doi.org/10.5772/49962

1. Introduction

The gastrointestinal tract has various functions including digestion, the production of hormones with local and systemic effects, a major role in immunological function, and acting as a barrier against antigens within its lumen. The intestinal microflora is an ecosystem which harbours over 400 bacterial species, predominantly anaerobes which outnumber facultative anaerobes. Most flora is present in the large bowel, mainly in the lumen and attached to the mucosa, but they do not normally penetrate the bowel wall. Intestinal bacteria form an important part of the enterohepatic circulation. Metabolites conjugated in the liver (including drugs and endogenous compounds) are excreted in bile to be deconjugated by bacterial enzymes in the intestine, so that they can then be absorbed across the intestine into the portal circulation and returned to the liver. Antibiotics that alter the intestinal flora can change the fecal excretion and the serum levels of these metabolites. Bacterial flora also increase fiber digestion and are believed to decrease the risk of gastrointestinal infections by interfering with gut pathogens. Our intestine harbours low concentrations of potentially pathogenic organisms (such as *Clostridium difficile).* Antibiotics that alter the normal intestinal flora can increase the risk of infection by exogenous pathogens or through the overgrowth of endogenous pathogens, like *Clostridium difficile.* If the bowel wall is damaged by trauma, burns or inflammation, intestinal bacteria may escape into the peritoneum to cause peritonitis and / or abscesses.[1]

Gastrointestinal dysfunction or gut failure frequently occurs in seriously ill patients and is responsible for bacterial translocation. This may in turn cause sepsis, with the initiation of a systemic inflammatory response syndrome (SIRS), multiple organ dysfunction syndrome (MODS), and / or death.[2] Gut dysfunction is also present in other conditions, including inflammatory bowel disease, *Clostridium difficile* infection, and liver cirrhosis. In this chapter, we investigate common conditions affecting the liver and the gut and their relation to sepsis, as well as investigating the role of gut decontamination and probiotics in stabilising the gut flora.

2. Sepsis in liver cirrhosis

Liver cirrhosis occurs in response to chronic liver injury and involves the development of regenerative nodules surrounded by fibrous bands in the liver parenchyma. This in turn causes distortion of the hepatic vasculature, leading to portal hypertension and end stage liver disease. Cirrhosis leads to shunting of portal and arterial blood into the hepatic central veins, thus compromising the exchange between hepatic sinusoids and hepatocytes. Cirrhosis causes an impaired hepatocyte activity, portal hypertension and an increased risk of hepatocellular carcinoma. Hepatic vascular alterations and portal hypertension will in turn cause splanchnic vasodilatation, vasoconstriction and decreased renal perfusion, water and salt retention and an increased cardiac output.[3]

The estimated prevalence of cirrhosis in the United States is 0.15% [4], though this may be an underestimate due to the high prevalence of undiagnosed cirrhosis in hepatitis C and Non-Alcoholic Steatohepatitis (NASH). Similar numbers have been reported from Europe, and numbers are even higher in most Asian and African countries where chronic viral hepatitis B or C are frequent. Since compensated cirrhosis is frequently not detected until routine investigations are performed, a reasonable estimate is that up to 1% of the world population may have histological cirrhosis. Alcoholic liver disease and hepatitis C are the commonest causes of cirrhosis in the Western world, while hepatitis B is the most common cause in most parts of Asia and sub-Saharan Africa. Cryptogenic cirrhosis (cirrhosis without a recognised cause) is nowadays rarely diagnosed, particularly after the identification of the hepatitis C virus in the late 1980s and with the identification of nonalcoholic steatohepatitis in obese and diabetic subjects.[3]

Bacteraemic infections are more frequent in patients with hepatic cirrhosis. 9% of the overall number of bacteraemic episodes in newly-admitted patients occur in cirrhotic patients [5] and 46% of cirrhotic patients have bacterial infections on admission.[6] Advanced cirrhotics are more likely to have the systemic inflammatory response syndrome. This syndrome correlates with bacterial infection at admission and has been shown to be associated with a poor outcome.[7] Animal studies have identified the gut as the principal source of infection in liver cirrhosis, mainly through bacterial overgrowth and translocation in the small bowel. However, cultures of small intestinal mucosal bacteria in cirrhotic patients have shown that these microbiota are qualitatively and quantitatively normal. This has shifted attention towards factors that decrease gut integrity, or alter the removal of translocating bacteria as causative factors of bacteraemia in cirrhosis.[8] It is hypothesized that in cirrhosis the intestine is more permeable, allowing bacteria easy access into the circulation through the gut mucosa with consequent macrophage activation. This permeability is further increased in patients with portal hypertension. Serum levels of interleukin-6 and soluble receptors of tumor necrosis factor were shown to be significantly higher in HIV-HCV co-infected and HCV mono-infected patients with decompensated cirrhosis when compared with those with compensated liver disease.[9] This susceptibility was also demonstrated in non-alcoholic steatohepatitis.[10] In patients with cirrhosis and severe sepsis, high production of pro-inflammatory cytokines seems to cause a deterioration in liver function and predisposes to the development of shock, renal failure, acute lung injury or acute respiratory distress syndrome, coagulopathy, or hepatic encephalopathy. Variants of the NOD2 gene (100fs and G908R) appear to increase bacterial translocation in cirrhotics and have been associated with spontaneous bacterial peritonitis in a recent study.[11] There is an increased risk for culture-positive spontaneous bacterial peritonitis and infected ascites in cirrhotic patients with these variants.[11]

The second theory is that patients with chronic liver disease tend to have impaired bacterial clearance. This was demonstrated when quantitative real-time polymerase chain reaction (PCR) using primers that amplify all known bacteria was used to measure bacteraemia following tooth-brushing. The investigators showed greater than 75% bacteraemia following tooth-brushing, but while control subjects were able to clear this bacteraemia, subjects with cirrhosis had prolonged bacteraemia, suggesting that cirrhotic patients may be more susceptible to sepsis because of ineffective bacterial clearance.[12]

The mortality rate of patients with liver cirrhosis is significantly higher than that of patients with other diseases when they develop bacteraemia, and underlying cirrhosis is an independent risk factor for mortality in bacteraemic patients. In-hospital mortality rate in patients with liver cirrhosis and sepsis was shown to be up to 30% [13-16], with another 30% dying by 1 year.[16] Factors which are significantly associated with in-hospital mortality are the presence of more than 1 site of infection, pneumonia, Child's C status and a model for end-stage liver disease (MELD) score of 17 or more. In-hospital mortality rate increases as the number of factors increases (7% with one factor, 21% with two factors, 87% with three factors and 100% with four factors).[13] The initial CRP level does not predict mortality secondary to sepsis in liver cirrhosis patients. However, serial CRP measurements during the first week of antimicrobial therapy may be a useful prognostic factor for mortality in cirrhotic patients.[14] In a nationwide Korean surveillance study comparing bacteraemia in patients with liver cirrhosis with bacteraemia in patients with other liver diseases, patients with cirrhosis were shown to be more likely to have *Klebsiella pneumonia* bacteraemia (20.1% vs 14.3%, P=0.018) but less likely to have coagulase-negative staphylococcal bacteraemia (5.1% vs 10.4%, P=0.028).[14]

One of the sequelae of cirrhosis is the development of ascites. Patients with ascites have an increased risk of developing spontaneous bacterial peritonitis (SBP) with a prevalence of 10-30%. Even with early diagnosis and management of spontaneous bacterial peritonitis, mortality is still 31% at 1 month and 66% at 12 months.[16] SBP is a very common bacterial infection in patients with cirrhosis and ascites.[17] Bacterial translocation is believed to be responsible for the first step in the pathogenesis of spontaneous bacterial peritonitis. Translocation is only possible because of the concurrent failure of the defensive mechanisms in cirrhosis. Research has confirmed an increased bacterial translocation in cirrhotic rats. There is also pronounced impairment of gastrointestinal tract motility in cirrhosis. A disturbance of the gut microflora thus occurs and this, in association with changes in the permeability of the gastrointestinal tract, causes the passage of microorganisms and endotoxins to the mesenteric lymph nodes.[18] The diagnosis of SBP is based on diagnostic paracentesis. Half the episodes of SBP are present on hospital admission while the rest are acquired during hospitalization.[19] SBP may present with peritonitic signs (abdominal pain, tenderness, vomiting, ileus), fever, elevated white cell counts, tachycardia, hypotension, worsening of liver function, hepatic encephalopathy, renal failure and gastrointestinal bleeding. However, cirrhotic patients with SBP may be completely asymptomatic. Empirical antibiotics should be started immediately following the diagnosis of SBP. The first line antibiotic treatment in SBP are the third generation cephalosporins, as the commonest causative organisms are Gram-negative aerobic bacteria.[20] Other options include co-amoxiclav, ciprofloxacin and ofloxacin (though quinolones should not be used in patients who are using these antibiotics for SBP prophylaxis, in areas where there is a high prevalence of quinolone resistance or in nosocomial SBP). Antibiotics are effective in the management of SBP in approximately 90% of patients. Failure of antibiotic therapy usually occurs due to bacterial resistance or because of missed secondary bacterial peritonitis. If secondary bacterial peritonitis has been excluded, the antibiotic needs to be changed according to the culture and sensitivity results of the isolated organisms, or else modified to an alternative empiric broad spectrum agent.[21]

Hepato-renal syndrome (HRS) refers to the rapid deterioration of renal function in patients with liver cirrhosis. It occurs in approximately 30% of patients with SBP treated with antibiotics alone and is associated with a very poor survival. Albumin administration (1.5 g/kg at diagnosis and 1 g/kg on day 3) decreases the frequency and mortality of HRS in cirrhotic patients with SBP. For this reason, the European Association for the Study of the Liver (EASL) guidelines recommend that all cirrhotic patients who develop SBP should be treated with intravenous albumin and empirical antibiotics.[21]

In patients at high risk of developing SBP, antibiotic prophylaxis is recommended.[21] Since it is hypothesised that SBP occurs following the translocation of enteric Gram negative bacteria from the gut to the circulation, the ideal prophylactic antibiotic needs to be effective at decreasing the amounts of these organisms in the gut without altering the protective anaerobic flora. The use of prophylactic antibiotics should be strictly restricted to patients at high risk of SBP to decrease the risk of developing resistance. These high-risk patient populations include cirrhotics with acute gastrointestinal hemorrhage, those with low total protein content in ascitic fluid and no prior history of SBP (primary prophylaxis) and patients with a previous history of SBP (secondary prophylaxis). In such high-risk patients, antibiotics should be started immediately (i.e. following upper gastrointestinal bleed, after a first episode of SBP or upon finding low total protein) and are recommended life-long, or until liver transplant is performed.

Bacterial infection is a major problem in cirrhotic patients with acute gastrointestinal hemorrhage, occurring in 25 - 65% of these patients.[22] Bacteraemia in patients with variceal hemorrhage is associated with a decreased ability to control bleeding [23], an increased rebleeding rate, and increased hospital mortality.[24] Antibiotic prophylaxis has been shown to prevent infection in patients with gastrointestinal bleeding and decrease the rate of rebleeding. A meta-analysis of five studies performed in patients with gastrointestinal bleeding [25-29] has shown that antibiotic prophylaxis significantly decreased both the incidence of severe infections (SBP and/or sepsis) and mortality. The preferred antibiotic for SBP prophylaxis is norfloxacin (400 mg/12 h orally for 7 days) which provides selective intestinal decontamination. Norfloxacin is a quinolone antibiotic with antibacterial activity against Gram-negative bacteria but not against Gram-positive cocci or anaerobic bacteria. However, in view of the increasing incidence of quinolone-resistant bacteraemia [30-32], and because a substantial number of infections in patients with gastrointestinal hemorrhage are caused by Gram-positive bacteria, ceftriaxone has been studied as a prophylactic agent in cirrhotics with gastrointestinal bleeding. A study comparing oral norfloxacin with intravenous ceftriaxone for the prophylaxis of bacterial infection in cirrhotic patients with gastrointestinal bleeding showed that ceftriaxone was more effective than norfloxacin in the prevention of infections.[33] The main disadvantage with ceftriaxone is that it must be given intravenously and is therefore limited to hospital use. Cirrhotic patients with low protein concentrations (<10 g/L) in their ascitic fluid and/or high serum bilirubin levels are at an increased risk of developing SBP.[34] Studies have shown that norfloxacin (400 mg/day) is effective as a prophylactic agent against SBP and improves survival in patients with low total protein in their ascitic fluid.[35-37] Following an episode of SBP, the cumulative recurrence rate at 1 year is approximately 70% [38], with a 1-year survival probability of 30–50% and a 2-year survival probability of 25–30%. Prophylactic norfloxacin (400 mg/day, orally) reduces the risk of recurrent SBP. Other antibiotics which may be used in SBP prophylaxis after the first episode of SBP include ciprofloxacin (750 mg once weekly, orally) or co-trimoxazole (800 mg sulfamethoxazole and 160 mg trimethoprim daily orally), but the evidence with these antibiotics is not as strong as with norfloxacin. The EASL guidelines also recommend that patients recovering from SBP should be considered for liver transplantation.[21] The American Association for the Study of the Liver and the British Society of Gastroenterology guidelines [39,40] have similar recommendations for the management of spontaneous bacterial peritonitis and its prophylaxis.

Terlipressin is a vasoactive agent used in patients with septic shock and which has a selective affinity to vascular V1 receptors. It is an effective pressor agent in patients with catecholamine-unresponsive septic shock. Additional studies are needed to identify the best time to start terlipressin, the efficacy and dosages of continuous infusion versus bolus administration as well as the safety and efficacy of this compound in comparison with other vasoactive drugs.[41,42]

3. Acute cholangitis

Acute cholangitis and biliary sepsis are severe infectious diseases, frequently observed in patients with obstructive jaundice. The presence of bacteria in the biliary tract increases in the presence of biliary obstruction, particularly in the presence of foreign bodies like stones, but also in the presence of malignant obstruction secondary to pancreatic head carcinoma or cholangiocarcinoma. Reflux of bacteria from the biliary tract to the systemic circulation is believed to be the primary etiologic factor in bacteraemia and the development of sepsis in cholangitis. Biliary tract obstruction is the initiating factor in the pathogenesis of acute cholangitis causing elevated intraluminal pressures, and subsequent infection of the normally sterile bile. Bacteria may infect bile retrogradely from the gut (through the ascending route), through the haematogenous route or via lymphatics. The presence of bacteria in the biliary tract (bactibilia) increases rapidly with the development of biliary obstruction, particularly in the presence of foreign bodies like stones. Biliary obstruction causes local and systemic changes in the host defenses. There is decreased bile passage into the small bowel and decreased secretory IgA from the gastrointestinal tract. This promotes changes in the gut bacterial flora which in turn cause loss of mucosal integrity, decreased endotoxin inactivation and bacterial overgrowth. These changes cause portal bacteremia, endotoxemia and increased translocation of endotoxins to the liver, resulting in sepsis and also decreasing the hepatic Kupffer cell function in these patients. In view of these pathophysiological changes, early biliary decompression is necessary to restore normal function of the Kupffer cells in the liver and thus prevent functional alterations in the liver because of chronic, long-standing obstruction and cholestasis. Early biliary decompression also decreases postoperative morbidity and mortality.[43] The increased expression of triggering receptor expressed on myeloid cells (TREM-1) in the peripheral blood mononuclear cells of sepsis patients with acute cholangitis suggests an important role of TREM-1 in the development of acute cholangitis.[44, 45]

The predominant pathogens cultured from bile specimens in patients with obstructive jaundice (samples obtained at endoscopic retrograde cholangiopancreatography (ERCP) or percutaneous transhepatic biliary drainage) were gram-negative bacteria (68%) followed by gram-positive bacteria (26%), anaerobes (3%) and Candida (3%).[46] The predominant gram-negative pathogens were *Eschericia coli*, *Acinetobacter baumani* complex, *Klebsiella pneumonia* and *Enterobacter cloacae*. The most effective antibiotics against the gram-negative bacteria were shown to be imipenem (susceptibility: 97.9%), cefoperazone/sulbactam (89.4%), piperacillin/tazobactam (85.1%) and cefepime(85.1%).[46] Another study on patients with acute cholangitis [47] confirmed that gram-negative organisms are responsible for most bacteraemias (95%), with the commonest ones being *Eschericia coli* (62%), and *Klebsiella pneumonia* (26%). This study found that bacteraemias caused by biliary tract infection represented 5.5% of all causes of bacteraemias. Thirty-day mortality among these patients was 14% with 57% of these patients dying secondary to septic shock.[47] The management of ascending cholangitis involves the use of appropriate antibiotics and drainage of the biliary tract. Treatment should target Enterobacteriaceae with a cephalosporin, and if the patient becomes hypotensive, an aminoglycoside effective against ESBL-producing *E. coli* or *Klebsiella pneumonia* should also be administered. Biliary drainage, by ERCP or percutaneous transhepatic cholangiography, is frequently needed for adequate biliary decompression.[47]

Patients undergoing ERCP tend to be at high risk of sepsis because of the underlying biliary obstruction which predisposes to cholangitis and because of the invasive nature of the procedure. The use of prophylactic antibiotics before ERCP is therefore recommended by all major international gastroenterological societies, especially in the presence of an obstructed biliary system.[48-50] The use of prophylactic antibiotics attempts to decrease or eliminate the incidence of cholangitis, sepsis and pancreatitis after the procedure.[48] During ERCP, bacteraemia is believed to occur because of the injection of contrast and the iatrogenic introduction of foreign substances in the bile of patients who already have underlying pathologies such as biliary obstruction or pancreatic pseudocysts. Bacteraemia during ERCP is relatively uncommon in patients who do not have evidence of biliary or pancreatic ductal obstruction.[49] Bacteraemia is however well recognised during ERCP for biliary obstruction with pancreatic or biliary infection occurring following 0.4–0.8% of endoscopic biliary procedures. These episodes must always be taken seriously because of the associated 8–20% mortality risk.[50] Biliary dilatation, the insertion of biliary stents, prolonged procedure time and hilar cholangiocarcinoma have been shown to give an increased risk of post-ERCP cholangitis.[51] The British Society of Gastroenterology and the American Society of Gastrointestinal Endoscopy have similar recommendations on the prophylactic use of antibiotics for ERCP.[52,53] Patients with ongoing cholangitis who will be needing therapeutic endoscopic intervention should always be on appropriate antimicrobial therapy upon admission to hospital. Additional pre-ERCP antimicrobial prophylaxis is not normally recommended for those who are already taking antibiotics therapeutically for cholangitis. Routine prophylaxis for ERCP is not usually necessary, unless it is not possible to adequately decompress the biliary system during the procedure, in which case a full antibiotic course is indicated until adequate drainage can be achieved. Indications for routine antibiotic prophylaxis during ERCP include specific biliary disorders, such as primary sclerosing cholangitis or hilar cholangiocarcinoma (where complete biliary drainage will be difficult or impossible to achieve during one procedure), patients with a history of liver transplantation, patients with pancreatic pseudocysts, patients with severe neutropenia and / or advanced haematological malignancy. When antibiotic prophylaxis for ERCP is given, oral ciprofloxacin or intravenous gentamicin is usually recommended.

4. Inflammatory bowel disease and sepsis

Bacteria play an important role in the pathogenesis of inflammatory bowel disease (IBD), its complications and its symptoms. In IBD, antibiotics can decrease tissue invasion and eliminate aggressive bacterial species. Antibiotics are also used in IBD to treat infective complications and for altering bacterial flora, which may result in specific anti-inflammatory effects. The antibiotics which are used most frequently in IBD are metronidazole and ciprofloxacin, which may be effective in Crohn's colitis and ileocolitis, perianal disease and pouchitis.[54]

The pathophysiology of both Crohn's disease (CD) and ulcerative colitis (UC) involves dysfunction of the intestinal barrier, which then causes leak flux diarrhoea and the facilitated uptake of noxious antigens into the systemic circulation. Barrier dysfunction in IBD involves a reduction in epithelial horizontal tight junctions (TJ) and an abnormal TJ protein expression. An increased incidence and frequency of apoptosis as well as erosions and ulcerations in the gastrointestinal mucosa can add to the leakiness of the gut. The dysfunction of the intestinal barrier occurs because of the increased expression of pro-inflammatory cytokines like Tumor Necrosis Factor alpha, Interferon gamma, Interleukin 1β, and Interleukin 13 in the chronically inflamed intestine. Chronic inflammation in IBD is believed to result from genetic polymorphisms which cause an inadequate immune response as well as changes in the intestinal microbiota. Probiotics may offer some benefit in

IBD by stabilising the barrier function through TJ protein expression and distribution.[55] In CD, an increased presence of *Campylobacter concisus* and *Escherichia coli* as well as a substantial decrease in the amount of the anti-inflammatory commensal *Faecalibacterium prausnitzii* has been reported, while it has been suggested that *Fusobacterium varium* can promote the development of UC.[56-60] Cultures of *Mycobacterium avium* subspecies paratuberculosis (MAP) in the peripheral blood of CD patients and controls have revealed that MAP is commoner in CD patients, thus suggesting that MAP may have a role in the aetiology of CD.[61] Smokers with CD have also been shown to have luminal microbiota that consist of significantly higher bacteroides (38.4%) than non-smokers (28.1%).[62] While these microbiota frequently do not cause sepsis, sepsis is significantly commoner in IBD, both in immunosuppressed patients and in patients who are newly diagnosed and not on immunosuppressive therapy.[63-64] An increased incidence of bacterial endocarditis in both UC and CD has also been reported.[65] Rifaximin appears to be a promising antibiotic in inducing remission of CD (69% in open studies and significantly better than placebo in double blind trials) and UC (76% in open studies and significantly better than placebo in controlled studies). It may also have a role in remission of UC and pouchitis.[56]

Genetic polymorphisms play a major role in the aetiology of inflammatory bowel disease (IBD). Major advances in the aetiology of CD came from the discovery of polymorphisms in the NOD2 (nucleotide-binding oligomerization domain containing 2), autophagy-related susceptibility genes ATG16L1 (Autophagy-related 16-like gene) and IRGM (Immunity-Related Guanosine Triphosphate) in patients. The identification of the presence of adherent-invasive *E. coli* (AIEC) which are able to resist killing by macrophages on the ileal mucosa was another step forward in understanding the aetiology of Crohn's disease.[66] Mutations in NOD2 gene which cause loss of function of NOD proteins are strongly associated with ileal Crohn's disease. NOD2 is one of the genes controlling microbiota in the intestine, with studies showing loss of regulation of microflora in the terminal ileum of NOD2-deficient mice. Paneth cells, which regulate ileal microbiota by the production of anti-microbial compounds, show an elevated expression of the NOD2 gene, and therefore ileal intestinal epithelial cells which lack NOD2 are unable to destroy bacteria effectively. NOD2 mutations in CD therefore appear to increase disease susceptibility by disrupting the interaction between mucosal immunity and the ileal microflora.[67] NOD2 appears to activate pro-inflammatory signalling cascades once bacterial muramyl dipeptide has been sensed by the epithelial cells. It also seems to be involved in antiviral and anti-parasitic defence programs.

On the other hand, ATG16L1 is a protein necessary for autophagosome formation once bacterial or parasitic components are introduced into cells. Gene polymorphisms resulting in dysregulated immune responses to invasive micro-organisms, including those in the NOD2 and ATG16L1 genes, facilitate microbial replication and loss of the functional integrity of the epithelial barrier with an increase in permeability. The access to sub-epithelial tissues by the invasive micro-organisms may cause local chronic inflammation and microbial dissemination which may result in systemic inflammatory responses. The associated impaired response of myeloid cells to this microbial insult also increases the risk of chronic, low grade infection and inflammation.

5. Pouchitis

Restorative proctocolectomy with ileal-pouch anal anastomosis is the operation of choice for UC patients requiring surgery. It is also used for patients with familial adenomatous polyposis (FAP). Chronic pouchitis is an important long-term complication following ileal-pouch anal anstomosis, accounting for 10% of pouch failures and occurring in 50% of patients after pouch formation for UC. It is however rarely seen in FAP, suggesting that pouchitis tends to occur because of the inflammatory process occurring in UC. Antibiotics are effective in reducing the symptoms of pouchitis, implicating bacteria in its development.[68] Studies have revealed that patients with pouchitis have different bacterial families (Peptostreptococcaceae, Clostridiaceae) from patients with normal pouches (Ruminococcaceae, Bifidobacteriaceae).[69] Bacterial species in pouchitis are important because of the benefit that some probiotics have been shown to offer to these patients, as indicated in the next section.

6. Immunosuppressants in IBD

The increased risk of sepsis and bacteraemia in IBD patients has already been established. The treatment of IBD frequently involves the use of potent immunosuppressing agents including steroids, azathioprine, 6-mercaptopurine, methotrexate and biological drugs including infliximab and adalimumab. Potential complications with the use of these agents in IBD patients include sepsis. A recent meta-analysis which reviewed early post-operative infectious complications in UC patients undergoing colectomy showed no significant difference in the rate of infectious complications between patients who were treated with infliximab and those who were not.[70] In an analysis of serious infections (defined as infections requiring hospital admission) among 489 IBD patients receiving anti-TNFα therapy across Australia and New Zealand, only 14 (2.2%) serious infections were reported. These infections included 3 cases of Varicella Zoster, 2 cases of *Pneumocystis jiroveci* pneumonia, 2 flu-like illnesses, two cases of *Staphylococcus aureus* bacteraemia and five other bacterial infections.[71] Another single-centre analysis on the safety of infliximab in CD, revealed that in 297 patients on infliximab there was a 2.7% rate of serious infection, with 0.33% resulting in fatal sepsis.[72] Case reports of sepsis in patients treated with biological therapy are also numerous.[73-77] Active sepsis is an absolute contraindication for anti-TNF therapy use, as this risks overwhelming sepsis. Reactivation or development of tuberculosis has been reported in 24/100,000 patients with rheumatoid arthritis on anti-TNF therapy, compared with 6/100,000 not receiving such treatment.[78,79]

Reports of severe sepsis in patients with IBD while taking Azathioprine have also been described.[80,81] Azathioprine and 6-mercaptopurine are used in patients with moderate to severe CD or UC. Azathioprine has a complex, heterogeneous thiopurine methyltransferase (TPMT) metabolism which may affect required dosages and may increase the risk for adverse events. Routine TPMT activity testing before starting Azathioprine may decrease the risk of early leukopenia and avoid potentially life-threatening myelotoxicity.[82] The risk of severe sepsis increases further if combination immunosuppressants (such as combinations of azathioprine and anti-TNFα agents) are used.[83] The TREAT registry showed that while unadjusted analysis indicated that Infliximab is associated with an increased risk of infection, multivariate logistic regression analysis suggested that Infliximab was not an independent predictor of serious infections and the increased risk was associated with disease severity and concomitant prednisone use.[84] The REACH study, evaluating the efficacy of Infliximab in children with moderate to severe CD refractory to immunomodulatory treatment, reported serious infections as the major adverse events with their frequency being higher with shorter treatment intervals. The combination of immunosuppressive medications appears to increase the risk of opportunistic infections.[85]

7. *Streptococcus gallolyticus* and colorectal tumours

Streptococcus gallolyticus, previously called *S.bovis* biotype I (Table 1) is a gram positive bacterium found in the colon of 10% of healthy individuals. It is an opportunistic pathogen as it can cause bacteraemia and endocarditis, especially in the presence of colorectal cancer (CRC). In the International Collaboration on Endocarditis Prospective Cohort Study, *S. gallolyticus* accounted for a very significant 12.5% of the cases of infective endocarditis in patients over 65 and 5.4% in those 18-65 years of age.[86] The association between *S.bovis* bacteraemia and colonic neoplasia was first reported in the literature in 1951 by McCoy and Mason.[87] In a recent meta-analysis [88], among the *S.bovis*-infected patients who underwent colonoscopy, 60% of patients had underlying adenomas or carcinomas. One hypothesis on the association between CRC and *S. gallolyticus* suggests that colorectal malignancy specifically allows for colonisation and translocation of the bacterium through the altered mucosa. An alternative theory proposes that the organism itself promotes carcinogenesis by interacting with the colonic mucosa. Several studies comparing faecal carriage of *S. gallolyticus* in patients with colorectal cancer or adenomatous polyps with normal controls failed to show a significant difference.[87,89,90] However, studies on patients with proven *S. gallolyticus* bacteraemia consistently showed that 25 to 80% of patients with the infection had colorectal tumours. Similarly, 18 to 62% of patients with *S. gallolyticus* endocarditis have been diagnosed with colonic neoplasia.[91]

Old nomenclature	Later nomenclature	Recent nomenclature
S. bovis biotype I	*S. gallolyticus*	*S. gallolyticus* subsp. *gallolyticus*
S. bovis biotype II/1	*S. infantarius* *S. infantarius* subsp. *coli*	*S. infantarius* subsp. *infantarius* *S. lutetiensis*
S. bovis biotype II/2	*S. pasteurianus* *S. macedonicus*	*S. gallolyticus* subsp. *pasteurianus* *S. gallolyticus* subsp. *macedonicus*

Table 1. Nomenclature of *Streptococcus gallolyticus*

7.1. Virulence factors and possible carcinogenic effect of *S. gallolyticus*

Boleij et al [92] reconstructed the route of infection in vitro on a continuous cell line of heterogenous human epithelial colorectal adenocarcinoma cells that can be synthesized into a monolayer and which simulate the intestinal epithelium. Cellular immune responses upon infection and bacterial biofilm formation were analysed. The *S. gallolyticus* strains have a relatively low adhesiveness and are unable to internalise epithelial cells. However, they are able to cross a differentiated epithelium without inducing an interleukin 8 or 1β response within the epithelium. The organism has a particular ability to form biofilms on collagen-rich surfaces (representing heart valves in vivo). The authors concluded that *S. gallolyticus* has the ability to evade the innate immune system of the intestinal epithelium and the potential to form vegetations over collagen-rich surfaces as is observed in vivo.

7.2. Association with liver disease and extracolonic malignancy

S. gallolyticus has also been associated with chronic liver disease. Tripodi et al prospectively studied 199 patients with infective endocarditis and found that 30 of these were attributable to *S. bovis* biotype I (*S. gallolyticus*).[93] 56.7% of these patients had advanced liver disease, compared with only 15.3% of patients with non-*S.bovis* endocarditis, while colonic adenomas were present in 46.7% of cirrhotics. Alazmi and his team [94] retrospectively analysed microbiology data from 46 patients (38 adult and 8 paediatric) with proven *S.gallolyticus* bacteraemia and found that 19% had end-stage liver disease while colonic neoplasia was found in 6 of 10 adult patients in whom colonoscopy was performed. 7 of the adult patients had AIDS while no significant association with gastrointestinal disease was found in the paediatric population. An association between *S. gallolyticus* and extracolonic malignancy is less well established. Gold et al [95] report a series of 45 patients with documented *S. gallolyticus* bacteraemia. Eight of these patients had malignant lesions arising within the gastrointestinal tract, and 5 patients had extraintestinal malignancies. Vergara-López et al looked at 93 patients with *S. gallolyticus* bacteraemia [96] and found that 25% of individuals had a colonic neoplasm while 14 patients (15%) were diagnosed with non-colonic neoplasms including biliary and pancreatic (6.5%) and esophagogastric (3.2%) neoplasms. In view of these observations, the authors recommend that in the absence of colonic neoplasms clinicians should do a thorough investigation of the gut with gastroscopy and appropriate imaging of the hepatobiliary system.

8. Conclusion

A considerable body of evidence links colonic neoplasms with *S.gallolyticus* bacteraemia but many unanswered questions remain about this association. Evaluation of the colon by colonoscopy is essential in all cases of *S. gallolyticus* bacteraemia. In view of the high incidence of chronic liver disease and extracolonic neoplasms in some studies, formal evaluation of the liver may be warranted with or without cross sectional imaging of the abdomen. In the future, biomarkers for this organism may allow early diagnosis of colonic neoplasia.

8.1. Selective decontamination of the digestive tract

In critical illness, sepsis plays a major role in morbidity and mortality. Bacterial translocation from the gut is believed to occur following loss of the barrier function of the intestinal mucosa. Selective decontamination of the digestive tract (SDD) involves the use of local and systemic antimicrobial agents to clear potentially pathogenic organisms from the gastrointestinal tract, especially Gram negative organisms, *Staphylococcus aureus* and yeasts, while avoiding agents that inhibit the anaerobic flora. Reduction of the Gram negative bacterial load would be followed by a decrease in sepsis and bacteraemia. However, in spite of the evidence in favour of SDD, it is still not in widespread use in intensive-care units (ICU).

SDD involves the combination of orally administered non-absorbed antibiotic and antifungal agents with an intravenous broad spectrum antibiotic. A regimen that has been used in several major studies consists of orally administered amphotericin-B, tobramycin and colistin.[97,98] Along with the topical agents, intravenous cefotaxime is also given for the first four days of ICU stay. The systemic antibiotics should cover both community-acquired organisms and hospital-acquired organisms while having minimal influence on the normal bowel flora and good penetration to bronchial secretions, making cefotaxime an ideal candidate.[99] The enteral non-absorbable antibiotics are intended to prevent secondary endogenous infections but they fail to cover resistant organisms such as MRSA. Silvestri et al [100] have added oral vancomycin to Polymyxin E, tobramycin and amphotericin B in an attempt to decrease the incidence of MRSA ventilator-associated pneumonias (VAP). This combination was effective in reducing the incidence of VAP and secondary carriage of MRSA with no reported cases of vancomycin-resistant Enterococci or vancomycin-intermediate *Staphylococcus aureus*. In most randomised controlled trials, SDD has been compared to Selective Oropharyngeal Decontamination (SOD) and standard care. SOD involves local application of non-absorbable antibiotics restricted to the oropharynx, usually applied in the form of a gel. The topical antimicrobial combination for SOD is usually similar to the combination used in SDD. Studies have shown that both SDD and SOD are useful in preventing sepsis in critically ill patients but few studies have analysed the effect of their use on the prevalence of resistant organisms within ICUs. This remains an area that needs further study and is a major issue that precludes the widespread use of SDD.[101]

8.2. The evidence on SDD

Many randomised controlled trials (RCT) have been performed over the last decade studying the benefits and risks of SDD. An important recent RCT studied the effect of SDD and SOD on 28-day mortality in ICU patients.[97] 5939 patients in 13 different ICUs in the Netherlands were enrolled to receive either standard care, SDD or SOD. SDD included the application of topical tobramycin, colistin and amphotericin B to the oropharynx and stomach along with the intravenous administration of cefotaxime for the first four days of ICU stay. 28-day mortality was marginally reduced from 27.5% in patients treated with standard care to 26.6% and 26.9% in the SDD and SOD groups respectively. Another RCT looked at the role of oropharyngeal and intestinal colonisation with gram-negative bacteria as a source of ICU-acquired bacteraemia.[102] This trial randomised a total of 6778 ICU patients to receive SDD, SOD or standard care. The outcomes measured included the incidence densities (episodes per 1000 ICU patient days) of ICU-acquired gram-negative bacteraemia and rectal colonisation with gram-negative bacteria. SOD gave a 33% reduction while SDD gave a 45% reduction in the incidence of Gram-ve bacteraemia.

In another study [103], 107 patients with more than 20% burns and/or suspected inhalation injury were randomised to receive SDD or placebo and mortality rates and incidence of pneumonias were measured. A similar antibiotic regimen to the one used in [97] was used but topical polymixin E substituted colistin. Results showed an ICU mortality of 27.8% in the placebo arm compared to 9.4% in the SDD arm. Rates of pneumonia were 30.8 and 17.0 per 1000 ventilator-days in the placebo and the SDD arms respectively. The authors also noted that MRSA infection was commoner in the SDD group amounting to 26.4% versus 20% in the placebo group. Various other trials have been summed up by three major meta-analyses (Table 2).[104-106]

Name and year of meta-analysis	Number of trials/number of patients	Clinical end points studied	Results	Conclusions
Silvestri et al 2007 [106]	51 trials 8065 patients	BSI Causative organisms Total mortality	Significantly reduced in SDD group OR 0.73 Significantly reduced G- BSI without increasing G+ BSI Reduced in SDD group	NNT to prevent 1 G- BSI is 20 NNT to prevent one death is 22
Silvestri et al 2008 [105]	54 trials 9473 patients	Carriage of G- bacteria Carriage of G+ bacteria G- RTI G- BSI	Significantly reduced Not significantly changed Significantly reduced Significantly reduced	SDD mainly targets G- bacteria and does not show a significant increase in G+ bacterial infections. SDD was better than SOD at reducing carriage of and severe infections due to G- bacteria
Liberati et al 2009 [104]	36 trials 6914 patients	Rate of RTI Mortality	Significantly reduced in both SOD and SDD groups Significantly reduced in SDD but not in SOD	SOD alone reduces RTI but not mortality while SDD reduces both

Table 2. Meta-analysis on benefits of SDD in preventing sepsis. (BSI blood stream infection, RTI respiratory tract infection, SDD selective decontamination of the digestive tract, SOD selective oropharyngeal decontamination, G+ gram positive, G- gram negative, NNT numbers needed to treat, OR odds ratio)

8.3. Prevention of Ventilator-Associated Pneumonia (VAP)

Pneumonia is a major cause of mortality in critically ill and ventilated patients. The incidence of VAP in different studies ranges between 7 and 40% while mortality ranges from 25 to 50%.[107] In an important meta-analysis carried out by Liberati et al [104], 36 RCTs studying the effects of different combinations of SDD and SOD in ICU patients on the incidence of VAP were analysed. This showed that in trials comparing combined topical and systemic antibiotics to controls, there was a significant reduction in both VAP and mortality in the treated group. In trials comparing topical antibiotics to controls, a significant reduction in VAP (but not in total mortality) was shown.[108] Methicillin-Resistant *Staphylococcus aureus* (MRSA) is a common cause of VAP. In a study by Silvestri et al [106], oropharyngeal vancomycin was applied along with standard SDD using only enteral non-absorbable antibiotics in a group of ventilated ICU patients. The rate of pneumonia due to MRSA was reduced in the vancomycin group when compared to controls who received only the topical SDD. Patients in this study were also investigated for the emergence of vancomycin-resistant Enterococci and vancomycin-intermediate *S. aureus* but these bacteria were not isolated. This suggests that the addition of topical glycopeptides to the SDD regimen may help reduce the rate of MRSA though further studies are needed before this approach can be recommended.

8.4. Evidence supporting use in surgical patients

Roos et al [109] studied the incidence of infections and anastomotic leakage 30 days following surgery in 289 patients receiving either topical SDD or placebo. Results show that 19.6% of the SDD group had infectious complications when compared to 30.8% in the placebo group. Anastomotic leakage was also reduced in the SDD group (6.3% vs 15.1%). In spite of this, there was no significant difference in mortality or hospital stay between the two groups. Melsen et al [110] compared the benefits of SOD and SDD in surgical and medical ICU patients. 2762 surgical and 3165 non surgical patients were randomised to receive SDD, SOD or standard care. Compared with standard care, mortality was comparable in SDD treated surgical and non surgical patients though the duration of ventilation, ICU and hospital stay were significantly reduced in the surgical patients. SOD failed to reduce mortality when compared to standard treatment in the surgical cohort while providing a reduced mortality by 16.6% in non-surgical patients. Patients undergoing liver transplant are very vulnerable to infection during the early post-operative period, particularly with gram-negative organisms. SDD has been studied in these patients in several RCTs [111-113] and meta-analyses [114]. The results have been conflicting and several small RCTs failed to show any benefit of SDD over standard care following liver transplant.

9. Conclusion and recommendations

The evidence so far shows a decrease in 28 day mortality and reduction in bacteraemia in high risk patients and suggests that SDD should be regularly used in ICU settings. However SDD is still not common practice in most ICUs as many intensivists still question its safety and efficacy. In a UK based survey of ICUs to document the use of SDD [106], 95% of British centres did not use SDD, mainly because of concerns regarding resistance. In addition there is a reluctance to use intravenous antibiotics in many of those who used SDD in intubated patients. Convincing the medical world of the effectiveness and safety of SDD will require more robust data about antibiotic resistance with SDD and SOD.

9.1. *Clostridium difficile* infection

Clostridium difficile is an anaerobic, spore-forming, gram-positive rod found in the intestines of 2-5% of the healthy human population [115] but responsible for 16-25% of hospital-acquired antibiotic-associated diarrhoea.[116] It has been recognised as an important cause of antibiotic-associated colitis since the introduction of clindamycin in 1977 when it was understood that the disturbance of bowel flora by antimicrobial agents allowed overgrowth and subsequent infection by *Clostridium difficile*.[117] Transmission occurs through the feco-oral route via contact with contaminated surfaces, with the hands of healthcare workers being potential routes of contamination. Vegetative bacterial cells produce spores in conditions of stress, making them resistant to commonly used techniques of surface disinfection such as alcohol handrubs, most disinfectants and antibiotics. It is however susceptible to chlorine-based antiseptics such as diluted bleach.[118] The spectrum of disease is wide and ranges from asymptomatic carriage to fulminant pseudomembraneous colitis which may be fatal.

Toxin synthesis by *C. difficile* mediates disease progression and the severity of illness. The potent exotoxins produced by *C. difficile* have been labelled A and B. They are both large monoglycosyltransferases that catalyse the glucosylation and inactivation of Rho-GTPases, the small regulatory proteins of the actin cell cytoskeleton, leading to disruption of the cell cytoskeleton and subsequent cell death. Some strains of *C.difficile* produce an unrelated binary toxin which consists of two separate components: CDTa and CDTb. CDTb mediates translocation of CDTa into cells which allows the disruption of cytoskeleton proteins through phosphorylation, ultimately causing cell death.[118] The virulence of different strains of *C. difficile* is related to the rate of toxin production. Hypervirulent strains such as the molecular type NAP1/027/BI, have been found to have more robust toxin production and show an earlier spore-formation than other strains thus causing more severe infections.[119] Excessive toxin production in this strain has been traced to a mutation in the Toxin B encoding gene sequence.[120] Another emerging strain is the PCR ribotype 078, which is associated with community-associated *C.difficile* infection and has been isolated in animal and food products.[121]

9.2. Epidemiology

The emergence of *C. difficile*-associated disease (CDAD) can be traced back to the start of the antibiotic era. Antibiotic-associated diarrhoea and colitis became well established and *C. difficile* was identified as the cause of most of these cases in 1978. The earliest cases were attributed to clindamycin but later, as the use of cephalosporins and wide spectrum peniclins increased, these antibiotics were increasingly implicated as causes of CDAD. An important outbreak in the US between 1989 and 1992 was traced to a strain of *C. difficile* with resistance to clindamycin.[122] Since 2003, an increase in the incidence of CDAD was observed, along with a decrease in their response to the standard antibiotic regimens. The hypervirulent strain NAP1/027/BI was identified as a cause of several outbreaks in North America and Europe and is believed to be related to the increase in use of fluoroquinolones, to which this strain is particularly resistant.[123,124]

9.3. Risk factors for CDAD

Antibiotic use is the strongest factor associated with CDAD. The most important mechanism involves the disruption of normal colonic commensal bacterial populations providing a niche for *C. difficile* to multiply and produce toxins. Resistance to antibiotics plays an important role in infections due to strains with increased virulence such as the NAP1/027/B1 strain.[125] Antibiotics commonly implicated include fluoroquinolones, clindamycin, broad-spectrum penicillins and cephalosporins. However, all antibiotics (including metronidazole and vancomycin) can predispose to *C.difficile* infection by disrupting the anaerobic gut flora. In fact it is hypothesised that the same antibiotics used for treating CDAD might be responsible for the recurrence of CDAD after treatment.[126] It has been shown that both the use of broad-spectrum antibiotics and prolonged courses of antimicrobials increase the risk of CDAD.[127,128] Advanced age is also an important risk factor associated with CDAD prevalence and severity. The increased frequency of comorbidities places elderly patients at higher risk of mortality and serious infections though compromised immune function also plays an important role.[126] The role of gastric acid suppression with proton pump inhibitors has also been implicated in the pathogenesis of CDAD though the evidence is equivocal.

9.4. Diagnosis and investigations

In most cases of suspected CDAD, the clinical presentation and microbiological evidence of toxin-producing *C. difficile* in stools is sufficient for diagnosis. The clinical picture may include bloody diarrhoea with abdominal pain and tenderness and ileus with abdominal pain, vomiting and reduced bowel motility. Pseudomembraneous colitis can be diagnosed by the visualisation of pseudomembranes at endoscopy while toxic megacolon presents with characteristic radiologic findings.[129] The markers of disease severity are outlined in Table 3. Microbiological evidence of infection is obtained from stool culture or assay for stool *C. difficile* toxin (CDT). Different tests can be used to detect the toxins. The most widely used test is the enzyme immunoassay (EIA) for toxin A, toxin B or both. The EIA CDT assay has sensitivities and specificities of 50-90% and 70-95%, respectively. Diagnostically, *C.difficile* cell culture cytotoxin assay remains the gold standard with sensitivity and specificity of 93% and 89%.[130]

Physical findings	Blood investigations	Imaging studies
Fever, rigors, haemodynamic instability (including vasodilatory or septic shock), signs of peritonitis, (including decreased bowel sounds, abdominal tenderness, rebound tenderness and guarding), signs of ileus (including vomiting and absent passage of stool). Admixture of blood with stools is rare in CDI and the correlation with severity of disease is uncertain	marked leukocytosis (leukocyte count > 15 X 10^9/L) marked left shift (band neutrophils >20% of leukocytes) rise in serum creatinine (>50% above the baseline) elevated serum lactate distension of large intestine	colonic wall thickening including low-attenuation mural thickening pericolonic fat stranding ascites not explained by other causes The correlation of haustral or mucosal thickening, including thumbprinting, pseudopolyps and plaques with severity of disease is unclear.

Table 3. Markers of severe disease [127]

9.5. Treatment

The management of CDAD is tailored to the severity of the condition. The treatment recommended by the ESCMID guidelines (2009) [129] is summarised in Table 4.

Degree of severity	Mild (stool frequency <4 times daily, no signs of colitis)	Moderate (no markers of severe disease)	Severe (any marker of severe disease)
Oral treatment possible	Stop antibiotics and observe closely	Metronidazole 500 mg tds orally for 10 days	Vancomycin 125 mg qds orally for 10 days (A-I)
Oral treatment not possible		Metronidazole 500 mg tds intravenously for 10 days (A-III)	Metronidazole 500 mg tds intravenously for 10 days (A-III) + intracolonic vancomycin 500 mg in 100 mL of normal saline every 4–12 h (C-III) and/or vancomycin 500 mg qds by nasogastric tube (C-III)

Table 4. Treatment of C.difficile infection [129]

Oral vancomycin may be replaced by teicoplanin 100mg twice daily. Other antibiotics have been shown to be effective in CDAD but are not as yet recommended for routine use. In a phase 3 clinical trial [131], fidaxomycin had a better response rate and a lower recurrence rate than standard dose vancomycin. Oral rifaximin was studied on comparatively smaller numbers. Neff et al [132] report three liver transplant patients with moderately severe CDAD who had relapsed after treatment with metronidazole and did not tolerate vancomycin. All three showed a good response after 28 days of rifaximin 400mg three times daily. In another small study [133], there was only one recurrence after treatment of 8 patients with rifaximin for ten days. If severe disease does not respond to medical therapy, surgical intervention may be necessary. Indications for colectomy include perforation of the colon and systemic inflammation with deteriorating clinical condition not responding to antibiotic therapy. This includes the clinical diagnoses of toxic megacolon and severe ileus. Colectomy should preferably be performed before colitis is very severe. Serum lactate may serve as a marker of severity with surgery ideally performed before lactate exceeds 5.0mmol/L.[127]

9.6. Recurrence and the role of fecal transplant

Recurrence of infection is defined as the recurrence of symptoms due to incomplete clearance of the initial infection. 15-30% of patients with CDAD experience recurrent infections in spite of seemingly adequate treatment.[134] Various combinations of antibiotics (Table 5) have been suggested for the management of recurrent infections as well as measures to normalise the intestinal flora using probiotics or fecal transplantation. Healthy donor fecal installation has been proposed as a way to restore normal bowel flora in patients with CDAD recurrence not responding to antibiotics. Several studies have been performed to date with most showing favourable results [135] but the lack of well designed RCTs makes the evidence weak and more studies are needed before it can be formally recommended in the guidelines.

First recurrence	Second recurrence	Third recurrence
Mild to moderate infection - Metronidazole at a dose of 500 mg orally three times daily for 10 to 14 days *Severe infection or unresponsive to or intolerant of metronidazole* - Vancomycin at a dose of 125 mg orally four times daily for 10 to 14 days	Prolonged vancomycin orally in tapered and pulsed doses, for example: 125 mg four times daily for 14 days 125 mg twice daily for seven days 125 mg once daily for seven days 125 mg once every two days for eight days (four doses) 125 mg once every three days for 15 days (five doses)	Vancomycin at a dose of 125 mg orally four times daily for 14 days, combined with any of the other options for recurrent infection (not evidence based): Intravenous immunoglobulin at a dose of 400 mg per kg body weight once every three weeks, for a total of two or three doses depending on effect. Vancomycin, followed by rifampicin at a dose of 400 mg twice daily for 14 days Healthy donor fecal implantation

Table 5. Management of CDAD recurrence [134]

10. Conclusion

International guidelines [136] have issued a list of evidence-based infection control measures intended to contain outbreaks of CDI within hospitals. Measures include the strict use of hand hygiene using soap and water, the use of gloves and gowns when approaching an infected patient, isolation of infected patients in single rooms and maintaining contact precautions for the duration of diarrhoea. Routine identification and treatment of carriers is not recommended. Identification of potential sources of infection, such as rectal thermometers, can help reduce the incidence of CDAD. Frequent use of chlorine-containing cleaning agents to disinfect the clinical area along with routine environmental screening for *C.difficile* are also recommended. Restricting the use of cephalosporins and clindamycin may also be useful. The frequency, duration of antibiotic courses and number of agents used should be as recommended by international guidelines. Implementing these recommendations was shown to be of benefit by the Centre for Disease Control and Prevention [137] in several hospitals in the USA with a decline in *C. difficile* infection (CDI) rate of 20% among 71 hospitals participating in the CDI prevention program, thus confirming that with *C. difficile* infections, prevention is better than cure.

10.1. Probiotics

The term *probiotic,* first introduced in 1965 by Lilly and Stillwell, describes bacterially-derived factors that stimulate the growth of other organisms. This definition was updated by Fuller in 1989 who defined probiotics as viable organisms with a beneficial effect on the host. Fermented ingredients containing no viable organisms but that still cause beneficial changes in the intestinal flora are termed *prebiotics,* while *symbiotics* are mixtures of pre- and probiotics. *Lactobacillus, Bifidobacterium, Eschericia coli, Saccharomyces cerevisae* and *Bacillus* species are the microflora most commonly used in probiotics.[138] The healthy human gut hosts a large community of microorganisms that interact with the host in a positive manner. Disruption of the normal gut flora by antibiotics or infections causes a change in bowel function, most frequently resulting in diarrhoea. It has been proposed that the normal commensal flora occupies most binding sites on the intestinal mucosa and out-competes potentially pathogenic organisms, thus providing a protective effect on the host. Probiotics are believed to function in a similar way to the normal commensal flora by colonising the intestinal contents so as to prevent the proliferation of potentially pathogenic organisms by competing for resources and intestinal binding sites. Probiotics may also lead to an improvement in intestinal barrier function, modulation of the immune system by induction of protective cytokines and modulation of pain perception.

Probiotics have been around for decades and are available in different formulations including capsules, powders and fermented milk products. However, evidence of their benefit has been relatively scarce until recently as most studies were hampered by poor standardisation in view of the different species and strains used. Species used vary widely as do the number of viable organisms and their resistance to gastric acid. Some examples of commercially available probiotics are: Erceflora (*Bacillus clausii*), Align® (*B. infantis*),

Bioflor® (*Saccharomyces boulardii*), Culturelle® (*L. rhamnosus* GG), DanActive® (*L. casei*), Mutaflor® (*E. coli* Nissle 1917), Florastor® (*Saccharomyces boulardii*), and VSL#3® (*Bifidobacterium breve, B. longum, B. infantis, Lactobacillus acidophilus, L. plantarum, L. paracasei, L. bulgaricus, Streptococcus thermophilus*). The evidence on the use of probiotics in inflammatory bowel disease and pouchitis has been described earlier.

10.2. Infectious diarrhoea

Infectious diarrhoea is a major cause of morbidity and mortality especially in third world countries. Most studies with probiotics analysing the effect on diarrhoea duration have been in paediatric patients and they show a significant benefit. In a meta-analysis [139] of 63 studies of which 56 involved infants and young children, there was a significant decrease in the mean duration of diarrhoea (mean difference 24.76 hours; n=4555, trials=35), diarrhoea lasting ≥4 days (risk ratio 0.41; n=2853, trials=29) and stool frequency on day 2 (mean difference 0.80; n=2751, trials=20). However, there was a wide variation in the probiotics used, patient characteristics and clinical settings. When probiotics are used in conjunction with rehydration therapy they appear to be safe and have clear benefits in shortening the duration of diarrhoea and reducing stool frequency in acute infectious diarrhoea.

4 randomised controlled trials (n=464) comparing specified probiotic agents with placebo or no treatment in children with persistent diarrhoea (diarrhoea lasting more than 14 days) [140] showed that probiotics reduced the duration of persistent diarrhoea by a mean of 4.2 days and significantly reduced stool frequency at day 5. In a randomised controlled trial that randomised 88 children younger than two years old with acute diarrhoea to receive *S.boulardii* or placebo there was an average reduction in the duration of diarrhoea of 1.44 days in the treatment arm along with a significant reduction in stool frequency at day 4.[141] The dose-dependent effect of administering *L. rhamnosus* on fecal shedding of rotavirus was analysed in another study. 23 children with acute rotavirus infection were randomised to placebo, low-dose or high-dose *L rhamnosus*.[142] This trial showed no significant reduction in viral shedding in the low dose group but a significant reduction in the high dose group suggesting that a minimum of 6×10^8 CFU (colony forming units) for 3 days has to be given to paediatric patients to achieve a good effect. Other studies [143] also suggest a definite but modest benefit in probiotic use in acute infectious diarrhoea, especially in rotavirus-induced diarrhoea.

10.3. Antibiotic-associated diarrhoea and *Clostridium difficile*-associated disease

Antibiotic-associated diarrhoea (AAD) occurs in about 25% of patients receiving antibiotics, with rates varying between different populations and according to the type of antibiotic used.[144] *Clostridium difficile* accounts for only 10-20% of cases and a causative agent is frequently not found. Diarrhoea may begin following a single dose of antibiotic or up to 6 weeks after treatment [145] and can range in severity from mild symptoms to the life-threatening colitis usually associated with *C. difficile*. Risk factors for AAD include oral broad-spectrum antibiotics, advanced age and prolonged hospital stay. Probiotics have been advocated to reduce the incidence of AAD since they help re-establish beneficial intestinal flora after disturbance by antibiotics. Probiotic organisms that have been studied for preventing AAD include *Lactobacillus acidophilus, Lactobacillus casei, Lactobacillus rhamnosus* GG and *Saccharomyces boulardii.*

Several meta-analysis have highlighted the positive effects of probiotics on AAD. In [146], 8 RCTs (n=1220) evaluating the effectiveness of probiotics in preventing AAD and CDAD were analysed. Probiotics used included *S. boulardii* in 3 studies and various strains of *Lactobacillus, Bifidobacterium bifidum* and *Streptococcus thermophilus* in different combinations in the other 5 studies. Results were found to be protective for AAD (Risk Ratio [RR]: 0.56; 95% CI, 0.44–0.71) as well as for CDAD (RR: 0.29; 95% CI 0.18–0.46). In [147], different strains of *Lactobacillus* as single agents in the prevention of AAD were analysed in 10 RCTs (n=1862). The total daily dose of *Lactobacillus* ranged from 2 x 10^9 to 4 x 10^{10} CFUs and was administered throughout the entire antibiotic treatment (5-14 days) for all patients. The combined RR of developing AAD was significantly lower with *Lactobacillus* when compared with placebo (RR 0.35, 95% CI 0.19-0.67). In a subgroup analysis, this benefit was seen among adult but not among pediatric patients (RR 0.24, 95% CI 0.08-0.75 and RR 0.44, 95% CI 0.18-1.08, respectively). Considerable evidence backs the use of probiotic agents (especially *Lactobacillus* species and *S. boulardii*) as an extra measure to prevent AAD and CDAD.

10.4. Probiotics in IBD

Probiotics alter the microbial concentrations of the intestines and may also be used to deliver microbial metabolic products which affect intestinal mucosal inflammation in IBD. There is little evidence of benefit with currently available probiotics in CD though newer probiotics composed of other micro-organisms may prove beneficial in the future. On the other hand, studies have shown a benefit of probiotics in recurrent and relapsing antibiotic sensitive pouchitis and in mild UC. In fact, recent practice guidelines [148] on the management of pouchitis suggest that in patients with prompt recurrence of pouchitis following antibiotic cessation, and in those with multiple recurrences of pouchitis despite antibiotics, either VSL#3™ or chronic use of antibiotics may be helpful. These guidelines however do not recommend probiotics in the acute treatment of pouchitis.[148]

Probiotics may prevent relapse in chronic pouchitis and ulcerative colitis, and may also prevent the development of pouchitis postoperatively. However, further studies are needed to identify optimal dosing, duration of therapy, delivery methods and whether blends of different strains of probiotics are superior to single strains.[149] Following a systematic review of studies using VSL#3™, *E.coli* Nissle 1917 and Yakult™, Mallon et al concluded that the addition of probiotics to conventional medical therapy had no effect in overall remission rate in mild to moderate UC.[150-152] Other randomized controlled trials have also shown conflicting results with some showing a higher rate of remission (with VSL#3 or a combination of a prebiotic and *B.longum*) [153-155] and others showing little or no benefit (with *E.coli* Nissle 1917).[156] There are no recommendations regarding the use of probiotics as maintenance therapy in UC. Few studies have been carried out using single or combined strain probiotics as maintenance therapy in UC with 3 of 4 single probiotic trials using *E.coli* strain Nissle 1917. The results from these reports showed that probiotics had similar efficacy to 5-aminosalicylates.[153,157-159] In children with active distal ulcerative colitis, decreased mucosal inflammation was noticed following rectal infusion of *Lactobacillus reuteri*.[160] Even non-living probiotic bacteria may prevent the onset of severe intestinal inflammation by strengthening the integrity of the intestinal barrier and stabilising the environment for gut microbiota.[161,162]

The risks of probiotic use are generally low, but cases of fungaemia in ICU patients on *S. boulardii* and a case of sepsis from a *Lactobacillus* strain in a UC patient have been reported.[163,164] An important consideration before starting probiotics is whether the patient is on immunosuppressing agents. There is no evidence for the use of probiotics in severe IBD and little clinical evidence on the safety of probiotics in severely immunocompromised IBD patients.

10.5. Mortality of preterm infants with necrotising enterocolitis

Necrotising Enterocolitis (NEC) is an important cause of morbidity and mortality in preterm and very low birth weight (<1500g) infants. There is strong evidence [165-167] that the administration of enteral probiotics plays an important role in establishing benign commensal flora and preventing NEC and its complications. In these studies, the most commonly used species were *Bifidobacterium* and *Lactobacillus* species.[168] Very few adverse events from probiotics have been reported and they are thus being recommended as evidence-based treatment.[169]

10.6. Irritable Bowel Syndrome

Irritable Bowel Syndrome (IBS) is a heterogeneous group of disorders characterised by functional bowel symptoms such as abdominal pain, bloating and changes in bowel habit in the absence of other pathologies which might explain these symptoms. IBS is typically difficult to treat as its aetiology is still poorly understood. Targeting the intestinal flora with probiotics has been an attractive potential treatment and has shown some promise in several meta-analyses.[170-174] These studies showed a modest improvement in the patients' symptoms when using strains like *S. boulardii* and *Lactobacillus rhamnosus* GG. Longer term studies with specific strains are warranted to clarify the most appropriate species and long-term effects with probiotics.

11. Conclusion

The emergence of probiotics as a popular type of alternative medicine has preceded by several decades their promotion as an evidence-based treatment. Their role in treatment or prevention for several important conditions namely NEC, UC, pouchitis and AAD is expected to fuel further research as many unanswered questions still remain. In spite of many large trials the data is still relatively weak to allow specific recommendations on which probiotics to prescribe in specific conditions. Optimum dose recommendations also remain to be clarified.

Author details

Neville Azzopardi*
Gastroenterology Department, Mater Dei Hospital, Malta

Manuel Fenech and Tonio Piscopo
Infectious Disease Department, Mater Dei Hospital, Malta

12. References

[1] Gorbach SL. Microbiology of the Gastrointestinal Tract. Medical Microbiology 1996. PMID: 21413258

[2] Puleo F, Arvanitakis M, Van Gossum A, Preiser JC. Gut failure in the ICU. Semin Respir Crit Care Med. 2011 Oct;32(5):626-38.

[3] Schuppan D, Afdhal NH. Liver Cirrhosis. Lancet 2008 march 8; 371(9615):838-851.

[4] Digestive diseases in the United States: Epidemiology and Impact. NIDDK; Bethesda, MD: 1994. NIH Publication No. 94-1447.

[5] Munita S, Araos B, Perez G, Alvarez V, Canals C, Conteras B, et al. Bacteraemia in patients with liver cirrhosis. Rev Chilena Infectol. 2011 Feb; 28(1):35-9.

[6] Mathurin S, Chapelet A, Spanevello V, Sayago G, Balparda C, Virga E, et al. Infections in hospitalized patients with cirrhosis. Medicina (B aires). 2009;69(2):229-38.

[7] Cazzaniga M, Dionigi E, Gobbo G, Fioretti A, Monti V, Salerno F. The systemic inflammatory response syndrome in cirrhotic patients: relationship with their in-hospital outcome. J Hepatol. 2009 Sep;51(3):475-82.

[8] Steed H, Macfarlane G, Blackett K, Macfarlene S, Miller M, Bahrami B, et al. Bacterial translocation in cirrhosis is not caused by an abnormal small bowel gut microbiota. FEMS Immunol Med Microbiol. 2011 Dec; 63(3):346-54.

[9] Montes-de-Oca M, Blanco MJ, Marquez M, Soto MJ, Fernandez-Gutierrez C, Rodriguez-Ramos C, et al. Haemodynamic derangement in human immunodeficiency virus-infected patients with hepatitis C virus-related cirrhosis: the role of bacterial translocation. Liver Int. 2011 Jul;31(6):850-8.

[10] Farhadi A, Gundlapalli S, Shaikh M, Frantzides C, Harrell L, Kwasny M, et al. Susceptibility to gut leakiness: a possible mechanism for endotoxaemia in non-alcoholic steatohepatitis. Liver Int. 2008 Aug;28(7):1026-33.

[11] Bruns T, Peter J, Reuken P, Grabe D, Schuldes S, Brenmoehl J, et al. NOD2 gene variants are a risk factor for culture-positive spontaneous bacterial peritonitis and monomicrobial bacterascites in cirrhosis. Liver Int. 2011 Jun 13.

* Corresponding Author

[12] Ashare A, Stanford C, Hancock P, Stark D, Lilli K, Birrer E, et al. Chronic liver disease impairs bacterial clearance in a human model of induced bacteraemia. Clin Transl Sci. 2009 Jun;2(3):199-205.
[13] Lim L, Tan X, Woo S, Dan Y, Lee Y, Lai V, et al. Risk factors for mortality in cirrhotic patients with sepsis. Hepatol Int. 2011 Sep;5(3):800-7.
[14] Ha Y, Kang C, Joo E, Joung M, Chung D, Peck K, et al. Usefulness of C-Reactive Protein for Evaluating Clinical outcomes in Cirrhotic Patients with Bacteraemia. Korean J Intern Med. 2011 June;26(2):195-200.
[15] Kang C, Song J, Chung D, Peck K, Yeom J, Ki H, et al. Liver cirrhosis as a risk factor for mortality in a national cohort of patients with bacteraemia.J Infect.2011 Nov; 63(5):336-43.
[16] Arvaniti V, D'Amico G, Fede G, Manousou P, Tsochatzis E, PleguezueloM, et al. Infections in patients with cirrhosis increase mortality four-fold and should be used in determining prognosis. Gastroenterology. 2010 Oct;139(4):1246-56.
[17] Wong F, Bernardi M, Balk R, Christman B, Moreau R, Garcia-Tsao G, et al; International Ascites Club. Sepsis in cirrhosis: report on the 7th meeting of the International Ascites Club. Gut 2005;54:718–725.
[18] Koulaouzidis A, Bhat S, Saeed A. Spontaneous bacterial peritonitis. World J Gastroenterol. 2009 Mar 7;15(9):1042-1049.
[19] Rimola A, Gracia-Tsao G, Navasa M, Piddock L, Planas R, Bernard B, et al. Diagnosis, treatment and prophylaxis of spontaneous bacterial peritonitis: a consensus document. International Ascites Club. J Hepatol 2000;32:142–153
[20] Xu H, Wang J, Tsai M, Wu K, Chiou S, Changchien C, et al. The effects of cefazolin on cirrhotic patients with acute variceal haemorrhage after endoscopic interventions. Surg Endosc. 2011 Sep;25(9):2911-8.
[21] EASL clinical practice guidelines on the management of ascites, spontaneous bacterial peritonitis, and hepatorenal syndrome in cirrhosis. Journal of Hepatology 2010;53:397–417
[22] Fasolato S, Angeli P, Dallagnese L, Maresio G, Zola E, Mazza E, et al. Renal failure and bacterial infections in patients with cirrhosis: epidemiology and clinical features. Hepatology 2007;45:223–229.
[23] Hou M, Lin H, Liu T, Kuo B, Lee F, Chang F, Lee S. Antibiotic prophylaxis after endoscopic therapy prevents rebleeding in acute variceal hemorrhage: a randomized trial. Hepatology 2004;39:746–753.
[24] Vivas S, Rodríguez M, Palacio M, Linares A, Alonso J, Rodrigo L. Presence of bacterial infection in bleeding cirrhotic patients is independently associated with early mortality and failure to control bleeding. Dig Dis Sci 2001;46:2752–2757
[25] Carbonell N, Pauwels A, Serfaty L, Fourdan O, Lévy V, Poupon R. Improved survival after variceal bleeding in patients with cirrhosis over the past two decades. Hepatology 2004;40:652–659.
[26] Rimola A, Bory F, Teres J, Pérez-Ayuso R, Arroyo V, Rodés J. Oral, nonabsorbable antibiotics prevent infection in cirrhotics with gastrointestinal hemorrhage. Hepatology 1985;5:463–467.

[27] Soriano G, Guarner C, Tomas A, Villanueva C, Torras X, González D, et al. Norfloxacin prevents bacterial infection in cirrhotics with gastrointestinal hemorrhage. Gastroenterology 1992;103:1267–1272.

[28] Blaise M, Pateron D, Trinchet J, Levacher S, Beaugrand M, Porriat J. Systemic antibiotic therapy prevents bacterial infection in cirrhotic patients with gastrointestinal hemorrhage. Hepatology 1994;20:34–38.

[29] Pauwels A, Mostefa-Kara N, Debenes B, Degoutte E, Levy V. Systemic antibiotic prophylaxis after gastrointestinal hemorrhage in cirrhotic patients with a high risk of infection. Hepatology 1996;24:802–806.

[30] Hsieh W, Lin H, Hwang S, Hou M, Lee F, Chang F, Lee S. The effect of ciprofloxacin in the prevention of bacterial infection in patients with cirrhosis after upper gastrointestinal bleeding. Am J Gastroenterol 1998;93:962–966.

[31] Dupeyron C, Mangeney N, Sedrati L, Campillo B, Fouet P, Leluan G. Rapid emergence of quinolone resistance in cirrhotic patients treated with norfloxacin to prevent spontaneous bacterial peritonitis. Antimicrob Agents Chemother 1994;38:340–344.

[32] Aparicio J, Such J, Pascual S, Arroyo A, Plazas J, Girona E, et al. Development of quinolone-resistant strains of Escherichia coli in stools of patients with cirrhosis undergoing norfloxacin prophylaxis: clinical consequences. J Hepatol 1999;31:277–283.

[33] Fernández J, Ruiz del Arbol L, Gómez C, Durandez R, Serradilla R, Guarner C, et al. Norfloxacin vs ceftriaxone in the prophylaxis of infections in patients with advanced cirrhosis and hemorrhage. Gastroenterology 2006;131:1049–1056.

[34] Llach J, Ginès P, Arroyo V, Rimola A, Titó L, Badalamenti S, et al. Prognostic value of arterial pressure, endogenous vasoactive systems and renal function in cirrhotic patients admitted to the hospital for the treatment of ascites. Gastroenterology 1988;94:482–487.

[35] Guarner C, Solà R, Soriano G, Andreu M, Novella M, Vila C et al. Risk of a first community-acquired spontaneous bacterial peritonitis in cirrhotics with low ascitic fluid protein levels. Gastroenterology 1999;117:414–419.

[36] Fernández J, Navasa M, Planas R, Montoliu S, Monfort D, Soriano G, et al. Primary prophylaxis of spontaneous bacterial peritonitis delays hepatorenal syndrome and improves survival in cirrhosis. Gastroenterology 2007;133:818–824.

[37] Terg R, Fassio E, Guevara M, Cartier M, Longo C, Lucero R, et al. Ciprofloxacin in primary prophylaxis of spontaneous bacterial peritonitis: a randomized, placebo-controlled study. J Hepatol 2008;48:774–779.

[38] Ginès P, Rimola A, Planas R, Vargas V, Marco F, Almela M, et al. Norfloxacin prevents spontaneous bacterial peritonitis recurrence in cirrhosis: results of a double-blind, placebo-controlled trial. Hepatology 1990;12:716–724.

[39] Runyon B. AASLD Practice Guidelines: Management of Adult Patients with Ascites Due to Cirrhosis: An Update. Hepatology. Jun 2009; 49(6): 2098-2103.

[40] Moore K, Aithal G. BSG Guidelines: Guidelines on the management of ascites in cirrhosis. Gut 2006;55;1-12.

[41] Morelli A, Ertmer C, Pietropaoli P, Westphal M. Terlipressin: a promising vasoactive agent in haemodynamic support of septic shock. Expert Opin Pharmacother. 2009 Oct;10(15):2569-75.
[42] Saner F, Canbay A, Gerken G, Broelsch C. Pharmacology, clinical efficacy and safety of terlipressin in esophageal varices bleeding, septic shock and hepatorenal syndrome. Expert Rev Gastroenterol Hepatol. 2007 Dec;1(2):207-17.
[43] Navaneethan U, Jayanthi V, Mohan P. Pathogenesis of cholangitis in obstructive jaundice-revisited. Minerva Gastroenterol Dietol. 2011 Mar;57(1):97-104.
[44] Liao R, Liu Z, Wei S, Xu F, Chen Z, Gong J. Triggering receptor in myeloid cells (TREM-1) specific expression in peripheral blood mononuclear cells of sepsis patients with acute cholangitis. Inflammation. 2009 Jun;32(3):182-90.
[45] Miao Y, Liu Z, Gong J, Wei S, Xu F, Chen Z. Expression of human triggering receptor expressed on myeloid cells 1 in peripheral blood mononuclear cells of patients with acute obstructive suppurative cholangitis. Nan Fang Yi Ked a Xue Xue Bao. 2009 Nov;29(11):2179-81
[46] Karpel E, Madej A, Buldak L, Dulawa-Buldak A, Nowakowska-Dulawa E, Labuzek K, et al. Bile bacterial flora and its in vitro resistance pattern in patients with acute cholangitis resulting from choledocholithiasis. Scand J Gastroenterol. 2011 Jul;46(7-8):925-30.
[47] Melzer M, Toner R, Lacey S, Bettany E, Rait G. Biliary tract infection and bacteraemia: presentation, structural abnormalities, causative organisms and clinical outcomes. Postgrad Med J. 2007 Dec; 83(986):773-776.
[48] Brand M, Bizos D, O'Farrell P. Antibiotic prophylaxis for patients undergoing elective endoscopic retrograde cholangiopancreatography. Cochrane Database Syst Rev. 2010 Oct 6;(10):CD007345.
[49] Nelson DB. Infectious disease complications of GI endoscopy: Part 1: endogenous infections. Gastrointest Endosc 2003;57:546–56.
[50] Alveyn CG. Antimicrobial prophylaxis during biliary endoscopic procedures. J Antimicrob Chemother 1993;31(Suppl B):101–5.
[51] Ertugrul I, Yuksel I, Parlak E, Cicek E, Ataseven H, Basar O, et al. Risk factors for endoscopic retrograde cholangiopancreatography-related cholangitis: A prospective study. Turk J Gastroenterol 2009 Jun; 20(2):116-121.
[52] Allison M, Sandoe J, Tighe R, Simpson I, Hall R, Elliott T. BSG Guidelines: Antibiotic prophylaxis in gastrointestinal endoscopy. Gut 2009;58:869–880.
[53] ASGE Guidelines: Antibiotic prophylaxis for GI endoscopy. Gastrointest Endosc 2008;67(6):791-8.
[54] Hammer H. Gut microbiota and inflammatory bowel disease. Dig Dis 2011;29(6):550-3.
[55] Hering N, Fromm M, Schulzke J. Determinants of colonic barrier function in inflammatory bowel disease and potential therapeutics. J Physiol. 2012 Mar 1;590(Pt 5):1035-44
[56] Guslandi M. Rifaximin in the treatment of inflammatory bowel disease. World J Gastroenterol. 200 Nov;17(42):4644-46.

[57] Man S, Zhang L, Day A, Leach S, Lemberg D, Mitchell H. Campylobacter concisus and other Campylobacter species in children with newly diagnosed Crohn's disease. Inflamm Bowel Dis. 2010;16:1008–1016.
[58] Schwiertz A, Jacobi M, Frick J, Richter M, Rusch K, Köhler H. Microbiota in pediatric inflammatory bowel disease. J Pediatr. 2010;157:240–244.e1.
[59] Sokol H, Pigneur B, Watterlot L, Lakhdari O, Bermúdez-Humarán L, Gratadoux J, et al. Faecalibacterium prausnitzii is an anti-inflammatory commensal bacterium identified by gut microbiota analysis of Crohn disease patients. Proc Natl Acad Sci USA.2008;105:16731–16736.
[60] Ohkusa T, Okayasu I, Ogihara T, Morita K, Ogawa M, Sato N. Induction of experimental ulcerative colitis by Fusobacterium varium isolated from colonic mucosa of patients with ulcerative colitis. Gut. 2003;52:79–83.
[61] Naser S, Ghobrial G, Romero C, Valentine J. Culture of Mycobacterium avium subspecies paratuberculosis from the blood of patients with Crohn's disease. Lancet. 2004 Sep 18-24;364(9439):1039-44.
[62] Benjamin J, Hedin C, Koutsoumpas A, Ng S, McCarthy N, Presctt N, et al. Smokers with active Crohn's disease have a clinically relevant dysbiosis of the gastrointestinal microbiota. Inflamm Bowel Dis 2011 Aug 29. [Epub ahead of print]
[63] Fata F, Myers P, Addeo J, Grinberg M, Nawabi I, Cappell M. Cyclic neutropoenia in Crohn's ileocolitis: efficacy of granulocyte colony-stimulating factor. J Clin Gastroenterol. 1997 Jun;24(4):253-6.
[64] Aguas M, Bastida G, Nos P, Beltran B, Grueso J, Grueso J. Septic thrombophlebitis of the superior mesenteric vein and multiple liver abscesses in a patient with Crohn's disease at onset. BMC Gastroenterol. 2007;7:22
[65] Kreuzpaintner G, Horstkotte D, Losse B, Strhmeyer G. An increased incidence of bacterial endocarditis in inflammatory bowel disease. Z Gastroenterol.1992 Jun;30(6):397-402.
[66] Caprilli R, Lapaquette P, Darfeuille-Michaud A. Eating the enemy in Crohn's disease: An old theory revisited. JCC Oct 2010: 4(4); 377-383.
[67] Biswas A, Petnicki-Ocwieja T, Kobayashi K. Nod2: a key regulator linking microbiota to intestinal mucosal immunity. J Mol Med (Berl). 2012 Jan;90(1):15-24.
[68] Landy J, Al-Hassi H, McLaughlin S, Knight S, Ciclitra P, Nicholls R, et al. Etiology of pouchitis. Inflamm Bowel Dis. 2011 Oct 21.
[69] Tannock G, Lawley B, Munro K, Lay C, Taylor C, Daynes C, et al. Comprehensive analysis of the bacterial contents of stool from patients with chronic pouchitis, normal pouches, or familial adenomatous polyposis pouches. Inflamm Bowel Dis. 2011 Nov.[Epub ahead of print]
[70] Ehteshami-Afshar S, Nikfar S, Rezaie A, Abdollahi M. A systematic review and meta-analysis of the effects of infliximab on the rate of colectomy and post-operative complications in patients with inflammatory bowel disease. Arch Med Sci. 2011 Dec;7(6):1000-1012.
[71] Lawrence I, Radford-Smith G, Bampton P, Andrews J, Tan P, Croft A, et al. Serious infections in patients with inflammatory bowel disease receiving anti-tumor-necrosis-

factor-alpha therapy: an Australian and New Zealand experience. J Gastroenterol Hepatol. 2010 Nov;25(11):1732-8.
[72] Hamzaoglu H, Cooper J, Alsahli M, Falchuk K, Peppercorn M, Farrell R. Safety of infliximab in Crohn's disease: A large single-center experience. Inflamm Bowel Dis. 16:2109-2116.
[73] Williams G, Khan A, Schweiger F. Listeria meningitis complicating infliximab treatment for Crohn's disease. Can J Infect Dis Med Microbiol. 2005 Sep;16(5):289-92.
[74] Bassetti M, Nicco E, Delfino E, Viscoli C. Disseminated Salmonella paratyphi infection in a rheumatoid arthritis patient treated with infliximab. Clin Microbiol Infect. 2010 Jan;16(1):84-5.
[75] Krishnamurthy R, Dincer H, Whittemore D. Strongyloides stercoralis hyperinfection in a patient with rheumatoid arthritis after anti-TNF-alpha therapy. J Clin Rheumatol. 2007 Jun;13(3):150-2.
[76] Goode S, Tierney G, Deighton C. Life threatening intra-abdominal sepsis in patients on anti-TNF-α therapy. Gut. 2006 Apr;55(4):590-591.
[77] Zimmer C, Beiderlinden M, Peters J. Lethal acute respiratory distress syndrome during anti-TNF-alpha therapy for rheumatoid arthritis. Clin Rheumatol. 2006 May;25(3):430-2
[78] Ljung T, Karlen P, Schmidt D, Hellström P, Lapidus A, Janczewska I et al. Infliximab in inflammatory bowel disease: clinical outcome in a population based cohort from Stockholm County. Gut 2004;53:849–53.
[79] Colombel J, Loftus E, Tremaine W, Egan L, Harmsen W, Schleck C et al. The safety profile of infliximab in patients with Crohn's disease: the Mayo clinic experience in 500 patients. Gastroenterology 2004;126:19–31
[80] Hizawa K, Nagata Y, Taniguchi M, Nakamori M, Matsumoto T, Iida M. Bacillus cereus bacteraemia in Crohn's disease with multiple ileal stricture on maintenance azathioprine therapy. Nihom Shokakibyo Gakkai Zasshi. 2009 Jan;106(1):56-60.
[81] Silva R, Jara J, Soto T, Sepulveda P. Severe disseminated tuberculosis in a patient on immunosuppressive treatment. Report of one case. Rev Med Chil. 2011 Jun;139(6):774-8.
[82] Levesque B, Loftus E. Initiating Azathioprine for Crohn's Disease. Clin Gastroenterol Hepatol. 2012 Feb 10. [Epub ahead of print]
[83] Marehbian J, Arrighi H, Hass S, Tian H, Sandborn W. Adverse events associated with common therapy regimens for moderate-to-severe Crohn's disease. Am J Gastroenterol. 2009 Oct;104(10):2524-33.
[84] Lichtenstein G, Feagan B, Cohen R, Salzberg B, Diamond R, Chen D, et al. Serious infections and mortality in association with therapies for Crohn's disease: TREAT registry. Clin Gastroenterol Hepatol. 2006 May;4(5):621-30.
[85] Veereman-Wauters G, de Ridder L, Veres G, Kolacek S, Fell J, Malmborg P, et al. Espghan ibd porto group commentary on risk of infection and prevention in pediatric ibd patients. J Pediatr Gastroenterol Nutr. 2012 Feb 10. [Epub ahead of print]
[86] Schlegel L, Grimont F, Collins M, Regnault B, Grimont PA, Bouvet A. Streptococcus infantarius sp. nov., Streptococcus infantarius subsp. infantarius subsp. nov and Streptococcus infantariu subsp. coli subsp. Nov. Isolated from humans and food. Int J Syst Evol Microbiol. 2000;50:1425-1434.

[87] McCoy W, Mason J. Enterococcal endocarditis associated with carcinoma of the sigmoid: report of a case. J Med Assoc State Ala. 1951;21:162-166.
[88] Boleij A, van Gelder M, Swinkels D, Tjalsma H. Clinical importance of Streptococcus gallolyticus infection among colorectal cancer patients: systematic review and meta-analysis. Clin Infect Dis. 2011 Nov;53(9):870-8.
[89] Dubrow R, Edberg S, Wikfors E, Callan D, Troncale F, Vender R, et al. Faecal carriage of Streptococcus bovis and colorectal adenomas. Gastroenterology. 1991 Sep;101(3):721-5.
[90] Potter M, Cunliffe N, Smith M, Miles R, Flapan A, Dunlop M. Prospective controlled study of the association of Streptococcus bovis with colorectal carcinoma. J Clin Pathol. 1998 Jun;51(6):473-4.
[91] Burns C, McCaughey R, Lauter C. The association of Streptococcus bovis fecal carriage and colon neoplasia: possible relationship with polyps and their premalignant potential. Am J Gastroenterol. 1985 Jan;80(1):423-6.
[92] Boleij A, Muytjens C, Bukhari S, Cayet N, Glaser P, Hermans P, et al. Novel clues on the specific association of Streptococcus gallolyticus subsp gallolyticus with colorectal cancer. J Infect Dis. 2011 Apr 15;203(8):1101-9.
[93] Tripodi M, Adinolfi L, Ragone E, Durante Mangoni E, Fortunato R, Iarussi D, et al. Streptococcus bovis endocarditis and its association with chronic liver disease: an underestimated risk factor. Clin infect Dis 2004; 38:1394-1400.
[94] Alazmi W, Bustamante M, O'Loughlin C, Gonzalez J, Raskin J. The association of Streptococcus bovis bacteraemia and gastrointestinal diseases: a retrospective analysis. Dig Dis Sci. 2006 Apr;51(4):732-6.
[95] Gold J, Bayar S, Salem R. Association of Streptococcus bovis BacteremiaWith Colonic Neoplasia and Extracolonic Malignancy. Arch Surg July 2004 139:760-765
[96] Vergara-López S, de Alarcón A, Mateos-Gómez A, Georgieva R, González-Nieto J, Guerrero Sánchez F, et al. Descriptive analysis of diseases associated with *Streptococcus bovis* bacteremia. Med Clin (Barc). 2011 Nov 12;137(12):527-32.
[97] de Smet A, Kluytmans J, Cooper B, Mascini E, Benus R, van der Werf T, et al. Decontamination of the digestive tract and oropharynix in ICU patients. N Engl J Med. 2009;360(1):20-31.
[98] de Jonge E, Schultz M, Spanjaard L, Bossuyt P, Vroom M, Dankert J, et al. Effects of selective decontamination of the digestive tract on mortality and acquisition of resistant bacteria in intensive care: a randomised controlled trial. Lancet 2003;362(9389):1011-6.
[99] Stoutenbeek C. The role of systemic antibiotic prophylaxis in infection prevention in intensive care by SDD. Infection Volume 17; 6:418-421.
[100] Silvestri L, van Saene H, Milanese M, Fontana F, Gregori D, Oblach L, Piacente N, Blazic M. Prevention of MRSA pneumonia by oral vancomycin decontamination: a randomised trial. Eur Respir J. 2004 Jun;23(6):921-6.
[101] Bastin A, Ryanna K. Use of selective decontamination of the digestive tract in United Kingdom intensive care units. Anaesthesia. 2009 Jan;64(1):46-49.
[102] Oostdijk E, de Smet A, Kesecioglu J. Dutch SOD-SDD Trialists Group. The role of intestinal colonisation with gram-negative bacteria as a source for intensive care unit-acquired bacteraemia. Crit Care Med. 2011 May;39(5):961-6.

[103] De La Cal M, Cerda E, Garcia-Hierro P, van Saene HK, Gomez-Santos D, Negro E, et al. Survival benefit in critically ill burned patients receiving selective decontamination of the digestive tract: a randomized, placebo-controlled, double-blind trial. Ann Surg. 2005 Mar;241(3):424-30.

[104] Liberati A, D'Amico R, Pifferi S, Torri V, Brazzi L, Parmelli E. Antibiotic prophylaxis to reduce respiratory tract infections and mortality in adults receiving intensive care. Cochrane Database Syst Rev. 2009 Oct 7;4:CD0000022

[105] Silvestri L, van Saene H, Casarin A, Berlot G, Gullo A. Impact of selective decontamination of the digestive tract on carriage and infection due to gram-negative and gram-positive bacteria: a systematic review of randomised controlled trials. Anaesth Intensive Care. 2008 May;36(3):324-38.

[106] Silvestri L, van Saene H, Milanese M, Gregori D, Gullo A. Selective decontamination of the digestive tract reduces bacterial bloodstream infection and mortality in critically ill patients. Systematic review of randomized, controlled trials. Hosp infect. 2007 Mar;65(3):187-203.

[107] Safdar N, Said A, Lucey M. The role of selective digestive decontamination for reducing infection in patients undergoing liver transplantation: a systematic review and meta-analysis. Liver transpl. 2004 Jul;10(7):817-27.

[108] Guidelines for the Management of Adults with Hospital-acquired, Ventilator-associated, and Healthcare-associated Pneumonia. Am. J. Respir. Crit. Care Med. 2005; 171: 388-416

[109] Roos D, Dijksman L, Oudemans-van Straaten H, de Wit L, Gouma D, Gerhards M. Randomized clinical trial of perioperative selective decontamination of the digestive tract versus placebo in elective gastrointestinal surgery. Br J Surg. 2011 Oct;98(10):1365-72.

[110] Melsen W, de Smet A, Kluytmans J, Bonten M; Dutch SOD-SDD Trialists' Group. Selective decontamination of the oral and digestive tract in surgical versus non-surgical patients in intensive care in a cluster-randomized trial. Br J Surg. 2012 Feb;99(2):232-7.

[111] Zwaveling J, Maring J, Klompmaker I, Haagsma E, Bottema J, Laseur M, et al. Selective decontamination of the digestive tract to prevent postoperative infection: a randomized placebo-controlled trial in liver transplant patients. Crit Care Med. 2002 Jun;30(6):1204-9.

[112] Maring J, Zwaveling J, Klompmaker I, van der Meer J, Slooff M. Selective bowel decontamination in elective liver transplantation: no improvement in endotoxaemia, initial graft function and post-operative morbidity. Transpl Int 2002 Jul;15(7):329-34

[113] Hellinger W, Yao J, Alvarez S, Blair J, Cawley J, Paya C, et al. A randomized, prospective, double-blinded evaluation of selective bowel decontamination in liver transplantation. Transplantation. 2002 Jun 27;73(12):1904-9.

[114] Safdar N, Said A, Lucey M. The role of selective digestive decontamination for reducing infection in patients undergoing liver transplantation: a systematic review and meta-analysis. Liver Transpl. 2004 Jul;10(7):817-27.

[115] Ryan K, Ray C (2004). Sherris Medical Microbiology (4th ed.). McGraw Hill; pp 322–4.

[116] Larson H, Price A, Honour P, Borriello S. *Clostridium difficile* and the aetiology of pseudomembranous colitis. Lancet 1978;1:1063–1066.

[117] Bartlett J. Clinical practice: Antibiotic-associated diarrhea. N Engl J Med 2002;346:334–349.

[118] Wilcox M, Fawley W, Wigglesworth N, Parnell P, Verity P, Freeman J. Comparison of the effect of detergent versus hypochlorite cleaning on environmental contamination and incidence of *Clostridium difficile* infection. J Hosp Infect. 2003 Jun;54(2):109-14.

[119] Merrigan M, Venugopal A, Mallozzi M, Roxas B, Viswanathan V, Johnson S, et al. Human hypervirulent *Clostridium difficile* strains exhibit increased sporulation as well as robust toxin production. 2010 Oct;192(19):4904-11.

[120] Stabler R, Dawson L, Phua L, Wren B. Comparative analysis of BI/NAP1/027 hypervirulent strains reveals novel toxin B-encoding gene (tcdB) sequences. J Med Microbiol. 2008 Jun;57(Pt 6):771-5.

[121] O'Donoghue C, Kyne L. Update on *Clostridium difficile* infection. Curr Opin Gastroenterol. 2011 Jan;27(1):38-47.

[122] Johnson S, Samore M, Farrow K, Killgore G, Tenover F, Lyras D, et al. Epidemics of diarrhea caused by a clindamycin-resistant strain of *Clostridium difficile* in four hospitals. N Engl J Med. 1999;341(22):1645.

[123] Pépin J, Saheb N, Coulombe M, Alary M, Corriveau M, Authier S, et al. Emergence of fluoroquinolones as the predominant risk factor for *Clostridium difficile*-associated diarrhea: a cohort study during an epidemic in Quebec. Clin Infect Dis. 2005;41(9):1254

[124] Goorhuis A, Van der Kooi T, Vaessen N, Dekker F, Van den Berg R, Harmanus C, et al. Spread and epidemiology of Clostridium difficile polymerase chain reaction ribotype 027/toxinotype III in The Netherlands. Clin Infect Dis. 2007;45(6):695

[125] Pépin J, Saheb N, Coulombe M, Alary M, Corriveau M, Authier S, et al. Emergence of fluoroquinolones as the predominant risk factor for *Clostridium difficile*-associated diarrhea: a cohort study during an epidemic in Quebec. Clin Infect Dis. 2005;41(9):1254

[126] Cocanour C. Best Strategies in Recurrent or Persistent *Clostridium difficile* Infection. Surg Infect (Larchmt). 2011 Jun;12(3):235-9

[127] Bignardi G. Risk factors for *Clostridium difficile* infection. J Hosp Infect. 1998;40(1):1.

[128] Stevens V, Dumyati G, Fine L, Fisher S, van Wijngaarden E. Cumulative antibiotic exposures over time and the risk of *Clostridium difficile* infection. Clin Infect Dis. 2011;53(1):42.

[129] Bauer M, Kuijper E, van Dissel J. European Society of Clinical Microbiology and Infectious Diseases (ESCMID): treatment guidance document for *Clostridium difficile* infection (CDI). Clin Microbiol Infect. 2009 Dec;15(12):1067-79.

[130] Alfa M, Swan B, Van Dekerkhove B, Pang P, Harding G. The diagnosis of *Clostridium difficile*-associated diarrhea: comparison of triage C. difficile panel, EIA for Toxin A/B and cytotoxin assays. Diagn Microbiol Infect Dis . 2002;43:257–263

[131] Louie T, Miller M, Mullane K, Weiss K, Lentnek A, Golan Y, et al. Fidaxomicin versus vancomycin for Clostridium difficile infection. N Engl J Med. 2011 Feb 3;364(5):422-3

[132] Neff G, Zacharias V, Kaiser T, Gaddis A, Kemmer N. Rifaximin for the treatment of recurrent *Clostridium difficile* infection after liver transplantation: A case series. N.Liver Transpl. 2010 Aug;16(8):960-3

[133] Rubin D, Sohi S, Glathar M, Thomas T, Yadron N, Surma B. Rifaximin Is Effective for the Treatment of *Clostridium difficile*-Associated Diarrhea: Results of an Open-Label Pilot Study.Gastroenterol Res Pract. 2011;2011:106978.

[134] van Nood E, Speelman P, Kuijper E, Keller J. Struggling with recurrent Clostridium difficile infections: is donor faeces the solution? Euro Surveill. 2009 Aug 27;14(34). pii: 19316

[135] Guo B, Harstall C, Louie T, Veldhuyzen van Zanten S, Dieleman L. Systematic review: faecal transplantation for the treatment of *Clostridium difficile*-associated disease. Aliment Pharmacol Ther. 2012 Feb 23. [Epub ahead of print]

[136] Cohen SH, Gerding DN, Johnson S, Kelly C, Loo V, McDonald L et al. Clinical practice guidelines for *Clostridium difficile* infection in adults: 2010 update by the society for healthcare epidemiology of America (SHEA) and the infectious diseases society of America (IDSA). Infect Control Hosp Epidemiol 2010;31:431–55

[137] Centers for Disease Control and Prevention (CDC). Vital Signs: Preventing *Clostridium difficile* Infections. MMWR Morb Mortal Wkly Rep. 2012 Mar 9;61:157-62

[138] Pham M, Lemberg D, Day A. Probiotics: sorting the evidence from the myths. MJA 2008; 188 (5): 304-308

[139] Allen S, Martinez E, Gregorio G, Dans L. Probiotics for treating acute infectious diarrhoea. Cochrane Database Syst Rev. 2010 Nov 10;(11):CD003048.

[140] Bernaola Aponte G, Bada Mancilla C, Carreazo Pariasca N, Rojas Galarza R. Probiotics for treating persistent diarrhoea in children. Cochrane Database Syst Rev. 2010 Nov 10;(11):CD007401

[141] Villarruel G, Rubio D, Lopez F, Cintioni J, Gurevech R, Romero G, et al. Saccharomyces boulardii in acute childhood diarrhoea: a randomized, placebo-controlled study. Acta Paediatr 2007; 96(4):538-41.

[142] Fang S, Lee H, Hu J, Hou S, Liu H, Fang H. Dose-dependent effect of Lactobacillus rhamnosus on quantitative reduction of faecal rotavirus shedding in children. J Trop Pediatr. 2009 Oct;55(5):297-301.

[143] Szajewska H, Mrukowicz J. Probiotics in the treatment and prevention of acute infectious diarrhea in infants and children: a systematic review of published randomized, double-blind, placebo-controlled trials. J Pediatr Gastroenterol Nutr. 2001;33 Suppl 2:S17.

[144] Cazzaniga M, Dionigi E, Gobbo G, Fioretti A, Monti V, Salerno F. The systemic inflammatory response syndrome in cirrhotic patients: relationship with their in-hospital outcome. J Hepatol. 2009 Sep;51(3):475-82.

[145] Wiström J, Norrby S, Myhre E, Eriksson S, Granström G, Lagergren L et al. Frequency of antibiotic-associated diarrhoea in 2462 antibiotic-treated patients: a prospective study. J Antimicrob Chemother 2001;47:43-50

[146] Avadhani A, Miley H. Probiotics for prevention of antibiotic-associated diarrhea and *Clostridium difficile*-associated disease in hospitalized adults-a meta-analysis. Am Acad Nurse Pract. 2011 Jun;23(6):269-74.

[147] Kale-Pradhan P, Jassal H, Wilhelm S. Role of Lactobacillus in the prevention of antibiotic-associated diarrhea: a meta-analysis. Pharmacotherapy. 2010 Feb;30(2):119-26.

[148] Pardi D, D'Haens G, Shen B, Campbell S, Gionchetti P. Clinical guidelines for the management of pouchitis. Inflamm Bowel Dis. 2009; 15:1421-1431.

[149] Mack D. Probiotics in Inflammatory Bowel Diseases and Asociated Conditions. Nutrients. 2011 Feb;3(2):245-264.

[150] Mallon P, McKay D, Kirk S, Gardiner K. Probiotics for induction of remission in ulcerative colitis. Cochrane Database Syst Rev. 2007;4:CD005573.

[151] Kato K, Mizuno S, Umesaki Y, Ishii Y, Sugitani M, Imaoka A, et al. Randomized placebo-controlled trial assessing the effect of bifidobacteria-fermented milk on active ulcerative colitis. Aliment. Pharmacol. Ther. 2004;20:1133-41.

[152] Tursi A, Brandimarte G, Giorgetti G, Forti G, Modeo ME, Gigliobianco A. Low-dose balsalazide plus a high-potency probiotic preparation is more effective than balsalazide alone or mesalazine in the treatment of acute-mild-to-moderate ulcerative colitis. Med. Sci. Monit. 2004;10:PI126-PI131.

[153] Rembacken B, Snelling A, Hawkey P, Chalmers D, Axon A. Non-pathogenic Eschericia coli versus mesalazine for the treatment of ulcerative colitis: a randomized trial. Lancet. 1999;354:635-639.

[154] Miele E, Pascarella F, Giannetti E, Quaglietta L, Baldassano R, Staiano A. Effect of a probiotic preparation (VSL#3) on induction and maintenance of remission in children with ulcerative colitis. Am J Gastroenterol. 2009;104:437-443.

[155] Fujimori S, Gudis K, Mitsui K, Seo T, Yonezawa M, Tanaka S, et al. A randomized controlled trial on the efficacy of symbiotic versus probiotic or prebiotic treatment to improve the quality of life in patients with ulcerative colitis. Nutrition. 2009;25:520-525.

[156] Sood A, Midha V, Makharia G, Ahuja V, Singal D, Goswami P, Tandon R. The probiotic preparation VSL#3 induces remission in patients with mild-to-moderately active ulcerative colitis. Clin Gastroenterol Hepatol. 2009;7:1202-1209.

[157] Matthes H, Krummerel T, Giensch M, Wolff C, Schulze J. Clinical trial: probiotic treatment of acute distal ulcerative colitis with rectally administered Eschericia coli Nissle 1917(ECN). BMC Complement. Altern. Med. 2010;10:13

[158] Kruis W, Fric P, Pokrotnieks J, Lukas M, Fixa B, Kascak M, et al. Maintaining remission of ulcerative colitis with the probiotic Escherichia coli Nissle 1917 is as effective as with standard mesalazine. Gut. 2004;53:1617–1623.

[159] Zocco M, dal Verme L, Cremonini F, Piscaglia A, Nista E, Candelli M, et al. Efficacy of Lactobacillus GG in maintaining remission of ulcerative colitis. Aliment Pharmacol Ther 2006;23:1567–1574.

[160] Ishikawa H, Akedo I, Umesmaki Y, Tanaka R, Imaoka A, Otani T. Randomized controlled trial of the effect of Bifidobacteria-fermented milk on ulcerative colitis. J Am Coll Nutr. 2003;22:56–63.

[161] Oliva S, Di Nardo G, Ferrari F, Mallardo S, Rossi P, Patrizi G, et al. Randomised clinical trial: the effectiveness of Lactobacillus reuteri ATCC 55730 rectal enema in children with active distal ulcerative colitis. Aliment Pharmacol Ther. 2012 Feb;35(3):327-34.

[162] Zakostelska Z, Kverka M, Klimesova K, Rossmann P, Mrazek J, Kopecny J, et al. Lysate of probiotic Lactobacillus casei DN-114 001 ameliorates colitis by strengthening the gut barrier function and changing the gut microenvironment. PLoS One. 2011;6(11):e27961. Epub 2011 Nov 22.

[163] Munoz P, Bouza E, Cuenca-Estrella M, Eiros J, Perez M, Sanchez-Somolinos M, et al. Saccharmoyces cerevisiae fungaemia: an emerging infectious disease. Clin Infect Dis 2005;40:1625-34.

[164] Farina C, Arosio M, Mangia M, Moioli F. Lactobacillus casei subsp. Rhamnosus sepsis in a patient with ulcerative colitis. J Clin Gastroenterol. 2001;33:251-252.

[165] Alfaleh K, Anabrees J, Bassler D, Al-Kharfi T. Probiotics for prevention of necrotizing enterocolitis in preterm infants. Cochrane Database Syst Rev. 2011 Mar 16;(3):CD005496

[166] Alfaleh K, Anabrees J, Bassler D. Probiotics reduce the risk of necrotizing enterocolitis in preterm infants: a meta-analysis. Neonatology 2010;97(2):93-9.

[167] Deshpande G, Rao S, Patole S, Bulsara M. Updated meta-analysis of probiotics for preventing necrotizing enterocolitis in preterm neonates. Pediatrics 2010;125(5):921-30.

[168] Braga T, da Silva G, de Lira P, de Carvalho L. Efficacy of Bifidobacterium breve and Lactobacillus casei oral supplementation on necrotizing enterocolitis in very-low-birth-weight preterm infants: a double-blind, randomized, controlled trial. Am J Clin Nutr. 2011 Jan;93(1):81-6.

[169] Tarnow-Mordi W, Wilkinson D, Trivedi A, Brok J. Probiotics reduce all-cause mortality and necrotizing enterocolitis: it is time to change practice. Pediatrics 2010;125(5):1068-70.

[170] Enck P, Klosterhalfen S, Martens U. Probiotic therapy of the irritable bowel syndrome. Dtsch Med Wochenschr. 2011 Feb;136(8):371-5

[171] McFarland L. Systematic review and meta-analysis of Saccharomyces boulardii in adult patients. World J Gastroenterol. 2010 May 14;16(18):2202-22.

[172] Hoveyda N, Heneghan C, Mahtani K, Perera R, Roberts N, Glasziou P. A systematic review and meta-analysis: probiotics in the treatment of irritable bowel syndrome. BMC Gastroenterol. 2009 Feb 16;9:15.

[173] Moayyedi P, Ford A, Talley N, Cremonini F, Foxx-Orenstein A, Brandt L, et al. The efficacy of probiotics in the treatment of irritable bowel syndrome: a systematic review. Gut. 2010 Mar;59(3):325-32

[174] McFarland L, Dublin S. Meta-analysis of probiotics for the treatment of irritable bowel syndrome. World J Gastroenterol. 2008 May 7;14(17):2650-61.

Chapter 4

Nerve Growth Factor and Sepsis

Ayse Belin Ozer and Mustafa Bayar

Additional information is available at the end of the chapter

http://dx.doi.org/10.5772/50532

1. Introduction

Neurotrophins are a family of growth factors that are polypeptide in structure and are necessary for the development and maintenance of the vertebrate nervous system. The first member of this family, nerve growth factor (NGF) was discovered in 1952 by an Italian group of scientists led by Rita Levi-Montalcini. She received a Nobel Prize in 1987 for her team's discovery. A few decades after the discovery of NGF, brain-derived neurotrophin factor (BDNF), neurotrophin-3 (NT-3), neurotrophin-4 (NT-4), and neurotrophin-5 (NT-5) were discovered, followed by neurotrophin-6 (NT-6) and neurotrophin-7 (NT-7) [1-3].

2. NGF Structure

There are two forms of NGF isolated from the short arm of human chromosome 1, a high molecular weight 7S NGF and a low molecular weight 2.5S NGF. The 7S form is a complex with three subunits (α, β and γ) and has a molecular weight of 130-140 kDa. Two beta subunits, each 118 amino acids long, are linked together by disulfide bonds and are responsible for the biological activity of NGF. The alpha and gamma subunits are members of the kallikrein protein family, and while the role of the alpha subunit is unknown, the gamma subunit is an epidermal growth factor (EGF) binding protein and has a role in the functions of the beta subunit. The 2.5S form has a molecular weight of 26 kDa and is formed by non-covalent interactions of two different subunits. NGF is synthesized and stored mostly in the mouse submandibular gland for reasons still unknown despite extensive research [3,4].

3. NGF receptors

Recently, it has been demonstrated that neurotrophins have many roles. Nerve growth factor has two receptors, p75NTR and tyrosine kinase A (Trk A), whose signaling pathways can be synergic, antagonistic or independent of each other [5].

The p75NTR receptor is a transmembrane glycoprotein with an extracellular domain and a member of the TNF receptor family; it has low affinity for NGF. The p75NTR is a pan-neurotrophin receptor and, in addition to NGF, binds to other neurotrophins, such as BDNF, NT-3, and NT-4/5. It induces the NFκB and c-Jun kinase transduction pathways with varying effects depending on the pathway. The p75 receptor has been shown to act as a co-receptor in the presence of high affinity receptors and as an antagonist in their absence. The p75NTR receptor is thought to act as a mediator in the pro-apoptotic process induced by NGF. p75NTR increases the production of ceramides and activates gene transcription or programmed cell death in cells [5,6].

Receptor protein-tyrosine kinases A, B, and C (Trk A, B, C) are specific, high-affinity neurotrophin receptors. Trk receptors have transmembrane, extracellular, and intracellular domains. The portion of the Trk receptor responsible for tyrosine kinase activity, and thus for signal transduction, is located in the cytosolic domain. While p75 receptors bind to all neurotrophins, the tyrosine kinase receptor family binds to different receptors with different affinities. The Trk A receptor binds with high affinity to NGF but also binds to NT-3, NT-4, and NT-5 with low affinity. The Trk B receptor binds to BDNF and NT-4 with high affinity and to NT-3 with lower affinity. In contrast, the Trk C receptor only binds to NT-3 [5,7]. The Trk A receptor only has high affinity for NGF, and most NGF activity takes place through Trk A receptors. Trk A is a 140 kDa transmembrane protein encoded by proto-oncogenes on chromosome 1. The binding of NGF to a Trk A receptor induces tyrosine kinase receptor autophosphorylation, leading to the activation of parts of signal transduction cascades. These cascades are mainly mitogen-activated protein kinase (MAPK)-Ras-Erk, phospholipase Cγ1, inositol triphosphate, and SNT pathways. Mutagenesis studies of the Trk A receptor showed that Trk A has significant effects on the development of the nervous system, and loss of Trk A results in neuronal loss. The Trk A receptor also induces gene transduction in cells [5,7].

4. Nerve growth factor and the nervous system

Neurotrophins are a group of structurally and functionally similar proteins that are secreted by a target tissue; they play a role in the development of the nervous system and in signal transmission. The largest concentrations of neurotrophins are found where major cholinergic pathways are present, such as in the hippocampus and cerebral cortex. In neonatal rats, when NGF is applied intracerebroventricularly, it increases the activity of choline acetyltransferase in the cortex and hippocampus. In addition, intracerebraventricular application of anti-NGF antibodies reduces the activity of choline acetyltransferase [7,8].

NGF plays a role in growth, differentiation, maintenance, regeneration, neurotransmitter function, neurotoxin resistance, and lesions in nerve cells [7,8]. Under normal conditions, neurons are largely responsible for the synthesis of NGF; however, brain damage can cause glial cells to produce NGF as well. The blockade of the glutamate receptors and/or stimulation of the GABAergic system reduces NGF mRNAs in hippocampus and NGF protein in hippocampus and septum [9]. The level of NGF in the nervous system and cerebrospinal fluid has been found to decrease with age [10,11]. During the fetal and early post-natal periods, neurons are NGF-dependent; however, at later stages, they become NGF-sensitive. NGF levels were found to be high in blood, tissue and cerebrospinal fluid of patients with pathological conditions, such as hypoxia, ischemia, age-related cerebral atrophy, and increased intracranial pressure [7,12].

The increase in NGF levels after cerebral injury is required for neuronal recovery. Many studies have shown that neurotrophic factors control cellular calcium homeostasis, regulate cerebral blood flow, reverse the effects of ischemia, and inhibit the formation of free radicals by increasing antioxidant enzyme levels. However, the underlying mechanism of the neuroprotective role of NGF is unknown [13, 14].

Neurotrophic factors were used in *in vivo* and *in vitro* studies of neurodegenerative diseases. Many of the neurotrophic factors were only used in primate models, while some were tested as treatment for human neurogenerative diseases. However, none of these studies provided satisfactory results due to technical problems, side effects, and insufficient activities. Studies have argued that, because of its beneficial effects, NGF may be a new potential therapeutic tool for the treatment of neurodegenerative diseases, especially Alzheimer's disease [15]. In addition, NGF has been shown to be involved in cognitive functions, especially learning [16].

5. Nerve growth factor and sepsis

Sepsis and associated clinical manifestations are the main causes of mortality and morbidity in intensive care units outside coronary intensive care units [17, 18]. Despite the high mortality, the pathophysiology of sepsis is not completely known. However, infection with a microorganism is known to be the first step in the development of sepsis. In order for the inflammatory response to occur, the activation of endogenous mediators is also required. There are numerous complex endogenous mediators, including the coagulation system, complements, kinins, cytokines, metabolites of arachidonic acid, myocardial depressant factor, endorphins, histamines, lysosomal enzymes, platelet activating factors, and free oxygen radicals. In addition to increased inflammation, mechanisms such as anti-inflammatory cytokine secretion, anergy, and apoptosis cause immunosuppression [18-21].

When interactions between NGF and the mechanisms involved in sepsis pathogenesis are examined, NGF is found to be associated with inflammatory events and apoptosis.

6. NGF and inflammation

In studies conducted before the interaction of neurotrophins with the inflammation process was discovered, interactions between neurotrophins and immune organs and immune cells were investigated. In recent decades, detailed studies on the cellular localization and tissue distribution of neurotrophins have been completed. These studies determined that neurotrophin and its receptors are present in all lymphoid organs, including the thymus and bursa of Fabricius [3, 22-25]. The first immune cell shown to associate with NGF was the mast cell, and its close localization to the nerve cells suggests the functional interaction between the nervous system and the immune system. Exogenous NGF was shown to activate mast cells in some peripheral tissues and to increase their number, size and degranulation [26, 27]. In addition to mast cells, NGF receptors are expressed in T and B lymphocytes, monocytes, macrophages, and granulocytes. Studies have shown that NGF is not only synthesized in immune cells, but also interacts with them [22,24,26].

Increased NGF serum and tissue levels were also found in patients with other inflammatory conditions, such as allergies, asthma, cystitis, immune diseases and cardiopulmonary bypass [28-33]. It was determined that, when NGF is administered systemically, the bronchial hyperactivity induced by histamines is increased, while bronchial hyperactivity is inhibited by anti-NGF application. NGF interacts with tachykinins causing the increase in bronchial hyperactivity [32]. Human fibroblast, airway smooth muscle, and lung epithelium A549 cells have the ability to synthesize NGF. Synthesis in this cells is induced by pro-inflammatory cytokines (IL-1β, TNF-α) and inhibited by glucocorticoids [34-39]. In mouse models of arthritis, stimulation with IL-1β has been demonstrated to increase the synthesis of NGF, which results in the increase of TNF-α [40]. According to some uncertain data, NGF has a causal role in inflammation, most likely in pro-inflammatory processes based on the interaction of NGF with pro-inflammatory cytokines, such as TNF-α and IL-1β.

On the other hand, application of NGF resulted in dramatic shrinkage or disappearance of lesions in chronic vasculitic ulcers and allergic encephalomyelitis, and accelerated wound healing, which suggested an anti-inflammatory role for NGF as well [41-44]. In studies which investigated NGF's interaction with anti-inflammatory cytokines, a strong interaction between NGF and IL-10 was found. In inflammatory processes, changes in the levels of NGF and IL-10 were correlated, each up-regulating the other. The effect of IL-10 on increasing the secretion of NGF is dose-dependent, and the application of anti-IL-10 blocks the secretion of NGF [42,45-47].

In addition to pro-inflammatory and anti-inflammatory cytokines, NGF has been noted to interact with Toll-like receptors (TLR), which are involved in the pathogenesis of sepsis, and other inflammatory mediators. In the conjunctival epithelial cells obtained from patients with vernal conjunctivitis, NGF has been shown to modulate the expression of TLR-4 and TLR-9 [48]. TLR-4 signaling in the dendritic cells may activate the p38MAPK and NFκB pathways and induce the expression of NGF and p75 [49]. The human leukocyte antigen-DR (HLA-DR), CD40, CD80, CD83, CD86, and CCR7 expression induced by LPS is thought to cause the secretion of IL-12p40 and pro-inflammatory cytokines, such as IL-1, IL-6, and TNF-α. In addition, NGF was noted to inhibit the degranulation of natural killer (NK) cells; however, NK cells are not the cause of NGF production [50].

In monocyte and microglial cell cultures induced by lipopolysaccharaide (LPS), LPS was shown to activate mRNA expression and protein release of NGF in a dose and time-dependent manner [51,52]. The use of NFκB inhibitor pyrrolidine dithiocarbamate was also shown to inhibit LPS-induced synthesis of NGF, and it was concluded that NFκB modulates expression of LPS-induced NGF [51]. The only study that showed the interaction between NGF and sepsis was conducted by Bayar et al [53]. In rats with sepsis experimentally induced by LPS, blood was obtained before the intervention, 2, 12, 24 and 72 hours after LPS injection, and serum NGF levels were measured using the Emax Immunoassay method. Twenty-four hours after LPS injection, NGF levels were significantly higher in sepsis-induced rats compared to the control group. It was observed that anti-NGF administered in the early period, one hour before induction of sepsis, reduced the level of NGF observed two hours after injection. However, administration of the same dose of anti-NGF after sepsis was induced did not result in any change in the NGF levels. The dose of anti-NGF might have been inadequate to reduce NGF levels, as NGF synthesis increases after sepsis begins.

The use of anti-NGF to eliminate the effects of NGF is a method employed in studies of the interaction between inflammation and NGF. While some studies have shown that NGF decreases inflammation in groups which have received anti-NGF [29,54], others have reported no change [55] or increased inflammation [56,57].

In one study, application of anti-NGF decreased the early allergic reaction in an experimental model of asthma induced by intratracheal administration of ovalbumin [54]. In a second study using a respiratory syncytial virus (RSV) infection model, high levels of NGF and NGF receptors were observed in both young and adult rats. In the same study, the inflammatory effect of NGF was shown to decrease with age. When NGF was administered exogenously, expression of the neurokinin 1 (NK1) receptor, which is a sign of neurogenic inflammation, increased in the lungs, and pre-treatment with anti-NGF antibody decreased the expression of NK1 and, thus, alleviated the neurogenic inflammation [58]. In the rat model of inflammation generated by inoculation of *Trisinella spiralis*, the application of anti-NGF prevented intestinal dysmotility in rats; however, it had no effect on inflammation [55].

When latent herpes simplex virus (HSV-1) infected rabbits were administered anti-NGF antibodies, the anti-NGF was shown to react with ocular HSV-1 [57]. In another study, in which colitis was induced using trinitrobenzene sulfonic acid, and damage was assessed four weeks later, pre-treatment with anti-NGF and anti-NT-3 increased the intensity of inflammation 2-3 folds [56]. In acute and chronic experimental colitis models, neuropeptides, such as substance P and CGRP, serve a protective function and are regulated by NGF; when neurotrophins are experimentally and selectively blocked, the inflammation is significantly increased [56]. Present studies suggest that NGF has more anti-inflammatory effects than inflammatory. In a study investigating the interaction between sepsis and anti-NGF, anti-NGF was applied and its effect on apoptosis was evaluated during both the early period, when no manifestations of sepsis are present, and the late period, when manifestations of sepsis are established [53].

Studies involving NGF and anti-NGF have reported that NGF has both pro-inflammatory and anti-inflammatory effects. The difference might be a result of using different models of inflammation, applying different NGF and anti-NGF doses, and/or using different administration techniques. However, at the 2002 NGF meeting, it was reported that NGF and Trk A weaken immune response primarily through inhibition; in other words, they mainly have immunosuppressant effects. Researchers argue that NGF is a potent and complier neuroimmunomodulator that secretes, and is secreted by, inflammatory mediators, and that, NGF's proinflammatory or anti-inflammatory role can change depending on the type and stage of inflammation [59].

7. NGF and apoptosis

The term apoptosis was used for the first time in 1972 by Kerr, Wyllie, and Curie and means the falling of leaves from a tree in Greek. Apoptosis is the genetically controlled programmed cell death mechanism used by organisms to harmlessly dispose of damaged or unnecessary cells. Numerous physiological, adaptive, and pathological events may occur after apoptosis in the organism [60,61].

Cell proliferation and cell death are balanced in tissues to provide continuity of tissue volume. In a 1992 study by Buchman et al., apoptosis was triggered in an experimental sepsis model induced by LPS [62]. In a postmortem study by Hotchkiss et al., cases that died from sepsis demonstrated that apoptosis occurred particularly in lymphocytes and intestinal epithelial cells. Although neutrophil apoptosis is known to be delayed overall during sepsis, a recent clinical study showed that neutrophil apoptosis increased in the earlier periods of sepsis. This phenomenon was explained as a mechanism to compensate for the inflammatory response [63]. Another study suggested that, among the immunosuppression mechanisms observed in sepsis, lymphocyte apoptosis is one of the most important and is a primary response, rather than a compensatory response [64].

The interaction between nerve growth factor and apoptosis was first suggested in 1952 by Rita Levi Montalcini. She demonstrated that, during the development of sympathetic and sensory neurons, NGF levels were half those of normal neurons. The increase in NGF-sensitive neurons, due to exogenous NGF application, and in neuronal death, due to anti-NGF administration, supported her data. At the same time, NGF had an effect on regulating cell death in the bursa of Fabricius of chickens and in human memory B lymphocytes [65-67]. Autocrine regulation of the cell cycle in vascular smooth muscle cells was attributed to NGF. The presence of NGF was detected in aortic endothelial cells. It was determined that NGF levels increased with pro-inflammatory cytokine IL-1ß, and after anti-NGF application, the cell count during S and G2/M phases and the ratio of hypodiploid cells were both increased [68]. In yet another study, the application of anti-NGF antibodies resulted in a 5-fold increase in the hypodiploid DNA of LPS-activated monocyte/macrophage cultures compared to the control group. Morphological changes, such as round-shaped dense chromatin and DNA fragmentation, were also observed in apoptotic cells [52]. It was determined that Trk A activity inhibited cell development in PC 12 pheochromocytoma and neuroblastoma cells, and high expression of Trk A was correlated with neuroblastoma prognosis [69,70]. In a recent study, NGF was shown to inhibit the induction of cyclins, as well as, cyclin interaction with corresponding cyclin-dependent kinases, thus, preventing progression through the G1 phase of the cell cycle [71]. Cell death induced in trigeminal ganglions by tunicamycin, another drug that stops the cell cycle at the G1 phase, is suppressed by NGF in mouse embryos [72].

In a study of normal and NGF transgenic mice that underwent middle cerebral artery occlusion (MCAO), investigators evaluated infarct volume and antioxidant enzyme activity in the tissue that caused the occlusion. They observed higher NGF protein level increases in the cortical regions after ischemic damage in transgenic mice compared to the controls. In addition, the infarct volume and density of apoptotic cells were lower in transgenic mice. As a result, it was concluded that NGF had antioxidant and antiapoptotic properties [73]. Yang et al. reported that NGF applied after MCAO reduced apoptosis, and NGF's neuroprotective effect lasted up to five hours [74]. NGF eye drops applied to a rat model of experimental glaucoma improved the long-term function of the optic nerve, widened the visual field, and inhibited apoptosis in retinal ganglion cells [75].

Nine people volunteered for a study in which erythemas were generated with UV radiation. Skin biopsies were performed afterwards, and by using anti-NGF dye, the number of NGF-positive melanocytes and keratinocytes were determined to have decreased [76]. In another study of rat peritoneal mast cell cultures, the effect of NGF on age-associated apoptosis was evaluated. It was determined that NGF prevents apoptosis in a dose-dependent manner, and when anti-NGF antibody is applied, NGF's antiapoptotic effect is completely blocked [77]. NGF has been reported to have a protective effect on respiratory syncytial virus (RSV)-induced apoptosis of airway epithelial cells, and therefore, it has been proposed as a new approach to the maintenance of respiratory tract infections [78].

Another study evaluated neurotrophins and their receptors on diffuse large B-cell lymphoma (DLBCL) cells with different rituximab sensitivities. NGF secretion was induced by DLBLC cell exposure to rituximab, and Trk-inhibitor K252a exposure produced additive cytotoxic effects to rituximab [79]. Using immunohistochemical staining, bevacizumab, a drug used in cancer treatment, was determined to decrease the level of NGF protein, and thus, via NGF down-regulation, bevacizumab increases apoptosis [80]. Diabetic rats subjected to treadmill exercise produce increased levels of NGF to suppress apoptotic cell death in muscles [81].

The hematoxylin-eosin, and other immunohistochemical stains, such as those for Bcl-2 and Bax, were used to stain liver, lung, and intestinal tissues in the above mentioned study which evaluated the effects of both early and late period anti-NGF application on apoptosis in experimental rat models of sepsis [53]. In this study, the increase in apoptosis was determined by H/E staining of all tissues from all sepsis groups. The ratio of apoptotic cells was more distinct in the sepsis group and in the group which received anti-NGF treatment in the early period. When the two groups were compared, rats from the early anti-NGF application group had distinctly increased levels of apoptosis in their liver and intestinal tissues. In addition, when early and late anti-NGF application groups were compared, the early anti-NGF application group exhibited a more prominent increase in apoptosis in the intestinal tissue compared to the late application group. When Bcl-2 staining of all tissues was compared, all sepsis groups were determined to have low Bcl-2 expression in the liver tissue compared to the control groups. When lung tissue was stained, all sepsis groups had low Bcl-2 expression compared to the control group. However, the results from the sepsis group without any treatment was significantly lower. In addition, when intestinal tissue was stained, all sepsis groups had low Bcl-2 expression compared to the control group. However, the results from the sepsis group without any treatment and the early NGF application groups were significantly lower. All groups with sepsis had increased Bax expression in the lung and intestinal tissues compared to the control group. In the liver tissue, all groups had increased Bax expression; however, the sepsis and early anti-NGF groups had had the highest levels of Bax expression. When the early and late NGF application groups were compared, Bax expression in all tissues was higher for the early NGF application group. The study concluded that early application of anti-NGF causes apoptosis at least as much as sepsis by itself; however, the application of anti-NGF after sepsis has been established causes less apoptosis compared to sepsis cases not treated with anti-NGF. The level of apoptosis was more distinct in the group with early anti-NGF application, which caused a prominent decrease in serum NGF levels. However, in the group with late application of anti-NGF and relatively stable NGF levels, less apoptosis was detected.

In conclusion, no clinical study addressing the role of NGF in the pathogenesis of sepsis has been completed to date. However, based on the last study, the application of anti-NGF before the start of inflammation increases inflammation and apoptosis. The application of anti-NGF after the start of inflammation causes less inflammation and apoptosis compared to sepsis cases which do not receive any anti-NGF treatment. Based on the data demonstrating that anti-NGF increases inflammation and apoptosis in sepsis, it can be suggested that NGF has anti-inflammatory and antiapoptotic properties in sepsis cases.

Author details

Ayse Belin Ozer and Mustafa Bayar
Firat University Medical School Department of Anesthesiology, Elazig, Turkey

8. References

[1] Levi-Montalcini R. Effects of mouse tumor transplantation on the nervous system. Ann N Y Acad Sci. 1952;55:330-44.

[2] http://www.nobelprize.org/nobel_prizes/medicine/laureates/1986/presentation-speech. The 1986 Nobel Prize in Physiology or Medicine for discoveries of growth factors

[3] Vega JA, Garcia-Suarez O, Hannestad J, Perez- Perez M, Germana A. Neurotrophins and the immune system. J Anat 2003;203:1-19

[4] Shooter EM. Early days of the nerve growth factor proteins. Annu. Rev. Neurosci. 2001; 24:601-629.

[5] Frossard N, Freund V, Advenier C. Nerve growth factor and its receptors in asthma and inflammation. Eur J Pharmacol 2004;500:453-465

[6] Rankin SL, Guy CS, Mearow KM. TrkA NGF receptor plays a role in the in the modulation of p75NTR expression. Neurosci Lett. 2005;383:305-10.
[7] Sofroniew MV, Howe CL, Mobley WC. Nerve growth factors signalling, neuroprotection and neural repair. Annu Rev Neurosci. 2001;24:1217-1281
[8] Castellanos MR, Aguiar J, Fernandez CI, Almaguer W, Mejias C, Varela A. Evaluation of the neurorestorative effects of the murine beta-nerve growth factor infusions in old rat with cognitive deficit. Biochem Biophys Res Commun. 2003;312:867-72
[9] Zafra F, Castrén E, Thoenen H, Lindholm D. Interplay between glutamate and gamma-aminobutyric acid transmitter systems in the physiological regulation of brain-derived neurotrophic factor and nerve growth factor synthesis in hippocampal neurons. Proc Natl Acad Sci U S A. 1991;88:10037-41.
[10] Xia YX, Ikeda T, Xia XY, Ikenoue T. Differential neurotrophin levels in cerebrospinal fluid and their changes during development in newborn rat. Neurosci Lett. 2000;280:220-2.
[11] Katoh-Semba R, Semba R, Takeuchi IK, Kato K. Age-related changes in levels of brain-derived neurotrophic factor in selected brain regions of rats, normal mice and senescence-accelerated mice: a comparison to those of nerve growth factor and neurotrophin-3. Neurosci Res. 1998;31:227-34.
[12] Hochhaus F, Koehne P, Schäper C, Butenandt O, Felderhoff-Mueser U, Ring-Mrozik E, Obladen M, Bührer C. Elevated nerve growth factor and neurotrophin-3 levels in cerebrospinal fluid of children with hydrocephalus. BMC Pediatr. 2001;1:2. (24 August 2001, doi: 10.1186/1471-2431-1-2)
[13] Zhou Z, Chen H, Zhang K, Yang H, Liu J, Huang Q. Protective effect of nerve growth factor on neurons after traumatic brain injury. J Basic Clin Physiol Pharmacol. 2003;14:217-24.
[14] Chiaretti A, Antonelli A, Genovese O, Fernandez E, Giuda D, Mariotti P, Riccardi R. Intraventricular nerve growth factor infusion improves cerebral blood flow and stimulates doublecortin expression in two infants with hypoxic-ischemic brain injury. Neurol Res. 2008;30:223-8.
[15] Salehi A, Delcroix JD, Swaab DF. Alzheimer's disease and NGF signaling. J Neural Transm 2004;111:323-45.
[16] Jakubowska-Dogru E, Gümüsbas U. Chronic intracerebroventricular NGF administration improves working memory in young adult memory deficient rats. Neurosci Lett. 2005;382:45-50.
[17] Balk RA. Severe sepsis and septic shock. Definitions, epidemiology, and clinical manifestations. Crit Care Clin. 2000;16:179-92.
[18] Mann EA, Baun MM, Meininger JC, Wade CE. Comparison of mortality associated with sepsis in the burn, trauma, and general intensive care unit patient: a systematic review of the literature. Shock. 2012;37:4-16.
[19] Remick DG. Pathophysiology of sepsis. Am J Pathol 2007;170:1435-44.
[20] Hotchkiss RS, Karl IE. The pathophysiology and treatment of sepsis. N Engl J Med 2003; 348:138-50

[21] Mitchell E, Whitehouse T. The pathophysiology of sepsis. Daniels R, Nutbeam T (eds). ABC of sepsis. Blacwell Publishing Ltd, 2010:20-28
[22] Ehrhard PB, Erb P, Graumann U, Otten U. Expression of nerve growth factor and nerve growth factor recetor tyrosine kinase Trk in activated CD4-positive T-cell clones. Immunology 1993;90:10984-8
[23] Laurenzi MA, Barbany G, Timmusk T, Lindgren JA, Persson H. Expression of mRNA encoding neurotrophins and neurotrophin receptors in rat thymus, spleen tissue and immunocompetent cells. Eur J Biochem 1994; 223:733-41
[24] Aloe L, Simone MD, Properzi F. Nerve growth factor: a neurotrophin with activity on cells of the immune system. Microsc. Res. Tech. 1999;45:285-91
[25] Simone MD, Santis SD, Vigneti E, Papa G, Amadori S, Aloe L. Nerve growth factor: a survey of activity on immune and hematopoietic cells. Hematol. Oncol. 1999;17:1-10
[26] Rost B, Hanf G, Ohnemus U, Otto-Knapp R, Groneberg DA, Kunkel G, Noga O. Monocytes of allergics and non- allergics produce, store and release the neurotrophins NGF, BDNF and NT-3. Regulatory Peptides 2005;124:19-25
[27] Tal M, Liberman R. Local injection of Nerve Growth Factor triggers degranulation of mast cells in rat paw. Neurosci Lett. 1997;221:129-32
[28] Manni L, Nikolova V, Vyagova D, Chaldakov GN, Aloe L. Reduced plasma levels of NGF and BDNF in patient with acute coronary syndromes. Int J Cardiol 2005;102:169-71
[29] Aloe L, Fiore M. Neuroinflammatory implications of Schistosoma mansoni infection: new information from the mouse model. Parasitology Today 1998;14:314-8
[30] Bonini S, Lambiase A, Bonini S, Levi-Schaffer F, Aloe L. Nerve growth factor: an important molecule in allergic inflammation and tissue remodelling. Int Arch Allergy Immunol 1999;118:159-62
[31] Oddiah D, Anand P, McMahon SB, Rattray M. Rapid increase of NGF, BDNF and NT- 3 mRNAs in inflamed bladder. NeuroReport 1998;9:1455-8
[32] Braun A, Lommatzsch M, Lewin GR, Virchow JC, Renz H. Neurotrophins: a link between airway inflammation and airway smooth muscle contractility in asthma? Int Arch Allergy Immunol. 1999;118:163-5.
[33] Barthel C, Yeremenko N, Jacobs R, Schmidt RE, Bernateck M, Zeidler H, Tak PP, Baeten D, Rihl M. Nerve growth factor and receptor expression in rheumatoid arthritis and spondyloarthritis. Arthritis Res Ther. 2009;11:R82. (2 June 2009, doi: 10.1186/ar2716)
[34] Pons F, Freund V, Kuissu H, Mathieu E, Olgart C, Frossard N. Nerve growth factor secretion by human lung epithelial A549 cells in pro-and anti-inflammatory conditions. Eur J Pharmacol 2001;428:365-9
[35] Freund V, Pons F, Joly V, Mathieu E, Martinet N, Frossard N. Upregulation of nerve growth factor expression by human airway smooth muscle cells in inflammatory conditions. Eur Respir J 2002;20:458-63
[36] Olgart C, Frossard N. Human lung fibroblasts secrete nerve growth factor: effect of inflammatory cytokines and glucocorticoids. Eur Respir J 2001;18:115-21

[37] Hattori A, Hayashi K, Kohno M. Tumor necrosis factor (TNF) stimulates the production of nerve growth factor in fibroblasts via the 55-kDa type 1 TNF receptor. FEBS Letters 1996;379:157-60
[38] Hattori A, Iwasaki S, Murase K, Tsujimoto M, Sato M, Hayashi K, Kohno M. Tumor necrosis factor is markedly synergistic with interleukin 1 and interferon-gamma_in stimulating the production of nerve growth factor in fibroblasts. FEBS Letters 1994;340:177-80
[39] Blasing H, Hendrix S, Paus R. Pro-inflammatory cytokines upregulate the skin immunoreactivity for NGF, NT-3, NT-4 and their receptor, p75NTR in vivo: a preliminary report. Arch Dermatol Res 2005;296:580-4.
[40] Mani L, Lundeberg T, Tirassa P, Aloe L. Role of cholecystokinin-8 in nerve growth factor and nerve growth factor mRNA expression in carrageenan-induced joint inflammation in adult rats. Rheumatology 2002;41:787-92.
[41] Tuveri M, Generini S, Matucci-Cerinic M, Aloe L. NGF, a useful tool in the treatment of chronic vasculitic ulcers in rheumatoid arthritis. The Lancet 2000;356:1739-40
[42] Micera A, Properzi F, Triaca V, Aloe L. Nerve growth factor antibody exacerbates neuropathological signs of experimental allergic encephalomyelitis in adult Lewis rats. J Neuroimmunol 2000;104:116-23
[43] Nithya M, Suguna L, Rose C. The effect of nerve growth factor on the early responses during the process of wound healing. Biochimica et Biophysica Acta 2003;1620:25-31
[44] Cellini M, Leonetti P, Campos EC. The use of nerve growth factor in herpetic keratitis: a case report. Journal of Medical Case Reports 2007; 1:124-6
[45] Miller LJ, Fischer KA, Goralnick SJ, Litt M, Burleson JA, Albertsen P, Kreutzer DL. Nerve growth factor and chronic prostatitis/chronic pelvic pain syndrome. Urology 2002;59:603-8.
[46] Brodie C. Differential effects of Th1 and Th2 derived cytokines on NGF synthesis by mouse astrocytes. FEBS Letters 1996;394:117-20
[47] Ma D, Wolvers D, Stanisz AM, Bienenstock J. Interleukin-10 and nerve growth factor have reciprokal upregulatory effects on intestinal epithelial cells. Am J Physiol Integr Comp Physiol 2003;284:R1323-9
[48] Micera A, Stampachiacchiere B, Normando EM, Lambiase A, Bonini S, Bonini S. Nerve growth factor modulates toll-like receptor (TLR) 4 and 9 expression in cultured primary VKC conjunctival epithelial cells. Mol Vis. 2009;15:2037-44.
[49] Jiang Y, Chen G, Zheng Y, Lu L, Wu C, Zhang Y, Liu Q, Cao X. TLR4 signaling induces functional nerve growth factor receptor p75NTR on mouse dendritic cells via p38MAPK and NF-kappa B pathways. Mol Immunol. 2008;45:1557-66
[50] Ralainirina N, Brons NH, Ammerlaan W, Hoffmann C, Hentges F, Zimmer J. Mouse natural killer (NK) cells express the nerve growth factor receptor TrkA, which is dynamically regulated. PLoS One. 2010;5:e15053. (1 December 2010, doi: 10.1371/journal.pone.0015053)
[51] Heese K, Fiebich BL, Bauer J, Otten U. NF-κB modulates lipopolysaccharide-induced microglial nerve growth factor expression. GLIA 1998;22:401-7

[52] Caroleo MC, Costa N, Bracci- Laudiero L, Aloe L. Human monocyte/macrophages activate by exposure to LPS overexpress NGF and NGF receptors. J Neuroimmunol 2001;113:193-201

[53] Bayar M, Özer B, Beştaş A, Çeribaşı S, Özercan İ. Effects of Anti-NGF on Apoptosis in Rats with Experimentally Induced Sepsis Model. Turkiye Klinikleri J Med Sci 2010;30: 1127-33

[54] Glaab T, Hoymann HG, Hecht M, Korolewitz R, Tschernig T, Hohlfeld JM, Krug N, Braun A. Effect of anti-nerve growth factor on early and late airway responses in allergic rats. Allergy 2003;58:900-4

[55] Torrents D, Torres R, De Mora F, Vergara P. Antinerve growth factor treatment prevents intestinal dysmotility in Trichinelle spiralis- infected rats. J Pharmacol Exp Ther. 2002;302:659-65

[56] Delafoy L, Raymond F, Doherty AM, Eschalier A, Diop L. Role of nerve growth factor in the trinitrobenzene sulfonic acid- induced colonic hypersensitivity. Pain 2003;105:489-97

[57] Hill JM, Garza HH, Helmy MF, Cook SD, Osborne PA, Johnson EM Jr, Thompson HW, Green LC, O'Callaghan RJ, Gebhardth BM. Nerve growth factor antibody stimulates reactivation of ocular herpes simplex virus type 1 in latently infected rabbits. J Neurovirol 1997;3:206-11

[58] Piedimonte G. Contribution of neuroimmune mechanisms to airway inflammation and remodeling during and after respiratory syncytial virus infection. Pediatr Infect Dis J 2003;22:S66-75

[59] Fainzilber M, Carter BD. From neurotrophins to immunotrophins. EMBO reports 2002;3:1029-34

[60] Kerr JF, Wyllie AH, Currie AR. Apoptosis: a basic biological phenomenon with wide-ranging implications in tissue kinetics. Br J Cancer. 1972;26:239-57.

[61] Elmore S. Apoptosis: a review of programmed cell death. Toxicol Pathol. 2007;35: 495-516.

[62] Buchman TG, Abello PA, Smith EH, Bulkley GB. Induction of heat shock response leads to apoptosis in endothelial cells previously exposed to endotoxin. Am J Physiol. 1993;265: 165-70.

[63] Hotchkiss RS, Swanson PE, Freeman BD, Tinsley KW, Cobb JP, Matuschak GM, Matuschak GM, Buchman TG, Karl IE. Apoptotic cell death in patients with sepsis, shock and multiple organ dysfunction. Crit Care Med 1999;27:1230-51

[64] Roth G, Moser B, Krenn C, Brunner M, Haisjackl M, Almer G, Gerlitz S, Wolner E, Boltz-Nitulescu G, Ankersmit HJ. Susceptibility to programmed cell death in T-lymphocytes from septic patients:a mechanism for lymphopenia and Th2 predominance. Biochem Biophys Res Commun 2003;308:840-6

[65] Jensen LM, Zhang Y, Shooter EM. Steady-state polypeptide modulations associated with nerve growth factor (NGF)-induced terminal differentiation and NGF deprivation-induced apoptosis in human neuroblastoma cells. J Biol Chem. 1992;267:19325-33.

[66] Goldstein RS, Avivi C, Geffen R. In vivo NGF treatment increases proliferation in the primary sympathetic ganglia of chick embryos. Dev Biol. 1997;181:116-20.

[67] Levi-Montalcini R. The nerve growth factor: thirty-five years later. EMBO J. 1987;6:1145-54.

[68] Tanaka A, Wakita U, Kambe N, Iwasaki T, Matsuda H. An autocrine function of nerve growth factor for cell cycle regulation of vascular endothelial cells. Biochem Biophys Res Commun 2004;313:1009-14

[69] Nakagawara A, Arima-Nakagawara M, Scavarda NJ, Azar CG, Cantor AB, Brodeur GM. Association between high levels of expression of the TRK gene and favorable outcome in human neuroblastoma. N Engl J Med. 1993;328:847-54.

[70] Nakagawara A, Arima-Nakagawara M, Azar CG, Scavarda NJ, Brodeur GM. Clinical significance of expression of neurotrophic factors and their receptors in neuroblastoma. Prog Clin Biol Res. 1994;385:155-61.

[71] Cragnolini AB, Volosin M, Huang Y, Friedman WJ. Nerve growth factor induces cell cycle arrest of astrocytes. Dev Neurobiol. 2011;20981. (26 September 2011, doi: 10.1002/dneu.20981)

[72] Ichikawa H, Zhao BR, Kano M, Shimizu Y, Suzuki T, Terayama R, Matsuo S, Sugimoto T. Tunicamycin-induced cell death in the trigeminal ganglion is suppressed by nerve growth factor in the mouse embryo. Cell Mol Neurobiol. 2010;30:461-7.

[73] Kent TA, Quast M, Taglialatela G, Rea C, Wei J, Tao Z, Perez-Polo JR. Effect of NGF treatment on outcome measures in a rat model of middle cerebral artery occlusion. J Neurosci Res 1999;55:357-69

[74] Yang JP, Liu HJ, Yang H, Feng PY. Therapeutic time window for the neuroprotective effects of NGF when administered after focal cerebral ischemia. Neurol Sci. 2011;32:433-41.

[75] Lambiase A, Aloe L, Centofanti M, Parisi V, Mantelli F, Colafrancesco V, Manni GL, Bucci MG, Bonini S, Levi-Montalcini R. Experimental and clinical evidence of neuroprotection by nerve growth factor eye drops: Implications for glaucoma. Proc Natl Acad Sci U S A. 2009;106:13469-74.

[76] Stefanato CM, Yaar M, Bhawan J, Phillips TJ, Kosmadaki MG, Botchkarev V, Gilchrest BA. Modulations of nerve growth factor and bcl-2 in ultraviolet-irradiated human epidermis. J Cutan Pathol 2003;30:351-7

[77] Kawamoto K, Okada T, Kanan Y, Ushio H, Matsumoto M, Matsuda H. Nerve growth factor prevents apoptosis of rat peritoneal mast cells through the trk proto-oncogene receptor. Blood 1995;86:4638-44

[78] Othumpangat S, Gibson LF, Samsell L, Piedimonte G. NGF is an essential survival factor for bronchial epithelial cells during respiratory syncytial virus infection. PLoS One. 2009;4:e6444. (31 July 2009, doi: 10.1371/journal.pone.0006444)

[79] Bellanger C, Dubanet L, Lise MC, Fauchais AL, Bordessoule D, Jauberteau MO, Troutaud D. Endogenous neurotrophins and Trk signaling in diffuse large B cell lymphoma cell lines are involved in sensitivity to rituximab-induced apoptosis. PLoS One. 2011;6:e27213. (4 November 2011, doi: 10.1371/journal.pone.0027213)

[80] Jee D, Lee WK. Inhibitory Effect of intravitreal Injection of Bevacizumab on Nerve Growth Factor. Curr Eye Res. 2011 (31 October 2011, doi: 10.3109/02713683.2011.632108)

[81] Chae CH, Jung SL, An SH, Jung CK, Nam SN, Kim HT. Treadmill exercise suppresses muscle cell apoptosis by increasing nerve growth factor levels and stimulating p-phosphatidylinositol 3-kinase activation in the soleus of diabetic rats. J Physiol Biochem. 2011;67:235-41

Chapter 5

Nicotinamide Phosphoribosyltransferase in Sepsis

Peixin Huang, Ding You Li, Daniel P. Heruth, Li Qin Zhang,
Dmitry N. Grigoryev and Shui Qing Ye

Additional information is available at the end of the chapter

http://dx.doi.org/10.5772/50236

1. Introduction

The word sepsis was derived from the Greek word: sêpsis, which means the state of putrefaction or decay. Sepsis is a potentially deadly medical condition that is characterized by a whole-body inflammatory state, called a systemic inflammatory response syndrome, and the presence of a known or suspected infection. The more critical subsets of sepsis are severe sepsis with acute organ dysfunction, hypoperfusion, or hypotension and septic shock with refractory arterial hypotension despite adequate fluid resuscitation [1, 2]. Because the molecular pathogenesis of sepsis is incompletely understood and its specific and effective therapies are lacking, sepsis is still a major cause of death in intensive-care units worldwide, with mortality rates that range from 20% for sepsis, through 40% for severe sepsis, to over 60% for septic shock [3, 4]. More knowledge of the pathophysiology of sepsis is needed if we are to develop better, more effective interventions to sepsis. It has been increasingly recognized that genetic factors influence individual susceptibility, severity and outcome in sepsis [5, 6]. Identification of new genetic factors in sepsis may hold promise for new mechanistic insights and new therapeutic modalities.

Nicotinamide phosphoribosyltransferase (NAMPT) is emerging as a risk factor in sepsis. NAMPT is a pleiotropic protein. It catalyzes the condensation of nicotinamide with 5-phosphoribosyl-1-pyrophosphate to yield nicotinamide mononucleotide, which is the key step in a salvage pathway of the mammalian NAD biosynthesis[7]. NAMPT was first cloned by Samal et al.[8]and it was originally named pre-B-cell colony enhancing factor (PBEF) because it can promote the maturation of pre-B-cells. NAMPT was also called visfatin because it is an adipokine highly produced by visceral fat and it displayed insulin mimetic functions [9] though the latter claim was disputed in literature. In this chapter, NAMPT and PBEF are used interchangeably in some parts. Jia et al. [10] from University of Toronto, Canada, first reported that NAMPT mRNA in neutrophils from critically ill septic patients was expressed at higher levels than those in controls. Our previous study at Johns Hopkins University, USA, discovered that a susceptible haplotype GC in the promoter of human NAMPT gene had a 4.84-fold higher risk of sepsis while a potential protective haplotype TT had a lower risk of sepsis in a Caucasian patient population [11]. Bajwa et al. [12] from Massachusetts General Hospital, Harvard University, USA, replicated and extended our findings that the NAMPT-1001T>G variant allele and related haplotype were associated with increased odds of developing acute respiratory distress syndrome (ARDS), which is frequently associated with severe sepsis, and increased hazard of intensive care unit mortality among at-risk patients, whereas the -1535C>T (originally labeled as -1543C>T) variant allele and related haplotype are associated with decreased odds of ARDS among patients with septic shock and better outcomes among patients with ARDS. Molecular mechanisms underlying these associations have been actively explored. The first part of this chapter introduces the physiological functions of the NAMPT gene. The second part of this chapter synopsize the clinical investigation and epidemiological studies of NAMPT in sepsis. The third part describes our current understanding of molecular mechanisms underlying NAMPT in sepsis. The final part of this chapter includes a brief summary and some perspectives on exploring *Terra Ignota* of NAMPT in sepsis.

2. Physiological functions of the NAMPT gene

This section briefly introduces the three major functions of the NAMPT: Growth Factor, Cytokine and Nicotinamide phosphoribosyltransferase [13]. Accumulating evidence suggests that NAMPT can function as a growth factor or a cytokine though the underlying molecular mechanisms remain to be established. It is beyond the dispute that NAMPT can function as a Nicotinamide phosphoribosyltransferase.

Growth Factor. Several studies indicate that NAMPT may function as a growth factor. Samal et al.[8] first found that conditional medium from COS7 or PA317 cells transiently expressing human NAMPT can significantly enhance the number of pre-B-cell colonies derived from normal human or mouse bone marrow by at least 70% in the presence of both IL-7 and stem cell factor. Similar observation was obtained using the antibody purified NAMPT protein. Thus, the authors first named this protein as pre-B-cell colony enhancing factor. Van der Veer et al.[14] reported that NAMPT can promote vascular smooth muscle cell maturation. They found that knockdown of endogenous NAMPT increased smooth muscle cell apoptosis and reduced the capacity of synthetic smooth muscle cells to mature to a contractile state. On the other hand, human smooth muscle cells transduced with the NAMPT gene had enhanced survival, an elongated bipolar morphology, and increased levels of h-caldesmon, smoothelin-A, smoothelin-B, and metavinculin. Fukuhara and co-workers [9] proposed NAMPT as a Visfatin, an adipokine produced by visceral fat that can engage and activate the insulin receptor. Although this publication was retracted because of questions regarding the reproducibility of the NAMPT/ insulin receptor interaction from different preparations of recombinant NAMPT protein[15]. Xie et al.[16] found that NAMPT exerts an insulin-like activity as a growth factor for osteoblasts. They used the recombinant human NAMPT provided by Axxora Life Sciences (San Diego, CA, USA) in their experiments. They noticed that the effects of NAMPT such as glucose uptake, proliferation, and type I collagen enhancement in cultured human osteoblast-like cells bore a close resemblance to those of insulin and were inhibited by hydroxy-2-naphthalenylmethylphosphonic acid tris-acetoxymethyl ester, a specific inhibitor of IR tyrosine kinase activity. They also unexpectedly found that NAMPT downregulated osteocalcin secretion from human osteoblast-like cells. These data indicate that the regulation of glucose uptake, proliferation, and type I collagen production by NAMPT in human osteoblasts involves insulin receptor phosphorylation, the same signal transduction pathway used by insulin.

Cytokine. NAMPT may be added to the list of cytokines. The first NAMPT cDNA was screened out using a degenerate oligonucleotide probe designed on the basis of the similarity in the coding sequences of five different cytokines: GM-CSF, IL-2, IL-1β, IL-6 and IL-13, at the signal peptidase processing site though the DNA or protein sequence of NAMPT bears no homology to other known cytokines[8]. Ognjanovic et al.[17] reported that lipopolysaccharide, IL-1β, TNF α and IL-6 all significantly increased the expression of NAMPT in a 4 h treatment of the amniotic epithelial cell line, WISH cells. The addition of dexamethasone to IL-1β and TNFα significantly reduced the response to these cytokines. They concluded that NAMPT is a cytokine expressed in the normal fetal membranes and up-regulated when they are infected. NAMPT expression is up-regulated in a variety of acute and chronic inflammatory diseases including sepsis[10], acute lung injury [11], rheumatoid arthritis [18], inflammatory bowel disease[19], and myocardial infarction [20] and plays a key role in the persistence of inflammation through its capacity to inhibit neutrophil apoptosis[10]. rhNAMPT treatment of WISH cells and fetal membrane explants significantly increased IL-6 and IL-8 gene expression[21]. We also found that an overexpression of NAMPT significantly augmented IL-8 secretion and mRNA expression in A549 cells, a human pulmonary carcinoma type II epithelial cell line and human pulmonary artery endothelial cells. It also significantly augmented IL-1β-mediated cell permeability. The opposite results were obtained with the knockdown of NAMPT expression. NAMPT expression also affected the expression of two other inflammatory cytokines (IL-16 and CCR3 genes) [22, 23]. Hong et al.[24] demonstrated recombinant human NAMPT as a direct rat neutrophil chemotactic factor in *in vitro* studies. They also demonstrated a marked increase in bronchoalveolar lavage leukocytes after the intratracheal injection of rhNAMPT into C57BL/6J mice. Thus, NAMPT behaves like a chemokine.

Nicotinamide phosphoribosyl transferase. The clue that PBEF could be a nicotinamide phosphoribosyl transferase was first obtained by the work of Martin et al.[25] in 2001. They demonstrated that the presence of the *nadV* gene allowed *A. pleuropneumoniae* to utilize nicotinamide mononucleotide as a precursor for NAD biosynthesis, and indicate that the enzyme encoded by this gene is a novel NAMPT. They found that the sequence of nadV gene is homologous to that of human NAMPT, suggesting that mammalian PBEF may also function as a NAMPT. Rongvaux et al.[26] verified that similarly to its microbial counterpart, PBEF is a NAMPT, catalyzing the condensation of nicotinamide with 5-phosphoribosyl-1-pyrophosphate to yield nicotinamide mononucleotide, an intermediate in the biosynthesis of NAD (Figure 1). The role of PBEF as a NAMPT was further confirmed by showing that the mouse gene was able to confer the ability to grow in the absence of NAD to a NAMPT-defective bacterial strain. Study by Revollo et al.[7] demonstrated that NAMPT catalyzes a rate-limiting step in a salvage pathway of the mammalian NAD biosynthesis. Van der Veer et al.[27] proved that it is due to the enhanced NAMPT activity of PBEF that cellular lifespan of human primary smooth muscle cells, human clonal smooth muscle cells, and fibroblasts derived from a patient with Hutchinson-Gilford progeria syndrome can be lengthened. Recent work by Revollo et al [33] revealed that NAMPT regulates insulin secretion in beta cells as a systemic NAD biosynthetic enzyme.

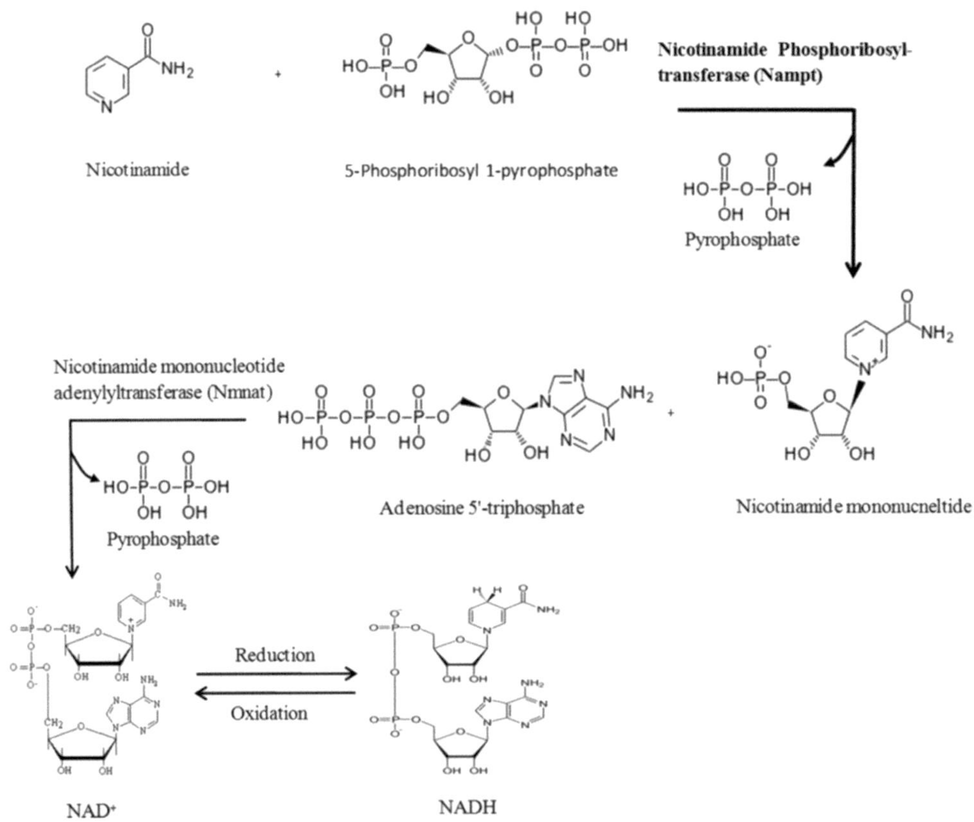

Figure 1. Mammalian salvage pathway of NAD⁺ synthesis mediated by nicotinamide phosphoribosyltransferase. Nicotinamide, either derived from the degradation of NAD^+ by NAD^+ consuming enzymes or provided in the diet, is condensed with 5-phosphoribosyl-1-pyrophosphate to yield nicotinamide mononucleotide under the catalysis of nicotinamide phosphoribosyltransferase. Nicotinamide mononucleotide is then adenylylated to form NAD^+, by Nicotinamide mononucleotide adenylyltransferase. NAD^+ and NADH can be interconverted by a reduction and a oxidation reaction, respectively. This figure is copied from Zhang et al. (7).

Because the salvage pathway of NAD synthesis is much more efficient and quicker one than that of de novo NAD synthesis, it is conceivable that NAMPT plays an important role in varieties of physiological processes in life via the synthesis of NAD. NAD is now regarded as a universal energy- and signal-carrying molecule[28, 29]. Recent research has unraveled an unexpectedly wide array of signaling pathways that involve nicotinamide adenine dinucleotide (NAD) and its phosphorylated form, NADP. NAD serves as substrate for protein modification including protein deacetylation and mono- and poly-ADP-ribosylation. Both NAD and NADP represent precursors of intracellular calcium-mobilizing molecules. It is now well accepted that NAD (P)-mediated signal transduction does not merely regulate metabolic pathways but might hold a key position in the control of fundamental cellular processes. In mammals, it has been shown recently that an NAD-dependent protein deacetylase, silent information regulator (SIR) T1/2, plays important roles in a variety of biological processes, such as stress and cytokine responses[30], by deacetylating transcriptional regulators. Endogenous mono-ADP-ribosylation in higher eukaryotes appears to modulate the immune response, cell adhesion, signal, and energy metabolism[31]. Recently, defensin-1, an antimicrobial arginine-rich protein secreted by immune cells, was demonstrated to lose its antimicrobial effect after its mono-ADP-ribosylation. Poly-ADP-ribosylation of proteins such as NFkB by poly-ADP-ribose polymerase can trigger the release of apoptosis-inducing factor from mitochondria and therefore effectively mediate apoptosis. Gerth et al.[32] demonstrated that NAD and ADP-ribose, generated from NAD by CD38, an NAD-glycohydrolase, induce the activation of a Ca^{2+} channel through a pathway that involves Ca^{2+} influx in human monocytes. Ca^{2+} ions play a critical role in variety of monocyte functions such as chemotaxis and production of cytokine (TNFα)[33]. Increased intracellular calcium in human monocyte-derived macrophages *in vitro* by loading with the basic calcium phosphate microcrystals was associated with secretion of proinflammatory cytokines (TNFα, IL-1β, and IL-8) capable of activating cultured endothelial cells and promoting capture of flowing leukocytes under shear flow[34].

3. Role of NAMPT in Sepsis

Because of its pleiotropic functions, NAMPT has been implicated in various human diseases[13] including sepsis. Increasing evidence indicates that NAMPT is a risk factor in sepsis. Jia et al. [10] determined the expression of PBEF in neutrophils harvested from 16 critically ill septic patients in an intensive care unit. They found that neutrophils from these patients showed marked expression of PBEF mRNA. PBEF expression was significantly greater in neutrophils from septic patients than in resting neutrophils or LPS-stimulated neutrophils from healthy volunteers. Lee et al. [35] determined the clinical correlates for elevated plasma PBEF upon intensive care unit admission for severe sepsis and the usefulness of NAMPT to predict sepsis mortality. Plasma collected within 24 h of intensive care unit admission was measured for NAMPT concentrations by enzyme-linked immunosorbent assay. They reported that elevated PBEF levels significantly correlated with higher Acute Physiology and Chronic Health Evaluation III scores (R(2) = 0.08, P = .003). The higher

Acute Physiology and Chronic Health Evaluation III score indicates more severe diseased status. Non-survivors had higher PBEF levels than survivors (2.53 ng/mL; interquartile range [IQR], 1.07-8.16 vs 1.44 ng/mL; IQR, 0.84-2.81; P = .02). They concluded that NAMPT was associated with sepsis mortality mainly due to its association with greater severity of illness on intensive care unit admission. Cekmez et al. [36] found that plasma NAMPT level was significantly higher in septic infants than in healthy ones. There was a positive correlation between NAMPT and other markers (white blood cells, *C-reactive protein*, procalcitonin and IL-6) for sepsis. A cut-off value of 10 ng/mL for NAMPT showed 92% sensitivity and 94% specificity in the diagnosis of sepsis. Thus, the authors proposed that NAMPT could be used as a diagnostic marker similar to *C-reactive protein*, procalcitonin and IL-6 in neonatal sepsis.

In our previous genetic epidemiological study [11], we determined the frequencies of minor alleles, genotypes and haplotypes of two human NAMPT gene promoter SNPs [-1001T>G and -1535C>T (originally labeled as -1543C>T)] in Caucasian septic patients and Caucasian healthy subjects. We found that the frequency of the minor G allele of the SNP -1001T>G was significantly higher (23%) in septic patients than in healthy subjects (12%, p=0.01). Similarly, the frequency of its genotype GT was significantly higher (44%) in septic patients than in healthy subjects (20%, p=0.004). The haplotype-weighted analysis of these two SNPs indicated that a susceptible haplotype GC had a 4.84-fold higher risk of sepsis while a potential protective haplotype TT had a lowest risk of sepsis in a Caucasian patient population among four haplotypes: GC, GT, TC and TT. Our findings were validated and extended in a different patient cohort by Bajwa et al. [12]. They genotyped the NAMPT T-1001G and C-1543T polymorphisms in 375 patients with ARDS, a frequent consequence of sepsis, and 787 patients at risk for developing ARDS. It was found that among the 397 patients with sepsis syndrome, the odds of developing ARDS were significantly increased by presence of T-1001G and among the 561 patients with septic shock, the odds of developing ARDS for patients with C-1543T were significantly decreased. Overall, the NAMPT T-1001G variant allele and related haplotype are associated with increased odds of developing ARDS and increased hazard of intensive care unit mortality among at-risk patients, whereas the C-1543T variant allele and related haplotype are associated with decreased odds of ARDS among patients with septic shock and better outcomes among patients with ARDS. These results support that NAMPT is a genetic risk factor for sepsis.

4. Molecular Mechanisms of NAMPT in Sepsis

Although the role of NAMPT in sepsis is still incompletely understood, accumulating evidence indicates that at least the following molecular mechanisms may in part underlie NAMPT in sepsis (Figure 2).

Augment expressions of other inflammatory cytokines. Sepsis is also known as a systemic inflammatory response syndrome caused by the body's response to infection [1]. Systemic inflammation is a hallmark of sepsis. During the early stage or mild inflammatory response phase of sepsis, a controlled production of proinflammatory cytokines triggers beneficial inflammatory responses to confine the infection and tissue damage. However, the protracted, excessive production of inflammatory cytokines causes capillary leakage, tissue

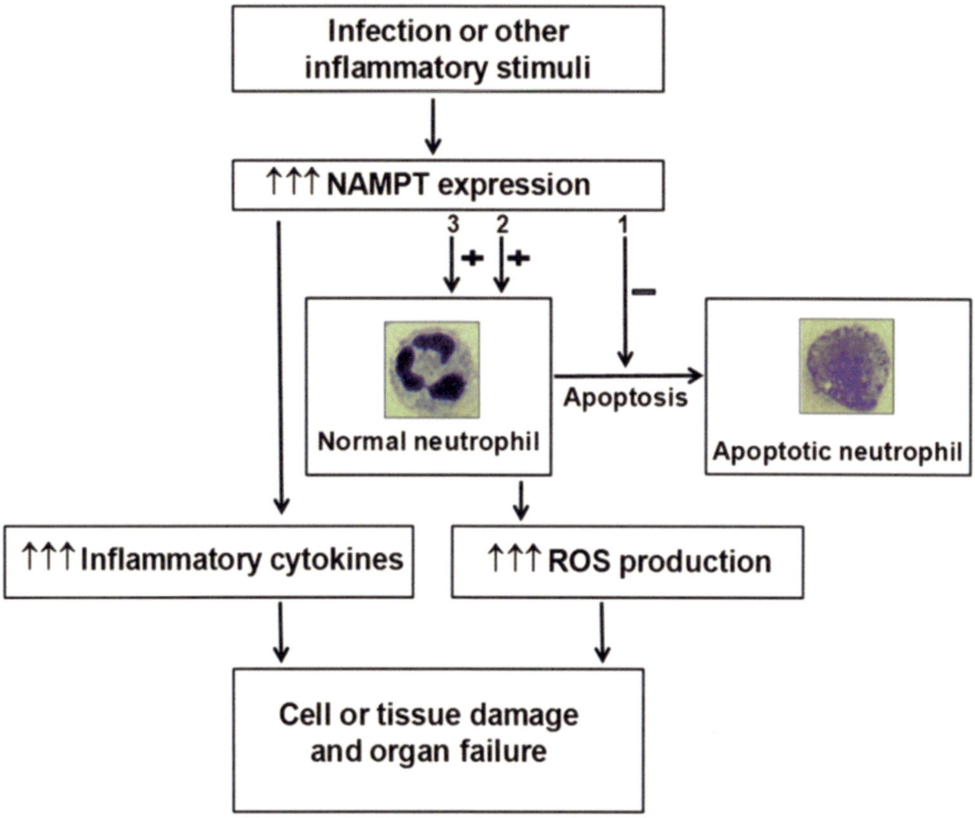

Figure 2. Working mechanisms underlying NAMPT in the pathogenesis of sepsis. During sepsis or prelude to sepsis, bacterial infection or other inflammatory stimuli excessively augment NAMPT expression, which in turn induces an excessive production of other inflammatory cytokines such as TNFα and IL1-β. Dysregulated NAMPT also affects the number and function of neutrophils in one of three ways: 1. inhibiting neutrophills' apoptosis and thus prolonging neutrophil's survival; 2. priming neutrophils for increased ROS generation; 3. acting as a chemotactic factor to neutrophils. Prolonged and increased neutrophils can lead to excessive ROS production. Both excessive expression of inflammatory cytokines and excessive generation of ROS contribute to unwanted side effects such as cell or tissue damage and organ failure in sepsis.

injury, and lethal multiple organ failure in severe sepsis [37]. NAMPT was considered as an inflammatory cytokine [21]. Elevated plasma NAMPT level was associated with sepsis mortality [10, 35]. Elevated NAMPT may augment expressions of other inflammatory cytokines and thus aggravate inflammation, which in part contribute to increased severity and mortality in patients with sepsis.

Besides sepsis, NAMPT expression is up-regulated in a variety of acute and chronic inflammatory diseases including acute lung injury, inflammatory bowel disease, myocardial infarction, and rheumatoid arthritis[13]. It have been demonstrated *in vitro*, that other inflammatory stimuli can increase the expression of NAMPT gene. Ognjanovic et al.[17] reported that lipopolysaccharide, IL-1β, TNF α and IL-6 all significantly increased the expression of NAMPT in a 4 h treatment of the amniotic epithelial cell line, WISH cells. The addition of dexamethasone significantly reduced the response to IL-1β and TNFα. They concluded that NAMPT is expressed in the normal fetal membranes and up-regulated when they are infected. NAMPT can also stimulate the expression of other inflammatory cytokines. The rhNAMPT treatment of WISH cells and fetal membrane explants significantly increased IL-6 and IL-8 gene expression[21]. We also found that an overexpression of NAMPT significantly augmented IL-8 secretion and mRNA expression in both human pulmonary carcinoma type II epithelial cell line (A549) and human pulmonary artery endothelial cells. It also significantly augmented IL-1β-mediated cell permeability. The opposite results were obtained with the knockdown of NAMPT expression. NAMPT expression also affected the expression of two other inflammatory cytokines (IL-16 and CCR3 genes)[23, 38]. Our further investigation found that PBEF stimulated expression of IL-8, IL-16, and CCR3 via its non-enzymatic activity. This effect is AP-1-dependent, in part via the p38 MAPK pathway and the JNK pathway[22]. From these results, it can be reasoned that infection in sepsis can induce the expression of NAMPT gene, which in turn stimulate the expression of other inflammatory cytokines, thus aggravating inflammation in sepsis.

Increase number of activated neutrophils. Neutrophils play important roles in host defense against all classes of infectious agents but, paradoxically, they are also involved in the pathology of various inflammatory conditions. Although destruction of infectious agents by neutrophils occurs intracellularly, release of cytotoxic molecules into the extracellular milieu can damage body tissues. Thus, neutrophils is a double-edged sword [39]. Neutrophilia is a prominent feature in sepsis and many lines of evidence link activated neutrophils to the organ injury of sepsis [40]. Jia et al. [10] reported that NAMPT plays a requisite role in the delayed neutrophil apoptosis of clinical and experimental sepsis. They found that transcription of the NAMPT gene is increased in neutrophils from septic patients; prevention of NAMPT translation through the use of an antisense oligonucleotide largely restores the normal kinetics of apoptosis. Moreover, the incubation of quiescent neutrophils from healthy volunteers with recombinant NAMPT results in dose-dependent inhibition of apoptosis, and antisense NAMPT prevents the inhibition of apoptosis that results from exposure to LPS or to a variety of host-derived inflammatory cytokines. They postulated that this prolonged survival of activated neutrophils may be linked to sustained inflammation and the organ injury of sepsis.

The potent antimicrobial activity by neutrophils is effected through proteolytic enzymes and the generation of reactive oxygen species (ROS). ROS released by neutrophils are also implicated in the bystander tissue injury that accompanies an inflammatory response. Malam et al. [41] demonstrated that NAMPT can prime neutrophils for increased ROS generation through the NADPH oxidase. NAMPT promoted membrane translocation of cytosolic NADPH oxidase subunits p40 and p47, but not p67, induced p40 phosphorylation on Thr154, and activated the small GTPase Rac. Priming, translocation, and phosphorylation were dependent on activation of p38 and ERK MAPKs, but not of PI3K. Priming by NAMPT occurred independently of its NAD-generating capacity because neither nicotinamide mononucleotide nor NAD could recapitulate the effects, and a specific inhibitor of NAMPT, APO-866, could not inhibit priming. This represents another molecular mechanism underlying NAMPT in the pathogenesis of sepsis, in which increased expression of NAMPT contributes to tissue damage by priming neutrophils to produce excessive ROS.

In a different study, Hong et al. [24] demonstrated recombinant human NAMPT as a direct rat neutrophil chemotactic factor in in vitro studies. They also demonstrated a marked increase in bronchoalveolar lavage leukocytes after the intratracheal injection of rhNAMPT into C57BL/6J mice in an acute lung injury model. Organ failure is frequently associated with severe sepsis. Chemoattractant property of NAMPT may also in part account for its role of increasing or activating neutrophils in sepsis.

5. Summary and perspective

Increasing evidence suggest that NAMPT is a risk factor in sepsis. NAMPT is highly up-regulated in sepsis and it has been proposed as a diagnostic marker in neonatal sepsis. It was associated with the severity and mortality of patients with sepsis. Genetic epidemiological studies found that a susceptible haplotype GC in the promoter of human NAMPT gene had a 4.84-fold higher risk of sepsis while a potential protective haplotype TT had a lower risk of sepsis in a Caucasian patient population. Those findings indicate that NAMPT is a potential genetic marker in sepsis. A few molecular mechanisms may underlie role of dysregulated NAMPT in the pathogenesis of sepsis. Infection in sepsis can induce the expression of NAMPT gene, which in turn stimulate the expression of other inflammatory cytokines, thus aggravate inflammation in sepsis. Prolonged survival of activated neutrophils by NAMPT via its inhibition of neutrophil apoptosis may be linked to sustained inflammation and the organ injury during sepsis. NAMPT can act as a chemoattractant to neutrophils. Increased expression of NAMPT in sepsis may also contribute to tissue damage by priming neutrophils to produce excessive ROS.

It remains to be fully elucidated that role of NAMPT in sepsis may be a "double-edged sword". Although accumulated evidence as synopsized in this chapter and summarized in the above paragraph indicates that excessive up-regulation of NAMPT expression in sepsis contributes to excessive inflammation and tissue damage in sepsis, emerging evidence also suggests that a modest increase of NAMPT expression in early phase may be of beneficial value. A recent study by Liu et al. [42] suggested that TLR signaling might increase cellular NAD+ by inducing Nampt expression, which could thereby provide substrate for SIRT1 deacetylase activity. SIRT1 deacetylates RelA/p65 lysine 310 and nucleosomal histone H4 lysine 16 to promote termination of NFκB-dependent transcription, which results in the attenuation of inflammatory response. Thus, Nampt activity promotes endotoxin tolerance.

Therapeutic potential of NAMPT inhibitions to sepsis has not been pursued clinically though several basic and translational studies pointed to the possibility. Jia et al. [10] demonstrated that the NAMPT antisense oligonucleotide prevented the LPS or other inflammatory cytokines' induced neutrophil apoptosis. In neutrophils of patients with sepsis, addition of PBEF antisense oligonucleotide resulted in a greater than twofold increase in rates of apoptosis. This study indicated that the antisense oligonucleotide to NAMPT could effectively inhibit PBEF expression. Ye et al. [11] reported a successful knockdown of NAMPT expression by more than 70% in human pulmonary vascular endothelial cells using three NAMPT stealth siRNAs in combination or individually. Our group also showed that a NAMPT antibody can block the function of NAMPT in a mouse model [24]. Several chemical inhibitors of NAMPT such as FK866 (also called APO866 or WK175, (E)-N-[4-(1-benzoylpiperidin-4-yl) butyl]-3-(pyridin-3-yl)) and related compounds have been tested to inhibit tumor cell growth [43] and in clinical trials as an anticancer agent [44]. Montecucco et al [45] recently showed that treatment with FK866 reduced myocardial infarct size, neutrophil infiltration and ROS generation within infarcted hearts in vivo in a mouse model of ischemia and reperfusion. It is of interest to explore the therapeutic potential of all these NAMPT inhibitory reagents to sepsis in the clinical setting.

It is anticipated that further elucidation of the role and mechanisms of NAMPT in sepsis will enhance our understanding of molecular pathogenesis underlying NAMPT in sepsis and lead to the development of the NAMPT based strategy and management of sepsis in the future.

Author details

Peixin Huang, Ding You Li, Daniel P. Heruth,
Li Qin Zhang, Dmitry N. Grigoryev and Shui Qing Ye
Department of Pediatrics, Children's Mercy Hospitals and Clinics,
University of Missouri School of Medicine, Kansas City, USA

Shui Qing Ye
Department of Biomedical and Health Informatics, Children's Mercy Hospitals and Clinics,
University of Missouri School of Medicine, Kansas City, USA

Acknowledgement

Some cited studies in this chapter were in part supported by NIH grants (R01HL080042 and RO1 HL080042-S1, SQY) as well as the start-up funds of Children's Mercy Hospitals and Clinics, University of Missouri (SQY).

6. References

[1] Levy MM, Fink MP, Marshall JC, Abraham E, Angus D, Cook D, Cohen J, Opal SM, Vincent JL, Ramsay G: 2001 SCCM/ESICM/ACCP/ATS/SIS International Sepsis Definitions Conference. *Crit Care Med* 2003, 31(4):1250-1256.

[2] Bone RC, Balk RA, Cerra FB, Dellinger RP, Fein AM, Knaus WA, Schein RM, Sibbald WJ: Definitions for sepsis and organ failure and guidelines for the use of innovative therapies in sepsis. The ACCP/SCCM Consensus Conference Committee. American

College of Chest Physicians/Society of Critical Care Medicine. *Chest* 1992, 101(6):1644-1655.

[3] Martin GS, Mannino DM, Eaton S, Moss M: The epidemiology of sepsis in the United States from 1979 through 2000. *N Engl J Med* 2003, 348(16):1546-1554.

[4] Dombrovskiy VY, Martin AA, Sunderram J, Paz HL: Rapid increase in hospitalization and mortality rates for severe sepsis in the United States: a trend analysis from 1993 to 2003. *Crit Care Med* 2007, 35(5):1244-1250.

[5] Wunderink RG, Waterer GW: Genetics of sepsis and pneumonia. *Curr Opin Crit Care* 2003, 9(5):384-389.

[6] Del Vecchio A, Laforgia N, Capasso M, Iolascon A, Latini G: The role of molecular genetics in the pathogenesis and diagnosis of neonatal sepsis. *Clin Perinatol* 2004, 31(1):53-67.

[7] Revollo JR, Grimm AA, Imai S: The NAD biosynthesis pathway mediated by nicotinamide phosphoribosyltransferase regulates Sir2 activity in mammalian cells. *J Biol Chem* 2004, 279(49):50754-50763.

[8] Samal B, Sun Y, Stearns G, Xie C, Suggs S, McNiece I: Cloning and characterization of the cDNA encoding a novel human pre-B-cell colony-enhancing factor. *Mol Cell Biol* 1994, 14(2):1431-1437.

[9] Fukuhara A, Matsuda M, Nishizawa M, Segawa K, Tanaka M, Kishimoto K, Matsuki Y, Murakami M, Ichisaka T, Murakami H *et al*: Visfatin: a protein secreted by visceral fat that mimics the effects of insulin. *Science* 2005, 307(5708):426-430.

[10] Jia SH, Li Y, Parodo J, Kapus A, Fan L, Rotstein OD, Marshall JC: Pre-B cell colony-enhancing factor inhibits neutrophil apoptosis in experimental inflammation and clinical sepsis. *J Clin Invest* 2004, 113(9):1318-1327.

[11] Ye SQ, Simon BA, Maloney JP, Zambelli-Weiner A, Gao L, Grant A, Easley RB, McVerry BJ, Tuder RM, Standiford T *et al*: Pre-B-cell colony-enhancing factor as a potential novel biomarker in acute lung injury. *Am J Respir Crit Care Med* 2005, 171(4):361-370.

[12] Bajwa EK, Yu CL, Gong MN, Thompson BT, Christiani DC: Pre-B-cell colony-enhancing factor gene polymorphisms and risk of acute respiratory distress syndrome. *Crit Care Med* 2007, 35(5):1290-1295.

[13] Zhang LQ, Heruth DP, Ye SQ: Nicotinamide Phosphoribosyltransferase in Human Diseases. *J Bioanal Biomed* 2011, 3:13-25.

[14] van der Veer E, Nong Z, O'Neil C, Urquhart B, Freeman D, Pickering JG: Pre-B-cell colony-enhancing factor regulates NAD+-dependent protein deacetylase activity and promotes vascular smooth muscle cell maturation. *Circ Res* 2005, 97(1):25-34.

[15] Fukuhara A, Matsuda M, Nishizawa M, Segawa K, Tanaka M, Kishimoto K, Matsuki Y, Murakami M, Ichisaka T, Murakami H *et al*: Retraction. *Science* 2007, 318(5850):565.

[16] Xie H, Tang SY, Luo XH, Huang J, Cui RR, Yuan LQ, Zhou HD, Wu XP, Liao EY: Insulin-like effects of visfatin on human osteoblasts. *Calcif Tissue Int* 2007, 80(3):201-210.

[17] Ognjanovic S, Bao S, Yamamoto SY, Garibay-Tupas J, Samal B, Bryant-Greenwood GD: Genomic organization of the gene coding for human pre-B-cell colony enhancing factor and expression in human fetal membranes. *J Mol Endocrinol* 2001, 26(2):107-117.

[18] Brentano F, Schorr O, Ospelt C, Stanczyk J, Gay RE, Gay S, Kyburz D: Pre-B cell colony-enhancing factor/visfatin, a new marker of inflammation in rheumatoid arthritis with proinflammatory and matrix-degrading activities. *Arthritis Rheum* 2007, 56(9):2829-2839.

[19] Tilg H, Moschen AR: Role of adiponectin and PBEF/visfatin as regulators of inflammation: involvement in obesity-associated diseases. *Clin Sci (Lond)* 2008, 114(4):275-288.

[20] Dahl TB, Yndestad A, Skjelland M, Oie E, Dahl A, Michelsen A, Damas JK, Tunheim SH, Ueland T, Smith C *et al*: Increased expression of visfatin in macrophages of human unstable carotid and coronary atherosclerosis: possible role in inflammation and plaque destabilization. *Circulation* 2007, 115(8):972-980.

[21] Ognjanovic S, Bryant-Greenwood GD: Pre-B-cell colony-enhancing factor, a novel cytokine of human fetal membranes. *Am J Obstet Gynecol* 2002, 187(4):1051-1058.

[22] Liu P, Li H, Cepeda J, Xia Y, Kempf JA, Ye H, Zhang LQ, Ye SQ: Regulation of inflammatory cytokine expression in pulmonary epithelial cells by pre-B-cell colony-enhancing factor via a nonenzymatic and AP-1-dependent mechanism. *J Biol Chem* 2009, 284(40):27344-27351.

[23] Li H, Liu P, Cepeda J, Fang D, Easley RB, Simon BA, Zhang LQ, Ye SQ: Augmentation of Pulmonary Epithelial Cell IL-8 Expression and Permeability by Pre-B-cell Colony Enhancing Factor. *J Inflamm (Lond)* 2008, 5:15.

[24] Hong SB, Huang Y, Moreno-Vinasco L, Sammani S, Moitra J, Barnard JW, Ma SF, Mirzapoiazova T, Evenoski C, Reeves RR *et al*: Essential role of pre-B-cell colony enhancing factor in ventilator-induced lung injury. *Am J Respir Crit Care Med* 2008, 178(6):605-617.

[25] Martin PR, Shea RJ, Mulks MH: Identification of a plasmid-encoded gene from Haemophilus ducreyi which confers NAD independence. *J Bacteriol* 2001, 183(4):1168-1174.

[26] Rongvaux A, Shea RJ, Mulks MH, Gigot D, Urbain J, Leo O, Andris F: Pre-B-cell colony-enhancing factor, whose expression is up-regulated in activated lymphocytes, is a nicotinamide phosphoribosyltransferase, a cytosolic enzyme involved in NAD biosynthesis. *Eur J Immunol* 2002, 32(11):3225-3234.

[27] van der Veer E, Ho C, O'Neil C, Barbosa N, Scott R, Cregan SP, Pickering JG: Extension of human cell lifespan by nicotinamide phosphoribosyltransferase. *J Biol Chem* 2007, 282(15):10841-10845.

[28] Berger F, Ramirez-Hernandez MH, Ziegler M: The new life of a centenarian: signalling functions of NAD(P). *Trends Biochem Sci* 2004, 29(3):111-118.

[29] Ziegler M: New functions of a long-known molecule. Emerging roles of NAD in cellular signaling. *Eur J Biochem* 2000, 267(6):1550-1564.

[30] Yeung F, Hoberg JE, Ramsey CS, Keller MD, Jones DR, Frye RA, Mayo MW: Modulation of NF-kappaB-dependent transcription and cell survival by the SIRT1 deacetylase. *EMBO J* 2004, 23(12):2369-2380.
[31] Corda D, Di Girolamo M: Functional aspects of protein mono-ADP-ribosylation. *EMBO J* 2003, 22(9):1953-1958.
[32] Gerth A, Nieber K, Oppenheimer NJ, Hauschildt S: Extracellular NAD+ regulates intracellular free calcium concentration in human monocytes. *Biochem J* 2004, 382(Pt 3):849-856.
[33] MacIntyre JP, Pope BL: The involvement of protein kinase C, calcium, and 5-lipoxygenase in the production of tumor necrosis factor by a cloned interleukin-3 dependent cell line with natural cytotoxic activity. *Int J Immunopharmacol* 1991, 13(2-3):175-184.
[34] Nadra I, Mason JC, Philippidis P, Florey O, Smythe CD, McCarthy GM, Landis RC, Haskard DO: Proinflammatory activation of macrophages by basic calcium phosphate crystals via protein kinase C and MAP kinase pathways: a vicious cycle of inflammation and arterial calcification? *Circ Res* 2005, 96(12):1248-1256.
[35] Lee KA, Gong MN: Pre-B-cell colony-enhancing factor and its clinical correlates with acute lung injury and sepsis. *Chest* 2011, 140(2):382-390.
[36] Cekmez F, Canpolat FE, Cetinkaya M, Aydinoz S, Aydemir G, Karademir F, Ipcioglu OM, Sarici SU: Diagnostic value of resistin and visfatin, in comparison with C-reactive protein, procalcitonin and interleukin-6 in neonatal sepsis. *Eur Cytokine Netw* 2011, 22(2):113-117.
[37] Cai B, Deitch EA, Ulloa L: Novel insights for systemic inflammation in sepsis and hemorrhage. *Mediators Inflamm* 2010, 2010:642462.
[38] Liu P, Li H, Cepeda J, Zhang LQ, Cui X, Garcia JG, Ye SQ: Critical role of PBEF expression in pulmonary cell inflammation and permeability. *Cell Biol Int* 2009, 33(1):19-30.
[39] Smith JA: Neutrophils, host defense, and inflammation: a double-edged sword. *J Leukoc Biol* 1994, 56(6):672-686.
[40] Brown KA, Brain SD, Pearson JD, Edgeworth JD, Lewis SM, Treacher DF: Neutrophils in development of multiple organ failure in sepsis. *Lancet* 2006, 368(9530):157-169.
[41] Malam Z, Parodo J, Waheed F, Szaszi K, Kapus A, Marshall JC: Pre-B cell colony-enhancing factor (PBEF/Nampt/visfatin) primes neutrophils for augmented respiratory burst activity through partial assembly of the NADPH oxidase. *J Immunol* 2011, 186(11):6474-6484.
[42] Liu TF, Yoza BK, El Gazzar M, Vachharajani VT, McCall CE: NAD+-dependent SIRT1 deacetylase participates in epigenetic reprogramming during endotoxin tolerance. *J Biol Chem* 2011, 286(11):9856-9864.
[43] Hasmann M, Schemainda I: FK866, a highly specific noncompetitive inhibitor of nicotinamide phosphoribosyltransferase, represents a novel mechanism for induction of tumor cell apoptosis. *Cancer Res* 2003, 63(21):7436-7442.

[44] Holen K, Saltz LB, Hollywood E, Burk K, Hanauske AR: The pharmacokinetics, toxicities, and biologic effects of FK866, a nicotinamide adenine dinucleotide biosynthesis inhibitor. *Invest New Drugs* 2008, 26(1):45-51.
[45] Montecucco F, Bauer I, Braunersreuther V, Bruzzone S, Akhmedov A, Luscher TF, Speer T, Poggi A, Mannino E, Pelli G *et al*: Inhibition of nicotinamide phosphoribosyltransferase (Nampt) reduces neutrophil-mediated injury in myocardial infarction. *Antioxid Redox Signal* 2012.

Chapter 6

Neural Reflex Control of Inflammation During Sepsis Syndromes

Ricardo Fernandez and Claudio Acuña-Castillo

Additional information is available at the end of the chapter

http://dx.doi.org/10.5772/50283

1. Introduction

"Healthy organs behave as 'biological oscillators', which couple to one another, and this orderly coupling is maintained through a communication network, including neural, humoral, and cytokine components" (Godin & Buchman, 1996). The nervous system –acting through the autonomic nervous system (ANS)– coordinates the fine-tuning of cardiorespiratory interplay, to maintain an appropriate oxygen delivery to the tissues (Abboud & Thames, 1983; Eyzaguirre *et al.*, 1983). Autonomic (sympathetic-parasympathetic) balance is maintained by several reflex arcs, like arterial baroreflexes (Kirchheim, 1976), central chemoreflexes, peripheral arterial chemoreflexes, and pulmonary stretch reflexes (Liljestrand, 1958). These reflexes represent the major components of blood pressure and breathing regulation. Therefore, the interactions among these reflexes are of special clinical interest, since the overactivity of a single reflex, occurring pathophysiologically in several disorders, can lead to the suppression of opposite reflex responses (Schmidt *et al.*, 2001).

Sepsis syndromes (SS), which include systemic inflammatory response syndrome (SIRS) and its consequences, severe sepsis and septic shock, involve many pathological processes like systemic inflammation, coagulopathies, hemodynamic abnormalities, and multiple organ dysfunction syndrome (MODS) (Riedemann *et al.*, 2003). The progression of MODS associated to systemic inflammation is mainly due to an uncontrolled release of pro-inflammatory mediators, which damage parenchymatous organs. Additionally, sepsis activates and/or depress numerous other systems within the body, including neural, hormonal, and metabolic pathways (Carre & Singer, 2008; Singer *et al.*, 2004). Thus, systemic inflammation would initiates disruption of communication and uncoupling, and subsequent MODS would reflects the progressive uncoupling of 'biological oscillators' that can become irremediable.

Increasing evidences here summarized shown that a particular neural reflection, the carotid body chemoreflexes, not only serves as a chemoreceptor for respiratory reflex responses, as traditionally accepted, but also as a sensor for the immune status, as modulator of autonomic balance tending to coordinate cardiorespiratory interplay, devoted to maintain oxygen homeostasis in different pathologies, and as a protective factor during sepsis and MODS.

2. Sepsis syndromes prevalence and current therapies

Sepsis is defined as "the systemic inflammatory response that occurs during infection" (Bone *et al.*, 1992). It involves the evidence of infection and two or more of the following conditions: fever or hypothermia, tachycardia, tachypnea or a respiratory frequency resulting in an arterial PCO_2 below 32 mm Hg, and altered white blood cells count; *severe sepsis*, sepsis associated with organ dysfunction, hypoperfusion or hypotension including lactic acidosis, oliguria, or acute alteration in mental state; *septic shock*, sepsis-induced hypotension despite adequate fluid resuscitation, and sustained perfusion abnormalities; and *multiple organ dysfunction syndrome (MODS)*, by the presence of altered organ function in an acutely ill patient such that homeostasis cannot be maintained without intervention (Riedemann *et al.*, 2003).

Significant demographic variation exists in the risk of developing sepsis. For example, from the standpoint of gender, the incidence of sepsis is higher in men, and the mean age at which men develop sepsis is younger. Case fatality rates also increase with age (Martin *et al.*, 2006). The overall burden of severe sepsis is also increasing, in terms of both the number of patients who develop the syndrome and the extent and intensity of care that they require (Angus *et al.*, 2001). Sepsis also poses a significant burden of disease in pediatric patients, where the incidence is highest in infants, mainly in children younger than one year of age (Watson & Carcillo, 2005). Maternal sepsis and neonatal sepsis are of particular concern. Maternal sepsis is responsible for at least 75,000 deaths annually, disproportionately affecting low-income countries (van Dillen *et al.*, 2010). In the United States, studies of neonatal sepsis have documented rates as high as 170 cases per 1000 live births (Thaver & Zaidi, 2009). The average costs per case are US$22,100. Costs are higher in infants, non-survivors, intensive care unit patients, surgical patients, and patients with more organ failure. The incidence was projected to increase by 1.5% per annum (Angus *et al.*, 2001). The international costs associated with sepsis and its management are reviewed in Chalupka & Talmor (2012).

Instead of many efforts and significant advances in maintaining therapies, SS and MODS, are the main cause of death between critical care patients (Martin *et al.*, 2003). Increased morbi-mortality associated to SS is due to the absence of a really effective therapy (Riedemann *et al.*, 2003). Thus, the knowledge of molecular mechanisms and pathophysiology of sepsis help us to improve current therapies (for a Review see Barochia *et al.*, 2010) and to identify new pharmacological therapeutic targets.

Treatments of sepsis and septic shock involves antibiotic administration, intravenous fluids (crystalloids or colloids), vasopressors and/or inotropes (adrenergic agents), packed red blood cells (PRBC) transfusions, and corticosteroids (Barochia *et al.*, 2010). Sepsis care bundles increase patients' survival. Numerous studies have demonstrated improved outcomes in life-threatening infections with early administration of appropriate antibiotics. Hemodynamic support with fluids and vasopressors is as important as antibiotic in reducing mortality (Natanson *et al.*, 1990), but there are great differences among different patient populations. A considerable variation in the ranges of central venous pressure and mean arterial pressure prompted physicians to suggest that "*the usage should be individualized to different patients, based on their own underlying medical conditions*" (Perel, 2008).

Administration of PRBC decreases inotropes use (Nguyen *et al.*, 2007), but the efficacy of administration in patients with sepsis is unclear. The usage of low-dose corticosteroids is variable between patient populations. However, as questions persist regarding the risk and benefits of these therapies for sepsis, they continue to undergo investigation (Misset *et al.*, 2010). Although the use of these agents may be beneficial for some septic patients, the Surviving Sepsis Campaign guidelines (Dellinger *et al.*, 2004) gave a weak recommendation for use these therapies, even the inclusion of some patients, until the knowledge of individual components that could modify the expected results. It is clear that the course of sepsis and therapies outcomes depend largely from host predisposition factors and response.

The serial evaluation of the SOFA score helps to predict outcome in critically ill patients. SOFA score can help assess organ dysfunction or failure over time and are useful to evaluate morbidity and mortality, by evaluating respiratory, coagulation, liver, cardiovascular, central nervous system (CNS), and renal variables (Peres *et al.*, 2002). However, in spite of SOFA score assessment, "*It is more important to know what sort of person this disease has, than what sort of disease this person has*" (William Osler, 1849-1919).

3. Pathophysiology of sepsis and multiple organ dysfunction syndrome

As it was mentioned, the progression of MODS is due to an uncontrolled release of pro-inflammatory mediators, which damage parenchymatous organs. However, it is still unknown why sepsis progresses to MODS in only certain individuals or what the exact pathway is that leads to this. But, it is clear that if the inflammatory process becomes self-sustained and progressive, MOD results. In addition, because of marked hypotension and tissue hypoperfusion, oxygen delivery fails to meet tissue oxygen demands, which results in a compensatory increase in oxygen extraction. If the imbalance between oxygen delivery and consumption is not corrected, tissue 'dysoxia' progress to an anaerobic metabolism and lactate production (Nguyen *et al.*, 2004). Persistent serum lactate elevation is an important marker of decreased tissue perfusion –even in the absence of arterial hypotension (Howell *et al.*, 2007)–, and is strongly associated with mortality rate in critically ill patients (Meregalli *et al.*, 2004). Thus, during sepsis an extraordinarily complex and intricate cascade of inflammatory mediators, extra- and intra-cellular signaling pathways are activated, resulting in microvascular dysregulation and/or mitochondrial dysfunction ('cytopathic hypoxia') (Crouser, 2004), which culminate in MODS and death.

To avoid tissue dysoxia, early in the course of sepsis, cardiac output (CO) rises to maintain blood pressure and organ perfusion in the face of reduced peripheral vascular resistance ('hyperdynamic sepsis'). As sepsis progresses, CO is frequently reduced ('hypodynamic sepsis'), which has a poor prognosis. Cardiac dysfunction *per se* is apparent in up to 44% of critically ill septic patients, with the etiological agents suspected to be circulating depressant factors (Singh & Evans, 2006). Elevated cardiac biomarkers (*e.g.*, Troponin I (ver Elst *et al.*, 2000; Yucel *et al.*, 2008)) in conjunction with electrocardiographic (ECG) changes are valuable in the diagnostic of sepsis and in the assessment of progression. Raised Troponin I levels in patients with sepsis result from various mechanisms, including hypoperfusion or direct extension of infection to cardiac tissue. Electrocardiographic changes in sepsis are not as well described. Some of them include loss of QRS amplitude, increase in corrected QT (QTc) interval, bundle branch blocks, and development of narrowed QRS intervals with deformed, positively deflected J waves (Martinez *et al.*, 2009).

Contradictory evidences from animal studies suggest that such hypoperfusion does not invariably lead to heart dysfunction and death. But, our preliminary results (unpublished data) reveal many other ECG and vectorcardiographic changes in rats injected intraperitoneally (i.p.) with 15 mg/kg lipopolysaccharide (LPS), which are strongly associated with cardiac dysfunction and, almost certainly, left vetricular hypoperfusion and ischemia. Briefly, LPS administration decreases RR interval (RRI) and R amplitude. Also, sepsis increases QTc interval and ST height. Strikingly, when both carotid/sinus nerves are sectioned (bilateral carotid neurotomy (BCN) prior to LPS administration, the changes in the parameters mentioned above are greater than control condition (with intact carotid chemo- and baro-sensory innervations). In addition, BCN decreases QRS duration, increases JT interval and T amplitude. On the other hand, the cardiac vector is significantly decreased (from *ca.* 65º to *ca.* 15º)

As it was mentioned, the major task toil of autonomic nervous system (ANS) is the fine-tuning of the cardiorespiratory interplay, in order to maintain an appropriate oxygen delivery to the tissues. However, the neural regulation of cardiorespiratory function and the role-played by peripheral reflexes during sepsis, in which organ communications networks are disrupted, is poorly understood. In addition to plasma or urinary levels of neurotransmitters or their metabolites, there are three methods to evaluate autonomic function: a) analysis of heart rate variability (HRV); b) baroreflex sensitivity (BRS); and c) cardiac chemoreflex sensitivity (CCRS).

The analysis of HRV gives a clear idea about the neural (autonomic) control of cardiorespiratory function and interaction. Decreased HRV is consistent with the pathogenesis of MODS, which involves the physiological uncoupling of vital organ systems. In fact, HRV decreases in response to human endotoxemia (Godin *et al.*, 1996; Rassias *et al.*, 2005), and is a good index of cardiac mortality (Schmidt *et al.*, 2001). Moreover, patients with sepsis (Barnaby *et al.*, 2002) and MODS (Korach *et al.*, 2001;

Schmidt *et al.*, 2005) have an impaired sympatho-vagal balance. In fact, some evidences describe a sustained sympatho-excitation during sepsis, which accompanies the fall in blood pressure. Baroreceptors and chemoreceptors denervation accelerated the fall in mean blood pressure and increases sympathetic tone (Vayssettes-Courchay *et al.*, 2005). Thus, under altered baro- and chemo-reflexes pathways, the sympathetic output from the *medulla* appears to play a key role in the correlation between heart rate and sympathetic nerve activity. On the other hand, decreased parasympathetic tone is a good predictor of risk of death in patients with sepsis (Chen *et al.*, 2008). Altogether, these data suggest that reflex arcs involved in maintaining the autonomic balance are altered during sepsis.

Vayssettes-Courchay *et al.* (2005) shown that baro- and chemo-reflexes are not inhibited during sepsis, and they give them a minor importance in the sympathetic activation and in the blood pressure modifications. Nevertheless, recently we described the first functional evidence of chemoreceptors inflammation and dysfunction during sepsis. In cats, local or systemic administration of LPS induces a significant reduction in chemoreceptor activity, ventilatory chemoreflexes, and ventilator chemosensory drive (Fernandez *et al.*, 2008). In fact, LPS-induced tachypnea is prevented by prior bilateral carotid neurotomy.

Our results (unpublished data) shown that the i.p. administration of 15 mg/kg LPS to rats, decreases HRV and increases sympathetic tone, assessed by HRV frequency bands and low frequency/high frequency (LF/HF) quotient. Bilateral carotid neurotomy previous to LPS administration evokes a greater decrease in HRV and increase in LF/HF ratio than animals with intact carotid/sinus nerves. As it was mentioned, both decreased HRV and increased sympathetic tone are good markers of morbi-mortality. In fact, BCN prior to LPS administration increases the relative risk of death (Table 1). In addition, rats submitted to peripheral chemodenervation prior to the intravenous (i.v.) administration of high doses of LPS, show a smaller survival time (Tang *et al.*, 1998).

	SHAM		BCN	
	saline	LPS	saline	LPS
Relative Risk (RR) (IC 95%)	1 (n=8)	1.2 (0.9 – 1.6) (n=12)	1.3 (0.9 – 1.8) (n=9)	2.6 (1.5 – 4.5)[a] (n=21)
Plasma Cortisol (ng/mL) (Mean ± SD)	536.5 ± 383.3 (n=7)	1552.0 ± 940.5[b] (n=7)	637.5 ± 397.0 (n=6)	321.5 ± 153.2[c] (n=6)

[a], $p=0.0033$ vs. SHAM-saline. Fisher's exact test

[b], $p<0.05$ vs. SHAM-saline. Kruskal-Wallis ANOVA, Dunn's post test.

[c], $p<0.01$ vs. SHAM-LPS. Kruskal-Wallis ANOVA, Dunn's post test.

Table 1. Summary of observations in rats submitted to bilateral carotid neurotomy (BCN) or simulated surgery (SHAM) prior to the i.p. administration of 15 mg/kg LPS (LPS) or vehicle (saline). The data were assessed 90-min after LPS or vehicle administration. Table prepared from part of the data presented in Reyes *et al.*, 2012 (In press. Adv Exp Med Biol)

Baroreflex sensitivity describes ANS capacity to increase vagal activity and to decrease sympathetic activity after a sudden increase in blood pressure. Baroreflex activation counteract sympathetic activation (Somers *et al.*, 1991). BRS is altered in rats treated with a lethal dose of LPS (Shen *et al.*, 2004). Rougaush *et al.* reported an increased BRS after bacterial sub-pyrogenic dose of endotoxin. The change in sensitivity may underlie necessary adjustments to altered blood flow distribution after LPS administration (Rogausch *et al.*, 2000). However, Schmidt *et al.* reported a marked decrease in BRS during MODS (Schmidt *et al.*, 2005). Thus, there is no consensus about the role played by arterial baroreceptors during sepsis. Classically, the stimulation of peripheral chemoreceptors evokes respiratory and cardiovascular effects and a sympatho-excitatory response (Alanis *et al.*, 1968; Montarolo *et al.*, 1976). Cardiac chemoreflex sensitivity (CCRS) allow us to estimate the sympathetic influence upon cardiorespiratory responses (Schmidt *et al.*, 1999). Hyperoxia decreases autonomic function –*i.e.*, decreased CCRS– and increases BRS. CCRS gives an important component of the cardiorespiratory interactions in patients with MODS. Severity of illness is the more pronounced determinant of impaired CCRS (Schmidt *et al.*, 2004). Recently, Schueller *et al.* described a reduced CCRS in critical ill patients (sepsis or cardiogenic shock). Moreover, there is a close negative correlation between the CCRS and the SOFA-score (Schueller *et al.*, 2008).

In summary, there is consensus that uncoupling of the autonomic, respiratory and cardiovascular systems occurs over both short- and long-range time scales during sepsis and MODS. However, the origin from these altered reflex arcs is not well described.

4. Inflammatory mediators during sepsis

The development of sequential organ failure in critically ill patients with sepsis is strongly predictive of mortality. However, the mechanisms involved in the dynamic interaction between different organ systems are dictated by the intricate interplay of homodynamic, oxygen transport, and metabolic disturbances. Genetic predisposition is almost certainly relevant in upregulating the expression of inflammatory mediators [*e.g.*, tumor necrosis factor (TNF), interleukin (IL)-1, IL-6, high mobility group box (HMGB) 1], thereby influencing adversely the anti-/pro-inflammatory balance.

Mammals are continuously exposed to different pathogens, like Gram-negative bacteria and/or its components, such as LPS (endotoxin). LPS exerts many different biological effects. While low-doses could be beneficial, by inducing immunostimulation and by increasing resistance to infection (Schletter *et al.*, 1995), larger-doses of LPS in plasma evoke many pathophysiological reactions, like fever, leucopenia, tachycardia, tachypnea, hypotension, disseminated intravascular coagulation, MODS, and death (Patel *et al.*, 2003; Hotchkiss & Karl, 2003; Pinsky, 2004). The systemic inflammatory response induced by LPS is due to host cells stimulation (monocytes/macrophages, endothelial, and polymorphonuclear cells) to produce and release endogenous mediators like reactive oxygen species (ROS) and pro-inflammatory cytokines (Schletter *et al.*, 1995). Inflammatory mediators and ROS are believed to disrupt communication pathways between organs, which precedes organ failure. Indeed, endothelial dysfunction has been proposed as a common pathway for organ dysfunction in sepsis (Simon & Fernandez, 2009). During systemic inflammation, many physiological functions of endothelial cells are disrupted, contributing to multiple organ failure (Volk & Kox, 2000).

During the last decade, there has been a rapid progress in understanding innate immune response to pathogens or their component. The early concept supposed a nonspecific recognition. But, the discovery of Toll-like receptors (TLRs) showed that recognition by the innate immune system is specific (Akira *et al.*, 2001). TLR-4 is identified as the long-sought receptor that respond to bacterial LPS (Akira *et al.*, 2006). TLR4 forms a complex with MD-2 on the cell surface. Additional proteins such as the soluble plasma protein LPS-binding protein (LBP) and either soluble or membrane-anchored CD14 are also involved in LPS binding (Akashi-Takamura & Miyake, 2008). LPS transfer to the LPS-binding receptor (TLR-4/MD-2) (da Silva *et al.*, 2001), activates nuclear factor-κB (NF-κB), a transcription factor involved in the synthesis and release of immune system-related cytotoxic factors, by stimulation of pro-inflammatory and immunoregulatory molecules synthesis in mononuclear cells (monocytes /macrophages and neutrophils), like IL-1, IL-6, TNF-α, IL-10, and transforming growth factor (TGF)-β (Medvedev *et al.*, 2000;Sanlioglu *et al.*, 2001). Increased plasma levels of TNF-α, IL-1 and IL -6, γ-interferon (IFN-γ), and TGF-β are present in patients with different pathological conditions (Schletter *et al.*, 1995), but a particular cytokine, TNF-α, seems to play a pivotal role during sepsis and MODS (Tracey *et al.*, 1986).

Tumor necrosis factor-α has been implicated as an important mediator of the lethal effect of endotoxin. Several publications have shown that by reducing the activity or the expression of TNF-α significantly decrease the endotoxin-induced damages. The amount of TNF-α in serum can be associated with the degree of tissue damage because of the stagnant blood capillary (Yang *et al.*, 2007). TNF-α is a well-known cytotoxic cytokine for certain tissue cells. In fact, plasma levels of several biophysical damage indicators are increased during sepsis, like liver alanine aminotransferase, aspartate aminotransferase, and bilirrubin; heart and other possible organ (such as muscle) lactic dehydrogenase and creatine phosphokinase; ureic nitrogen (BUN, renal function); and pancreatic alkaline phosphatase and amylase.

5. Reflex control of inflammation: Part I – Brain-to-immune communication

Inflammation is a localized protective response to infection or injury. It evokes many different effects upon the organisms tending to solve the inflammatory focus, like humoral factors which increase the blood flow or attract specific immune cells (Libert, 2003). As it was mentioned above, TNF-α, plays a pivotal role during systemic inflammation. Excessive inflammation and TNF-α synthesis increase morbi-mortality in SS. In consequence, highly conserved endogenous mechanisms normally regulate the magnitude of innate immune response and prevent excessive inflammation (Wang *et al.*, 2003).

The CNS regulates systemic inflammatory responses to endotoxin through neural and humoral mechanisms. Evidence accumulated over the last 30 years suggests that norepinephrine (NE), the main neurotransmitter of the sympathetic nervous system, fulfills the criteria for neurotransmitter/neuromodulator in lymphoid organs: i) primary and secondary lymphoid organs receive extensive sympathetic/noradrenergic innervation; ii) under stimulation, NE is released from the sympathetic nerve terminals in these organs; and iii) the target immune cells, including lymphocytes and macrophages, express adrenergic receptors (AR). Adrenoceptors are G-protein coupled receptors that can be divided into two subgroups: the α- and β-AR, which can be further subdivided into different subtypes. Neutrophils, mononuclear, and natural killer cells, also T- and B-lymphocytes express α- and β-AR. The most important adrenoceptor –in terms of the immune system– is the β2-AR. Activation of β2-AR results in an increase in cAMP concentrations, which can modulate cytokine expression, *i.e.*, decreasing TNF-α and increasing IL-8 (Elenkov & Chrousos, 1999). However, recently was described that α2A-AR stimulation increases TNF-α gene expression in Kupffer cells and plasma TNF-α during sepsis (Miksa *et al.*, 2009). Thus, through AR stimulation, locally released NE, or circulating catecholamines, affect lymphocyte traffic, circulation, and proliferation, and modulate cytokine production and the functional activity of different lymphoid cells (Elenkov *et al.*, 2000), just as they control heart rate and other vital functions. Serum levels of sympatoadrenergic transmitters –*i.e.*, Neuropeptide-Y, ATP, and vanillyl mandelic acid (VMA, as an indirect measurement of catecholamine levels)–, are also increased during sepsis (Donoso *et al.*, 2008).

A growing body of literature is aimed at studying β-blockade as a treatment of sepsis. Their effects on metabolism and glucose homeostasis, cytokine expression, and myocardial function may be beneficial in the setting of sepsis. Sepsis induces an overall catabolic state, mainly due to excessive adrenergic stimulation (Bergmann *et al.*, 1999). β-Blockade has been proposed as a strategy to counteract the devastating consequences of this hyperadrenergic state. But treating a potentially hypotensive condition with a drug with antihypertensive properties may initially seem detrimental (Novotny *et al.*, 2009). Peripheral (i.p.) β1-AR blockade prior to endotoxemia increases survival time, reduces hepatic expression of pro-inflammatory cytokines, decreases protein expression of cardiac dysfunction markers, and preserves arterial blood pressure and left ventricular contractility (Ackland *et al.*, 2010). Surprisingly, few studies report overall mortality in the published β-blocker trials in sepsis. Interestingly, of those investigators that do report mortality in sepsis models, one out of four show increased mortality in β-blockade groups.

Vasopressor and inotropic therapies for sepsis employ adrenergic support. In fact, a recent publication about the "*Efficacy and Safety of Dopamine Versus Norepinephrine in the Management of Septic Shock*" showed that NE treatment decreases 28-day mortality and has a lower risk of sinus tachycardia and arrhythmias than dopamine (DA) (Patel *et al.*, 2010). This work concludes that arrhythmias are significant predictors of sepsis morbi-mortality, and that "*patients receiving DA should be monitored for the development of cardiac arrhythmias*", but does not consider a potential increase of MOD indicators induced by DA infusion, since high doses of DA (> 20 μg/kg/min) has a predominant α-AR effect, a potent immunostimulator (Povoa & Carneiro, 2010). Recently De Baker *et al.* reported that DA administration is associated with greater mortality and a higher incidence of arrhythmic events compared to NE administration (De Backer *et al.*, 2012).

It should be noted that different cathecholamines used to treat patients with septic shock, have relative α- and β-AR effects (depending on the dose). Thus, in addition to individual differences, it is necessary to consider the fine-tuning of both, immune system and cardiovascular effects of adrenergic drugs used for sepsis treatment.

The CNS can also rapidly inhibit the release of macrophage TNF-α, and attenuate systemic inflammatory responses acting through the vagus (parasympathetic) nerve. This physiological mechanism, termed the 'cholinergic anti-inflammatory pathway (Borovikova *et al.*, 2000)' has major implications in immunology and in therapeutics (Rosas-Ballina & Tracey, 2009). The main vagal neurotransmitter, acetylcholine (ACh), inhibits LPS-induced TNF-α, IL-1β and IL-6 release, but not anti-inflammatory cytokine IL-10, in LPS stimulated *in vitro* cultured human macrophages (Borovikova *et al.*, 2000; Wang *et al.*, 2003). In addition, peripheral vagus nerve electrical stimulation inhibits liver TNF-α production, attenuates peak serum TNF-α amounts, and prevents the development of shock, during lethal endotoxemia in rats (Borovikova *et al.*, 2000).

Recent work on the anatomical basis of the cholinergic anti-inflammatory pathway indicates that the spleen is required for vagus nerve control of inflammation (Huston *et al.*, 2006). The spleen is the major source of serum TNF-α during endotoxemia (Mignini *et al.*, 2003). In splenectomized rats injected with endotoxin, serum TNF-α is reduced by 70%, and vagus nerve stimulation fails to further suppress TNF-α. The celiac branches of the vagus terminate in the celiac-superior mesenteric plexus and not in the spleen (Berthoud & Powley, 1996). The spleen is innervated by the splenic nerve, which originates in celiac-superior mesenteric plexus. The splenic nerve is composed mainly by catecholaminergic fibers, which terminate in close apposition to immune cells (Felten *et al.*, 1987). Thus, attenuation of TNF-α production by spleen macrophages induced by vagus nerve stimulation is mediated by norepinephrine released from splenic nerve endings. These data confirms the importance of the adrenergic transmitters in the regulation of immune response. It must be noted that immune cells have all the essential components of a non-neuronal cholinergic system and that ACh synthesized and released from lymphocytes acts as an immunomodulator via both muscarinic (mAChR) and nicotinic ACh receptors (nAChR) (Kawashima & Fujii, 2000; Kawashima & Fujii, 2003). Most evidences points towards a crucial role for the α7 nAChR in the cholinergic regulation of macrophage activity (Wang *et al.*, 2003). Nicotine exerts anti-inflammatory effects through α7 nAChR (Ulloa, 2005). Acetylcholine (and nicotine), also has cardiorespiratory effects (Fernandez *et al.*, 2002; Zapata *et al.*, 2002). Acting through the peripheral arterial chemoreceptors, ACh, nicotine, and epibatidine (a selective agonist for neuronal nAChRs) increases tidal volume and blood pressure in anesthetized cats (Zapata *et al.*, 2003; Reyes *et al.*, 2007), which support the idea that cholinergic nicotinic treatment can also improve cardiorespiratory performance during sepsis, and prevent tissue dysoxia, lactic acidosis and MODS. In addition, nicotine inhibit cardiac apoptosis induced by LPS in rats (Suzuki *et al.*, 2003).

Finally, both endotoxin and cytokines, stimulates HPA anti-inflammatory responses, either by adrenal glucocorticoids (Turnbull & Rivier, 1999) or by inhibiting prolactin secretion, a potent regulator of humoral and cellular immune response during physiological and pathological states (Freeman *et al.*, 2000). Thus, it is clear that the nervous system reflexively regulates the inflammatory response in real time, just as it controls heart rate and other vital functions.

6. Reflex control of inflammation: Part II – Immune-to-brain communication

Much less is known about the effect of the immune system on the CNS. Immune system-derived signals act on the CNS through four different pathways: i) by saturable transport across the blood–brain barrier (BBB) (Banks & Kastin, 1987); ii) by brain circumventricular organs (CVOs) (Stitt, 1990); iii) by cytokine binding to brain endothelial cells, which evokes paracrine mediators release (Fabry *et al.*, 1993; Cao *et al.*, 1998); and iv) by the activation of peripheral sensory nerves (i.e., vagus nerve) (Goehler *et al.*, 1997).

The role of peripheral sensory nerves in immunomodulation is controversial. It is believed that chemosensory transduction begins in immune cells, which release inflammatory mediators to activate neural elements, including vagal paraganglia (Goehler *et al.*, 1997; Goehler *et al.*, 1999) and primary afferent neurons located in sensory ganglia, which evokes host defense reflexes. Two cell types compose vagal paraganglia: type I (glomus) cells and type II (sustentacular) cells (Berthoud *et al.*, 1995). Vagal glomus cells (GC) are innervated by vagal afferent neurons, whose cell bodies are located in the nodose ganglion, and their central projection end primarily within the dorsal vagal complex (DVC) of the *medulla oblongata*. Thus, immunosensory inputs could initiate local cardiorespiratory reflexes and carry information about the state of inflammation.

In spite of the interleukin-1 (IL-1) receptor expression in vagal GC (Goehler *et al.*, 1997), IL-1β (and TNF-α), had no significant effect on the frequency of action potentials recorded from single fibers from isolated superfused rat GC obtained from vagal nerve paraganglia (Mac Grory *et al.*, 2010). In addition, in rodents exposed to i.p. LPS or IL-1β, bilateral subdiaphragmatic vagotomy prevents sickness manifestations and activation of *nucleus tractus solitarii* (NTS), *locus coeruleus* (LC), and hypothalamus (Bluthe *et al.*, 1994; Bret-Dibat *et al.*, 1995; Gaykema *et al.*, 1995; Watkins *et al.*, 1995; Hansen & Krueger, 1997; Borsody & Weiss, 2005). Thus, immune chemosensory inputs and incoming neural signals could be originated from other receptors, such as the peripheral arterial chemoreceptors neural pathway: the carotid body (CB) and its sensory ganglion.

The DVC consists of the NTS, the dorsal motor nucleus of the vagus (DMN), and the *area postrema* (AP) (Berthoud & Neuhuber, 2000). The DMN is the main site of origin of preganglionic vagus efferent fibers; while cardiovascular vagal efferences originate within the medullar *nucleus ambiguus* (NA). The AP, which lacks of BBB, is an important CVO and an important site for humoral immune-to-brain communication. The main portion of vagal sensory input is received by neurons in the NTS, which coordinate autonomic function and interaction with the endocrine system. Ascending projections from the NTS reach hypothalamic paraventricular nucleus (PVN), an important structure in the HPA axis activation. Synaptic contacts also exist between the neurons in the NTS and rostral ventrolateral *medulla* (RVM), which occupies an important role in control of cardiovascular and respiratory homeostasis. The neurons from RVM project to the *locus coeruleus* (LC), which innervates higher brain sites, like hypothalamus and PVN. Neuronal projections emanate from the RVM and LC to sympathetic preganglionic neurons in the spinal cord. There are also descending pathways from the PVN to the RVM and NTS (Pavlov *et al.*, 2003). Thus, these ascending and descending connections provide a neuronal substrate for interaction between HPA axis and the ANS as an immunomodulatory mechanism.

In response to plasma levels of TNF-α, vagal immunosensory activity increases (Emch *et al.*, 2000) or decreases (Emch *et al.*, 2002) vagal motor activity. Transection of abdominal vagal trunks suppresses fever and hyperalgesia caused by i.p. LPS but has little effect on the febrile response to i.v. or intramuscular LPS. To elucidate the importance of visceral afferent innervation on the response to LPS, Wan *et al.* studied the expression of the immediate early gene c-fos in the hypothalamus and brain stem of the rat following peripheral –either i.v. or i.p.– injection of LPS. Subdiaphragmatic vagotomy completely blocked the induction of c-Fos protein following i.p. injection of LPS; however, vagotomy had a minimal effect on c-Fos protein induction following i.v. LPS administration (Wan *et al.*, 1994). In addition, c-Fos activation of NTS neurons induced by LPS persists after cervical bilateral vagotomy (Hermann *et al.*, 2001). Both subdiaphragmatic and cervical bilateral vagotomy abolition of CNS c-Fos activation induced by i.p. LPS are controversial, since it could be due to the section of neurons from the abdominal region that mediate the response to LPS *per se* or, merely, because of the role played by the vagus efferent fibers –perhaps those within the celiac branches– in LPS transport from the peritoneal cavity to the blood. Thus, when these fibers are cut, LPS escape to systemic circulation is limited, and systemic responses to LPS would be diminished (*e.g.*, c-Fos protein induction in the CNS) (Lenczowski *et al.*, 1997; Romanovsky *et al.*, 2000).

The number of neurons within the DVC that expressed c-Fos activation after peripheral administration of LPS is correlated with plasma levels of TNF-α. Thus, the activation of DVC neurons did not require intact vagal pathways, suggesting that TNF-α generated peripherally could acts directly on these neurons, because DVC exhibits the characteristics of CVOs (*i.e.*, fenestrated capillary network and absence of functional BBB) (Hermann *et al.*, 2001) or, more probably, through another neural afferent pathway. In consequence, it is possible to suggest that prominent CNS manifestations of endotoxemia are apparently caused by incoming neural signals provided by other peripheral receptors, distinct from vagal paraganglia, like the carotid arterial chemoreceptors, which function is intact after bilateral cervical vagotomy. Our results shown that LPS-induced c-Fos activation in NTS neurons and plasmatic cortisol increases in septic rats (treated i.p. with 15 mg/kg LPS) are suppressed by bilateral carotid neurotomy (Reyes *et al.*, 2012. Adv Exp Med Biol. *In press*) (Table 1).

Seen from an anatomical standpoint, the carotid body (CB) is the largest paraganglia in the body (Mascorro & Yates, 1980), and like other paraganglia, it receives sensory innervation, and has specialized glomus cells with abundant synapses with the sensory nervous fibers (Verna, 1997).

7. The arterial chemoreceptors in neuroimmunomodulation

The CB is the main peripheral chemoreceptor responsible for the detection of blood oxygen levels. The CB consists of groups of glomus (type I) cells arranged around capillaries, ensheathed by sustentacular (type II) cells, and surrounded by connective tissue. It receives profuse sensory innervation from the carotid (sinus) nerve (CSN), a branch of the glossopharyngeal nerve, whose sensory nerve endings are in close contact with glomus cells (GC) (Hess & Zapata, 1972). CB innervation is essentially by sensory neurons residing mainly in the petrosal ganglion (Kalia & Davies, 1978; Berger, 1980). Interestingly, the first synapsis at the CNS for afferent CSN fibers occurs in the NTS (Donoghue *et al.*, 1984; Finley & Katz, 1992). Thus, inflammation-derived sensory input originated from arterial chemoreceptors (Zapata *et al.*, 2011) can be differentially processed in the peripheral chemoreceptor *per se*, in the sensory ganglion, and/or in the brainstem, and modify cardiorespiratory chemoreflexes, endocrine, and autonomic functions, like the neural control on the immune system. In rats, petrosal ganglion is a constituent of a ganglion complex, composed by nodose, petrosal and jugular ganglia, the nodose-petrosal-jugular ganglion complex (NPJgc).

Many reports allow us to propose that peripheral arterial chemoreceptors play a pivotal role in afferent signaling during sepsis. Recently, we demonstrated that i.v. administration of LPS to pentobarbitone-anesthetized cats evokes similar symptoms to those observed in patients with severe sepsis and septic shock, with tachycardia, tachypnea and hypotension, and that the increased respiratory frequency is prevented by bilateral section of the carotid and aortic nerves (Fernandez *et al.*, 2008). In addition, LPS enhances tonic CB chemosensory activity (measured by recording the frequency of chemosensory discharges) but reduces its responsiveness to transient excitatory (hypoxia and nicotine) or depressant (pure oxygen) stimuli. Diminished ventilatory responses to moderate and severe hypoxia in cats reproduces the diminished ventilatory responses to hypoxia observed in unanesthetized newborn piglets subjected to *Escherichia coli* endotoxin infusion (McDeigan *et al.*, 2003), as well as in rats, in a process that is in part mediated by an inhibitory effect of endothelial nitric oxide on the respiratory control mechanisms (Ladino *et al.*, 2007). Apoptosis studies carried out in CB excised from endotoxemic cats discard that CB diminished chemosensory activity observed in LPS-treated animals resulted from a reduction of functional tissue (Fernandez *et al.*, 2008), and suggest the participation of systemic soluble factors (*e.g.*, cytokines), or locally produced by either resident monocytes/macrophages (Dvorakova *et al.*, 2000), or parenchyma cells.

Lipopolysaccharide administration increases cytokine plasma levels in many species, including rats (Waage, 1987), bovines (Ohtsuka *et al.*, 1997) and cats (Otto & Rawlings, 1995). Thus, by using *in vitro* experiments, where the carotid artery is perfused and the entire preparation (including the CB) is superfused, the frequency of carotid nerve discharges recorded under normoxic conditions was not significantly modified by TNF-α, but the enhanced CB chemosensory discharges recorded along responses to hypoxic stimulation was transiently diminished, in a dose-dependent manner (Fernandez *et al.*, 2008). The cat CB expresses both type-1 and type-2 TNF-α receptor mRNA. Immunohistochemical studies with specific antibodies, determined that TNF-R1 protein is located mainly in the GC. In addition, a strong positive TNF-α protein immunoreactivity was also found in the GC cytoplasm (Fernandez *et al.*, 2008). These observations suggest that locally or systemically produced and secreted TNF-α, acting in an autocrine or paracrine fashion, could modify GC function.

Apart from the presence of TNF-α and TNF-R1, it is known that GC from rat CB express IL-1 receptor type I (Wang *et al.*, 2002) and IL-6 receptor α (Wang *et al.*, 2006), and that GC respond to IL-1β application with depolarization and a transient rise in intracellular calcium (Shu *et al.*, 2007). On the other hand, i.p. administration of IL-1β evokes IL-1 receptor type I and tyrosine hydroxylase (TH) up-regulation in the rat CB (Zhang *et al.*, 2007). The fact that pro-inflammatory cytokines and their receptors are functionally expressed in the CB type I cells, suggests that inflammatory mediators may have different functional roles in the activation of neurons in the NPJgc, even in the absence of sepsis syndromes –*e.g.*, exerting a tonic control of cardiorespiratory, endocrine, autonomic, and/or immune functions–. In fact, hypoxia, the natural stimulus for peripheral arterial chemoreceptors upregulates the expression and function of proinflammatory cytokines in the rat CB (Lam *et al.*, 2008), and the adaptation to chronic hypoxia involves immune cell invasion and increased expression of inflammatory cytokines in rat CB (Liu *et al.*, 2009). Thus, it is possible to suggest that local or systemic pro-inflammatory cytokines, recognized by membrane receptors located in the GC, modify CB chemosensory activity and, through afferent pathways projecting to the NTS, stimulate or inhibit specific components of the systemic inflammatory response. It must be noted that, regarding the source of immune signals, neural pathways provide faster and more precise information than humoral pathways.

In view of data mentioned above, we tested whether LPS-induced systemic inflammation exerts a direct effect upon CB chemoreceptors. We determined that the rat CB and NPJgc constitutively express the mRNAs for TLR4, MyD88, TNF-α and its receptors (TNF-R1 and TNF-R2). Intraperitoneal administration of 15 mg/kg LPS evokes IKκB degradation, and subsequent NF-κB p65 translocation into the nucleus from GC and NPJgc chemosensory neurons. LPS also evokes p38 MAPK and ERK phosphorylation. Consistently, LPS treatment increases both mRNA and protein levels of TNF-α, TNF-R2, and TH. Double-labeling studies show that TLR4, TNF-α, and TNF-R1 are localized in TH-containing GC and neurons from CB and NPJgc, respectively, suggesting that the expression was confined to the chemoafferent neural pathway. TNF-R2 is also present surrounding GC clusters within the CB and in chemosensitive neurons. TNF-α, and TNF-R2 expression are increased in the carotid chemoreceptors from endotoxemic rats (Fernandez *et al.*, 2011). Thus –in addition to systemic LPS effect– our results suggest that LPS acting directly through TLR-4 modifies TNF-α and its receptors expression on chemosensory cells of the carotid chemoreceptors neural pathway. These results show a novel afferent pathway to the CNS during physiological conditions and endotoxemia, and could be relevant in understanding sepsis pathophysiology and therapy.

Thus, it is very interesting to highlight that during sepsis syndromes, LPS acting directly upon carotid chemoreceptors, modify TNF-α expression. In addition systemic or local inflammatory mediators could change arterial chemoreceptors function and afferent signaling through TNF-α receptors, whose expression is also modified during sepsis (our results), or through IL-1 and/or IL-6 receptors (Figure 1). Interestingly, TNF-α stimulates c-Fos activation of neurons in the NTS (Hermann *et al.*, 2001). Results here obtained would imply that arterial chemoreflexes, not only serves as a chemoreceptor for respiratory reflex responses, as traditionally accepted, but also as a sensor for the immune status, as modulator of autonomic balance tending to coordinate cardiorespiratory interplay devoted to maintain oxygen homeostasis in different pathologies, and as a protective factor during sepsis and MODS.

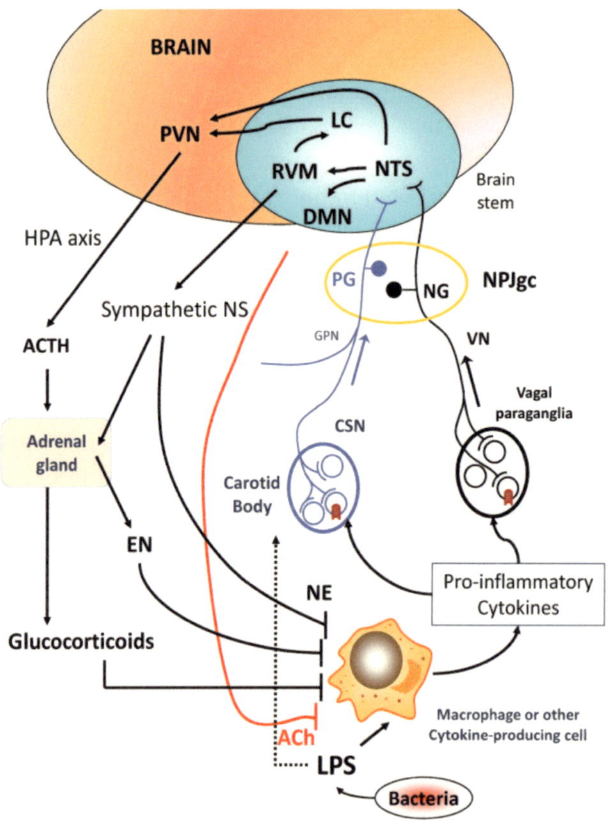

Figure 1. Proposed model for neural reflex control of inflammation during sepsis syndromes. Lypopolysaccharide (LPS) acting through macrophages or other cytokine-producing cell, increases plasma levels of pro-inflammatory cytokines (*e.g.*, TNF-α) which in activates immunosensory inputs from vagal paraganglia or carotid body (CB) chemoreceptors. Immunosensory signals reach the *nucleus tractus solitarii* (NTS) neurons. The dorsal motor nucleus (DMN) is the main site of origin of preganglionic vagus efferent fibers, activating the cholinergic anti-inflammatory reflex, by secreting acetylcholine (ACh), which decreased immune response. The main portion of vagal sensory inputs received by NTS neurons coordinates autonomic function and interaction with the endocrine system. Ascending projections from the NTS reach hypothalamic paraventricular nucleus (PVN), activating the hypothalamic-pituitary-adrenal (HPA) axis for glucocorticoids production and immunosupression. Synaptic contacts with the rostral

ventrolateral *medulla* (RVM) and subsequent projection to the *locus coeruleus* (LC) innervates higher brain sites, like PVN. Also, neuronal projections emanate from the RVM and LC to sympathetic preganglionic neurons in the spinal cord, which in turn activates adrenal epinephrine (EN) secretion and norepinephrine (NE), reducing pro-inflammatory activity. Thus, these ascending and descending connections provide a neuronal substrate for interaction between HPA axis and the ANS as an immunomodulatory mechanism. PG, petrosal ganglion; NG, nodose ganglion; CSN, carotid/sinus nerve; VN, vagus nerve; GPN, glossopharyngeal nerve; NS, nervous system; ACTH, adrenocorticotrophic hormone.

The disruption of continuous detection of the 'inflammatory status' of the body exerted by carotid chemoreceptors could be responsible for modifying the activity of the ANS, thus altering the control exerted by the nervous system on the immune system, and evoking an uncontrolled cytokine production. This excessive and uncontrolled systemic inflammatory response and dysautonomy could be responsible for subsequent neural uncoupling of the vital organs and MODS.

8. Conclusion

Sepsis syndromes are the main cause of death between critical care patients. They result from neural, cardiovascular, respiratory, and immune systems uncoupling. Multiple organ dysfunction syndrome (MODS) is due to an uncontrolled release of pro-inflammatory mediators, which damage parenchymatous organs. However, it is still unknown why sepsis progresses to MODS in only certain individuals.

The effects of sepsis therapies are controversial and strongly dependent of individual components, like individual response and genetic predisposition. Thus, the course of sepsis and therapies outcomes depends largely from host factors.

Increasing evidences shown that peripheral carotid chemoreceptors act as sensor for the immune status, as modulator of autonomic balance tending to coordinate cardiorespiratory interplay devoted to maintain oxygen homeostasis in different pathologies, and as a protective factor during sepsis and MODS.

As result of the autonomic and immune imbalance originated from carotid chemoreceptors, neural and cytokine communication networks between healthy organs are disrupted. So, the impaired autonomic function would decrease cardiorespiratory function, oxygen delivery to the tissues, and the reflex control of inflammation. The heterostasis induced by systemic inflammation worsens the uncoupling of biological oscillators, what would lead to MODS and death.

Author details

Ricardo Fernandez*

Departamento de Ciencias Biologicas,

Facultad de Ciencias Biologicas y Facultad de Medicina, Universidad Andres Bello, Chile

* Corresponding author

Claudio Acuña-Castillo
Centro de Biotecnologia Acuicola y Departamento de Biologia,
Facultad de Quimica y Biologia, Universidad de Santiago de Chile, Chile

Acknowledgement

Ricardo Fernandez is supported by FONDECYT 1120976 and UNAB DI-40-11/R.

Claudio Acuña-Castillo is supported by FONDECYT 1110734.

9. References

Abboud FM & Thames MD. Interaction of cardiovascular reflexes in circulatory control. Sheperd, J. T, Abboud, F. M, Geiger, S. R, and Bethesda, M. D. [3], 675-752. 1983. American Physiological Society. Handbook of Physiology.

Ackland GL, Yao ST, Rudiger A, Dyson A, Stidwill R, Poputnikov D, Singer M, & Gourine AV (2010). Cardioprotection, attenuated systemic inflammation, and survival benefit of beta1-adrenoceptor blockade in severe sepsis in rats. *Crit Care Med* 38, 388-394.

Akashi-Takamura S & Miyake K (2008). TLR accessory molecules. *Curr Opin Immunol* 20, 420-425.

Akira S, Takeda K, & Kaisho T (2001). Toll-like receptors: critical proteins linking innate and acquired immunity. *Nat Immunol* 2, 675-680.

Akira S, Uematsu S, & Takeuchi O (2006). Pathogen recognition and innate immunity. *Cell* 124, 783-801.

Alanis J, Defillo B, & Gordon S (1968). Changes in the efferent discharges of sympathetic and parasympathetic cardiac nerves provoked by activation of carotid chemoreceptors. *Arch Int Physiol Biochim* 76, 214-235.

Angus DC, Linde-Zwirble WT, Lidicker J, Clermont G, Carcillo J, & Pinsky MR (2001). Epidemiology of severe sepsis in the United States: analysis of incidence, outcome, and associated costs of care. *Crit Care Med* 29, 1303-1310.

Banks WA & Kastin AJ (1987). Saturable transport of peptides across the blood-brain barrier. *Life Sci* 41, 1319-1338.

Barnaby D, Ferrick K, Kaplan DT, Shah S, Bijur P, & Gallagher EJ (2002). Heart rate variability in emergency department patients with sepsis. *Acad Emerg Med* 9, 661-670.

Barochia AV, Cui X, Vitberg D, Suffredini AF, O'Grady NP, Banks SM, Minneci P, Kern SJ, Danner RL, Natanson C, & Eichacker PQ (2010). Bundled care for septic shock: an analysis of clinical trials. *Crit Care Med* 38, 668-678.

Berger AJ (1980). The distribution of the cat's carotid sinus nerve afferent and efferent cell bodies using the horseradish peroxidase technique. *Brain Res* 190, 309-320.

Bergmann M, Gornikiewicz A, Sautner T, Waldmann E, Weber T, Mittlbock M, Roth E, & Fugger R (1999). Attenuation of catecholamine-induced immunosuppression in whole blood from patients with sepsis. *Shock* 12, 421-427.

Berthoud HR, Kressel M, & Neuhuber WL (1995). Vagal afferent innervation of rat abdominal paraganglia as revealed by anterograde DiI-tracing and confocal microscopy. *Acta Anat (Basel)* 152, 127-132.

Berthoud HR & Neuhuber WL (2000). Functional and chemical anatomy of the afferent vagal system. *Auton Neurosci* 85, 1-17.

Berthoud HR & Powley TL (1996). Interaction between parasympathetic and sympathetic nerves in prevertebral ganglia: morphological evidence for vagal efferent innervation of ganglion cells in the rat. *Microsc Res Tech* 35, 80-86.

Bluthe RM, Walter V, Parnet P, Laye S, Lestage J, Verrier D, Poole S, Stenning BE, Kelley KW, & Dantzer R (1994). Lipopolysaccharide induces sickness behaviour in rats by a vagal mediated mechanism. *C R Acad Sci III* 317, 499-503.

Bone RC, Balk RA, Cerra FB, Dellinger RP, Fein AM, Knaus WA, Schein RM, & Sibbald WJ (1992). Definitions for sepsis and organ failure and guidelines for the use of innovative therapies in sepsis. The ACCP/SCCM Consensus Conference Committee. American College of Chest Physicians/Society of Critical Care Medicine. *Chest* 101, 1644-1655.

Borovikova LV, Ivanova S, Zhang M, Yang H, Botchkina GI, Watkins LR, Wang H, Abumrad N, Eaton JW, & Tracey KJ (2000). Vagus nerve stimulation attenuates the systemic inflammatory response to endotoxin. *Nature* 405, 458-462.

Borsody MK & Weiss JM (2005). The subdiaphragmatic vagus nerves mediate activation of locus coeruleus neurons by peripherally administered microbial substances. *Neuroscience* 131, 235-245.

Bret-Dibat JL, Bluthe RM, Kent S, Kelley KW, & Dantzer R (1995). Lipopolysaccharide and interleukin-1 depress food-motivated behavior in mice by a vagal-mediated mechanism. *Brain Behav Immun* 9, 242-246.

Cao C, Matsumura K, Yamagata K, & Watanabe Y (1998). Cyclooxygenase-2 is induced in brain blood vessels during fever evoked by peripheral or central administration of tumor necrosis factor. *Brain Res Mol Brain Res* 56, 45-56.

Carre JE & Singer M (2008). Cellular energetic metabolism in sepsis: the need for a systems approach. *Biochim Biophys Acta* 1777, 763-771.

Chalupka AN & Talmor D (2012). The economics of sepsis. *Crit Care Clin* 28, 57-76, vi.

Chen WL, Chen JH, Huang CC, Kuo CD, Huang CI, & Lee LS (2008). Heart rate variability measures as predictors of in-hospital mortality in ED patients with sepsis. *Am J Emerg Med* 26, 395-401.

Crouser ED (2004). Mitochondrial dysfunction in septic shock and multiple organ dysfunction syndrome. *Mitochondrion* 4, 729-741.

da Silva CJ, Soldau K, Christen U, Tobias PS, & Ulevitch RJ (2001). Lipopolysaccharide is in close proximity to each of the proteins in its membrane receptor complex. transfer from CD14 to TLR4 and MD-2. *J Biol Chem* 276, 21129-21135.

De Backer D, Aldecoa C, Njimi H, & Vincent JL (2012). Dopamine versus norepinephrine in the treatment of septic shock: a meta-analysis*. *Crit Care Med* 40, 725-730.

Dellinger RP, Carlet JM, Masur H, Gerlach H, Calandra T, Cohen J, Gea-Banacloche J, Keh D, Marshall JC, Parker MM, Ramsay G, Zimmerman JL, Vincent JL, & Levy MM (2004).

Surviving Sepsis Campaign guidelines for management of severe sepsis and septic shock. *Crit Care Med* 32, 858-873.

Donoghue S, Felder RB, Jordan D, & Spyer KM (1984). The central projections of carotid baroreceptors and chemoreceptors in the cat: a neurophysiological study. *J Physiol* 347, 397-409.

Donoso V, Gomez CR, Orriantia MA, Perez V, Torres C, Coddou C, Nelson P, Maisey K, Morales B, Fernandez R, Imarai M, Huidobro-Toro JP, Sierra F, & Acuna-Castillo C (2008). The release of sympathetic neurotransmitters is impaired in aged rats after an inflammatory stimulus: a possible link between cytokine production and sympathetic transmission. *Mech Ageing Dev* 129, 728-734.

Dvorakova M, Hohler B, Vollerthun R, Fischbach T, & Kummer W (2000). Macrophages: a major source of cytochrome b558 in the rat carotid body. *Brain Res* 852, 349-354.

Elenkov IJ & Chrousos GP (1999). Stress Hormones, Th1/Th2 patterns, Pro/Anti-inflammatory Cytokines and Susceptibility to Disease. *Trends Endocrinol Metab* 10, 359-368.

Elenkov IJ, Wilder RL, Chrousos GP, & Vizi ES (2000). The sympathetic nerve--an integrative interface between two supersystems: the brain and the immune system. *Pharmacol Rev* 52, 595-638.

Emch GS, Hermann GE, & Rogers RC (2002). Tumor necrosis factor-alpha inhibits physiologically identified dorsal motor nucleus neurons in vivo. *Brain Res* 951, 311-315.

Emch GS, Hermann GE, & Rogers RC (2000). TNF-alpha activates solitary nucleus neurons responsive to gastric distension. *Am J Physiol Gastrointest Liver Physiol* 279, G582-G586.

Eyzaguirre C, Fitzgerald RS, & Lahiri S. Arterial Chemoreceptors. Sheperd, J. T, Abboud, F. M, Geiger, S. R, and Bethesda, M. D. [3], 557-662. 1983. American Physiological Society. Handbook of Physiology. Ref Type: Serial (Book,Monograph)

Fabry Z, Fitzsimmons KM, Herlein JA, Moninger TO, Dobbs MB, & Hart MN (1993). Production of the cytokines interleukin 1 and 6 by murine brain microvessel endothelium and smooth muscle pericytes. *J Neuroimmunol* 47, 23-34.

Felten DL, Ackerman KD, Wiegand SJ, & Felten SY (1987). Noradrenergic sympathetic innervation of the spleen: I. Nerve fibers associate with lymphocytes and macrophages in specific compartments of the splenic white pulp. *J Neurosci Res* 18, 28-21.

Fernandez R, Gonzalez S, Rey S, Cortes PP, Maisey KR, Reyes EP, Larrain C, & Zapata P (2008). Lipopolysaccharide-induced carotid body inflammation in cats: functional manifestations, histopathology and involvement of tumour necrosis factor-alpha. *Exp Physiol* 93, 892-907.

Fernandez R, Larrain C, & Zapata P (2002). Acute ventilatory and circulatory reactions evoked by nicotine: are they excitatory or depressant? *Respir Physiol Neurobiol* 133, 173-182.

Fernandez R, Nardocci G, Simon F, Martin A, Becerra A, Rodriguez-Tirado C, Maisey KR, cuna-Castillo C, & Cortes PP (2011). Lipopolysaccharide signaling in the carotid chemoreceptor pathway of rats with sepsis syndrome. *Respir Physiol Neurobiol* 175, 336-348.

Finley JC & Katz DM (1992). The central organization of carotid body afferent projections to the brainstem of the rat. *Brain Res* 572, 108-116.

Freeman ME, Kanyicska B, Lerant A, & Nagy G (2000). Prolactin: structure, function, and regulation of secretion. *Physiol Rev* 80, 1523-1631.

Gaykema RP, Dijkstra I, & Tilders FJ (1995). Subdiaphragmatic vagotomy suppresses endotoxin-induced activation of hypothalamic corticotropin-releasing hormone neurons and ACTH secretion. *Endocrinology* 136, 4717-4720.

Godin PJ & Buchman TG (1996). Uncoupling of biological oscillators: a complementary hypothesis concerning the pathogenesis of multiple organ dysfunction syndrome. *Crit Care Med* 24, 1107-1116.

Godin PJ, Fleisher LA, Eidsath A, Vandivier RW, Preas HL, Banks SM, Buchman TG, & Suffredini AF (1996). Experimental human endotoxemia increases cardiac regularity: results from a prospective, randomized, crossover trial. *Crit Care Med* 24, 1117-1124.

Goehler LE, Gaykema RP, Nguyen KT, Lee JE, Tilders FJ, Maier SF, & Watkins LR (1999). Interleukin-1beta in immune cells of the abdominal vagus nerve: a link between the immune and nervous systems? *J Neurosci* 19, 2799-2806.

Goehler LE, Relton JK, Dripps D, Kiechle R, Tartaglia N, Maier SF, & Watkins LR (1997). Vagal paraganglia bind biotinylated interleukin-1 receptor antagonist: a possible mechanism for immune-to-brain communication. *Brain Res Bull* 43, 357-364.

Hansen MK & Krueger JM (1997). Subdiaphragmatic vagotomy blocks the sleep- and fever-promoting effects of interleukin-1beta. *Am J Physiol* 273, R1246-R1253.

Hermann GE, Emch GS, Tovar CA, & Rogers RC (2001). c-Fos generation in the dorsal vagal complex after systemic endotoxin is not dependent on the vagus nerve. *Am J Physiol Regul Integr Comp Physiol* 280, R289-R299.

Hess A & Zapata P (1972). Innervation of the cat carotid body: normal and experimental studies. *Fed Proc* 31, 1365-1382.

Hotchkiss RS & Karl IE (2003). The pathophysiology and treatment of sepsis. *N Engl J Med* 348, 138-150.

Howell MD, Donnino M, Clardy P, Talmor D, & Shapiro NI (2007). Occult hypoperfusion and mortality in patients with suspected infection. *Intensive Care Med* 33, 1892-1899.

Huston JM, Ochani M, Rosas-Ballina M, Liao H, Ochani K, Pavlov VA, Gallowitsch-Puerta M, Ashok M, Czura CJ, Foxwell B, Tracey KJ, & Ulloa L (2006). Splenectomy inactivates the cholinergic antiinflammatory pathway during lethal endotoxemia and polymicrobial sepsis. *J Exp Med* 203, 1623-1628.

Kalia M & Davies RO (1978). A neuroanatomical search for glossopharyngeal efferents to the carotid body using the retrograde transport of horseradish peroxidase. *Brain Res* 149, 477-481.

Kawashima K & Fujii T (2000). Extraneuronal cholinergic system in lymphocytes. *Pharmacol Ther* 86, 29-48.

Kawashima K & Fujii T (2003). The lymphocytic cholinergic system and its biological function. *Life Sci* 72, 2101-2109.

Kirchheim HR (1976). Systemic arterial baroreceptor reflexes. *Physiol Rev* 56, 100-177.

Korach M, Sharshar T, Jarrin I, Fouillot JP, Raphael JC, Gajdos P, & Annane D (2001). Cardiac variability in critically ill adults: influence of sepsis. *Crit Care Med* 29, 1380-1385.

Ladino J, Bancalari E, & Suguihara C (2007). Ventilatory response to hypoxia during endotoxemia in young rats: role of nitric oxide. *Pediatr Res* 62, 134-138.

Lam SY, Tipoe GL, Liong EC, & Fung ML (2008). Chronic hypoxia upregulates the expression and function of proinflammatory cytokines in the rat carotid body. *Histochem Cell Biol* 130, 549-559.

Lenczowski MJ, Van Dam AM, Poole S, Larrick JW, & Tilders FJ (1997). Role of circulating endotoxin and interleukin-6 in the ACTH and corticosterone response to intraperitoneal LPS. *Am J Physiol* 273, R1870-R1877.

Libert C (2003). Inflammation: A nervous connection. *Nature* 421, 328-329.

Liljestrand A (1958). Neural control of respiration. *Physiol Rev* 38, 691-708.

Liu X, He L, Stensaas L, Dinger B, & Fidone S (2009). Adaptation to chronic hypoxia involves immune cell invasion and increased expression of inflammatory cytokines in rat carotid body. *Am J Physiol Lung Cell Mol Physiol* 296, L158-L166.

Mac Grory B, O'Connor ET, O'Halloran KD, & Jones JF (2010). The effect of pro-inflammatory cytokines on the discharge rate of vagal nerve paraganglia in the rat. *Respir Physiol Neurobiol* 171, 122-127.

Martin GS, Mannino DM, Eaton S, & Moss M (2003). The epidemiology of sepsis in the United States from 1979 through 2000. *N Engl J Med* 348, 1546-1554.

Martin GS, Mannino DM, & Moss M (2006). The effect of age on the development and outcome of adult sepsis. *Crit Care Med* 34, 15-21.

Martinez JD, Babu RV, & Sharma G (2009). Escherichia coli septic shock masquerading as ST-segment elevation myocardial infarction. *Postgrad Med* 121, 102-105.

Mascorro JA & Yates RD (1980). Paraneurons and paraganglia: histological and ultrastructural comparisons between intraganglionic paraneurons and extra-adrenal paraganglion cells. *Adv Biochem Psychopharmacol* 25, 201-213.

McDeigan GE, Ladino J, Hehre D, Devia C, Bancalari E, & Suguihara C (2003). The effect of Escherichia coli endotoxin infusion on the ventilatory response to hypoxia in unanesthetized newborn piglets. *Pediatr Res* 53, 950-955.

Medvedev AE, Kopydlowski KM, & Vogel SN (2000). Inhibition of lipopolysaccharide-induced signal transduction in endotoxin-tolerized mouse macrophages: dysregulation of cytokine, chemokine, and toll-like receptor 2 and 4 gene expression. *J Immunol* 164, 5564-5574.

Meregalli A, Oliveira RP, & Friedman G (2004). Occult hypoperfusion is associated with increased mortality in hemodynamically stable, high-risk, surgical patients. *Crit Care* 8, R60-R65.

Mignini F, Streccioni V, & Amenta F (2003). Autonomic innervation of immune organs and neuroimmune modulation. *Auton Autacoid Pharmacol* 23, 1-25.

Miksa M, Das P, Zhou M, Wu R, Dong W, Ji Y, Goyert SM, Ravikumar TS, & Wang P (2009). Pivotal role of the alpha(2A)-adrenoceptor in producing inflammation and organ injury in a rat model of sepsis. *PLoS One* 4, e5504.

Misset D, Martin C, Cariou A, Carlet J, Brun-Buisson C, & Annane D. Activated Protein C and Corticosteroids for Human Septic Shock (APROCCHS). 2010. 2010. Ref Type: Internet Communication

Montarolo PG, Passatore M, & Raschi F (1976). Carotid chemoreceptor influence on the cardiac sympathetic nerve discharge. *Experientia* 32, 480-481.

Natanson C, Danner RL, Reilly JM, Doerfler ML, Hoffman WD, Akin GL, Hosseini JM, Banks SM, Elin RJ, MacVittie TJ, & . (1990). Antibiotics versus cardiovascular support in a canine model of human septic shock. *Am J Physiol* 259, H1440-H1447.

Nguyen HB, Corbett SW, Steele R, Banta J, Clark RT, Hayes SR, Edwards J, Cho TW, & Wittlake WA (2007). Implementation of a bundle of quality indicators for the early management of severe sepsis and septic shock is associated with decreased mortality. *Crit Care Med* 35, 1105-1112.

Nguyen HB, Rivers EP, Knoblich BP, Jacobsen G, Muzzin A, Ressler JA, & Tomlanovich MC (2004). Early lactate clearance is associated with improved outcome in severe sepsis and septic shock. *Crit Care Med* 32, 1637-1642.

Novotny NM, Lahm T, Markel TA, Crisostomo PR, Wang M, Wang Y, Ray R, Tan J, Al-Azzawi D, & Meldrum DR (2009). beta-Blockers in sepsis: reexamining the evidence. *Shock* 31, 113-119.

Ohtsuka H, Ohki K, Tanaka T, Tajima M, Yoshino T, & Takahashi K (1997). Circulating tumor necrosis factor and interleukin-1 after administration of LPS in adult cows. *J Vet Med Sci* 59, 927-929.

Otto CM & Rawlings CA (1995). Tumor necrosis factor production in cats in response to lipopolysaccharide: an in vivo and in vitro study. *Vet Immunol Immunopathol* 49, 183-188.

Patel GP, Grahe JS, Sperry M, Singla S, Elpern E, Lateef O, & Balk RA (2010). Efficacy and safety of dopamine versus norepinephrine in the management of septic shock. *Shock* 33, 375-380.

Patel GP, Gurka DP, & Balk RA (2003). New treatment strategies for severe sepsis and septic shock. *Curr Opin Crit Care* 9, 390-396.

Pavlov VA, Wang H, Czura CJ, Friedman SG, & Tracey KJ (2003). The cholinergic anti-inflammatory pathway: a missing link in neuroimmunomodulation. *Mol Med* 9, 125-134.

Perel A (2008). Bench-to-bedside review: the initial hemodynamic resuscitation of the septic patient according to Surviving Sepsis Campaign guidelines--does one size fit all? *Crit Care* 12, 223.

Peres BD, Melot C, Lopes FF, Nguyen B, V, & Vincent JL (2002). The Multiple Organ Dysfunction Score (MODS) versus the Sequential Organ Failure Assessment (SOFA) score in outcome prediction. *Intensive Care Med* 28, 1619-1624.

Pinsky MR (2004). Dysregulation of the immune response in severe sepsis. *Am J Med Sci* 328, 220-229.

Povoa P & Carneiro AH (2010). Adrenergic support in septic shock: a critical review. *Hosp Pract (Minneap)* 38, 62-73.

Rassias AJ, Holzberger PT, Givan AL, Fahrner SL, & Yeager MP (2005). Decreased physiologic variability as a generalized response to human endotoxemia. *Crit Care Med* 33, 512-519.

Reyes EP, Abarzua S, Martin A, Rodriguez J, Cortes PP & Fernandez R (2012) LPS-induced c-Fos activation in NTS neurons and plasmatic cortisol increases in septic rats are suppressed by bilateral carotid chemodenervation. *Adv Exp Med Biol*. In Press.

Reyes EP, Fernandez R, Larrain C, & Zapata P (2007). Carotid body chemosensory activity and ventilatory chemoreflexes in cats persist after combined cholinergic-purinergic block. *Respir Physiol Neurobiol* 156, 23-32.

Riedemann NC, Guo RF, & Ward PA (2003). The enigma of sepsis. *J Clin Invest* 112, 460-467.

Rogausch H, Vo NT, Del RA, & Besedovsky HO (2000). Increased sensitivity of the baroreceptor reflex after bacterial endotoxin. *Ann N Y Acad Sci* 917, 165-168.

Romanovsky AA, Ivanov AI, Berthoud HR, & Kulchitsky VA (2000). Are vagal efferents involved in the fever response to intraperitoneal lipopolysaccharide? *J Therm Biol* 25, 65-70.

Rosas-Ballina M & Tracey KJ (2009). Cholinergic control of inflammation. *J Intern Med* 265, 663-679.

Sanlioglu S, Williams CM, Samavati L, Butler NS, Wang G, McCray PB, Jr., Ritchie TC, Hunninghake GW, Zandi E, & Engelhardt JF (2001). Lipopolysaccharide induces Rac1-dependent reactive oxygen species formation and coordinates tumor necrosis factor-alpha secretion through IKK regulation of NF-kappa B. *J Biol Chem* 276, 30188-30198.

Schletter J, Heine H, Ulmer AJ, & Rietschel ET (1995). Molecular mechanisms of endotoxin activity. *Arch Microbiol* 164, 383-389.

Schmidt H, Muller-Werdan U, Hoffmann T, Francis DP, Piepoli MF, Rauchhaus M, Prondzinsky R, Loppnow H, Buerke M, Hoyer D, & Werdan K (2005). Autonomic dysfunction predicts mortality in patients with multiple organ dysfunction syndrome of different age groups. *Crit Care Med* 33, 1994-2002.

Schmidt H, Muller-Werdan U, Nuding S, Hoffmann T, Francis DP, Hoyer D, Rauchhaus M, & Werdan K (2004). Impaired chemoreflex sensitivity in adult patients with multiple organ dysfunction syndrome--the potential role of disease severity. *Intensive Care Med* 30, 665-672.

Schmidt HB, Heinroth K, & Werdan K (1999). Autonomic dysfunction in critically ill patients. In *Yearbokk of Intensive Care and Energency Medicine*, ed. Vincent JL, pp. 519-536. Springer, New York.

Schmidt HB, Werdan K, & Muller-Werdan U (2001). Autonomic dysfunction in the ICU patient. *Curr Opin Crit Care* 7, 314-322.

Schueller PO, Steiner S, Hennersdorf MG, & Strauer BE (2008). Cardiac chemoreflex sensitivity in critically ill patients. *J Physiol Pharmacol* 59 Suppl 6, 623-627.

Shen FM, Guan YF, Xie HH, & Su DF (2004). Arterial baroreflex function determines the survival time in lipopolysaccharide-induced shock in rats. *Shock* 21, 556-560.

Shu HF, Wang BR, Wang SR, Yao W, Huang HP, Zhou Z, Wang X, Fan J, Wang T, & Ju G (2007). IL-1beta inhibits IK and increases [Ca2+]i in the carotid body glomus cells and increases carotid sinus nerve firings in the rat. *Eur J Neurosci* 25, 3638-3647.

Simon F & Fernandez R (2009). Early lipopolysaccharide-induced reactive oxygen species production evokes necrotic cell death in human umbilical vein endothelial cells. *J Hypertens* 27, 1202-1216.

Singer M, De S, V, Vitale D, & Jeffcoate W (2004). Multiorgan failure is an adaptive, endocrine-mediated, metabolic response to overwhelming systemic inflammation. *Lancet* 364, 545-548.

Singh S & Evans TW (2006). Organ dysfunction during sepsis. *Intensive Care Med* 32, 349-360.

Somers VK, Mark AL, & Abboud FM (1991). Interaction of baroreceptor and chemoreceptor reflex control of sympathetic nerve activity in normal humans. *J Clin Invest* 87, 1953-1957.

Stitt JT (1990). Passage of immunomodulators across the blood-brain barrier. *Yale J Biol Med* 63, 121-131.

Suzuki J, Bayna E, Dalle ME, & Lew WY (2003). Nicotine inhibits cardiac apoptosis induced by lipopolysaccharide in rats. *J Am Coll Cardiol* 41, 482-488.

Tang GJ, Kou YR, & Lin YS (1998). Peripheral neural modulation of endotoxin-induced hyperventilation. *Crit Care Med* 26, 1558-1563.

Thaver D & Zaidi AK (2009). Burden of neonatal infections in developing countries: a review of evidence from community-based studies. *Pediatr Infect Dis J* 28, S3-S9.

Tracey KJ, Beutler B, Lowry SF, Merryweather J, Wolpe S, Milsark IW, Hariri RJ, Fahey TJ, III, Zentella A, Albert JD, & . (1986). Shock and tissue injury induced by recombinant human cachectin. *Science* 234, 470-474.

Turnbull AV & Rivier CL (1999). Regulation of the hypothalamic-pituitary-adrenal axis by cytokines: actions and mechanisms of action. *Physiol Rev* 79, 1-71.

Ulloa L (2005). The vagus nerve and the nicotinic anti-inflammatory pathway. *Nat Rev Drug Discov* 4, 673-684.

van Dillen J, Zwart J, chutte J, & an RJ (2010). Maternal sepsis: epidemiology, etiology and outcome. *Curr Opin Infect Dis* 23, 249-254.

Vayssettes-Courchay C, Bouysset F, & Verbeuren TJ (2005). Sympathetic activation and tachycardia in lipopolysaccharide treated rats are temporally correlated and unrelated to the baroreflex. *Auton Neurosci* 120, 35-45.

ver Elst KM, Spapen HD, Nguyen DN, Garbar C, Huyghens LP, & Gorus FK (2000). Cardiac troponins I and T are biological markers of left ventricular dysfunction in septic shock. *Clin Chem* 46, 650-657.

Verna A (1997). The Mammalian Carotid Body: morphological data. In *The Carotid Body Chemoreceptors*, ed. González C, pp. 1-29. Springer, New York.

Volk T & Kox WJ (2000). Endothelium function in sepsis. *Inflamm Res* 49, 185-198.

Waage A (1987). Production and clearance of tumor necrosis factor in rats exposed to endotoxin and dexamethasone. *Clin Immunol Immunopathol* 45, 348-355.

Wan W, Wetmore L, Sorensen CM, Greenberg AH, & Nance DM (1994). Neural and biochemical mediators of endotoxin and stress-induced c-fos expression in the rat brain. *Brain Res Bull* 34, 7-14.

Wang H, Yu M, Ochani M, Amella CA, Tanovic M, Susarla S, Li JH, Wang H, Yang H, Ulloa L, Al-Abed Y, Czura CJ, & Tracey KJ (2003). Nicotinic acetylcholine receptor alpha7 subunit is an essential regulator of inflammation. *Nature* 421, 384-388.

Wang X, Wang BR, Duan XL, Zhang P, Ding YQ, Jia Y, Jiao XY, & Ju G (2002). Strong expression of interleukin-1 receptor type I in the rat carotid body. *J Histochem Cytochem* 50, 1677-1684.

Wang X, Zhang XJ, Xu Z, Li X, Li GL, Ju G, & Wang BR (2006). Morphological evidence for existence of IL-6 receptor alpha in the glomus cells of rat carotid body. *Anat Rec A Discov Mol Cell Evol Biol* 288, 292-296.

Watkins LR, Goehler LE, Relton JK, Tartaglia N, Silbert L, Martin D, & Maier SF (1995). Blockade of interleukin-1 induced hyperthermia by subdiaphragmatic vagotomy: evidence for vagal mediation of immune-brain communication. *Neurosci Lett* 183, 27-31.

Watson RS & Carcillo JA (2005). Scope and epidemiology of pediatric sepsis. *Pediatr Crit Care Med* 6, S3-S5.

Yang FL, Li CH, Hsu BG, Tsai NM, Lin SZ, Harn HJ, Chen HI, Liao KW, & Lee RP (2007). The reduction of tumor necrosis factor-alpha release and tissue damage by pentobarbital in the experimental endotoxemia model. *Shock* 28, 309-316.

Yucel T, Memis D, Karamanlioglu B, Sut N, & Yuksel M (2008). The prognostic value of atrial and brain natriuretic peptides, troponin I and C-reactive protein in patients with sepsis. *Exp Clin Cardiol* 13, 183-188.

Zapata P, Larrain C, & Fernandez R (2002). Nicotine-evoked ventilatory reflexes in cats: sites of origin and afferents. *J Anat* 200, 204.

Zapata P, Larrain C, Fernandez R, & Reyes EP (2003). Cholinergic actions on carotid chemosensory system. *Adv Exp Med Biol* 536, 277-283.

Zapata P, Larrain C, Reyes P, & Fernandez R (2011). Immunosensory signalling by carotid body chemoreceptors. *Respir Physiol Neurobiol* 178, 370-374.

Zhang XJ, Wang X, Xiong LZ, Fan J, Duan XL, & Wang BR (2007). Up-regulation of IL-1 receptor type I and tyrosine hydroxylase in the rat carotid body following intraperitoneal injection of IL-1beta. *Histochem Cell Biol* 128, 533-540.

Section 3

Biomarkers in Sepsis

Chapter 7

Early Detection of Sepsis, MOF and Outcome Prediction in Severely Traumatized Patients

Zeljko Lausevic and Mirjana Lausevic

Additional information is available at the end of the chapter

http://dx.doi.org/10.5772/52347

1. Introduction

Trauma is the most common cause of death in developed countries among the population under 40 and the fourth overall cause of death in the general population. In the USA 4.6% of all deaths per year are due to accidental injuries. The hospital expenses for injured patients are higher compared to the expenses for patients hospitalized due to other causes.[1] Injury-induced anergy is one of the key factors contributing to trauma victims' high susceptibility to sepsis. Patients are mostly young and it is therefore essential to be able to predict as accurately as possible the development of septic complications so that the appropriate treatment could be provided. Multiple organ failure (MOF) is the leading cause of late death following trauma.[2] The term defines an "all-or-nothing" event and represents only the extreme points of a continuous dynamic process of organ function deterioration. Nowadays the concept of MOF could be revisited as a transient state of metabolic shutdown analogous to hibernation. Avoiding the detrimental effects of inappropriate and counter-adaptive iatrogenic interventions is an important cornerstone of therapeutic management.[3] Severity of injury, late or inadequate resuscitation, inadequate surgical intervention, persistent inflammatory focus, previous organ damage, chronic disease and age over 65 may affect the presentation and the outcome of MOF. Studies demonstrate that the degree of an initial injury is important in determining the patient's susceptibility to post-traumatic complications, but the issue of secondary surgical procedures acting as additional inflammatory insults (second hit) and a genetic predisposition are suspected to be responsible for different outcomes.[4] These factors can explain why some patients develop serious post-traumatic complications and others do not, despite the same injury severity scores. It is still not possible to identify the risk group when efficient intervention could be undertaken. There is a tight correlation between the cytokin plasma level, the development of MOF and the mortality rate.[5] Immunological system plays a major role in an inflammatory response to trauma, which leads to the negative outcome without a direct connection to the severity of trauma or quality of the initial treatment.

INTECH
open science | open minds

The development of immunomonitoring would help in the selection of patients at risk of post-traumatic complications and, thereby, the choice of the most appropriate treatment protocols for severely injured patients.[6]

Trauma triggers a complex cascade of post-traumatic events that are important when predicting the outcome in the first few days after the trauma.[7] Mediators play an important role in the development of the systemic inflammatory response syndrome (SIRS), multiple organ dysfunction (MODS) and multiple organ failure (MOF), the last two associated with high mortality. In critically injured patients who underwent resuscitation early, non-infective SIRS develops. A severe trauma can provoke serious SIRS, although mild SIRS can be useful and helpful in patient recovery. The objectives of the therapy should be pointed towards modulating early SIRS. [8,9]

Interleukin 6 (IL-6) plasma level could be the marker of cytokine's cascade activity and might show the severity of injury. In patients with an obscure sepsis syndrome, IL-6 plasma levels are well correlated to the later sepsis development and consecutive mortality.[10,11,12] The experiments in vitro showed that human monocytes produce interleukin 10 (IL-10) after lipopolysacharide stimulation, later compared to the production of the tumor necrosis factor (TNF)-α, IL-1, IL-6, or IL-8. The presence of anti IL-10 blocking antibodies in the cell culture results in production increase of these cytokines, implicating on the regulatory function of IL-10. IL-10 plasma levels are significantly increased in critically injured patients, especially in patients with sepsis, suggesting that this cytokine is an important inflammation mediator.[13,14]

Infection is identified as the essence of the major cause of multiple organ dysfunction in critically injured patients. [15,16] The course of patophysiological events, especially in the early post-traumatic period, is very important in predicting the outcome.[17,18]

The objectives of the study were to:

1. determine blood levels of C reactive protein (CRP), immunoreactive phospholypase A_2 group II (PLA_2-II), IL-6 and IL-10 concentration as quantifiable parameters of the outcome for critically injured patients;
2. evaluate prognostic values of the Simplified Acute Physiology Score (SAPS II), Injury Severity Score (ISS) score values and multiple organ failure (MOF) signs;
3. construct early predictive models for the outcome prediction.

2. Material and methods

A prospective 65- subject- study was performed at the Intesive Care Unit (ICU) of the Clinical Center of Serbia. The atients met the following criteria: ISS > 18, aged 16-65 , admittance in the first 24 hours after the trauma, survival longer than 48 hours. Patients with the leading neurosurgical trauma were excluded.

Mediators of inflammation were determined in all patients within the first 24 hours, on the second, third, seventh and tenth day of hospitalization. CRP concentration was determined by immunonephelometry on «Behring» laser nephelometer (normal value <9 mg/mL). Phospholipase A_2-II concentration was determined with enzyme-linked immunoadsorbent assay (ELISA), Boehringer Mannheim GmbH, Germany. Interleukin concentration was determined with Immunotech test based on «sandwich» enzyme immunodetermination. The reference range for IL-6 was 0 - 8 pg/mL and for IL-10 0 - 10 pg/mL.

We applied the MOF score, in which the presence of organic damages is defined by the presence of one or more characteristics.[19,20] Lung dysfunction is defined as mandatory mechanical ventilation, for at least 72 hours, PO_2/FiO_2 < 37,3 kPa, positive end expiratory pressure greater than 8 cm H_2O, ARDS verified using X-ray, or respiratory frequence ≤ 5/min or ≥ 49/min. Liver insufficiency is defined as bilirubinaemya >51 μmol/L, at least for 48 hours; heart insufficiency is defined as cardiac index <3,0 L x min^{-1} x m^{-2}, mandatory use of inotropic drugs, heart frequency ≤ 54/min, the presence of ventricular tachycardia and/or fibrilation, mean arterial pressure ≤ 49 mm Hg or pH ≤ 7,24; renal insufficiency is defined as blood level of serum creatinine >177 μmol/ L; haemathologic insufficiency is thrombocytopenia (<20000 cells/mm^3) or leucocytopenia (<1000 cells/ mm^3). All these analyses were conducted daily. The worst value was taken into account when defining the presence of organic insufficiency (the presence of only one of these listed meant the presence of insufficiency).

The criteria for defining the presence of the SIRS were: body temperature >38 or <36 °C, heart frequency greater than 90 bpm, tachypnea (>20 respiration per minute at room temperature or $PaCO_2$ <4.3 Kpa), WBC >12000 cells/mm^3 or < 4000 cells/mm^3, or presence of more than 10% immature neutrofils (bands). [21]

Simplified Acute Physiology Score (SAPS II) is made out of 17 variables: 12 of them are physiological, age, type of treatment (urgent surgery, planned surgery or non-operative treatment) and three variables are connected to the existence of chronic commorbidities, such as AIDS, metastatic cancer or hematologic malignancy. Each of these variables was given a certain number of points ranging from 0 to 3 (for body temperature) or from 0 to 26 (for the Glasgow Comma Scale). For 12 physiologic variables we took the worst values (with the highest number of points) during the first 24 hours after admission in ICU.[22]

ISS was calculated in a standard manner, by squaring the highest individual values for three body regions in the first 24 hours: $ISS = AIS^2 + AIS^2 + AIS^2$. [23,24]

The Chi^2 test was used for estimating the difference of frequency for categories that behaved according to the nominal scale. The differences between numerical charactistics were tested using the t-test. The Mann Whitney U test or Wilcoxon's test of pairs were used if the distribution was significantly different from normal. Each variable was assessed individually with the univariate analysis as a resulting variable for survival. The parameters that were found to be statistically significant predictors with the univariate analysis were included in the multivariate model. The logistic regression coefficient was used to analyse the correlation between the daily average CRP, IL-6, IL-10 and PLA_2-II concentrations and mortality. Values $p<0.05$ or $p<0,01$ were considered significant.

3. The results

Sixty five patients (52 male and 13 female), average age 47.13 ± 15.03 years, were included in this study. This can be explained by a greater exposure of men to trauma. There is a signifficant age difference among groups with MOF and without MOF (t= - 2.058, p=0.044) and survived and deceased patients group (t = - 3.26; p= 0.002). The most frequent was blunt trauma (51 patient, 78.1%), 14 patients (21.9%) had open wounds. Fourty three (66.1%) patients underwent surgical intervention, while 22 (33.9%) patients were treated non-operatively. The overall hospital stay was 23.85 ± 5.94 days, ranging from two days (which is a minimal entry criterion for this study) to 131 days. The overall mortality rate was 50.76% (33 died, 32 survived). After a severe trauma MOF developed in 36 patients, while 29 were with no MOF signs. The mortality rate in the group of patients with MOF was 75%. Concerning the outcome, there is a significant difference between the groups with and without MOF (Pearson –20,571 (b), p=,000).

The average CRP daily values, in both survived and deceased patients, are shown in the Table 1. There was a significant difference, with the highest value for the seventh day of hospitalization (Mann – Whitney U test). The level of correlation of serum concentrations and the survival rate is very high for the third and seventh day of hospitalization, and it is significant for the first (R_1), second (R_2) and tenth day (R_{10}) of hospital stay (R_3 = 0,4355, R_7 = 0,5460, R_1= 0,3246, R_2 = 0,3610, R_{10} = 0,3517). The average IL-6 values for each day of the two observed groups are shown in Table 1. There is a highly significant difference in IL-6 average values between the two observed groups for the four initial days of hospitalization, especially in the first three days. There is also a significant correlation between serum concentration and the overall survival, especially in two starting days (R_1 = 0,4278, R_2 = 0,4338), but with remaining significance for the third and seventh day, (R_3 = 0,4018, R_7 = 0,3082). There is a highly significant difference for the IL-10 concentration for the first three days and also for the tenth day of hospitalization. But, there is a high degree of correlation for the serum concentration of this cytokine and the negative outcome for the second day of hospitalization (R_2 = 0,2491).

We also compared average PLA_2 group II serum concentrations in the two observed groups, in the same manner and at the same time as described previously.

There is a substantial difference in average PLA_2 II levels in the first four measurments related to the outcome. There is a strong correlation between its values and the outcome, especially for the measurments conducted on the first, second, third and seventh day (R_1 = 0,3188, R_2 = 0,2766, R_3 = 0,2911, R_7 = 0,2977).

There is a signifficant difference in the number of positive SIRS characteristics for the day 1, 4. and 5 between the observed groups. There is also a huge statistically significant correlation between the SIRS charactersistics and the survival rate for the first, second, fourth and fifth day of hospitalization (Table 2).

Days		CRP	IL-10	IL-6	PLA_2
1.	S	129,83±13,44**	144,90±46,30**	256,59±75,34**	42,69±8,61
	D	212,83±18,29	285,96±64,28	804,33±96,62	120,68±19,94
2.	S	148,66±14,40**	64,95±14,31**	189,69±57,71**	57,42±11,90
	D	256,03±22,00	244,20±64,02	655,41±86,82	126,25±18,39
3.	S	141,99±14,59**	47,31±13,56**	106,81±26,87**	51,48±9,49
	D	257,28±18,27	161,50±53,28	437,18±79,55	119,80±19,62
7.	S	127,57±13,41**	34,75±14,93**	72,75±19,96**	41,75±9,00
	D	274,20±18,53	153,50±53,57	373,14±109,0	125,87±27,88
10.	S	163,71±25,69**	32,14±15,09	96,57±44,42	78,79±21,28
	D	275,38±26,33	86,83±45,69	151,66±44,76	109,48±32,45

C-reactive protein - CRP in mg/l
interleukin (IL) 6 (pg/mL)
IL-10 (pg/mL)
phospholipase A_2 (PLA_2 in ng/L)
survived (S) ,deceased (D)
* p<0,05
**p<0,01

Table 1. Average C-reactive protein, interleukin 6, interleukin 10 and phospholipase A_2 in survived (S) and deceased (D) patients following severe trauma (Mann Whitney U test).

days	SIRS1	SIRS2	SIRS3	SIRS4	SIRS5	SIRS6	SIRS7
S	2,31±0,06	2,31±0,09	2,13±0,12	2,04±0,10	1,85±0,15	2,25±0,13	2,30±0,15
D	2,71±0,03	2,56±0,08	2,54±0,10	2,62±0,13	2,87±0,12	2,70±0,16	2,76±0,18
p	**<0,01**	>0,05	>0,05	**<0,01**	**<0,01**	>0,05	>0,05
pR	**<0,01**	**<0,01**	**<0,05**	**<0,01**	**<0,01**	>0,05	>0,05

p – derived from t-test
pR – derived from logistic regression coefficient

Table 2. Number of positive systemic inflammatory response (SIRS) variables per hospital days in survived (S) and deceased (D)patients

SAPS II values in both groups are higly different (t = - 5.805; p<0.000), Table 3. The degree of correlation shows a considerable significance for the method of logistic regression (R = 0.4811; p<0.000). The prognostic power of this score considering the outcome is 78.13% in our series.

The anatomic score model for injury severity, ISS, in the group of survivors (27,62 ± 5,31 SD) and the group of deceased are highly different (t= - 4.103; p<0.0001), Table 3. Its predictive power in our series was 75%. The method of logistic regression shows a highly significant correlation between the severity of the injury (ISS) and the survival rate (R = 0.3627).

	ISS	SAPS2
S	27,62±5,09 (SD)	31,39±9,24 (SD)
D	33,34±6,01 (SD)	47,31±11,8 (SD)
R	0,3627	0.4811
p	<0,01	<0,01

R- logistic regression coefficient
p - derived from t-test

Table 3. The Injury Severity Score (ISS) and Simplified Acute Physiology Score (SAPS II) values in survived (S) and deceased (D) patients

The mutual effect of all significant variables obtained by the univariate analysis is examined by the multivariate logistic regression model, estimating that the most important predictors of the outcome were the values of SAPS II and the CRP values for day 2 (CRP 2), mutually combined. This model shows the predictive power of 88.50% (Table 4).

	B	**S.E.**	**Wald**	**sign**	**R^2**
SAPS II	0,122	0,035	12.316	0,0001***	0,341
CRP 2	0,008	0,003	5.083	0,024*	0,410
Const.	-6.179	1.461	17.896	0,0001	Ø

Table 4. Multivariate logistic regression model 1

$$Y=-6.179 + 0,122 \times \text{SAPS II} + 0,008 \times \text{CRP 2}$$

The second model includes CRP values for the second day of hospitalization, the numbers of positive SIRS criteria for the day 1 (SIRS.1) and the values of SAPS II score. This model shows the predicitve power of 80.70% (Table 5).

	B	**S.E.**	**Wald**	**s**	**R**
SIRS-1	1,9609	0,8401	5,4486	0,0196	0,2095
SAPS II	0,1306	0,0451	8,2631	0,0040	0,2833
CRP 2	0,0066	0,0035	3,5060	0,0611	0,1384
Const.	-11,4242	3,3775	11,4410	0,0007	Ø

Table 5. Multivariate logistic regression model 2

$$Y=-11,4242 + 1,96 \times \text{SIRS1} + 0,13 \times \text{SAPS II} + 0,007 \times \text{CRP 2}$$

The same significance has the predicitve model that takes into account the MOF development and the CRP values for the second day, again in mutual combination (Table 6).

	B	**S.E.**	**Wald**	**s**	**R**
MOF	2,6426	0,9643	7,5103	0,0061	0,3178
CRP 2	0,0132	0,0053	6,1129	0,0134	0,2746
Const.	-3,9805	1,3985	8,1014	0,0044	Ø

Table 6. Multivariate logistic regression model 3

$$Y=-3,98 + 2,64 \times MOF + 0,013 \times CRP$$

4. Discussion

The mortality rate is higher in the group of patients with a greater number of positive SIRS criteria. SIRS duration can play an important role. In other words, persistent SIRS probably assumes a high risk level. [25,26,27] The number of SIRS characteristics during the several initial days of hospitalization (for days 1 and 3) and SIRS duration are significantly related to the outcome. In our study the number of SIRS characteristcs is a better outcome predictor, than the SIRS duration. Three or more positive SIRS characteristics for the first and second day in our series are associated with a high risk of intrahospital death. Nowadays, the development of resuscitation and reanimation has decreased the mortality rate. One decade ago, a similar approach to sepsis included an early goal – directed therapy. The properly timed application of enteral nutrition, prevention of nosocomial infection, decubitus, mechanical ventilation, or haemodialysis, have a greater significance than previously thought.[28,29]

The predictive significance of physiological scoring systems is mostly expressed as «daily risk». We used the simple acute physiological score, second version, because of its simplicity of taking and calculating, and positive criticism.[22] The values of this score ranged from 17 to 75, with the average value of 39 points. There is a highly significant difference between the two groups related to the outcome. The overall predicting accuracy of intrahospital mortality in our series is very good (near 80%), greater than the ISS. SAPS II, using the method of multivariate logistic regression, entered as one of the most important variables into the model of regression for the outcome prediction. We feel that this data shows the usefulness of the physiological scoring systems application in the assessment of the patient's response to trauma and in outcome predicting. The best accuracy is obtained when combining physiological and anatomical scores, with the determination of specific inflammation markers, which is the recommendation of many researchers.[30,31]

The peak of IL-6 serum levels is related to surgical trauma, with the surgical procedure duration and blood loss.[43] Stratification of injured patients according to injury severity and the outcome, takes into account the cytokine status. [11,33] According to cytokine serum levels, patients are divided into four groups, with prognostic significance. The number of patients with the worst prognostic group, the third (over 250 pg/L) and the fourth (over 500 pg/L) in our series is very high (over 45%); there is a highly significant difference among the patients related to the outcome ($p=0.0000$). In deceased patients high levels persists in the form of plateau and decrease minimally (in case of death). Significantly high values for the first and second day are found, but the majority indicate that the window is closed after three days, meaning that values after that period have no predictive power.

Clinical IL-10 application was disappointing and its administration immediately after the trauma or surgical intervention didn't improve the survival rate. Also, this cytokine failed to decrease the level of other proinflammatory cytokines (TNF, IL-1, IL-8) in serum and fail in blocking the neutrophil accumulation in the lungs.[36] The IL-10 administration increase mice mortality during endotoxaemia, while blocking IL-10 activity decreased mortality in the Klebsiella and Candida infected mice.[34] In patients with an inevitable negative outcome (extensive combustions, critically injured patients), IL-10 serum levels are the highest. On the other hand, in patients with clinical signs of ARDS, the low IL-10 levels in the bronchalveolar lavage are associated with the increased mortality. These results pose a question when it would be the problem to have too little or too much IL-10; in other words, when IL-10 can be taken as a relevant marker or a mediator. The ratio of IL-6 to IL-10 may be a predictive factor in SIRS.[33] In our study we partially confirmed the disappointing overwhelming reports on a possible protective role of IL-10 in human sepsis.[34] The kinetics of its concentration is very similar to the IL-6 kinetics and appears to be more realistic in describing the illness severity and the outcome, than in playing a protective role in critically injured patients. Based upon our results, IL-10 kinetics and its high serum levels in the groups with the poorer outcome are not in favor of its protective role as a cytokine, but it can be used as a good predictor of injury course and the outcome for some group of patients.[14, 37,38]

A signifficant correlation between non-pancreatic PLA_2 levels and the development of respiratory insufficiency and hypotension in sepsis was found.[39] There is an obvious increase in non-pancreatic PLA_2 levels in relation to mortality. There are several contradictory results on the correlation of this enzyme plasma concentration with some diseases, their course and the outcome. It was found in patients with multiple trauma that PLA_2 group II might be considered as an important predictor of injury severity the outcome, and it was shown in several studies that its concentrations and kinetics are well correlated to the course and the outcome of septic syndrome.[40] On the other hand, the role of PLA_2 II in different conditions (multiple injuries, acute pancreatitis, sepsis) was studied and it was shown that in case of critical injuries (ISS average value was 41) the PLA_2 levels correlate well to the illness severity and the outcome.[41,42] In our series, average PLA_2 II values for each day have been compared to the septic syndrome and multiorganic insufficiency development and the outcome. The highest signifficance exists in average serum concentrations on the second and third day, related to the outcome. On the seventh day there is a peak value in patients with a negative outcome, while serum levels on the 10th and 14th day decreased. We created three models concerning the outcome. Al the models included CRP values for the second day of hospitalization. In the first model SAPS II values were added. Because of the availability of the needed data and the fact that it can be calculated on the second day of the hospitalization, this is the model we would like to emphasize. The second model includes the number of SIRS characteristics on the first day, SAPS II values and CRP values on second day of hospitalization. The third model that points out the probability of intrahospital death, except the CRP value for the second day, takes into account the presence of MOF (MOF present – 1; MOF absent – 0). Although the accuracy of this model is very high, the calculating of MOF score can be very complicated, and the MOF presence itself is a serious prognostic sign that decreases the predictive power of this model. We think that the utilization of these models in our practice would be very interesting and would test its value in the best way.

5. Conclusion

In our study the number of positive SIRS characteristics is related to the outcome. SAPS II values are significantly different in the survived and deceased groups. ISS enables very good quantification of the patients' injuries and represents a precise outcome predictor. It is possible to predict the outcome based on CRP kinetics from Day 1 to Day 10. IL-6 kinetics in the first seven days, before the clear appearance of clinical symptoms, can point to the possible outcome. A high average IL-10 serum level in the initial 24 hours after the injury, the second and the third day announce a negative course and injury outcome. PLA_2 in our series reflects the injury severity and systemic response, and its average daily concentrations with high probability can divide patients into groups of the survived and the deceased. It is possible to create predictive models based on our results considering the outcome. The most important parameters are SAPS II values and CRP values on day 2 combined.

Author details

Zeljko Lausevic*
Emergency Center, Clinical Center of Serbia, Serbia
School of Medicine, University of Belgrade, Belgrade, Serbia

Mirjana Lausevic
Clinic of Nephrology, Clinical Center of Serbia, Serbia
School of Medicine, University of Belgrade, Belgrade, Serbia

6. References

[1] Wilson C.W, Grande M.C and Hoyt B.D. (2007) Trauma, Emergency Resuscitation, Perioperative Anesthesia and Surgical Management. Informa Healthcare USA

[2] Waydhas C, Nast-Kolb D, Trupka A, et al. Posttraumatic inflammatory response, secondary operations, and late multiple organ failure. *J Trauma.* 1996; 40(4):624-31

[3] Mongardon N, Dyson A, Singer M. Is MOF an outcome parameter or a transient, adaptive state in critical illness? Curr Opin Crit Care. 2009 October; 15(5): 431–436.

[4] Moore FA, Sauaia A, et al. Postinjury multiple organ failure: a bimodal phenomenon. *J Trauma.* 1996; 40(4):501-12

[5] Hildebrand F, Pape HC, Krettek C. The importance of cytokines in the posttraumatic inflammatory reaction. Unfallchirurg. 2005; 108(10): 793-803

[6] Vincent JL. Prevention and Therapy of Multiple Organ Failure. World J. Surg. 1996;20(4): 465-70

[7] Sauaia A, Moore FA, Moore EE, Norris JM, Lezotte DC, Hamman RF. Multiple organ failure can be predicted as early as 12 hours after injury. The Journal of Trauma Injury, Infection, and Critical Care 1998; 45(2):291-303

* Corresponding Author

[8] Bone RC. Toward a theory regarding the pathogenesis of the systemic inflammatory response syndrome: What we know and do not know about cytokine regulation. *Crit Care Med* 1996; 24(1):162-72

[9] Ogawa M. Systemic Inflammatory Response Syndrome - A Concept for Avoiding Organ Dysfunction Induced by a "Second Attack". *Surgery Today* 1998; 28(7):679-81

[10] Frink M, Van Griensven M, Kobbe P, Brin T, Zeckey C, Vaske B, Krettek C, Hildebrand F. IL-6 predicts organ dysfunction and mortality in patients with multiple injuries. Scand J Trauma Resusc Emerg Med. 2009; 17: 49.

[11] Pileri D, Accardo Palomb A, D'Amelio L, Conte C. Concentrations of Cytokines Il-6 and Il-10 in Plasma of Burn Patients: Their Relationship to Sepsis and Outcome. Ann Burns Fire Disasters. 2008 ; 21(4): 182–185.

[12] Borden EC, Chin P. Interleukin-6: a cytokine with potential diagnostic and therapeutic roles. J Lab Clin Med. 1994; 123 (6):824-9

[13] A. Marchant, J.L. Vincent, M.Goldman. The protective role of interleukin-10 in sepsis; Yearbook of intensive care and emergency medicine 1994; 42-47

[14] Remick D.G., Gard S.J., Newcomb D.E., et al: Exogenous interleukin-10 fails to decrease the mortality or morbidity of sepsis. Crit. Care Med. 1998; 26:895-904

[15] Nasraway SA. Sepsis research: We must change course. Crit Care Med 1999; 27:427-30

[16] Cohen NH. Reduced mortality from septic shock – Lessons for the future. Crit Care Med 1998; 26:1956-8

[17] Guirao X, Lowry SF. Biologic control of injury and inflammation: Much more than too little or too late. World J Surgery. 1996; 20(4):437-46

[18] Keel M, Trentz O. Pathophysiology of polytrauma. Injury. 2005; 36(6): 691-709

[19] Vincent JL, Moreno R, Takala J, et al. The SOFA (sepsis-related organ failure assessment) score to describe organ dysfunction/failure. Intensive Care Med 1996; 22:707-710.

[20] Marshall JC, Cook DJ, Christou NV, Bernard GR, Sprung CL, Sibbald WJ. Multiple organ dysfunction score: a reliable descriptor of a complex clinical outcome. Crit Care Med 1995; 23:1638-1652.

[21] Members of the American College of Chest Physicians / Society of Critical Care Medicine Consensus Conference Committee: American College of Chest Physicians/Society of Critical Care. Medicine Consensus Conference: Definitions for sepsis and organ failure and guidelines for the use of innovative therapies in sepsys. Crit Care Med 1992; 20:864-74

[22] Auriant I et al. Simplified acute physiology Score II for measuring severity of illness in intermediate care units. Crit Care Med 1998; 26:1368-1372.

[23] Champion HR, Sacco WJ, Lepper RL, et al: An anatomic index of injury severity. J Trauma 20:197, 1980

[24] Champion HR, Copes WS, Sacco WJ, et al: Improved predictions from a severity characterization of trauma (ASCOT) over trauma and injury severity score (TRISS): Results of an independent evaluation. J Trauma 40:42, 1996

[25] Marshal J: Both the disposition and the means of cure: "Severe SIRS," "sterile shock," and the ongoing challenge of description. Crit-Care-Med. 1997 Nov; 25(11): 1765-6

[26] Rixen D. et al.: "Sepsis/SIRS," physiologis slassification, severity stratification, relation to cytokine elaboration and outcome prediction in posttrauma critical illness. The Journal of Trauma: Injury, Infection, and Critical Care 1996; 4:581-598.
[27] Michio Ogawa. Systemic Inflammatory Response Syndrome - A Concept for Avoiding Organ Dysfunction Induced by a "Second Attack". Surgery Today 1998; 28:679-681.
[28] Dellinger RP, Levy MM, Carlet JM, et al. Surviving Sepsis Campaign: International guidelines for management of severe sepsis and septic shock: 2008. Crit Care Med;36(1):296-327
[29] Cannon CM, for the Multicenter Severe S, Septic Shock Collaborative G. The GENESIS Project (GENeralisation of Early Sepsis Interventions): A Mulzicenter Quality Improvement Collaborative. Acad Emerg Med. 2010;17(11);1258
[30] Gorra AS, Clark DE, Mullins RM. Using Hospital Outcomes to Predict 30-Day Mortality Among Injured Patients Insured by Medicare.Arch Surg. 2011;146(2):195-200.
[31] Jack E. Zimmerman, MD et al.: Severity stratification and outcome prediction for multisystem organ failure and dysfunction. World J. Surg 1996; 20:401-405.
[32] Marecaux G, Pinsky MR, Dupont E, Kahn RJ, Vincent JL. Blood lactate levels are better prognostic indicators than TNF and IL-6 levels in patients with septic shock. Intensive Care Med. 1996. May 22:5 404-8
[33] Miyaoka K, Iwase M, Suzuki R, et al. Clinical evaluation of circulating interleukin-6 and interleukin-10 levels after surgery-induced inflammation J Surg Res. 2005;125 (2): 144-50
[34] Osuchowski F.M, Welch K, Siddiqui J, Remick D.G. Circulating Cytokine/Inhibitor Profiles Reshape the Understanding of the SIRS/CARS Continuum in Sepsis and Predict Mortality. The Journal of Immunology 2006 ; 177(3) 1967-1974.
[35] Parsons PE. Interleukin-10: The ambiguity in sepsis continues. Crit Care Med 1998; 26:818-9
[36] Parsons PE, Moss M, Vannice JL, et al: Circulating IL-1ra and IL-10 levels are increased but do not predict the development of acute respiratory distress syndrome in at-risk patients. Am J Respir Crit Care Med. 1997; 155:1469-73
[37] Gomes-Jimenes J, Martin MC, Sauri R, et al. Interleukin-10 and the monocytic/macrophage-induced inflammatory response in septic shock. Journal of Infectious Diseases 1995;711:472-5
[38] Donnelly SC, Strieter RM, Reid PT, et al: The association between mortality rates and decreased concentrations of IL-10 and IL-1ra in the lung fluids of patients with the adult respiratory distress syndrome. Ann Intern Med 1996; 125: 191-6
[39] Vadas P, Pruzanski W, Stefanski E, et al. Pathogenesis of hipotension in septic shock: correlation of circulating phospholipase A2 levels with circulatory collapse. Crit. Care Med. 1988;16(1): 1-7
[40] Waydhas C, Nast-Kolb D, Duswald KH, Lehnert P, Schweiberer L. Prognostic Value of Serum Phospholipase A in the Multitraumatized Patient. Klin Wochenschr 1989; 67(3):203-6.
[41] Buchler M, Deller A, Malfertheiner P, et al. Serum Phospholipase A2 in Intensive Care Patients with Peritonitis, Multiple Injury, and Necrotizing Pancreatitis. Klin Wochenschr 1989; 67(3):217-2

[42] Juha M. Grönroos, MD, et al. Group II phospholipase A_2 in serum in critically ill surgical patients. *Crit Care Med* 1994; 22:956-960.

[43] Giannoudis-PV, Smith-MR, Evans-RT, Bellamy-MC, Guillou-PJ: Serum CRP and IL-6 levels after trauma. Not predictive of septic complications in 31 patients. Acta-Orthop-Scand. 1998 Apr; 69(2): 184-8

Chapter 8

New Biomarkers for Sepsis

Lixin Xie

Additional information is available at the end of the chapter

http://dx.doi.org/10.5772/50197

1. Introduction

Sepsis is the most important cause of morbidity and mortality in the intensive care unit (ICU), but it lacks specific clinical manifestations. As a result, sensitive and specific indicators of infection that can be collected easily and that accurately reflect infection severity and prognosis are highly coveted and are clinically important. Currently, common clinical indicators of infection include pyrexia, white blood cell (WBC) counts, C-reactive protein (CRP), and procalcitonin (PCT). However, in clinical settings, the limitation of CRP and PCT for assessing the severity and predicting prognosis may affect the clinician's ability to effectively evaluate the change in septic patients' general condition that would indicate deterioration and even impending death. Therefore, looking for new biomarkers with high sensitivity and specificity is one of the main research fields in sepsis. The objective of this paper is to review new biomarkers that are ....

2. TREM-1

Triggering receptor expressed on myeloid cells-1 (TREM-1) is a recently discovered member of the immunoglobulin superfamily of receptors that is expressed on polymorphonuclear granulocytes and mature monocytes. Bacterial or fungal infections may induce its expression.

2.1. Soluble TREM-1

sTREM-1 is a soluble form of TREM-1 that may be released into body fluids upon the upregulated expression of TREM-1(Bouchon A,et al. 2001). An increasing number of studies indicate that there are increased levels of sTREM-1 in body fluid samples for the following diseases and conditions: sepsis, pneumonia, pleural effusion, septic arthritis, meningitis, peritonitis, and uterine cavity infection (Gibot S, et al. 2004) (Gibot S, et al. 2004) (Liu CL, et al. 2007) (Collins CE,et al. 2009) (Determann RM, et al. 2006) (Kusanovic JP, et al.2010)

(Determann RM, et al. 2009). This suggests that sTREM-1 may be a valuable diagnostic indicator for making distinctions between infectious and non-infectious diseases. It has also been found that septic shock patients have high levels of serum sTREM-1 that are closely related to the severity of infection, and sTREM-1 has a good positive correlation with the Sequential Organ Failure Assessment (SOFA) score (Gibot S, et al. 2004) (Dimopoulou I, et al. 2009). With regard to sepsis prognosis, dynamic changes in serum sTREM-1 may provide warnings concerning the life or death of patients (Zhang J, et al. 2011) (Gibot S, et al. 2005).

Urine sTREM-1 is more sensitive than WBC counts, serum CRP, and serum PCT for the early diagnosis of sepsis, as well as for dynamic assessments of severity and prognosis. It can also provide an early warning of possible secondary acute kidney injury (AKI) in sepsis patients (Su LX, et al. 2011).

In terms of diagnostic value for ventilator-associated pneumonia (VAP), the combination of sTREM-1 plus Clinical Pulmonary Infection Score (CPIS) improved the ability to diagnose VAP. Moreover, logistic regression analysis showed that sTREM-1 is an independent risk factor for VAP (Su LX, et al. for publication). We also found that sTREM-1 is of no use in determining bacteremia-caused, new fever in ICU patients, but sTREM-1 levels correlate with the prognosis of patients with bacteremia (Su LX, et al. for publication).

2.2. Genetics and TREM-1

More and more studies have confirmed that sepsis is caused by factors both environmental and genetic and that from the pathological point of view, genetic factors outweigh environmental factors. Therefore, clarification of how genetic factors are associated with sepsis may increase the awareness of susceptibility and prognosis concerning the disease. A study investigating an association between TREM-1 gene polymorphisms and severe sepsis concluded that 3 studied common polymorphisms within the TREM-1 gene (rs7768162, rs9471535, and rs2234237) may not play a major role in the predisposition to severe sepsis in a Chinese Han cohort (Chen Q, et al. 2008). However, Jung et al (Jung ES,et al. 2011) proved that TREM-1 SNPs (rs7768162, rs9471535, and rs2234237) may play a significant role in the development of intestinal Behcet's disease and may have modest effects on disease severity. Recently, in our study, we found that 2 variations (rs2234246 and rs2234237) within the TREM-1 gene are not correlated with susceptibility to sepsis. However, the TREM-1 rs2234237 polymorphism is associated with high 28-day mortality among sepsis patients, constituting a risk factor affecting prognosis (Su LX, et al. for publication). Therefore, TREM-1 could be a fairly ideal genetic biomarker for the diagnosis and prognosis of sepsis.

3. CD163

CD163 is a transmembrane molecule, hitherto only discovered on the membrane of mononuclear phagocytes. As a specific scavenger receptor for hemoglobin/heme inside the body, it is capable of specific recognition of the hemoglobin-haptoglobin complex. Studies in recent years have found that CD163 regulates the expression of anti-inflammatory molecules, such as Interleukin-10 (IL-10) and Hemeoxigenase-1 (HO-1) (Moestrup SK, et al.2004) (Graversen JH, et al.2002).

3.1. Soluble CD163

Soluble CD163 (sCD163) comes from CD163 molecules that peel off the membrane of mononuclear cells (Moestrup SK, et al.2004) (Hogger P, et al. 2001). Blood levels of sCD163 have prognostic value for several inflammatory diseases and may have use in clinical applications as a biomarker of inflammatory diseases. Our prospective, clinical study confirmed that the serum sCD163 level might have potential value for the diagnosis of sepsis and severe sepsis, and its performance was superior to PCT and CRP levels. sCD163 also would have advantages for the dynamic monitoring of sepsis development and prognosis and have favorable prospects for use in clinical applications (Feng L, et al. for publication).

3.2. Soluble CD163 and sepsis prognosis

We compared sTREM-1, sCD163 and other clinical parameters for their assessment value for sepsis (Su LX, et al, for publication). On the day of ICU admission, the sepsis group displayed higher levels of serum sTREM-1, sCD163, PCT, and CRP than the Systemic Inflammatory Response Syndrome (SIRS) group ($P<.05$). Although PCT, sTREM-1 and SOFA score were good markers to identify the severity of sepsis, sTREM-1 was the most reliable of these 3 markers. That is because serum sTREM-1 was a risk factor related to sepsis (OR=1.089, 95% confidence interval [CI] 1.045–1.136, $P<.001$). Its area under the Receiver Operating Characteristics (ROC) curve, meant for diagnosis, was 0.978 (95% CI, 0.958–0.997), and that for severity evaluation was 0.9 (95% CI, 0.823–0.977). Sensitivity and specificity were 0.91 and 0.87 respectively. On observation days 1, 3, 5, 7, 10, and 14, serum sCD163, sTREM-1, PCT and SOFA score continued to climb among non-survivors, while WBC and CRP levels decreased. In contrast, various indicators from the survivors showed a tendency to decline. The curves show that the non-survivors registered higher serum sTREM-1, sCD163, WBC and PCT levels, as well as SOFA score over an observation period of 14 days. Both sCD163 and SOFA score were independent factors impacting the survival time (sCD163 hazard ratio =1.09, 95% CI, 1.035–1.154, $P<.001$; SOFA score hazard ratio=1.23, 95% CI, 1.126–1.335, $P<.001$). Their areas under the ROC curve, denoting prognosis, measured 0.696 (95% CI, 0.593-0.799) and 0.794 (95% CI, 0.705–0.833), respectively. With 2.84 mg/L as the cutoff point for sCD163, sensitivity measured 0.535 and specificity was 0.789. In summary, the serum sCD163 level could be the most useful diagnostic value indicator for dynamic assessment of sepsis prognosis (Su LX, et al, for publication) .

3.3. Soluble CD163 and kidney disease

Some studies in patients with bacteremia report high serum sCD163 expression, which has prognostic value (Gaini S, et al. 2008) (Moller HJ, et al. 2006), and high serum sCD163 expression also occurs in people with chronic kidney diseases (Axelsson J, et al. 2006). The

CD163-hemoglobin scavenger receptor plays an important role in the process of the clearance and conversion of hemoglobin/heme in chronic kidney disease (Simoni J, et al. 2006). At present, it is unknown whether sCD163 can be detected in urine and what value it may possess for sepsis and secondary AKI. Recently, our team evaluated for the first time the potential value of urine sCD163 for sepsis and secondary AKI diagnosis, as well as for early assessment of prognosis. Our results demonstrated in an indirect manner the causes behind urine phagocyte increase and revealed a possible mechanism therein (Su LX, et al. for publication). Perhaps this new discovery of a noninvasive detection index may have potential clinical value for sepsis-related multiple organ dysfunction.

4. microRNAs

MicroRNAs (miRNAs) are a type of endogenous non-coding small RNAs that are about 22 nucleotides in length (Lagos-Quintana et al. 2001) (Ambros 2004). They play important biological roles by inhibiting the expressions of messenger RNAs (mRNAs) (Krutzfeldt et al. 2006). As with mRNAs, some miRNAs are differentially expressed among tissues or developmental stages. Unlike some widely expressed miRNAs, these tissue- or developmental stage-specific miRNAs likely play key roles in regulating specific processes involved in the development or function of individual tissues (Etheridge et al. 2011). The liver-specific miR-122 has been applied in lipid and cholesterol metabolism, which are both known to be important functions of the liver (Bolmeson et al. 2011; Fernandez-Hernando et al. 2011). Because of their unique expression profiles, these miRNAs hold promise as diagnostic markers or therapeutic targets for many diseases. For example, miR-122 is required in hepatitis C virus (HCV) replication (Cermelli et al. 2011) and reagents that can modulate the level of miR-122 have moved into clinical development for HCV treatment (Pan et al. 2007; Said 2010; Zhang et al. 2010). miRNAs play an essential role in many physical and biological processes; thus, altered miRNA expression levels are associated with the occurrence and progression of disease.

4.1. Circulating miRNAs

A significant number of miRNAs have been observed outside of cells, within various body fluids. These cell-free miRNAs in body fluids are stable under harsh conditions including boiling, low or high pH and multiple freeze-thaw cycles (Chen et al. 2008; Mitchell et al. 2008). At present, there are 2 possible hypotheses for the stability and origin of circulating miRNAs. One hypothesis is that passive release occurs during tissue injury. For example, miRNA-216a was differentially expressed in the plasma of a pancreatic injury model in rat (Kong et al. 2010). miR-122 was also a biomarker for drug-induced liver injury (Wang et al. 2009). Alternatively, miRNAs are contained in small particles and are, therefore, protected against RNase activity. Recently, it has been shown that a transfer of mRNA and miRNA between cells can be accomplished through microvesicles (Valadi et al. 2007). These are small particles, which are derived from the cell plasma membrane into the extracellular space and released into the circulation (Caby et al. 2005; van Niel et al. 2006). Microvesicles are derived from various cell types, e.g. reticulocytes, dendritic cells, B and T cells and mast cells (Escola et al. 1998; Valenti et al. 2006; Brase et al. 2010). And in the peripheral blood, two-thirds of microvesicles are derived from platelets. Platelet-derived microvesicles play a role in angiogenesis and the metastatic spread of cancers (Janowska-Wieczorek et al. 2005). Platelet-derived microvesicles induce an immune response upon regulating gene expression in hematopoietic, endothelial, and monocytic cells (Setzer et al. 2006; Majka et al. 2007). Notably, platelet-derived microvesicle subpopulations are increased in patients with sepsis (Janiszewski et al. 2004). However it is currently unknown whether microvesicle content changes in these diseases (Hunter et al. 2008).

4.2. What do we know about the miRNAs as biomarkers for sepsis?

4.2.1. miRNAs as prognostic biomarkers for sepsis

Circulating miRNAs have been recently identified as biomarkers for sepsis. miR-150 was firstly identified as a prognostic marker for sepsis, and levels of miR-150, as detected by microarrays, were significantly different between the leukocytes of healthy controls and sepsis patients. In sepsis patients' plasma, levels of miR-150 were correlated with the level of SOFA score, and the plasma level ratio for miR-150/interleukin-18 can be used to evaluate sepsis severity (Vasilescu et al. 2009). A recent study demonstrated that miR-150 differentially controls the development of natural killer (NK) and invariant NKT cell (iNKT) lineages by targeting the transcription factor c-Myb (Bezman et al. 2011). Few other functional studies about miR-150 in sepsis have been published. However, it has been demonstrated that the coding genes of tumor necrosis factor alpha (TNF-a), interleukin-10 (IL-10), and interleukin-18 (IL-18) have sequence complementarity to miR-150 (Vasilescu, Rossi et al. 2009). This finding suggests that miR-150 might be correlated with some of the immune system dysfunctions in sepsis patients, and it provides a new potential pathogenetic mechanism of sepsis. Hence, additional functional studies of miR-150 are required.

Sepsis is a complex disease that involves various tissues and organs. A simple screen for miRNAs differentially expressed in leukocytes may have missed many miRNAs secreted by other cell types. Hence, a genome-wide method was used to screen for differentially expressed miRNAs between the surviving and non-surviving groups of sepsis patients. Then, two novel prognostic biomarkers, miR-297 and miR-574-5p, were identified by microarray screening and quantitative real-time reverse transcription polymerase chain reaction (qRT-PCR) confirmation (Wang et al. 2012). miR-297 was more closely correlated with survival from sepsis, whereas miR-574-5p was correlated with death from sepsis. After analysis in a multivariable logistic regression model, results showed that a combination of sepsis stage, SOFA scores, and miR-574-5p were correlated with the death of sepsis patients. The predictive capability of these 3 combined variables was analyzed by a ROC curve; the area under the curve was 0.932 (95% CI, 0.887-0.977). When the cutoff point was set at 0.288, these 3 combined variables provided 78.13% sensitivity and 91.84% specificity.

In summary, a genome-wide scan of sepsis patients' sera demonstrated that 2 miRNAs, miR-297 and miR-574-5p, might be related to the prognosis of sepsis in a genetic way. Identification of these miRNAs could provide more therapeutic targets for sepsis.

4.2.2. miRNAs as diagnostic biomarkers for sepsis

As diagnostic biomarkers for sepsis, levels of these markers should be not only differentially expressed between sepsis patients and healthy controls, but also between sepsis patients and SIRS patients. Levels of miR-146a and miR-223 in sepsis patients' sera were significantly decreased compared to SIRS patients and healthy controls. These levels were evaluated by qRT-PCR in 50 sepsis patients and 30 SIRS patients. The areas under the ROC curve for miR-146a and miR-223 were 0.858 and 0.804, respectively, which were both higher than IL-6 with an AUC of 0.785 (Wang et al. 2010). miR-146a regulates a pathway that promotes the binding of transcription repressor RelB to the TNF-α promoter, which generates facultative heterochromatin to silence acute proinflammatory genes (El Gazzar et al. 2011). This mechanism was proved in the THP-1 sepsis cell model of bacterial LPS/endotoxin tolerance. During LPS tolerance, transcriptional- and translation-repressive events combine to tightly regulate proinflammatory genes, which was a common feature of severe systemic inflammation (El Gazzar and McCall 2010). Hence, miR-146a was an important regulator during sepsis. Although the source and the release mechanism of miR-146a remain unknown, its clinical value is undeniable.

miR-15a and miR-16 are also newly identified diagnostic markers for sepsis. Levels of these 2 miRNAs in sepsis and SIRS patients were both significantly higher than in normal controls. And miR-15a can be used to distinguish sepsis patients from SIRS patients. The area under the ROC curve for miR-15a was 0.858, which was much higher than the curves for CRP and PCT. These results were obtained from 166 sepsis patients and 32 SIRS patients (Wang et al, 2012). miR-15a and miR-16 were initially identified as tumor suppressors, and the dysregulation of these two miRNAs has been found to occur in many types of cancer (Calin et al. 2002; Bottoni et al. 2005; Bhattacharya et al. 2009; Yang et al. 2010; Bandi and Vassella 2011). Recently, decreases in miR-15a, miR-16 and miR-223 were found to be associated with the innate immune system by targeting IκB kinase alpha (IKKα) mRNA, which is involved in the non-canonical NF-κB signaling pathway (Li et al. 2010). IκB kinase (IKK) is an enzyme complex that is part of the upstream NF-κB pathway. IκBα (inhibitor of kappa B) protein can inactivate NF-κB, and IKK can phosphorylate the inhibitory IκBα protein. Besides that, there is still no direct evidence for the correlations between miR-15a and miR-16 and sepsis. Hence, more functional studies of miR-15a and miR-16 need to be done.

For sepsis patients, timely diagnosis and early treatment are very important factors to improve their prognosis. miRNAs are newly identified as the main regulators of the immune system, and altered expression profiles in circulation can be used as diagnostic and prognostic biomarkers for sepsis. Although the functions of these miRNAs are not completely understood, their clinical value has been confirmed. New biomarkers also mean novel treatment targets. Hence, target genes of these miRNAs may emerge as potential treatment targets for sepsis patients.

5. SNPs

A single nucleotide polymorphism (SNP) is the most common type of stable genetic variation in the population. Thus, SNPs explain different sequence alternatives (alleles) existing at single base pair positions in genomic DNA in normal individuals in some populations. They are distinguished from rare variations by a requirement for the least abundant allele to have a frequency of 1% or more.(Brookes 1999)

A SNP occurs in approximately 1 of 1000 base pairs, with the most frequent being a C to T substitution. Polymorphisms, which occur both in the coding and non-coding genome regions, involve replacement of a nucleotide with another one, or insertion or deletion of 1 or more nucleotides. Because of a higher degree of preservation of exons to assure the functionality of genes, the frequency of polymorphisms in the non-coding regions is much higher compared with the coding ones. But changes in non-coding regions interfere with the structure and process of transcription and gene expression; thus, polymorphisms and mutations in non-coding regions may also produce a marked effect on phenotype presentations.(Prucha et al. 2008)

5.1. Categories of SNPs

SNPs are divided into two main categories, linked SNPs and causative SNPs. Linked SNPs (also called indicative SNPs) are located outside genes and do not affect protein function. Nevertheless, they are associated with a particular drug response or with the risk for getting a certain disease.

Causative SNPs affect the function of protein, correlating with a disease or influencing a person's response to medication. There are 2 forms of causative SNPs, coding SNPs (cSNPs) and non-coding SNPs. Coding SNPs, located in the coding region of a gene, can change the amino acid sequence of a gene's protein product; this type of SNP attracts more research than non-coding SNPs. Non-synonymous cSNPs (nsSNPs), which change the amino acid sequence of proteins and are likely to affect the structure and function of the proteins, are good candidates for disease-modifying alleles.(Jegga et al. 2007) And non-coding SNPs, located in the gene's regulatory sequences, also can change the level of gene expression. Because only about 3% to 5% of a person's DNA sequence codes for the production of proteins, most SNPs are found outside of coding sequences.

5.2. Influence of SNPs

Single nucleotide substitutions may influence complex diseases by a variety of mechanisms. First, the amino acid sequence of some proteins whose functions include DNA binding, catalytic activity and receptor–ligand contact may be reduced or abolished by SNPs. Second, SNPs can interfere with the initiation or the termination codon or introduce errors in the reading frameshift. Third, mutations in known promoter motifs that alter DNA binding of transcription factors have the potential for decreasing or increasing gene expression. Finally, RNA cleavage-polyadenylation mutants in the untranslated region of the 5' UTR are thought to play a role in controlling mRNA translation while sequence variants in the 3' UTR control RNA cleavage, stability, export and intracellular localization.(Wjst 2004) It is reported that only 10% of all gene-based SNPs have sequence-predicted functional relevance making them a primary target for genotyping in association studies. (Wjst 2004) There has been an effort to explain the potential causal relationship between the genetic changes and the development and course of diseases in order to modulate a patient's response to administration of drugs.(Sachidanandam et al. 2001)

5.3. Researches in SNPs

Genome-wide association (GWA) studies have been used to compare patient populations. The International HapMap Project and the arrival of technologies that type more than 100,000 SNPs in a single experiment have made genome-wide single nucleotide polymorphism (GW-SNP) assay a realistic endeavor. (Gibbs and Singleton 2006)

5.4. SNPs as biomarkers for sepsis

More than 20 years ago, Sorensen and colleagues reported that if one of an adult adoptee's biologic parents died of infection before the age of 50, the adoptee had a 5.81-fold increased risk of dying from infection.(Sorensen et al. 1988) Current sepsis-related polymorphism studies have most commonly focused on one or more polymorphisms for specific genes whose protein products are elements of biologic pathways implicated in sepsis. Many of these studies are association studies where various proinflammatory cytokines and their receptors, novel biomarkers, enzymes and mediators were compared with the development and clinical outcomes of sepsis, severe sepsis and organ dysfunction. In particular, identification of genetic variation in the Toll-like receptors (TLRs) and proinflammatory cytokines has provided valuable insights into the influence of genetic heterogeneity on the response to bacterial infection. And sometimes, different conclusions were given in researching the same SNP. Analyzing the variation in genes and associated differences in response to infection may contribute to the development of new gene diagnosis and therapeutic interventions that will improve outcome in this patient population.

5.4.1. TLRs

Expressed by macrophages, dendritic cells, neutrophils, and other cell populations, TLRs play a central role in the innate immune response to infection through the recognition of distinct bacterial antigens. (Leulier and Lemaitre 2008) TLR4 is crucial for the recognition of lipopolysaccharide (LPS), while TLR2 is essential in the recognition of Gram-positive bacterial components.(Martin 2000; Opal and Huber 2002) In an American research study, human subjects with 2 TLR mutations (299 Asp→Gly and 399 Thr→Ile) were compared to subjects with TLR4 wild type for response to inhaled toxins. The changes in 299 Asp→Gly, but not 399 Thr→Ile, significantly reduced nuclear levels of NF-kB in LPS-stimulated THP-1 cells. The 299/399 polymorphisms had reduced levels of IL-1a associated with hyporesponsiveness to inhaled endotoxin in humans. (Arbour et al. 2000) Patients with septic shock with the TLR4 Asp299Gly/Thr399Ile alleles had a higher prevalence of gram-negative infections.(Lorenz et al. 2002) Furthermore, the TLR4 299 polymorphism has been reported to be associated with severe sepsis, septic shock and a higher mortality in septic patients with SIRS. (Lorenz, Mira et al. 2002; Child et al. 2003; Barber et al. 2004) Some studies illustrate that TLR2 753 Arg→Gln and 677 Arg→Trp may predispose individuals to certain gram-positive infections such as tuberculosis or leprosy.(Ben-Ali et al. 2004; Ogus et al. 2004)

5.4.2. Cytokines

A key role in the pathogenesis of sepsis is the balance or imbalance of pro- and anti-inflammatory cytokines. Disorders of coagulation are common in sepsis, and 30% to 50% of patients have the more severe clinical form, disseminated intravascular coagulation.(Levi et al. 2000)

TNF-α

TNF-α, a pleiotropic cytokine mainly produced by activated monocytes and macrophages, plays a key role in the inflammatory response, and its overexpression can lead to the progression of inflammatory and autoimmune diseases.(Locksley et al. 2001; O'Shea et al. 2002) But the association between TNF gene polymorphisms and morbidity or clinical outcome of sepsis was not so clearly defined. An association between development of sepsis, but not mortality from sepsis, and the TNF2 genotype in the overall population was found.(Teuffel et al. 2010) An Austrian study discovered that peak values of inflammatory and coagulation markers were not different between wild-type TNF-α -308 individuals (GG) and carriers of the TNF-α -308 mutant allele (GA and AA).(Kovar et al. 2007)

IL-1 and receptor

The interleukin-1 (IL-1) receptor-associated kinase 1 (IRAK1) is believed to play an important role in TLR2- and TLR4-induced activation of NF-κB, a critical event in the transcriptional regulation of many sepsis-associated proinflammatory mediators.(Arcaroli et al. 2006) Alleles A2, B2 and RN2 in the IL-1 gene might be important high-risk genetic markers for sepsis.(Ma et al. 2002) IRAK1 might be a genetic risk factor for the occurrence and development of sepsis in the Chinese population. (Arcaroli, Silva et al. 2006)

IL-10

Interleukin-10 (IL-10) is an anti-inflammatory cytokine produced by macrophages and T-helper-type II (TH2) lymphocytes that can downregulate inflammatory production, which plays a very important role in the process of induction of immunoparalysis. (Nicod et al.

1995; Thomassen et al. 1996) Three SNPs (–1082, –819, and –592) were found in the regulatory region of the IL-10 gene. The A allele of the -1082 polymorphism in the IL-10 gene promoter is associated with late blood stream infections in ventilated, very low-birth-weight infants and with sepsis susceptibility, whereas the G allele is associated with higher stimulated IL-10 production and increased mortality in severe sepsis.(Shu et al. 2003; Stanilova et al. 2006) Otherwise, the -1082G/G genotype has been associated with lower mortality and organ failure among the subjects with acute respiratory distress syndrome.(Gong et al. 2006) The A allele of the single nucleotide polymorphism at -592 base pairs was associated with higher mortality in sepsis.(Lowe et al. 2003)

Sepsis, an increasing cause of mortality in patients with infectious diseases, especially in seriously ill patients in the ICU, requires rapid diagnosis and treatment. Because SNPs occur frequently throughout the genome and tend to be relatively stable genetically, they can be used as excellent biological markers in sepsis. Depending on rapid advances in technology and informatics, the primary goal in the management of sepsis may change from rapid treatment to prevention for those most at risk. The health care cost savings from such changes could be substantial.

6. Conclusion

In conclusion, the search for new biomarkers for assessing the severity of sepsis patients and predicting prognosis is very important, interesting, and challenging work, providing new insights to confront sepsis.

Author details

Lixin Xie
Department of Respiratory Medicine, Hainan Branch of Chinese PLA General Hospital, China
Vice Director of Department of Respiratory Medicine, Chinese PLA General Hospital, China

7. References

Bouchon A, Facchetti F, Weigand MA, Colonna M, (2001) TREM-1 amplifies inflammation and is a crucial mediator of septic shock. Nature 410: 1103-1107

Gibot S, Kolopp-Sarda MN, Bene MC, Cravoisy A, Levy B, Faure GC, Bollaert PE, (2004) Plasma level of a triggering receptor expressed on myeloid cells-1: its diagnostic accuracy in patients with suspected sepsis. Ann Intern Med 141: 9-15

Gibot S, Cravoisy A, Levy B, Bene MC, Faure G, Bollaert PE, (2004) Soluble triggering receptor expressed on myeloid cells and the diagnosis of pneumonia. N Engl J Med 350: 451-458

Liu CL, Hsieh WY, Wu CL, Kuo HT, Lu YT, (2007) Triggering receptor expressed on myeloid cells-1 in pleural effusions: a marker of inflammatory disease. Respir Med 101: 903-909

Collins CE, La DT, Yang HT, Massin F, Gibot S, Faure G, Stohl W, (2009) Elevated synovial expression of triggering receptor expressed on myeloid cells 1 in patients with septic arthritis or rheumatoid arthritis. Ann Rheum Dis 68: 1768-1774

Determann RM, Weisfelt M, de Gans J, van der Ende A, Schultz MJ, van de Beek D, (2006) Soluble triggering receptor expressed on myeloid cells 1: a biomarker for bacterial meningitis. Intensive Care Med 32: 1243-1247

Kusanovic JP, Romero R, Chaiworapongsa T, Mittal P, Mazaki-Tovi S, Vaisbuch E, Erez O, Gotsch F, Than NG, Edwin SS, Pacora P, Jodicke C, Yeo L, Hassan SS, (2010) Amniotic fluid sTREM-1 in normal pregnancy, spontaneous parturition at term and preterm, and intra-amniotic infection/inflammation. J Matern Fetal Neonatal Med 23: 34-47

Determann RM, van Till JW, van Ruler O, van Veen SQ, Schultz MJ, Boermeester MA, (2009) sTREM-1 is a potential useful biomarker for exclusion of ongoing infection in patients with secondary peritonitis. Cytokine 46: 36-42

Gibot S, Kolopp-Sarda MN, Bene MC, Bollaert PE, Lozniewski A, Mory F, Levy B, Faure GC, (2004) A soluble form of the triggering receptor expressed on myeloid cells-1 modulates the inflammatory response in murine sepsis. J Exp Med 200: 1419-1426

Dimopoulou I, Orfanos SE, Pelekanou A, Kotanidou A, Livaditi O, Augustatou C, Zervou M, Douka E, Theodorakopoulou M, Karagianni V, Douzinas E, Armaganidis A, Giamarellos-Bourboulis EJ, (2009) Serum of patients with septic shock stimulates the expression of Trem-1 on U937 monocytes. Inflamm Res 58: 127-132

Zhang J, She D, Feng D, Jia Y, Xie L, (2011) Dynamic changes of serum soluble triggering receptor expressed on myeloid cells-1 (sTREM-1) reflect sepsis severity and can predict prognosis: a prospective study. BMC Infect Dis 11: 53

Gibot S, Cravoisy A, Kolopp-Sarda MN, Bene MC, Faure G, Bollaert PE, Levy B, (2005) Time-course of sTREM (soluble triggering receptor expressed on myeloid cells)-1, procalcitonin, and C-reactive protein plasma concentrations during sepsis. Crit Care Med 33: 792-796

Su LX, Feng L, Zhang J, Xiao YJ, Jia YH, Yan P, Feng D, Xie LX, (2011) Diagnostic value of urine sTREM-1 for sepsis and relevant acute kidney injuries: a prospective study. Crit Care 15: R250

Long-xiang Su KM, Xin Zhang, Hui-juan Wang, Peng Yan, Yan-hong Jia, Dan Feng, Li-xin Xie, Diagnostic Value of sTREM-1 and Procalcitonin Serum Levels and Pulmonary Infection Score for Ventilator-associated Pneumonia among ICU Sepsis Patients

Long-xiang Su B-cH, Li-ling Liang, Zhao-xu Jiang, Jie Deng, Yan-hong Jia, Dan Feng, Li-xin Xie, Value of Soluble TREM-1, Procalcitonin, and C-reactive Protein Serum Levels as Markers for Detecting Bacteremia among Sepsis Patients with New Fever in Intensive Care Units

Chen Q, Zhou H, Wu S, Wang H, Lv C, Cheng B, Xie G, Fang X, (2008) Lack of association between TREM-1 gene polymorphisms and severe sepsis in a Chinese Han population. Human immunology 69: 220-226

Jung ES, Kim SW, Moon CM, Shin DJ, Son NH, Kim ES, Lee HJ, Hong SP, Kim TI, Kim WH, Cheon JH, (2011) Relationships between genetic polymorphisms of triggering receptor expressed on myeloid cells-1 and inflammatory bowel diseases in the Korean population. Life sciences 89: 289-294

Long-xiang Su Z-xJ, Xin Zhang, Dan Feng, Li-xin Xie, Dynamic changes of serum soluble triggering receptor expressed on myeloid cells-1 (sTREM-1) and its gene polymorphisms are associated with sepsis prognosis

Lin Feng XZ, Long-Xiang Su,Dan Feng,Yan-Hong Jia,Li-Xin Xie, Clinical Significance of Soluble Hemoglobin Scavenger Receptor CD163 (sCD163) inSepsis, a Prospective Study

Long-xiang Su LF, Qing Song, Hong-jun Kang, Xin-gang Zhang, Zhi-xin Liang, Yan-hong Jia, Dan Feng, Li-xin Xie, Determining the Best Diagnostic Biomarker for Sepsis and Prognosis Assessment

Moestrup SK, Moller HJ, (2004) CD163: a regulated hemoglobin scavenger receptor with a role in the anti-inflammatory response. Annals of medicine 36: 347-354

Graversen JH, Madsen M, Moestrup SK, (2002) CD163: a signal receptor scavenging haptoglobin-hemoglobin complexes from plasma. The international journal of biochemistry & cell biology 34: 309-314

Hogger P, Sorg C, (2001) Soluble CD163 inhibits phorbol ester-induced lymphocyte proliferation. Biochemical and biophysical research communications 288: 841-843

Gaini S, Pedersen SS, Koldkaer OG, Pedersen C, Moestrup SK, Moller HJ, (2008) New immunological serum markers in bacteraemia: anti-inflammatory soluble CD163, but not proinflammatory high mobility group-box 1 protein, is related to prognosis. Clinical and experimental immunology 151: 423-431

Moller HJ, Moestrup SK, Weis N, Wejse C, Nielsen H, Pedersen SS, Attermann J, Nexo E, Kronborg G, (2006) Macrophage serum markers in pneumococcal bacteremia: Prediction of survival by soluble CD163. Critical care medicine 34: 2561-2566

Axelsson J, Moller HJ, Witasp A, Qureshi AR, Carrero JJ, Heimburger O, Barany P, Alvestrand A, Lindholm B, Moestrup SK, Stenvinkel P, (2006) Changes in fat mass correlate with changes in soluble sCD163, a marker of mature macrophages, in patients with CKD. American journal of kidney diseases : the official journal of the National Kidney Foundation 48: 916-925

Simoni J, Simoni G, Griswold JA, Moeller JF, Tsikouris JP, Khanna A, Roongsritong C, Wesson DE, (2006) Role of free hemoglobin in 8-iso prostaglandin F2-alpha synthesis in chronic renal failure and its impact on CD163-Hb scavenger receptor and on coronary artery endothelium. ASAIO J 52: 652-661

Long-xiang Su LF, Zhao-xu Jiang, Ming Li, Kun Xiao, Peng Yan, Dan Feng, Li-xin Xie, Diagnostic value of urine sCD163 for sepsis and relevant acute kidney injuries: a prospective study

Ambros, V. (2004).The functions of animal microRNAs. *Nature* VOL.431, NO.7006, (2004): PP. 350-355, ISSN 1476-4687.

Bandi, N. and E. Vassella (2011).miR-34a and miR-15a/16 are co-regulated in non-small cell lung cancer and control cell cycle progression in a synergistic and Rb-dependent manner. *Mol Cancer* VOL.10, (2011): PP. 55, ISSN 1476-4598.

Bezman, N. A., T. Chakraborty, et al. (2011).miR-150 regulates the development of NK and iNKT cells. *J Exp Med* VOL.208, NO.13, (2011): PP. 2717-2731, ISSN 1540-9538.

Bhattacharya, R., M. Nicoloso, et al. (2009).MiR-15a and MiR-16 control Bmi-1 expression in ovarian cancer. *Cancer Res* VOL.69, NO.23, (2009): PP. 9090-9095, ISSN 1538-7445.

Bolmeson, C., J. L. Esguerra, et al. (2011).Differences in islet-enriched miRNAs in healthy and glucose intolerant human subjects. *Biochem Biophys Res Commun* VOL.404, NO.1, (2011): PP. 16-22, ISSN 1090-2104.

Bottoni, A., D. Piccin, et al. (2005).miR-15a and miR-16-1 down-regulation in pituitary adenomas. *J Cell Physiol* VOL.204, NO.1, (2005): PP. 280-285, ISSN 0021-9541.

Brase, J. C., D. Wuttig, et al. (2010).Serum microRNAs as non-invasive biomarkers for cancer. *Mol Cancer* VOL.9, (2010): PP. 306, ISSN 1476-4598.

Caby, M. P., D. Lankar, et al. (2005).Exosomal-like vesicles are present in human blood plasma. *Int Immunol* VOL.17, NO.7, (2005): PP. 879-887, ISSN 0953-8178.

Wang H. J., Meng, et al. (2012). Evidence for serum miR-15a and miR-16 levels as bimarkers that distinguish sepsis from SIRS in human subjects. *Clin Chem and Lab Med.* VOL.50, NO.8, (2012).

Calin, G. A., C. D. Dumitru, et al. (2002).Frequent deletions and down-regulation of micro-RNA genes miR15 and miR16 at 13q14 in chronic lymphocytic leukemia. *Proc Natl Acad Sci U S A* VOL.99, NO.24, (2002): PP. 15524-15529, ISSN 0027-8424.

Cermelli, S., A. Ruggieri, et al. (2011).Circulating microRNAs in patients with chronic hepatitis C and non-alcoholic fatty liver disease. *PLoS One* VOL.6, NO.8, (2011): PP. e23937, ISSN 1932-6203 .

Chen, X., Y. Ba, et al. (2008).Characterization of microRNAs in serum: a novel class of biomarkers for diagnosis of cancer and other diseases. *Cell Res* VOL.18, NO.10, (2008): PP. 997-1006, ISSN 1748-7838.

El Gazzar, M., A. Church, et al. (2011).MicroRNA-146a regulates both transcription silencing and translation disruption of TNF-alpha during TLR4-induced gene reprogramming. *J Leukoc Biol* VOL.90, NO.3, (2011): PP. 509-519, ISSN 1938-3673.

El Gazzar, M. and C. E. McCall (2010).MicroRNAs distinguish translational from transcriptional silencing during endotoxin tolerance. *J Biol Chem* VOL.285, NO.27, (2010): PP. 20940-20951, ISSN 1083-351X.

Escola, J. M., M. J. Kleijmeer, et al. (1998).Selective enrichment of tetraspan proteins on the internal vesicles of multivesicular endosomes and on exosomes secreted by human B-lymphocytes. *J Biol Chem* VOL.273, NO.32, (1998): PP. 20121-20127, ISSN 0021-9258.

Etheridge, A., I. Lee, et al. (2011).Extracellular microRNA: a new source of biomarkers. *Mutat Res* VOL.717, NO.1-2, (2011): PP. 85-90, ISSN 0027-5107.

Fernandez-Hernando, C., Y. Suarez, et al. (2011).MicroRNAs in lipid metabolism. *Curr Opin Lipidol* VOL.22, NO.2, (2011): PP. 86-92, ISSN 1473-6535.

Hunter, M. P., N. Ismail, et al. (2008).Detection of microRNA expression in human peripheral blood microvesicles. *PLoS One* VOL.3, NO.11, (2008): PP. e3694, ISSN 1932-6203.

Janiszewski, M., A. O. Do Carmo, et al. (2004).Platelet-derived exosomes of septic individuals possess proapoptotic NAD(P)H oxidase activity: A novel vascular redox pathway. *Crit Care Med* VOL.32, NO.3, (2004): PP. 818-825, ISSN 0090-3493.

Janowska-Wieczorek, A., M. Wysoczynski, et al. (2005).Microvesicles derived from activated platelets induce metastasis and angiogenesis in lung cancer. *Int J Cancer* VOL.113, NO.5, (2005): PP. 752-760, ISSN 0020-7136.

Kong, X. Y., Y. Q. Du, et al. (2010).Plasma miR-216a as a potential marker of pancreatic injury in a rat model of acute pancreatitis. *World J Gastroenterol* VOL.16, NO.36, (2010): PP. 4599-4604, ISSN 1007-9327.

Krutzfeldt, J., M. N. Poy, et al. (2006).Strategies to determine the biological function of microRNAs. *Nat Genet* VOL.38 Suppl, (2006): PP. S14-19, ISSN 1061-4036.

Lagos-Quintana, M., R. Rauhut, et al. (2001).Identification of novel genes coding for small expressed RNAs. *Science* VOL.294, NO.5543, (2001): PP. 853-858, ISSN 0036-8075.

Li, T., M. J. Morgan, et al. (2010).MicroRNAs modulate the noncanonical transcription factor NF-kappaB pathway by regulating expression of the kinase IKKalpha during macrophage differentiation. *Nat Immunol* VOL.11, NO.9, (2010): PP. 799-805, ISSN 1529-2916.

Majka, M., J. Kijowski, et al. (2007).Evidence that platelet-derived microvesicles may transfer platelet-specific immunoreactive antigens to the surface of endothelial cells and CD34+ hematopoietic stem/ progenitor cells--implication for the pathogenesis of immune thrombocytopenias. *Folia Histochem Cytobiol* VOL.45, NO.1, (2007): PP. 27-32, ISSN 0239-8508.

Mitchell, P. S., R. K. Parkin, et al. (2008).Circulating microRNAs as stable blood-based markers for cancer detection. *Proc Natl Acad Sci U S A* VOL.105, NO.30, (2008): PP. 10513-10518, ISSN 1091-6490.

Pan, Q. W., S. D. Henry, et al. (2007).New therapeutic opportunities for hepatitis C based on small RNA. *World J Gastroenterol* VOL.13, NO.33, (2007): PP. 4431-4436, ISSN 1007-9327.

Said, E. A. (2010).The Need for New Anti-Hepatitis C Virus Therapeutic Strategies: Targeting the cellular micro-ribonucleic acids? *Sultan Qaboos Univ Med J* VOL.10, NO.3, (2010): PP. 312-317, ISSN 2075-0528.

Setzer, F., V. Oberle, et al. (2006).Platelet-derived microvesicles induce differential gene expression in monocytic cells: a DNA microarray study. *Platelets* VOL.17, NO.8, (2006): PP. 571-576, ISSN 0953-7104.

Valadi, H., K. Ekstrom, et al. (2007).Exosome-mediated transfer of mRNAs and microRNAs is a novel mechanism of genetic exchange between cells. *Nat Cell Biol* VOL.9, NO.6, (2007): PP. 654-659, ISSN 1465-7392.

Valenti, R., V. Huber, et al. (2006).Human tumor-released microvesicles promote the differentiation of myeloid cells with transforming growth factor-beta-mediated suppressive activity on T lymphocytes. *Cancer Res* VOL.66, NO.18, (2006): PP. 9290-9298, ISSN 0008-5472.

van Niel, G., I. Porto-Carreiro, et al. (2006).Exosomes: a common pathway for a specialized function. *J Biochem* VOL.140, NO.1, (2006): PP. 13-21, ISSN 0021-924X.

Vasilescu, C., S. Rossi, et al. (2009).MicroRNA fingerprints identify miR-150 as a plasma prognostic marker in patients with sepsis. *PLoS One* VOL.4, NO.10, (2009): PP. e7405, ISSN 1932-6203.

Wang, H., K. Meng, et al. (2012).Serum miR-574-5p: A Prognostic Predictor of Sepsis Patients. *Shock* VOL.37, NO.3, (2012): PP. 263-267, ISSN 1540-0514.

Wang, J. F., M. L. Yu, et al. (2010).Serum miR-146a and miR-223 as potential new biomarkers for sepsis. *Biochem Biophys Res Commun* VOL.394, NO.1, (2010): PP. 184-188, ISSN 1090-2104.

Wang, K., S. Zhang, et al. (2009).Circulating microRNAs, potential biomarkers for drug-induced liver injury. *Proc Natl Acad Sci U S A* VOL.106, NO.11, (2009): PP. 4402-4407, ISSN 1091-6490.

Yang, Y., X. Li, et al. (2010).The role of microRNA in human lung squamous cell carcinoma. *Cancer Genet Cytogenet* VOL.200, NO.2, (2010): PP. 127-133, ISSN 1873-4456.

Zhang, G., Q. Wang, et al. (2010).Therapeutics Based on microRNA: A New Approach for Liver Cancer. *Curr Genomics* VOL.11, NO.5, (2010): PP. 311-325, ISSN 1875-5488.

Arbour, N. C., E. Lorenz, et al. (2000).TLR4 mutations are associated with endotoxin hyporesponsiveness in humans. *Nat Genet* VOL.25, NO.2, (2000): PP. 187-191, ISSN 1061-4036.

Arcaroli, J., E. Silva, et al. (2006).Variant IRAK-1 haplotype is associated with increased nuclear factor-kappa B activation and worse outcomes in sepsis. *American Journal of Respiratory and Critical Care Medicine* VOL.173, NO.12, (2006): PP. 1335-1341, ISSN 1073-449X.

Barber, R. C., C. C. Aragaki, et al. (2004).TLR4 and TNF-alpha polymorphisms are associated with an increased risk for severe sepsis following burn injury. *J Med Genet* VOL.41, NO.11, (2004): PP. 808-813, ISSN 1468-6244.

Ben-Ali, M., M. R. Barbouche, et al. (2004).Toll-like receptor 2 Arg677Trp polymorphism is associated with susceptibility to tuberculosis in Tunisian patients. *Clin Diagn Lab Immunol* VOL.11, NO.3, (2004): PP. 625-626, ISSN 1071-412X.

Brookes, A. J. (1999).The essence of SNPs. *Gene* VOL.234, NO.2, (1999): PP. 177-186, ISSN 0378-1119.

Child, N. J., I. A. Yang, et al. (2003).Polymorphisms in Toll-like receptor 4 and the systemic inflammatory response syndrome. *Biochem Soc Trans* VOL.31, NO.Pt 3, (2003): PP. 652-653, ISSN 0300-5127.

Gibbs, J. R. and A. Singleton (2006).Application of genome-wide single nucleotide polymorphism typing: simple association and beyond. *PLoS Genet* VOL.2, NO.10, (2006): PP. e150, ISSN 1553-7404.

Gong, M. N., B. T. Thompson, et al. (2006).Interleukin-10 polymorphism in position -1082 and acute respiratory distress syndrome. *Eur Respir J* VOL.27, NO.4, (2006): PP. 674-681, ISSN 0903-1936.

Jegga, A. G., S. Gowrisankar, et al. (2007).PolyDoms: a whole genome database for the identification of non-synonymous coding SNPs with the potential to impact disease. *Nucleic Acids Res* VOL.35, NO.Database issue, (2007): PP. D700-706, ISSN 1362-4962.

Kovar, F. M., C. Marsik, et al. (2007).The tumor necrosis factor alpha -308 G/A polymorphism does not influence inflammation and coagulation response in human endotoxemia. *Shock* VOL.27, NO.3, (2007): PP. 238-241, ISSN 1073-2322.

Leulier, F. and B. Lemaitre (2008).Toll-like receptors--taking an evolutionary approach. *Nat Rev Genet* VOL.9, NO.3, (2008): PP. 165-178, ISSN 1471-0064.

Levi, M., E. de Jonge, et al. (2000).[Disseminated intravascular coagulation]. *Ned Tijdschr Geneeskd* VOL.144, NO.10, (2000): PP. 470-475, ISSN 0028-2162.

Locksley, R. M., N. Killeen, et al. (2001).The TNF and TNF receptor superfamilies: integrating mammalian biology. *Cell* VOL.104, NO.4, (2001): PP. 487-501, ISSN 0092-8674.

Lorenz, E., J. P. Mira, et al. (2002).Relevance of mutations in the TLR4 receptor in patients with gram-negative septic shock. *Arch Intern Med* VOL.162, NO.9, (2002): PP. 1028-1032, ISSN 0003-9926.

Lowe, P. R., H. F. Galley, et al. (2003).Influence of interleukin-10 polymorphisms on interleukin-10 expression and survival in critically ill patients. *Crit Care Med* VOL.31, NO.1, (2003): PP. 34-38, ISSN 0090-3493.

Ma, P., D. Chen, et al. (2002).[Genomic polymorphism within interleukin-1 family cytokines influences the outcome of septic patients]. *Zhonghua Yi Xue Za Zhi* VOL.82, NO.18, (2002): PP. 1237-1241, ISSN 0376-2491.

Martin, T. R. (2000).Recognition of bacterial endotoxin in the lungs. *Am J Respir Cell Mol Biol* VOL.23, NO.2, (2000): PP. 128-132, ISSN 1044-1549.

Nicod, L. P., F. el Habre, et al. (1995).Interleukin-10 decreases tumor necrosis factor alpha and beta in alloreactions induced by human lung dendritic cells and macrophages. *Am J Respir Cell Mol Biol* VOL.13, NO.1, (1995): PP. 83-90, ISSN 1044-1549.

O'Shea, J. J., A. Ma, et al. (2002).Cytokines and autoimmunity. *Nat Rev Immunol* VOL.2, NO.1, (2002): PP. 37-45, ISSN 1474-1733.

Ogus, A. C., B. Yoldas, et al. (2004).The Arg753GLn polymorphism of the human toll-like receptor 2 gene in tuberculosis disease. *Eur Respir J* VOL.23, NO.2, (2004): PP. 219-223, ISSN 0903-1936.

Opal, S. M. and C. E. Huber (2002).Bench-to-bedside review: Toll-like receptors and their role in septic shock. *Crit Care* VOL.6, NO.2, (2002): PP. 125-136, ISSN 1364-8535.

Prucha, M., R. Zazula, et al. (2008).Genomic polymorphism and sepsis--is there a reason for optimism? *Prague Med Rep* VOL.109, NO.2-3, (2008): PP. 113-126, ISSN 1214-6994.

Sachidanandam, R., D. Weissman, et al. (2001).A map of human genome sequence variation containing 1.42 million single nucleotide polymorphisms. *Nature* VOL.409, NO.6822, (2001): PP. 928-933, ISSN 0028-0836.

Shu, Q., X. Fang, et al. (2003).IL-10 polymorphism is associated with increased incidence of severe sepsis. *Chin Med J (Engl)* VOL.116, NO.11, (2003): PP. 1756-1759, ISSN 0366-6999.

Sorensen, T. I., G. G. Nielsen, et al. (1988).Genetic and environmental influences on premature death in adult adoptees. *N Engl J Med* VOL.318, NO.12, (1988): PP. 727-732, ISSN 0028-4793.

Stanilova, S. A., L. D. Miteva, et al. (2006).Interleukin-10-1082 promoter polymorphism in association with cytokine production and sepsis susceptibility. *Intensive Care Med* VOL.32, NO.2, (2006): PP. 260-266, ISSN 0342-4642.

Teuffel, O., M. C. Ethier, et al. (2010).Association between tumor necrosis factor-alpha promoter -308 A/G polymorphism and susceptibility to sepsis and sepsis mortality: a systematic review and meta-analysis. *Crit Care Med* VOL.38, NO.1, (2010): PP. 276-282, ISSN 1530-0293.

Thomassen, M. J., L. T. Divis, et al. (1996).Regulation of human alveolar macrophage inflammatory cytokine production by interleukin-10. *Clin Immunol Immunopathol* VOL.80, NO.3 Pt 1, (1996): PP. 321-324, ISSN 0090-1229.

Wjst, M. (2004).Target SNP selection in complex disease association studies. *BMC Bioinformatics* VOL.5, (2004): PP. 92, ISSN 1471-2105.

Chapter 9

The Role of Procalcitonin in the Early Diagnosis of Septic and Non-Septic Complications in the Immediate Postoperative Setting After Orthotopic Liver Transplantation

Aristotelis Perrakis, Volker Müller, Werner Hohenberger and Roland S. Croner

Additional information is available at the end of the chapter

http://dx.doi.org/10.5772/50242

1. Introduction

Very good survival rates have been achieved in patients with end stage liver disease after orthotopic liver transplantation (OLT), but in the MELD (model of end stage liver disease) era, the gap between patients in the need of OLT and available grafts has widened, leading to acceptance of marginal organs. This is one of the most important reasons for a complicated postoperative course, having a greater risk of graft or multiorgan dysfunction and systemic infection. The result of these factors is the increase of posttransplant morbidity and mortality [1].

Sepsis is the most common cause of mortality, especially in patients undergoing an immunsuppressive therapy and in these after a major surgical treatment. Despite the development and administration of new antimicrobial therapeutic modalities, the mortality rate of sepsis remains high over the last decades because of the high co morbidity and often because of delayed establishment of the diagnosis and treatment [1-4].

1.1. Sepsis and systemic inflammatory response syndrom

Sepsis and systemic inflammation response syndrome (SIRS) induce rapid and profound changes in endothelial function. The endothelial cells from their side trigger the immune response and activate the coagulation system. Endothelial cells cover the surface of blood vessels and are directly in tight contact with solid organs. This is the reason, why endothelial activation and damage leads to organ dysfunction. The endothelium plays also an important role in local and systemic immune responses; it is considered both as source of and as target for inflammation [5]. In cases of local activation of the endothelium there is an isolation of infectious procedures. On the other side and in cases of systemic activation the results are capillary leakage, hypotension and microvascular thrombosis. These aspects result in tissue hypoxia, and organ dysfunction [6– 10].

In cases of inflammation, systemic infection and sepsis there is a constant exposure of these endothelial cells to the circulating endotoxins and proinflammatory cytokines such as interleucin 6 (IL-6), interleucin 1 (IL-1), interleucin 8 (IL-8), tumor necrosis factor α (TNF α) and this leads to an activation of the endothelium and expression of endothelial leucocyte adhesion molecule (ELAM-1), intercellular adhesion molecule (ICAM-1) and vascular cell adhesion molecule (VCAM-1, 8). In cases of severe systemic inflammation and sepsis there is a significant level increase of these adhesion molecules and they could have a very good prognostic and diagnostic power, on the other side with a low specificity as far as the origin of the inflammation is concerned (infectious, non-infectious).

1.2. Markers for sepsis

Markers of sepsis and endothelial activation could potentially play a role in prediction and early diagnosis of onset and severity of the systemic inflammation and through differentiation between infectious and non-infectious causes of the SIRS.

The endothelial adhesion molecules (ELAM-1, ICAM-1 and VCAM1) are not sufficiently investigated and due to lack of specificity do not play a role in the clinical area.

A milestone in the sepsis era was the introduction of IL-6. IL-6, produced by various cell types, such as macrophages, monocytes and endothelial cells, can be stimulated be through bacteria, viruses, polysaccharides, TNF-α, interferons (especially interferon γ) and platelet derivated growth factor (PDGF). Through its very high sensitivity there was a reasonable euphoria, as many thought that the "ideal sepsis marker" was found. However and after introduction of the study of Habarth et al [11,12], who examined combined the diagnostic relevance of IL-6 and PCT in terms of sepsis, it was shown that the diagnostic accuracy of IL-6 is impaired through inflammation procedures independent of infection. On the other hand PCT seemed to have a better correlation to septic episodes and infection.

1.3. Sepsis and SIRS in hepatic dysfunction and after OLT

Liver transplant recipients often manifest a systemic inflammatory response syndrome (SIRS), because of various surgical and non surgical procedures, such as induction of the immunsuppressive therapy and reperfusion during transplantation, independently of the presence of an infectious focus. The clinical signs of infection and routine laboratory tests are not specific and are sometimes misleading. The lack of specific early markers of infection might be responsible in part for delaying of a targeted antimicrobial treatment in this patient population. Moreover, the uncontrolled use of wide spectrum antimicrobial agents as "prophylactic therapy" without use of terms of the pre-emptive therapy is leading to bacterial translocation and the presence of multiresistant microorganisms, which further impairs the patients' outcome [13-20].

Patients with impaired hepatic function are susceptible to an infectious episode because of immunologic deficits in the period before OLT. Impaired immunologic mechanisms resulting from the hepatic function deficit such as decreased hepatic production of complement, impaired Kupffer cell function, impairment of neutrophil chemotaxis, and of inflammatory cytokines [15-20]. Due to the immunological deficit there is also a decreased activity of immunoglobulins as answer to the circulation of gram-negative pathogens [20]. In the presence of structural and functional impairment of the liver, there is a damage of filtering by impaired macrophage mobilization and diminished killing of bacteria [20]. These described deficits lead to an increased risk for systemic infection in the early posttransplant setting and this fact is the most frequent and dangerous complication occurring after OLT. Mora et al, Singh et al and Lee et al reported in their studies the relevance of the early and late bacteriemia in liver transplant recipients, the higher mortality rates in comparison to other patient populations, such as surgical patients and the great importance of the early diagnosis and the early onset of a targeted antimicrobial therapy in order to achieve an acceptable posttransplant outcome [21-24]. Kim et al. reported also similar risk factors in their study about bacteriemia in living donor liver transplant recipients (LDLT) [25]. Several authors reported in their studies an increased infection risk in LDLT because of the small graft size, which might lead to an increased portal venous pressure with impaired bowel motility with consecutive bacterial translocation, which increases the risk for a bacterial infection [26,27]. Igekami et al reported in a large study with LDLT recipients that late enteral nutrition and great blood loss during operative procedure were significant and independent risk factors for a bacterial sepsis in the posttransplant setting [28]. The early start of enteral nutrition could be effective in transplant patients, because of the stimulating effect in terms of bile flow, the enterohepatic circulation and portal blood flow, preventing an atrophia of the intestinal mucosa and a bacterial translocation [28]. Furthermore high MELD score and the co morbidity of recipients seem to have a significant effect on the onset of bacteriemia and septic complications after OLT.

Bacteriemia accounts for up to 30% of all major infections after liver transplantation with an considerable mortality risk of 20% to 39% [21-28]. The main sources for bacteriemia and systemic infection, occurring within the first 3 months after OLT, are infected vascular catheter sited, pneumonia and infections of the biliary tract in terms of cholangitis following a biliary disorder(stenosis, ITBL, presence of biliodigestive anastomosis) [29]. Several authors examining blood stream infections in the posttransplant setting in their studies have shown that gram negatives, particularly, Klebsiella and Pseudomonas, tend to be the predominant species [30]. Furthermore Karvellas et al reported in a large study that the predominant species was enterococcus. Significantly more patients in the infected group had a biliodigestve anastomosis [30].

As underlined before, several studies have examined the risk factors and the onset of post-transplantation bacterial and fungal sepsis in patients undergoing OLT. Clinical signs of an infection (dysregulation of temperature, tachycardia) are either absent or nonspecific [4,13 31-44]. Various authors underlined the great importance of early initiation of a targeted antimicrobial therapy or the preemptive therapy in high-risk patients in order to achieve acceptable outcomes by preventing generalized sepsis, septic shock and multiorgan dysfunction.

Especially bacterial sepsis has a significant impact on the survival of patients who undergo a transplant proceeding because of the surgical trauma and the need for immunosuppression [1-4].

Furthermore, commonly used biochemical markers, such as C-reactive protein (CRP) or leucocyte count, cannot be considered to be specific inflammation markers in the early postoperative setting in order to establish a definite diagnosis [42].

2. Body

2.1. Procalcitonin; background

Calcitonin, a 32-amino-acid amidated hormone, is initially biosynthesized as a precursor, named preprocalcitonin [45] This protein is processed into several calcitonin precursors. In adults and children, infection and sepsis have been found to be associated with increased serum levels of calcitonin precursors [46-53]. These concentrations were shown to be positively correlated with a subsequent mortality rate [45]. Circulating calcitonin precursors, including procalcitonin, are raised in severe bacterial infections, but remain in low or normal ranges in viral infections and non-specific inflammatory diseases.(38,45,46).

Procalcitonin (PCT) is a precursor protein of the hormone calcitonin with a molecular weight of approximately 13 kDa. PCT is induced in the plasma of patients with severe bacterial or fungal infections or sepsis [38,40-54]. Local bacterial infections, viral infections, autoimmune and allergic disorders do not induce PCT. At present, it is not clear whether PCT is predominantly influenced merely by inflammation induced by microbial infections, or also by the severity of multiple organ dysfunctions secondary to the systemic inflammatory response.

Procalcitonin (PCT) is identified as a diagnostic marker for infectious or septic processes and correlates better with its severity as CRP [5, 44-57]. PCT is an acute phase protein, composed of 116 amino acids and is the precursor of calcitonin. In healthy individuals, PCT serum concentrations are very low (<0,5mg/dl). The half-life of PCT is approximately 26 to 30 hours [38-40]. Neuroendocrine cells of solid organs (lung, kidney, pancreas, adrenal gland, and liver) might be the source of PCT during an inflammatory procedure. A further role might play extrathyroid cells, such macrophages, monocytes and liver cells in the PCT production during sepsis [40, 41]. The main hypothesis as far as the PCT induction is concerned, presents that the stimulation for PCT elevation is a result of a systemic challenge of the organism with bacterial endotoxin and bacterial polysaccharides [39]. Overall the exact pathophysiology is still an open matter. [38,40].

2.2. PCT after liver surgery and in hepatic dysfunction

Procalcitonin (PCT) is a well established marker indicating a complication such as inflammation or sepsis among surgical patients. PCT rises 24–48 hours before and correlates better with the severity of sepsis and infection than CRP. In uncomplicated liver surgery cases, PCT peaks at 24 hours after the Pringle maneuver (clamp of the hepatoduodenal ligament) with a half-life of 24–30 hours. It has been reported that the liver has a primary role as the source of PCT production during endotoxin shock [24] In cirrhotic patients with impaired hepatic synthetic function, PCT levels were not lower, displaying the same predictive power for infection as in patients without cirrhosis [44].

2.3. PCT in trauma and surgery

Meissner et al emphasizing the differences in the kinetics of the main inflammation markers (PCT, CRP) after trauma and surgery, reported in their study that unlike CRP, PCT values typically declined rapidly after trauma. The rapid decline of the initial induction of PCT after trauma or surgery compared with the long-lasting increase of CRP promises an earlier use of PCT as a marker of sepsis and infection than of CRP in the postoperative /posttraumatic phase. He also demonstrates that the CRP level in trauma patients is not a valid parameter to gather more information about the severity of systemic inflammation, complications, and prognosis of the patient. PCT and clinical score systems are superior to CRP for risk stratification of the patient. On the contrary, the diagnostic use of CRP after trauma is limited because of its slow kinetics [35, 37, 39, 54, 55]. Other studies emphasize the major role of early changes of PCT levels for predicting the final outcome of septic patients. Any decrease of serum PCT within the first 48 hours by 30% or its persistence at levels within the normal ranges was an indicator of favorable outcome. On the contrary, any increase of serum PCT after 48 hours or any minimal decrease is a sign for insufficient antimicrobial therapeutic strategy. This finding applied both for patients with sepsis and for patients with severe sepsis/shock. It was a factor related to final outcome independently from disease severity.

2.4. PCT in OLT

However, the prognostic value of procalcitonin in liver transplant recipients, undergoing immunsuppression and showing severe co morbidities remains to be determined. Initially high PCT levels do not necessarily indicate a poor prognosis as do continuous or secondarily rising levels or elevations in the later postoperative course [42, 43]. In the posttransplant setting, elevated PCT levels are observed in the first 2-3 days after OLT [1]. Initially high PCT levels, however, do not necessarily indicate a poor prognosis as do continuous or secondarily rising levels [32,42]. Cardiac arrest and infection, but not PCT level in the donor, are associated with high post- OLT PCT levels in the recipient [43]. In patients with impaired hepatic synthesis, PCT levels were not lower; displaying the same predictive relevance for infection as in septic patients without cirrhosis or impairment of the liver function [44]. PCT has been shown to increase among OLT patients with infections, but it fails to predict an acute rejection episode. Furthermore, PCT rises in all patients undergoing OLT owing to the perioperative distress.

Coelho et al reported in a study with pediatric liver transplant recipients that it was possible to differentiate between bacterial infection and rejection by PCT measurement. In all patients with bacterial infection, an increase in PCT was to register. On the other hand patients suffering from acute graft rejection and these having an uneventful posttransplant course did not show an increase of PCT [56].

Furthermore an ATG (antithymocyte globulin)-based immunosuppressive therapy is a stimulus for synthesis and further elevation of PCT [53]. This fact presents the major limitation of PCT's diagnostic power. Additionally the presence of viral infection did not stimulate a PCT elevation and cannot be diagnosed through this inflammation marker [32,37-60].

Van den Broek et al [32] in a large study with 135 patients (LDLT and deceased donor recipients) examined the diagnostic and prognostic accuracy of PCT in cases of critical systemic infections in comparison to other traditional inflammation markes such as CRP and leucocyte count (LC). In this study peak PCT was found not to be an independent factor for occurrence of serious infections and septic episodes. On the other hand the authors underlined the importance of CRP, as it was found to be an independent risk factor for a critical systemic infection. Eyraud et al [43] investigated also the relevance of PCT in the posttransplant setting after OLT. The results of this study could not confirm them of previous studies [58,59] reporting that peak PCT could have its origin either from an infection of the recipient or from cardiac arrest of the donor. In this study the clinical characteristics of the donor are emphasized: the initial PCT of recipient has its origin from donor's cardiac arrest and it could not be predictive of graft dysfunction or postoperative complications after OLT. Furthermore graft preservation, graft flushing and type of reperfusion are factors, which have a significant influence on initial PCT values and this is one of the main bias as far as the sensitivity of PCT in the early posttransplant phase is concerned. Therefore Fazakas et al proposed standard procedures for graft harvesting, timing and technique of graft flushing in order to avoid the pathophysiological conditions, which lead to this bias [59].

The most significant value as far as the diagnostic power of PCT is concerned is the fact, that PCT levels increase far less than CRP levels, and the period of unspecific induction is much shorter [54].

2.5. PCT in MODS

In another large study with critically ill patients Meissner and colleagues indicate that PCT concentrations are associated with the severity of multiorgan dysfunction (MODS) during sepsis as assessed by the SOFA (sepsis-related organ failure assessment) score [39]. PCT has several advantages in severely ill patients compared with CRP. The most striking one, demonstrated in his study, is the enormous range of PCT reactivity resulting in a marked increase in PCT plasma levels, especially during severe stages of MODS and systemic inflammation. On the other hand, PCT concentrations are quite low when only a moderate organ dysfunction or a weak systemic inflammatory response is present. In contrast, CRP levels are often found to be already increased to maximal concentrations in patients with low SOFA scores. Thus, CRP cannot provide information as to further increases in organ dysfunction and the inflammatory progress, respectively, since it is already increased to its maximum values during a less severe stage of disease. Further advantages of PCT are its more rapid kinetics; PCT reacts faster than CRP both during an increase or decrease of inflammation. Regarding the prognosis of the disease, the course of PCT after day 4 from the onset of systemic inflammation was able to distinguish survivors from non-survivors. In summary, PCT compared with CRP is characterized by its ability to be induced to very high serum concentrations also during advanced stages of MODS and severe systemic inflammation, respectively, whereas CRP is often already in the upper concentration range, even in patients with low severity scores, and exhibits no such further dynamics during the course of MODS and systemic inflammation. PCT more rapidly declines to the normal range during the recovery of the patient compared with CRP, and thus provides more information in patients with MODS and sepsis of various etiologies than CRP.

Therefore the examination and the careful evaluation of postoperative PCT values are the most important stages for the early diagnosis of sepsis and infection after surgery.

Various authors and we emphasize the fact that the diagnostic accuracy of procalcitonin is completely dependent on use of a sensitive assay in an appropriate clinical setting. The clinical signs, physical examination and the clinical setting cannot be substituted by procalcitonin. They must be seen as complementary tools for early establishment of diagnosis. [38,42]

2.6. PCT: Our observations during liver transplantation

Aim of our research was to evaluate PCT as an early prognostic marker within 48 hours after OLT for subsequent postoperative complications and to assess the prognostic accuracy of PCT as marker for infectious and non infectious postoperative complications, septic episodes and as predict factor as far as the in hospital mortality is concerned. Our research included a retrospective study in a cohort liver transplant recipients underwent 32 liver transplantations [42] and a prospective part including patients underwent 75 OLT.

Patients with irreversible end-stage liver disease that was life threatening and refractory to other forms of conventional medical or surgical therapy who had no contraindications for transplantation were regarded as eligible for OLT. The organs were allocated according to the Model of End Stage Disease (MELD) [61]

For each recipient, the following were recorded: age, gender and PCT serum concentration before, 6 hours after reperfusion and then daily during the stay in the ICU after OLT.

Blood samples were obtained for routine testing (biochemical parameters), and for each patient, serum aliquots were used for PCT determination. The procalcitonin levels were measured by an immunoluminometric LUMItest PCT kit (Brahms; Diagnostica, Berlin, Germany) ; the normal range detected was from 0.1 to 0.5 ng/mL.

Postoperative clinical course was prospectively analyzed from admission to discharge according to main clinical data: infectious/non infectious complications, septic episodes, graft disorders, acute rejection episodes, renal failure, multiorgan failure and need for re-transplantation. Complications were graded according to the classification of Dindo et al [62].

2.6.1. *Definitions for our protocol*

Graft dysfunction was defined as the occurrence of at least one of the following criteria: the need for retransplantation (primary non function, PNF), a rise in aminotransferases of above 2,000 UI/L, impairment of factor V (<30%) with synchronous increase of bilirubin without a retrospective need for retransplantation, serum bilirubin greater than 10 mg/ml; PT of at least 17 sec; hepatic encephalopathy [63]. Mortality was defined as death from any cause occurring during the hospital stay.

Pulmonary complication was defined as the need for mechanical ventilation.

Acute renal failure was defined as plasma creatinemia of greater than 2mg/dl and urine output of less than 0.5 mL/hour. Renal complication was defined as the need for dialysis after OLT or greater than 100% of creatinine levels compared with preoperative values.

Postoperative complication was defined as hepatic dysfunction, infection, or pulmonary or renal complication or other surgical complication such as bleeding, hepatic artery thrombosis (HAT), thrombosis of the portal or cava vein and biliary complication such as insufficiency, stenosis, ITBL(ischemic type biliary lesion).

The definition of clinical infection was standardized with criteria proposed by the Centers for Disease Control and Prevention and included pulmonary, bloodstream, or intra-abdominal infections accompanied by clinical symptoms proven by microbiological, radiological, or surgical findings and reacting to instituted therapy.

Infection was diagnosed if clinical; biochemical or radiologic signs of infection were evident. Chest X-rays, ultrasound examinations were performed on daily basis during the ICU stay and computed tomography (CT) scans when a clinical infection was suspected, and on the basis of these examinations, prompt therapy was initiated. In cases where samples from the suspected site of infection were positive, a proven infection could be defined.

Sepsis was defined by the presence of infection and SIRS (systemic inflammatory response syndrome). The criteria for SIRS were met if more than one of the following signs occurred: a body temperature greater than 38°C or less than 36°C, a heart rate greater than 100 beats per minute, hyperventilation as evidenced by a respiratory rate greater than 20 breaths per minute or a partial pressure of carbon dioxide in the arterial blood less than 32 mm Hg, and an LC greater than 10.000 cells/µl or less than 4.000 cells/µl.5 Severe sepsis was defined as sepsis complicated by organ dysfunction [64]

2.6.2. *Immunsuppression protocol and antibiotic prophylaxis*

All patients were initially treated with tacrolimus, starting 36 hours after transplantation at 0.1 mg/kg twice daily and 500 mg methylprednisolone in the anhepatic phase. All patients received basiliximab (Simulect, 20 mg) in the anhepatic phase followed by a second administration (20mg), 4 days after transplantation. Mycophenolate mofetil (500 mg twice daily, intravenous or per oral) was administered starting on the 5th postoperative day. Acute rejection was diagnosed based on the histopathological examination after liver biopsy according to BANFF criteria [65]. In patients with tacrolimus neurotoxicity and other Tacrolimus triggered side effects, a conversion of the immunsuppressive regimen to Ciclosporin- based immunsuppression was performed. All recipients received broad-spectrum antimicrobial prophylaxis, consisting of antibacterial, antiviral, and antimycotic agents: with piperacilline-tazobactam for 7 days aciclovir and anidulafungin/posaconazole. Selective digestive decontamination consisted of 200mg of oral amphotericin B 3 times daily until the 21st postoperative day. Furthermore, high-risk patients, recipients of a cytomegalovirus (CMV) – positive donor received preemptive antiviral treatment with ganciclovir/ valganciclovir adjusted to renal function over a 6-week course. The standard laboratory workup included hematologic and biochemical parameters. The CMV status (viral load, pp65 antigen) was examined twice a week. Cytomegalovirus (CMV) infection was defined by the appearance of CMV antigen polymerase chain reaction in the blood. X-Ray examinations of the chest and ultrasounds of the graft were performed daily.

2.6.3. *Liver transplantation*

The donor organ was always retrieved as part of a multiorgan donation. Either University of Wisconsin (UW) or histidine-tryptophan-Ketoglutarate (HTK) solution was used for preservation. Liver transplantation was performed by using either the retrocaval resection technique or the piggyback technique. We performed either simultaneous portoarterial reperfusion or a portal reperfusion of the graft in a ratio 1:1. All patients were indicated for OLT because of end stage liver disease. Indications for OLT were: 1. acute liver failure, 2. hepatocellular carcinoma inside the Milan criteria, 3. hepatitis C induced liver cirrhosis, 4. hepatitis B induced liver cirrhosis , 5. nutritive toxic liver cirrhosis , 6. hemochromatosis , 7. autoimmunhepatitis . The median MELD score was 33 and 33 OLT were performed after acceptance of a request for high urgency (HU) liver transplantation

2.6.4. *Statistics and results*

Linear regression was used in univariate analysis to identify predictors of elevated PCT concentrations. Multivariate analysis was carried out using a logistic regression model. All of the tests performed were two-sided. Significant predictors in univariate analysis were included in a multivariate linear regression model, with a stepwise variable selection method. Potential associations between infectious complications or overall complications and surgical, clinical or biological parameters were tested with univariate procedures, using students' paired t-test for continuous variables and Pearson's chi-square test for categorical variables. P-values of less than 0.05 were considered to be statistically significant.

Statistical analysis was done with SPSS (SPSS v19.0, Chicago, IL, USA).

In the retrospective part of our research 32 adult patients with end-stage liver disease underwent OLT.

In 29 patients the peak-PCT occurred within 48 hours after OLT. A rapidly rising PCT was observed in 2 patients associated with subsequent fatal outcomes. Among the 10 patients with peak-PCT values less than 5 ng/mL, 9 displayed uneventful postoperative courses. PCT values more than 5 ng/mL were observed among 22 patients with 23 OLT, including 12 with 13 OLT who suffered more than 1 complications. The odds ratio (OR) for a complicated course in the presence of an initial PCT more than 5 ng/mL was calculated to be 11.7 (95% Confidence interval, 11.3–12.1; $P < .025$) with risk ratio of 5.65. The risk of renal failure requiring hemofiltration was independent of a PCT more than 5 ng/mL (OR 8.25; $P < 0\ .04$). Total bilirubin was significantly higher among patients with an initial PCT more than 5 ng/mL until day 7, compared with patients with a PCT less than 5 ng/mL. GOT was significantly higher on days 2 and 3 in these groups, but peak values for GOT and total bilirubin correlated significantly on univariate analysis . CRP did not show any significant difference between the complication and non-complication groups. The immunosuppression regimen was not significantly different regarding the occurrence of a complication or the occurrence of a peak-PCT of 5 ng/mL.

In the prospective part of our research patients with end-stage liver disease patients underwent 75 OLT. In this part we examined the clinical significance of the occurrence of a 2nd PCT peak, after the initial PCT peak, which occurs in the immediate post transplant setting.

In 65 patients the initial peak-PCT occurred within 72 hours after OLT. Patients with initial PCT values >5 ng/mL had a significantly higher risk to suffer more than 1 complications (infectious, non-infectious).

Overall 42 complications (infectious, non-infectious) were registered and there was a significant relevance with the occurrence of a 2nd PCT peak to register. In patients with a graft dysfunction, including acute rejection episodes, there was a significant PCT elevation with the occurrence of a 2nd peak. However in some patients there was a coincidence of an infectious focus to register. This fact was without statistical significance Among patients with a PNF and the need of re-transplantation, there was a significant elevation of PCT with the occurrence of a 2nd peak. On the contrary in patients with a HAT a 2nd PCT peak could not be registered.

Patients with biliary complications did not show an elevation of PCT or a 2nd peak. Patients which displayed an acute renal failure after OLT with the intermittent need for CVVH (continuous veno-venous hemofiltration), but there was no relevance between this complication and the PCT course. Furthermore the risk of renal failure requiring hemofiltration was independent of an initial PCT > 5 ng/mL

Furthermore we register that there was no relevance between the 1st peak-PCT and the further postoperative course or the occurrence of complications (infectious or non-infectious, $p=0.442$).

Patients, in which a 2nd PCT peak was occurred, had a significantly higher risk for a complicated course, for a complicated sepsis course with multiorgan dysfunction, for a non infectious complication ($p<0.0001$) and for in-hospital mortality ($p<0.0001$).

2.6.5. Interpretation of our findings

However, the peak value of PCT, usually occurring 2nd or 3rd postoperative day, was not an independent factor for a fatal outcome according to the present series. An initially high PCT has been described to not indicate a poor prognosis when followed by an adequate decline. A rapidly rising PCT without a decline after the 3rd postoperative day is associated with a fatal outcome correlating with a bacterial or fungal infection. In contrast to earlier studies where an elevation of PCT was seen only in infectious complications, we also observed a greater number of noninfectious complications. The high PCT did not predict the type or severity of the complication in general practice, but among transplant patients a further elevation was seen only in bacterial infections and not in rejection episodes or local inflammation. We observed a rise of PCT in respiratory failure and sepsis, but not in occurrence of ascites, pleural effusion, acute rejection episodes, or bleeding, as reported by other authors.

An initially high PCT has been described not to indicate a poor prognosis. Furthermore it is generally accepted that ischemic times as well as reperfusion produce a proinflammatory response of impaired liver function. Owing to tissue damage which predisposes to generalized infection and postoperative sepsis. In addition, elevated PCT values did not suggest a graft rejection process.

Furthermore our results show that OLT recipients with infectious and some non infectious complications had significantly higher values of PCT, in the majority of cases with a 2nd peak value after the initial PCT peak, in comparison to recipients with an uncomplicated post transplant course. The 1st peak PCT was not an independent risk factor in LTx recipients, while the occurrence of a 2nd peak was a significant independent factor for protracted septic course, for any complication overall (infectious or non infectious) and for post transplant mortality. The fact that the 1st PCT peak does not play a diagnostic and prognostic role underlined also Eyraud et al [43]. In this study was stated that PCT level in the donor and early PCT peak in the recipient have not a predictive value as far as post-OLT hepatic dysfunction or other complications are concerned. Cardiac arrest and infection in the donor seem to be associated with high post- OLT PCT levels in the recipient. As underlined before a major limitation as far as the diagnostic accuracy of PCT is concerned stated Zazula et al, who reported the ATG-stimulated elevation of PCT [53]. This aspect was not a limitation of our research, as we prefer ATG-free immunsuppressive regimens.

The occurrence of a 2nd PCT peak and of an eventful post transplant setting was significant in patients with a severe sepsis, bacterial or fungal infection and graft dysfunction overall (PNF and AR). In AR alone there was not a prognostic value of PCT to register. What this matter is concerned our results confirmed our first reports, as far the relevance between the 1st PCT peak and the AR is concerned [42].

In contrast to earlier studies where an elevation of PCT was seen only in infectious complications we also observed a greater number of non infectious complications when the PCT was elevated or showed a 2nd peak.

Our research included an acceptable cohort of deceased donor OLT recipients and showed that PCT was an independent risk factor for infectious and some non-infectious complications and that the occurrence of a 2nd peak was an independent factor for a complicated postoperative outcome and for mortality. Furthermore we registered a high prognostic value, due to its occurrence before clinical onset of the complications and clinical impairment of the patients.

Various studies have demonstrated that PCT is a useful diagnostic marker for bacterial and fungal infections and sepsis in different patient groups with superior diagnostic accuracy in comparison with CRP [34, 44, 55, 57]. Furthermore PCT was described in some small cohort studies as an accurate marker for any complication in the post transplant setting [57,58,60], which could not be fully confirmed by other study groups and by the present series [32,42,43].

However this research reports the significance of the role of PCT as independent factor as far as its course and the 2nd peak are concerned. We have to admit that PCT must not be regarded to be the only reliable diagnostic parameter. Postoperative complications after liver transplantation may result from multifactorial processes [66,67], which cannot be monitored by only 1 marker.

3. Conclusions

OLT is a complex procedure with a great and very important physiological and pathophysiological background and many parameters and biochemical pathways, which have to be taken into consideration after the operating procedure. The most common complication after OLT is the occurrence of systemic infection and sepsis. The great operative stress, the immunsupression and other parameters, such as the reperfusion injury of the graft lead to a higher risk for occurrence of a septic complication with high morbidity and mortality rates. Therefore the sufficient monitoring of this patient population, the early diagnosis and the immediate treatment of an infectious complication are of great importance. During the last years several studies and research have been performed in order to find the "ideal infectious marker" with high sensitivity and specificity for the early establishment of an infectious complication. Common inflammation markers such as LC and CRP cannot be considered as sufficient markers in order to diagnose quickly an infectious complication in the posttransplant setting. IL-6 has advantages and disadvantages and is not enough investigated, especially in the clinical area and the endothelial adhesion molecules (ICAM-1, VCAM-1, ECAM-1) have not been proofed. PCT is nowadays a well established sepsis marker. However PCT must not be regarded to be the only reliable diagnostic parameter. Postoperative complications after liver transplantation may result from multifactorial processes, which cannot be monitored by only 1 marker. However, the values and especially the trend after the peak value of PCT seem to be important diagnostic tools to detect serious infectious complications. Based on our results we believe that the value of PCT and of the occurrence of a 2nd peak seem to be important diagnostic tools for the early detection of serious infectious complications. Of great importance is to examine the correlation between PCT course, clinical course and CRP. This must be regarded as the basis of the post transplant management of a liver recipient. Furthermore our clinical research revealed that patients experienced great benefit from prophylactic and preemptive antibacterial, antifungal, and antiviral therapy.

The relevance and the importance of PCT and its course during the post transplant setting should be further examined in randomized controlled studies on multicenter basis. Furthermore we believe that inflammation markers such as IL-6 should be further examined e.g. in combination with PCT, because IL-6 is an extremely sensitive marker and could fill the "diagnostic gap" of PCT as far as viral infections are concerned. Endothelial adhesion molecules, which have the best sensitivity among the inflammation markers, are until today not examined and in our opinion have still a role to play.

Author details

Aristotelis Perrakis*, Volker Müller, Werner Hohenberger and Roland S. Croner
Surgical Department, Department of Hepatobiliary and Transplant Surgery,
University of Erlangen-Nuremberg, Erlangen, Germany

4. References

[1] Iida T, Kaido T, Yagi S et al.Posttransplant bacteremia in adult living donor liver transplant recipients. Liver Transpl. 2010 Dec;16(12):1379-85.
[2] Mora NP, Husberg BS, Gonwa TA, et al.The impact of the different severe infections on the outcome of liver transplantation. A study of 150 patients. Transpl Int 1992;5:S209–S210.
[3] Singh N, Paterson DL, Gayowski T, et al.Predicting bacteremia and septic mortality in liver transplant recipients. Liver Transpl 2000;6:54–61.

* Corresponding Author

[4] Lee SO, Kang SH, Abdel-Massih RC,et al. Spectrum of early- onset and late-onset bacteremias after liver transplantation: implications for management. Liver Transpl 2011; 17(6):733-41.

[5] Hack CE, Zeerleder S. The endothelium in sepsis: Source of and a target for inflammation. Crit Care Med 2001; 29(Suppl): S21–S27

[6] Mavrommatis AC, Theodoridis T, Orfanidou A, et al. Coagulation system and platelets are fully activated in uncomplicated sepsis. Crit Care Med 2000; 28:451–457

[7] Bernard GR, Vincent JL, Laterre PF, et al. Efficacy and safety of recombinant human activated protein C for severe sepsis. N Engl J Med 2001; 344:699–709

[8] Croner RS, Hohenberger W, Jeschke MG. Hepatic gene expression during endotoxemia. J Surg Res.2009 Jun 1;154(1):126-34

[9] Tschaikowsky K, Sagner S, Lehner N, et al. Endothelin in septic patients: Effects on cardiovascular and renal function and its relationship to proinflammatory cytokines. Crit Care Med 2000; 28:1854–1860

[10] Brauner JS, Rohde LE, Clausell N. Circulating endothelin-1 and tumor necrosis factor alpha: Early predictors of mortality in patients with septic shock. Intensive Care Med 2000; 26:305–313

[11] Reinhart K, Menges T, Gardlund B, et al. Randomized, placebo-controlled trial of the anti-tumor necrosis factor antibody fragment afelimomab in hyperinflammatory response during severe sepsis: The RAMSES Study. Crit Care Med 2001; 29:765–769

[12] Reinhart K, Wiegand-Löhnert C, Grimminger F, et al. The MAK 195F Sepsis Study Group. Assessment of the safety and efficacy of the monoclonal anti-tumor necrosis factor antibody-fragment, MAK 195F, in patients with sepsis and septic shock: A multicenter, randomized, placebo-controlled, dose-ranging study. Crit Care Med 1996; 24:733–742

[13] Castelli GP, Pognani C, Meisner M, et al. Procalcitonin and C-reactive protein during systemic inflammatory response syndrome, sepsis and organ dysfunction. Crit Care 2004;8 (4):234-42.

[14] Adams HG, Jordan C. Infections in the alcoholic. Med Clin North Am 1984;68:179-200.

[15] Wyke RJ. Problems of bacterial infection in patients with liver disease. Gut 1987;28:623-41.

[16] Johnson DH, Cunha BA. Infections in cirrhosis. Infect Dis Clin North Am 2001;15:363-71

[17] Campbell AC, Dronfield MW, Toghill PJ, et al. Neutrophil function in chronic liver disease. Clin Exp Immunol 1981;45:81-9.

[18] Fierer J, Finley F. Deficient bactericidal activity against Escherichia coli in patients with cirrhosis of the liver. J Clin Invest 1979;63:912.

[19] Liu YK. Effects of alcohol on granulocytes and lymphocytes. Semin Hematol 1980;17:130-6.

[20] Fortun J, Martin-Davila P, Moreno S, et al. Risk factors for invasive aspergillosis in liver transplant recipients. Liver Transpl 2002;8: 1065-70.

[21] Singh N, Wagener MM, Obman A, et al. Bacteremias in liver transplant recipients: shift toward gram-negative bacteria as predominant pathogens. Liver Transpl 2004;10:844-9

[22] Mora NP, Husberg BS, Gonwa TA, et al. The impact of the different severe infections on the outcome of liver transplantation.A study of 150 patients. Transpl Int 1992;5:209–210.

[23] Singh N, Paterson DL, Gayowski T, et al. Predicting bacteremia and septic mortality in liver transplant recipients. Liver Transpl 2000;6:54–61.

[24] Lee SO, Kang SH, Abdel-Massih RC, et al. Spectrum of early and late-onset bacteremia after liver transplantation: Implications for management. Liver Transpl 2011;17:733–741

[25] Kim SI, Kim YJ, Jun YH, et al. Epidemiology and risk factors for bacteremia in 144 consecutive living-donor liver transplant recipients.Yonsei Med J 2009;50:112–121

[26] Kiuchi T, Onishi Y, Nakamura T. Small-for-size graft: not defined solely by being small for size. Liver Transpl 2010;16:815–817

[27] Shimada M, Ijichi H, Yonemura Y, et al. Is graft size a major risk factor in living-donor adult liver transplantation? Transpl Int 2004;17:310–316

[28] Igekami T, Shirabe K, Yoshiya S, et al. Bacterial Sepsis after LivingDonor Liver Transplantation: The Impact of Early Enteral Nutrition. J Am Coll Surg;214;3;288-295

[29] Soejima Y, Taketomi A, Yoshizumi T, et al. Feasibility of left lobe living donor liver transplantation between adults: an 8-year, single-center experience of 107 cases. Am J Transplant 2006;6:1004–1011.

[30] Karvellas CJ, McPhail M, Pink F, et al. Bloodstream infection after elective liver transplantation is associated with increased mortality in patients with cirrhosis. Journal of Critical Care ; 2011 26, 468–474

[31] Kornberg A, Grube T, Wagner T, et al. Differentiated therapy with prostaglandin E1 (alprostadil) after orthotopic liver transplantation: the usefulness of procalcitonin (PCT) and hepatic artery resistive index (RI) for the evaluation of early graft function and clinical course. Clin Chem Lab Med 2000 Nov;38(11):1177-80

[32] van den Broek M AJ, Damnik S W M.O, Winkens B, et al. Procalcitonin as a Prognostic Marker for infectious complications in Liver Transplant Recipients in an Intensive Care Unit. Liver Transpl 2010;16:402-410

[33] Saner FH, Olde Damink SW, Pavlakovic G, et al. Pulmonary and blood stream infections in adult living donor and cadaveric liver transplant patients. Transplantation 2008; 85:1564-1568.

[34] Kuse ER, Langefeld I, Jaeger K, et al. Procalcitonin in fever of unknown origin after liver transplantation: a variable to differentiate acute rejection from infection. Crit Care Med 2000;28:555-559.

[35] Meisner M, Tschaikowsky K, Hutzler A, et al. Postoperative plasma concentrations of procalcitonin after different types of surgery. Intensive Care Med 1998;24:680-684.

[36] Morgenthaler NG, Struck J, Chancerelle Y, et al. Production of procalcitonin (PCT) in non-thyroidal tissue after LPS injection. Horm Metab Res 2003, 35:290-295.

[37] Meisner M, Tschaikowsky K, Schmidt J, et al. Procalcitonin (PCT)-indications for a new diagnostic parameter of severe bacterial infection and sepsis in transplantation,

immunosuppression and cardiac assist devices. Cardiovascular Engineering 1996, 1:67-76

[38] Assicot M, Gendrel D, Carsin H, et al. High serum procalcitonin concentrations in patients with sepsis and infection. Lancet 1993;341:515-518.

[39] Meisner M, Tschaikowsky K, Palmaers T, et al. Comparison of procalcitonin (PCT) and C-reactive protein (CRP) plasma concentrations at different SOFA scores during the course of sepsis and MODS. Crit Care 1999;3(1):45-50.

[40] Arkader R, Troster EJ, Lopes MR, et al. Procalcitonin does discriminate between sepsis and systemic inflammatory response syndrome. Arch Dis Child 2006;91(2):117-20

[41] Brunkhorst FM, Heinz U, Forycki ZF. Kinetics of procalcitonin in iatrogenic sepsis. Intensive Care Med 1998, 24:888-889.

[42] Perrakis A, Yedibela S, Schellerer V, et al. Procalcitonin in the setting of complicated postoperative course after liver transplantation. Transplant Proc. 2010; 42(10):4187-90

[43] Eyraud D, Ben Ayed S, Tanguy ML, et al. Procalcitonin in liver transplantation: are high levels due to donors or recipients? Crit Care 2008;12: R85.

[44] Bota DP, Van Nuffelen M, Zakariah AN,et al. Serum levels of C-reactive protein and procalcitonin in critically ill patients with cirrhosis of the liver. J Lab Clin Med. 2005;146(6):347-51.

[45] Becker KL, Nylén ES, Cohen R, et al. Calcitonin gene family of peptides. In: Principles and Practice of Endocrinology and Metabolism. Becker KL (Ed). Second Edition. Philadelphia, JB Lippincott, 1995, pp 474-483

[46] Mallet E, Lanse X, Devaux AM, et al. Hypercalcitoninaemia in fulminant meningococcaemia in children. Lancet 1983; i:294

[47] Chesney RW, McCarron DM, Haddad JG, et al. Pathogenic mechanisms of the hypocalcemia of the staphylococcal toxic-shock syndrome. J Lab Clin Med 1983; 101:576-585

[48] Becker KL, Silva OL, Snider RH, et al. The pathophysiology of pulmonary calcitonin. In: The Endocrine Lung in Health and Disease. Becker KL, Gazdar AF (Eds). Philadelphia, WB Saunders, 1984, pp 277-279

[49] Lind L, Bucht E, Ljunghall S. Pronounced elevation in circulating calcitonin in critical care patients is related to the severity of illness and survival. Intensive Care Med 1995; 21:63-66

[50] Gendrel D, Assicot M, Raymond J, et al. Procalcitonin as a marker for the early diagnosis of neonatal infection. J Pediatr 1996; 128:570-573

[51] de Werra I, Jaccard C, Corradin SB. Cytokines, nitrite/nitrate, soluble tumor necrosis factor receptors, and procalcitonin concentrations: Comparisons in patients with septic shock, cardiogenic shock, and bacterial pneumonia. Crit Care Med 1997; 25:607-613

[52] Gérard Y, Hober D, Assicot M, et al. Procalcitonin as a marker of bacterial sepsis in patients infected with HIV-1. J Infect 1997; 35:41-46

[53] Zazula R, Prucha M, Tyll T, et al. Induction of procalcitonin in liver transplant patients treated with anti-thymocyte globulin. Crit Care. 2007; 11(6):R131.

[54] Meissner M, Adina H, Schmidt J. Correlation of procalcitonin and C-reactiv protein to inflammation, complications and outcome during intensive care unit course of multiple-trauma patients. Critical Care; 2006;10;1;1-10

[55] Meisner M, Müller V, Khakpour Z, et al. Induction of procalcitonin and proinflammatory cytokines in an anhepatic baboon endotoxin shock model. Shock. 2003;19(2):187-90.

[56] Coelho MCM, Tannuri U, Tannuri ACA, et al.Is procalcitonin useful to differentiate rejection from bacterial infection in the early post-operative period of liver transplantation in children? Pediatr Transplantation 2009: 13: 1004–1006.

[57] Simon L, Gauvin F, Amre DK, et al. Serum procalcitonin and c-reactive protein levels as markers of bacterial infection: a systematic review and meta-analysis. Clin Infect Dis 2004;39:206-217.

[58] Cooper D, Sharples L, Cornelissen J, et al. Comparison between procalcitonin, serum amyloid A, and C-reactive protein as markers of serious bacterial and fungal infections after solid organ transplantation. Transplant Proc 2001;33: 1808-1810

[59] Fazakas J, Gondos T, Varga M, et al. Analysis of systemic and regional procalcitonin serum levels during liver transplantation. Transpl Int 2003: 16: 465–470.

[60] Kunz D, Pross M, Konig W, et al. Diagnostic relevance of procalcitonin, IL-6 and cellular immune status in the early phase after liver transplantation. Transplant Proc 1998;30:2398-2399

[61] Wiesner R, Edwards E, Freeman R, et al. United Network for Organ Sharing Liver Disease Severity Score Committee Model for end-stage liver disease (MELD) and allocation of donor livers.Gastroenterology.2003; 124(1):91-6.

[62] Dindo D, Demartines N, Clavien PA. Classification of surgical complications: a new proposal with evaluation in a cohort of 6336 patients and results of a survey. Ann Surg. 2004; 240(2):205-13.

[63] Deschênes M, Belle SH, Krom RA,et al. Early allograft dysfunction after liver transplantation: a definition and predictors of outcome. National Institute of Diabetes and Digestive and Kidney Diseases Liver Transplantation Database.Transplantation. 1998 15; 66(3):302-10.

[64] Calandra T, Cohen J. International Sepsis Forum Definition of Infection in the ICU Consensus Conference The international sepsis forum consensus conference on definitions of infection in the intensive care unit. Crit Care Med. 2005; 33(7):1538-48.

[65] BANFF schema for grading liver allograft rejection: An international consensus document. Hepatology 1997: 25: 658– 663.

[66] Dogan S, Aslan M. Hepatic ischemia-reperfusion injury and therapeutic strategies to alleviate cellular damage. Hepatol Res. 2011;41(2):103-17

[67] Jaeschke H. Molecular mechanisms of hepatic ischemia reperfusion injury and preconditioning. Am J Physiol Gastrointest Liver Physiol 2003; 284:G15-G26.

Chapter 10

Microdialysis Monitoring of Biomarkers for Early Recognition of Intestinal Ischemia

Radha Swathe Priya M. and Emma P. Córcoles

Additional information is available at the end of the chapter

http://dx.doi.org/10.5772/50240

1. Introduction

The intestinal tract is commonly involved in ischemia and reperfusion events, resulting from illness or surgical procedures that might lead to haemorrhage or shock. Ischemia is recognised as a poor blood supply and it is specifically known as intestinal or mesenteric ischemia when the bowel is involved. An ischemic insult can develop further into inflammation and injury. The mechanisms involved are still subject of study, but in general, an increase in intestinal cell membrane permeability provokes bacterial translocation and this in turn results in sepsis and multiple organ failure (MOF). The role of intestinal ischemia in septic shock will be discussed in this chapter as well as techniques commonly used to monitor gastrointestinal (GI) perfusion. However, most of these techniques depend on technical operators thus limiting the diagnosis of intestinal ischemia, which in most surgical departments still relies on clinical symptoms and examination.

Monitoring metabolic biomarkers has allowed not only the study of metabolic rates of tissues and organs, but the rapid detection of life-threatening events. During episodes of low blood flow, metabolic needs of the gastrointestinal tissue are not met. Monitoring this metabolic imbalance has the potential to provide an early diagnosis and prevent the injury from developing further into sepsis. Biosensors have been widely used to study tissue metabolism, proteins and nucleic acids with a wide range of applications. Biosensors as a diagnosis tool for gastrointestinal pathology will be revised in this chapter. The use of biosensors in clinical settings is, however, limited by issues such as biocompatibility, sterilisability and immunoreactivity and despite the extensive studies to overcome the immune-defensive reactions and toxicity effects due to the direct tissue implantation, other techniques have been used as an interface. Microdialysis is an extracting technique widely used to sample extracellular fluid of different human tissues. The use of microdialysis for the monitoring of digestive organs will be revised and intestinal microdialysis to monitor ischemia further described. Commonly off-line microdialysis pitfalls such as time lag and misplacement of samples are exposed as well as the use of recent technologies to overcome these issues. The synergetic combination of microdialysis and biosensors is the main reason for the position of this technology in the forefront of invasive monitoring. Biocompatibility issues of biosensors are extremely simplified when coupled with microdialysis and in turn biosensors confer microdialysis with a temporal resolution that it otherwise lacks. Although the combination of these techniques is still in research process, it presents the potential of close monitoring in clinical settings and home care scenarios for early diagnosis of conditions that can lead to sepsis if otherwise missed.

2. Intestinal ischemia and its role in septic shock

A poor blood supply to the intestine, also recognised as intestinal or mesenteric ischemia, generally leads to inflammation and injury (1) and easily develops into hypoxia (deprivation of oxygen supply) causing death of cells and tissue necrosis. This in turn can lead to sepsis and end in shock. Conversely, following haemorrhage or shock, the intestinal tract is the main organ to experience an ischemic/reperfusion injury. Intestinal cell membrane permeability can increase due to mesenteric ischemia (2), provoking bacterial translocation and injury of the gut barrier that in turn leads to sepsis and MOF (3-5). Hence, the measurement of intestinal permeability has been used as a valuable diagnosis of diseases affecting the bowel (6, 7).

The intestinal barrier protects the gastrointestinal tract, which under normal conditions is colonised by the bacterial flora containing enough microorganism, bacteria, and endotoxins to kill the host (8). Epithelial cells covering the surface of the gastrointestinal tract forms this barrier that prevents the absorption of toxins, antigens, proteases and microorganism across the intestinal wall (9). However, bacteria penetrates the intestinal barrier with relative ease and it is a common occurrence in healthy patients. This bacterial translocation can lead to further damage, worsening the health situation in ill patients (8), hence, it is of utmost importance to control this translocation in patients with critical conditions. Some studies have focused their efforts on understanding the function and mechanism of the intestinal barrier (10, 11), however, these are unclear and the correlation between bacterial translocation and intestinal permeability has raised controversies. A correlation between the loss of intestinal barrier function and bacterial translocation was found out in rodents, but not in humans, where bacterial translocation could not be related to the increase of permeability of the atrophied villous (6). Seemingly, no correlation was found after major gastrointestinal surgery between failure of the gut barrier function and septic complication (11). Hence, some studies have proposed a primary mechanism of translocation in the absence of damaged mucosal barrier, where migration of organism across the bowel occurred by pinocytosis in epithelial cells (12-14). Nevertheless, other investigations have identified alterations in intestinal permeability in critically ill patients, where the loss of tight junctions and cells at the villous tip was suggested to be the primary cause of changes in intestinal permeability (15, 16).

During the first stage of the bacterial translocation process, bacteria adhere onto the enterocytes and cross the barrier via transcellular and paracellular mechanisms (12, 17, 18). Disrupted epithelial tight junctions ('leaky gut') are the cause of bacterial translocation in the paracellular route (19, 20). While, intracellular trafficking follows the endocytic uptake during the transcellular route (21) (Figure 1). Nevertheless, regardless of the type of mechanism, bacterial translocation is triggered by common injuries such as ischemia/reperfusion, oxidative stress and bacterial action. Typically, the immune system will attack the bacteria once across the barrier. However, if this fails, sepsis or endotoxemia occurs, and further damage will develop into MOF (8, 22). In fact, the bowel is the main organ involved in MOF and this typically occurs as a consequence of a systemic inflammatory response syndrome (SIRS).

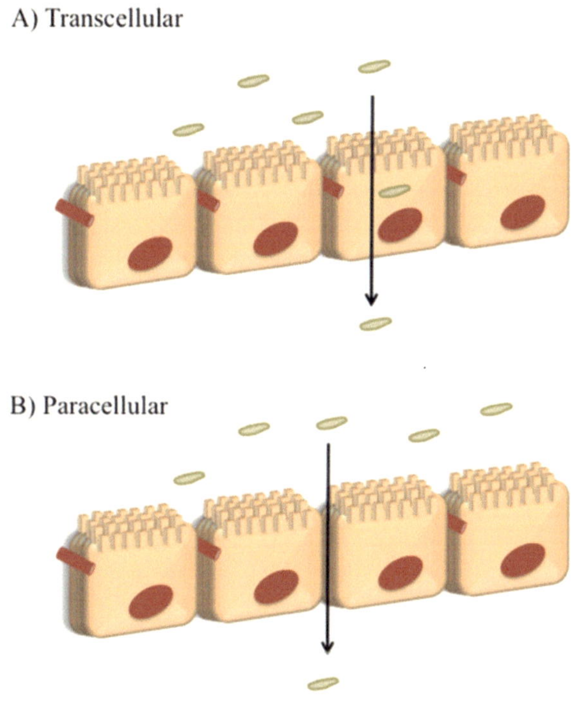

Figure 1. Schematic model of disrupted gut epithelial barrier. Ischemia and infection may be the initial cause of disruption allowing bacteria and other pathogens to cross the barrier and mix with the luminal content. A) Transcellular route occurs by intracellular trafficking; B) Paracellular route occurs due to the disruption of tight junctions.

Insults such as haemorrhage, ischemia/reperfusion, infection or trauma generally lead to an inflammatory response and this further develops into shock, if untreated. Toxins induce the release of cytokines, leukotrienes and platelets-activating factors (PAF), which play a major role in the initiation of shock (23-26). Hence, bacterial and toxin translocation have been suggested to be the main cause of all these intestinal dysfunctions (27, 28). The increase of membrane permeability has been related to bacterial translocation mechanisms and ischemic process in the intestine. In fact, translocation, vasoconstriction and hypoxic villi are common mechanisms occurring in the bowel due to the proximity of this to luminal bacteria and toxins (29). Reduction in blood flow is also a cause of initiation of shock, as well as activation of endotoxins, which release vasoactive substances and stimulate the formation of oxygen free radicals in the tissue (25, 27, 30, 31). The reduction of blood flow means a loss of plasma volume and hence a reduction of proteins into the interstitium space, which in turn leads to MOF (32-36). The sequence of shock varies with different pathologies (low perfusion, hypotension, hemoconcentration, vasocongestion), but the cause of death initiated due to the inflammatory response is very similar (37).

Certain diseases and common surgical procedures can lead to the weakness of blood vessels that with the continuous passage of blood can dilate forming an aneurysm. As the aneurysm expands, the risk of rupture increases and this can produce severe haemorrhage leading to other complications and ultimately to death. The most common abdominal aneurysm occurs in the aorta, hence the term abdominal aortic aneurysm (AAA). Ischemic colitis is the most common complication after abdominal aortic aneurysm surgery (38, 39) presenting a high impact in mortality rates (40-43). Another high risk postoperative complication is the leakage of a low rectal anastomosis connection, or the site where the two transacted bowel segments are joined again, closing the bowel lumen (44). Anastomosis leaks can easily develop into sepsis increasing the mortality toll. Although other variables contribute to the risk of anastomosis leakage, ischemia is the main factor related to anastomosis leak (45-47). During cardiac surgery with cardiopulmonary bypass (CPB), there is a high risk of patients developing intestinal mucosal ischemia. This may further lead to a disturbed mucosal integrity and increased intestinal permeability due to imbalance between splanchnic oxygen supply and demand which may contribute to systemic inflammation (48). Hence, an early diagnosis and the evaluation of an adequate splanchnic perfusion are crucial to improve outcome rates following surgical procedures such as aneurysm repair, anastomosis connections and CPB.

3. Gastrointestinal perfusion monitoring

The principal factors in the development of sepsis, systemic inflammatory syndrome and MOF are intestinal ischemia and gut barrier failure. These are also the main causes for the development of anastomosis leak and present a high rate of recurrence after AAA repair. During inadequate blood flow, the metabolic needs of the tissue are not met, leading to tissue injury. Consequently, ensuring both perfusion pressure and blood flow to maintain the necessary metabolic supply and demand are highly important to avoid diseases (49). It is in situations when blood flow has been partially compromised, where an early diagnosis could prevent the injury from developing further into organ dysfunction and death. In order to monitor these perfusion irregularities, several techniques have been used over the years. Human GI perfusion has been monitored by means of tonometry (50-52), laser Doppler flowmetry (53, 54), reflectance spectrophotometry (55), near-infrared spectroscopy (56), orthogonal polarisation spectral imaging, (57, 58), indocyanine green clearance (59), and measurements of plasma D-lactate (60). While the outcome of patients with septic shock can be predicted, these techniques cannot be compared to each other since they measure different constituents of GI perfusion (61). Alternatively, intestinal bleeding, which is undisputably an indication of organ damage, has been used to diagnose intestinal failure, however this fails to quantify the damage. Absorption markers of increasing permeability have also been extensively studied to assess gut functions, however, as they are highly invasive and require extensive nursing time, they are not appropriate for clinical monitoring in the intensive care unit (ICU). Gastrointestinal tonometry, due to its simplicity, is currently the most commonly used technique. It provides adequate information of GI perfusion and it is highly suitable for use in ICU. The technique consists of a silicone balloon inserted in the stomach that automatically infuses and samples gas every 10 minutes. The gas sample is analysed automatically using an infrared sensor within the measurement instrument (62, 63). However, it has several disadvantages as it does not provide a continuous measurement, presents long response time and leads to potential systematic errors as the gas samples are drawn from the catheter and analysed using an external measurement device. Furthermore, this method depends on the technical operator, compromising its reproducibility, and the effect of perfusion countercurrents changes on its sensitivity is still obscure (64). In addition, improvement of gastrointestinal perfusion has failed to prevent mucosal failure and otherwise, increasing the perfusion might have an effect on the metabolic rate, modifying the balance between oxygen demand and supply (61).

Currently, techniques most commonly used in clinical practices for the diagnosis of leaks are routine blood tests, colonoscopy, ultrasound and abdominal x-rays such as, CT scans, mesenteric angiography and MRIs and as a last resort, an exploratory abdominal surgery. Regardless of all advances in clinical technology, the monitoring of gastrointestinal perfusion is still limited and in most surgical departments, the diagnosis of intestinal ischemia relies on clinical symptoms and examination (65). However, subjectivity, the lack of precision and the delayed manifestation of the symptoms account for the unreliability of this procedure.

Research based on microcirculation and secretion during shock has been broadly explored at cellular and molecular level, however, there is a lack of information at the organ level (66). The mechanism of ischemia before shock and MOF begin, is not only an important area of research but one with plenty of room for exploration. Monitoring organ function and metabolism could be the ultimate mode of measuring gut perfusion (64), since there are evidences of the existence of localised biochemical changes in specific segments of the patient's gut (67).

Splanchnic hypoperfusion is generally associated with a poor outcome in critically ill patients. Moreover, despite presenting a hyperdynamic systemic circulation, the mucosa hypoperfusion in gastric, small intestine and colonic tissue commonly develops into sepsis (68). Gastrointestinal mucosa has been described as one of the highest metabolically active tissues under conditions of sepsis (69, 70) and although no clear association has been found, gut flow and metabolic changes appear to be heterogeneous (71-74). During compromised mucosal tissue, the reaction mechanism has been proposed as an increase of oxygen extraction (75). However, regardless of adequate oxygen delivery, the cells are unable to use oxygen during sepsis (76). During the initiation of intestinal ischemia, whatever the cause of injury (bowel strangulation, intestinal perforation or impaired blood flow), a rise in intracellular biomarkers occurs due to the increase of intestinal permeability (77). Therefore, metabolic levels are presented as useful measurements for the monitoring of intestinal ischemia.

During ischemia, a change from aerobic to anaerobic tissue metabolism occurs, which results in a decrease of glucose and pyruvate levels and increased lactate and glycerol levels. During anaerobic metabolism, the support of glucose from sphlanchnic circuit is inhibited causing pyruvate to accumulate in the tissue. Due to the lack of oxygen, pyruvate cannot be incorporated into the citric acid cycle, metabolising pyruvate to lactate. Monitoring the gut metabolic markers provides information on the variation from aerobic to anaerobic metabolism, the balance between oxygen supply and demand and therefore the ischemic degree of that tissue. In order to obtain a more accurate assessment of tissue metabolism, determination of lactate/pyruvate or lactate/glucose ratio is preferred compared to lactate alone. In addition, during sustained ischemia, a breakdown of the cellular plasma membrane occurs resulting in the release of phospholipids into the extracellular fluid, which are degraded to free fatty acids and glycerol. Hence, glycerol is another common metabolic product monitored during ischemic studies (78).

4. Biosensors as a diagnosis tool of gastrointestinal pathology

Over the past few decades, a large number of biosensors (a biological sensing element directly interfaced to a signal transducer) have been developed for the detection of various metabolites, proteins and nucleic acids with a wide range of applications, such as for medical diagnosis of gastrointestinal disorders.

Currently, the most common minimally invasive method to monitor the perfusion of the gastrointestinal tract in clinical settings is gastric tonometry. However, the technique only provides discrete measurements. In order to overcome this limitation, an optical fibre sensor was developed (79). This is based on the utilisation of a CO_2 sensing layer fixed at the end of an optical fibre catheter that is connected to an optoelectronic unit. The sensor allows the continous monitoring of the rapid changes in the gastric pCO_2 and hence provides a better understanding of gastrointestinal physiology (Figure 2).

Monitoring tissue adenosine triphosphate (ATP), in addition to other metabolic products, provides a further understanding of the cellular respiration rate. Furthermore, ATP has an important function within the immune system as a clotting signal molecule (80) and it is thought to regulate serotonin (5-HT) release and hence gastrointestinal motility (81-83). An ATP microelectrode biosensor with high long-term stability and selectivity was used to study the regulation of mucosal release mechanisms such as 5-HT based on the long-term in vitro variations of ATP release from isolated ileum and colon tissues (84).

Others have developed a microcapillary immunoassay, the Quantum-dot-Linked Immunosorbent Assay (QLISA), in order to differentiate between inflammatory bowel

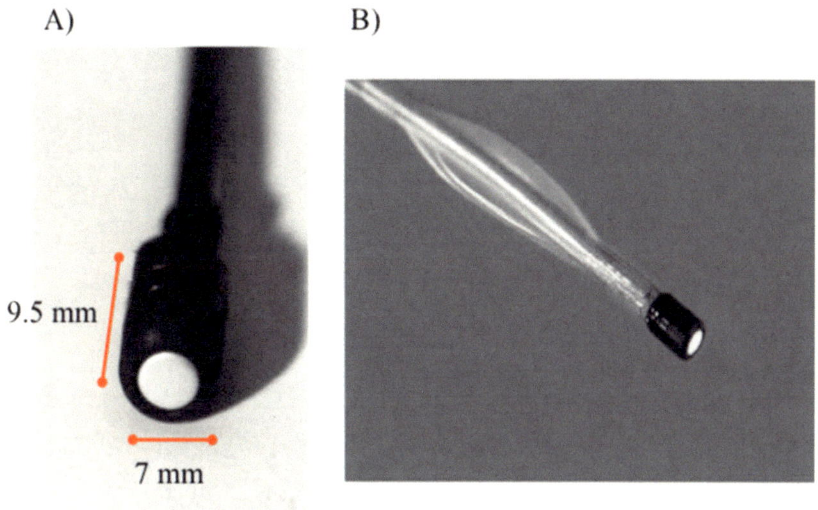

Figure 2. Optical probe for continuous monitoring of gastric carbon dioxide. A) Tip of the optical probe head; B) Optical probe mounted on a Tonocap catheter for gastric tonometry. Modified with permission from Elsevier (79).

diseases such as ulcerative colitis and Crohn's disease and irritable bowel syndrome (IBS). The fecal levels of the gastrointestinal inflammatory disease's biomarkers, myeloperoxidase and lactoferrin, could be quantified using this biosensor (85). In another study, a filter-paper-based strip was used to develop a bacterial whole-cell biosensor that allows optical on-site detection of a chemical signalling molecule in Gram-negative bacteria, which plays an important role in the pathogenesis of several gastrointestinal disorders (86). Differentiation of old blood and new blood for the surveillance of rebleeding occurrence was possible with an endoscopically implantable wireless biosensor designed to detect blood labelled with fluoroscein. This has the potential of immediate, real-time detection of upper gastrointestinal bleeding. Furthermore, the wireless signal can be transmitted to external computers that relay the data to the patient's cell phone or to an emergency response network allowing an early-warning remote surveillance system. In this way, the detection of rebleeding of endoscopically defined sources of GI hemorrhage during periods of high risk is possible (87) (Figure 3).

Studies with biosensors are still commonly performed in animal models or rely on collecting patients' fluids and tissue samples. Implantable biosensors still have problems associated with biocompatibility. Damage of the tissue surrounding the biosensor is believed to affect the measurement levels. In addition, implanted biosensors suffer the reaction of the tissue towards the foreign body, the so-called biofouling. A cascade signal is sent by the immune system that triggers the release of platelets and immune proteins as well as the formation of new blood vessels, which encapsulate the biosensor and hence impair the sensing layer (88-90). Therefore, alternative techniques have been explored to monitor gastrointestinal biomarkers.

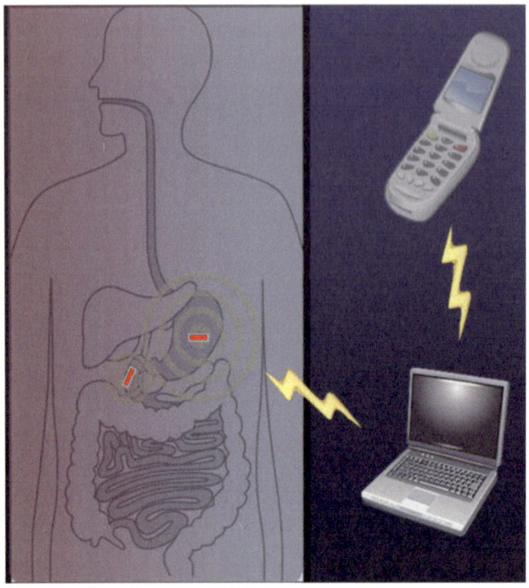

Figure 3. Scheme of wireless communication for gastric bleeding. Optical biosensor implanted endoscopically in the stomach transmits the signal wirelessly to external computers and to the patient's cell phone or other networks. Reprinted with permission from Elsevier (87).

5. Microdialysis monitoring

In the early seventies, Ungertstedt and Pycock (91) developed microdialysis, an extraction technique to measure interstitial substance in the brain without causing extensive tissue damage. The original concept for microdialysis was to mimic a blood capillary (92). Microdialysis is based on the passive diffusion of the molecules through a hollow fibre membrane (93). A sterile physiological solution (perfusate) is infused by a syringe pump at very low flow rates (typically 0.3-2 μl/min). Molecules present in the extracellular fluid diffuse to the lumen of the microdialysis (dialysate) and this is sampled through the outlet (Figure 4). The membrane cut-off confers selectivity to the technique, limiting the size of molecules diffusing through it. In clinical situation, this prevents the passage of virus into the dialysate and it eliminates problems associated with instability of metabolites due to sample preparation. Since the dialysate is free of proteins, this can be directly injected into analytical systems for analysis.

Since its beginning, microdialysis applications have broadened to the sampling of extracellular fluid of different human tissues including ear fluid (94), brain (95, 96), liver (97), heart (98), lungs, muscle (99) and bowel (78). The reader is directed to some of the reviews on microdialysis found in the literature (92, 100-103). Extensive studies have been carried out using microdialysis in the digestive system organs. This section describes some of the work published in stomach tissue, liver, pancreas and intestine.

Gastric microdialysis has been used to continuously monitor gastrin release to determine the response to food, acid blockage and acute vagal excitation (104). Microdialysis monitoring of

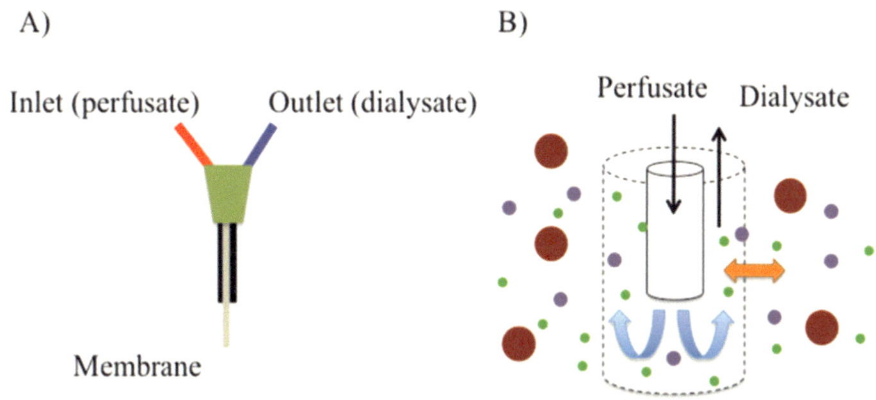

Figure 4. Scheme of a Microdialysis probe. A) Microdialysis membrane is depicted as a tip, which is connected via a shaft to the inlet and outlet tubings; B) The semipermeable membrane limits the diffusion of large molecules such as red blood cells, large proteins and virus.

gastric ischemia during temporary celiac artery occlusion in anesthetised rats showed a more remarkable response to ischemia in the relative changes of metabolic ratios of lactate/pyruvate and lactate/glucose compared to changes in the flow indicator of H_2O efflux and glycerol (105). Histamine release from enterochromaffin-like (ECL) cells during ischemia has been commonly sampled from the stomach submucosa with a single microdialysis probe (106-109). However, submucosal microdialysis sampling has been suggested to be unrepresentative of histamine levels released from ECL cells, since these are located in the mucosa layer, requiring a diffusion of histamine from the mucosa to the submucosa and finally to the probe (110). A more accurate sampling of stomach analytes was introduced using a multiple probe approach in which the probes were implanted in the stomach lumen, mucosa, submucosa and in the blood of a rat (111) (Figure 5). This four-probe microdialysis sampling was used to directly compare drug absorption between gastric ulcerated and healthy tissue in the same animal, where the dialysate was analysed using high performance liquid chromatography ultraviolet (HPLC-UV). The study showed a higher drug concentration in ulcer tissue, which was a function of ulcer size and thickness and probe location within the tissues when compared to healthy tissue (112). The reconstructed oesophagus of patients undergoing resection of carcinoma was monitored with microdialysis to investigate the risk of postoperative complications caused by ischemia. This study showed lactate/glucose ratio to be the most reliable parameter and sets microdialysis as a promising method for examination of free jejunal flaps (113).

Liver metabolism has also been studied using microdialysis sampling. A study in anaesthetised rats showed that of the stimulation of hepatic nerves result in glycogenesis via α-adrenergic mechanism and eicosanoids mediators (114). Other metabolites typically measured in the liver are glucose, lactate, pyruvate and glycerol. Dialysate concentrations of these analytes were measured in swine models during and after liver transplantation. The samples were collected and analysed at 20 minute intervals during both the donor operation and cold preservation, and 7 hours after reperfusion in the recipient (115).

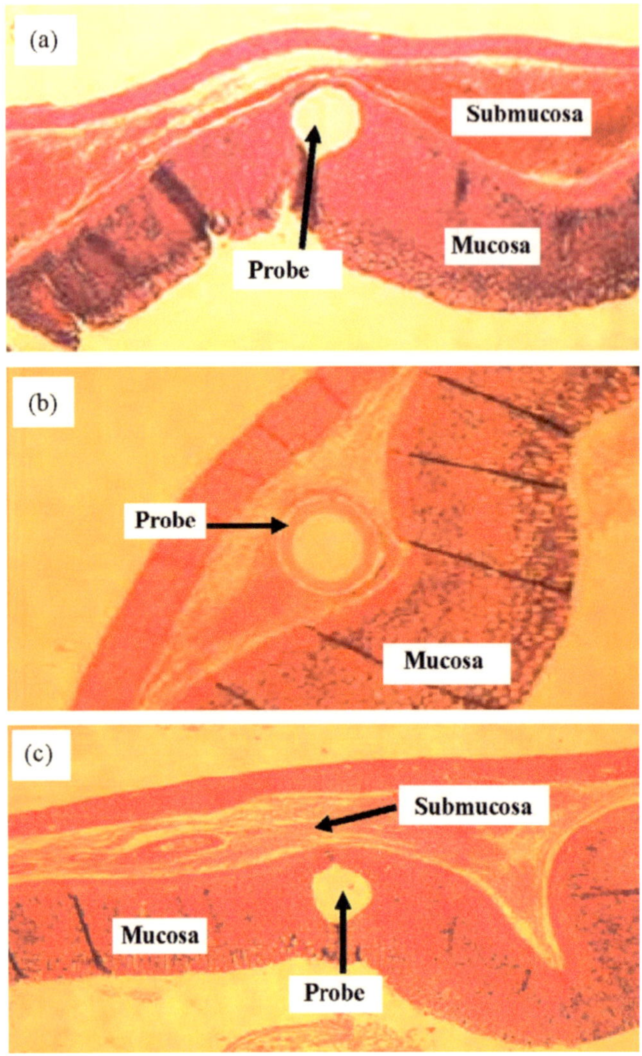

Figure 5. Histology images of microdialysis probe implantation (a) in the mucosa right after implantation, (b) in the submucosa 2 h post implantation and (c) in the mucosa 12 h post implantation (20x magnification). Reprinted with permission from Elsevier (111).

This led to the monitoring of metabolic changes in liver grafts in a clinical pilot study with 10 patients (116). Metabolic products were also monitored during ischemia-reperfusion injury in the rat liver using microdialysis and commercially available bedside kits (117). This study proved that microdialysis is applicable for human liver surgery by continuous intraoperative monitoring of intrahepatic metabolism (118). Alternatively, liver slices and microsomes have been used to carry out in vitro microdialysis studies of hypoxia (119), steroid enzymes activity (120) and drug metabolic processes (121).

As microdialysis collects only the unbound fraction (the pharmacologically active fraction) of the drug, it eliminates the need for unnecessary extensive sample preparation and enzyme degradation processes. This is highly advantageous during pharmacokinetic studies, such as the intraperitoneal monitoring of a drug active concentration in freely moving rodents (122). Other studies have used microdialysis to investigate the pathophysiology of brain activity among irritable bowel syndrome (IBS) patients and brain-gut interactions. In vivo brain microdialysis monitoring during colorectal distention in rats showed that noradrenaline is released in the hippocampus during the distention thus suggesting a possible correlation with behavioural changes (123).

5.1. Intestinal microdialysis

Microdialysis possesses the advantage of its applicability to other organs in which needle puncturing is possible including the stomach and intestines. On the other hand, the puncturing performed by the probe implantation, as seen in Figure 5, can inflict an acute inflammatory response that may influence the measurement levels and interpretation (124). A common solution has been to establish equilibration periods after probe implantation. Nevertheless, there is a critical need for smaller microdialysis probes to reduce the damage in surrounding tissue and local blood supply. This trauma caused by the implantation of the microdialysis probe is one of the main controversial issues when deciding the probe placement in gastrointestinal tissue.

Intraluminal probe placement could be a good approach, because the injury that occurs in the bowel causes a bigger damage to the mucosa than to the seromuscular layer, and therefore, biomarkers in the lumen rise early during the injury period (125). However, intraluminal metabolites measurements have been found to be extremely low and the detection is not feasible due to the resting phase of the intestine and to the high volume of contents in the lumen (126). A common approach is to place the microdialysis probe in the human peritoneal cavity (127-129). The assumption is that due to the high amount of intestinal anaerobic products metabolised by the liver, the metabolic markers of an impaired circulation are greater in the peritoneum than in blood (77). However, the ischemic biomarkers are diluted by non-ischemic markers and by the systemic circulation supplied to the peritoneum (78). Sommer et al. compared results from microdialysis probes inserted intraperitoneally, intramurally and intraluminally in the bowel of a swine model (126) (Figure 6). Insertion of the probe intramurally provides faster detection of metabolic changes than intraluminal and peritoneal microdialysis due to the proximity of the probe to the damaged tissue and the lack of dilution artifacts (130). However, this is more invasive and presents a difficult challenge for the clinician thus requiring intensive training. A recent approach has been to evaluate the insertion of the microdialysis probe in pancreatic tissue guided by an endoscopic ultrasound device (131), which has the potential to be used in other tissues. In addition, the microdialysis probe has a fragile tip, which can be broken during the probe implantation. It is increasingly recognised the need for the production of less fragile probes and alternative geometries.

Microdialysis monitoring can be divided into off-line and on-line microdialysis depending on the coupling method between the microdialysis outlet and the detection technique.

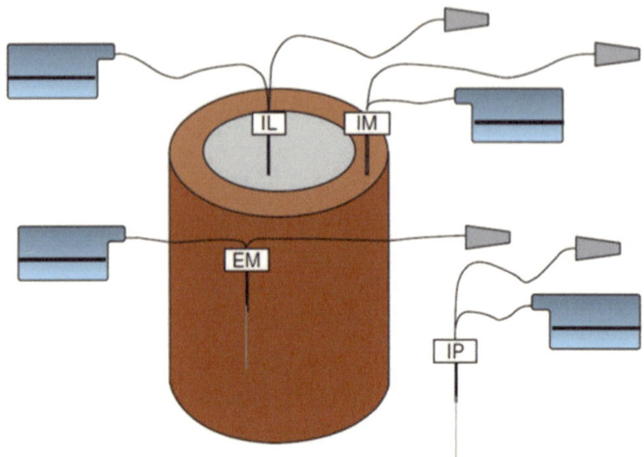

Figure 6. Microdialysis probe placement in the bowel. IL, intraluminal; IM, intramural; EM, extramural; IP, intraperitoneal. Reprinted with permission from John Wiley & Sons (126).

Off-line Microdialysis

Several studies have used in vivo microdialysis monitoring in animal models to investigate splanchnic metabolic disorders by measuring glucose, lactate/pyruvate ratio and glycerol both intraluminally (132-134) and in the intraperitoneal space (128). From these studies, microdialysis was suggested as a valuable tool for surgeons to detect early signs of mesenteric ischemia and the postoperative complications associated with this. In another study, microdialysis was used to monitor several episodes of ischemia in the pig intestine. The results showed lower dialysate levels of lactate during the second ischemic event compared with the first. This suggested that extended periods of ischemia triggered a mechanism of protection against hyperpermeability for later ischemic events (135).

Few have translated this technology to human subjects. Some pilot studies have used microdialysis for intraoperative monitoring. Intestinal luminal microdialysis and tonometry was used to monitor the rectal mucosa of patients undergoing elective cardiac surgery with cardiopulmonary bypass. This combination allowed the monitoring of both circulation and metabolism to indicate the adequacy of splanchnic perfusion in the colon (136). Others have used blood, urine and interstitial fluid microdialysis samples to investigate the phamacokinetic effect of antibiotic concentrations at the sites of infection during AAA open repair surgery (137). But, in general, studies in patients are carried out postoperatively. The safety of intraperitoneal microdialysis was evaluated to monitor metabolic and inflammatory changes in infants after surgery for necrotising enterocolitis (138). Peritoneal microdialysis was used postoperatively to assess the anastomosis leak rate in patients undergoing a low rectal resection due to cancer. In a medical trial for defunction stoma procedure, where patients were randomised, results showed that showed that defunctioning loop stoma decreased the probability of anastomosis leak (139). Another study distinguished a higher lactate/pyruvate ratio postoperatively in patients presenting anastomosis leakage before evidences of clinical symptom compared with those without (140).

From these clinical studies, scientists have agreed on the advantages of microdialysis as an early indication of intraoperative and postoperative complications compared with customary devices for the monitoring of splanchnic circulation. However, most of the microdialysis studies presented here used either bulky laboratory techniques such as liquid chromatography and electrophoresis or the commercially available bedside kit analyser from CMA/Microdialysis (141). Since the detection is off-line, samples are required to be collected in vials and manually stored in ice by a trained technician or the ward nurse. This time lag and the problem associated with sample misplacement are serious pitfalls of off-line microdialysis.

On-line Microdialysis

In order to have an early diagnosis, a tight monitoring is required. Metabolic events are rapid so a continuous monitoring is necessary. In recent years, compact instrumentation and microfluidic devices are being coupled online with microdialysis probes to overcome the temporal resolution of microdialysis. Lab-on-chip technology, such as microchip electrophoresis and liquid chromatography (142, 143) and microfluidic devices that increase temporal resolution by creating segmented nanolitres dialysate samples (144) are increasingly being investigated. However, the synergetic combination of microdialysis and biosensors has put this technology to the forefront of invasive monitoring. Sensitivity and biocompatibility of the biosensors increased when coupled to microdialysis and in turn biosensors enhance the temporal resolution of microdialysis to the millisecond scale (145, 146). This technology plays an important role in both point-of-care testing and home care (147).

Some studies placed the biosensors inside the microdialysis tubing (148-150), while others use connectors (151-153) or flow injection analysis systems (95, 154, 155). Alternatively, miniaturised flow-through biosensors have been fabricated for the connection with microdialysis (156).

An on-line rapid sampling microdialysis biosensor system has been used to monitor ischemia at the bowel level. The system couples selectively glucose and lactate electrochemical biosensors on-line with the microdialysis probe using a flow injection analysis (FIA) system. This allows in vivo monitoring of metabolic substrates changes in the colon at a high time resolution, every 30 seconds, without the need for extensive manipulation, running by itself during 24 hours up to 5 days (Figure 7).

Rapid sampling microdialysis was used to monitor rapid changes of glucose and lactate levels in patients undergoing an elective colectomy, most typically due to cancer. The microdialysis probe was inserted in the seromuscular layer of the colon and sutured to ensure fixation and allow the surgeon to proceed with the resection. A stabilisation period of 10-15 minutes was allowed before the transection of the main feeding artery, where glucose and lactate levels decrease and increase, respectively. These metabolic changes were not immediate as expected, but after an average interval of 12 minutes, attributed to the colon collateral flow, however, these agreed with the mechanism of blood flow reduction

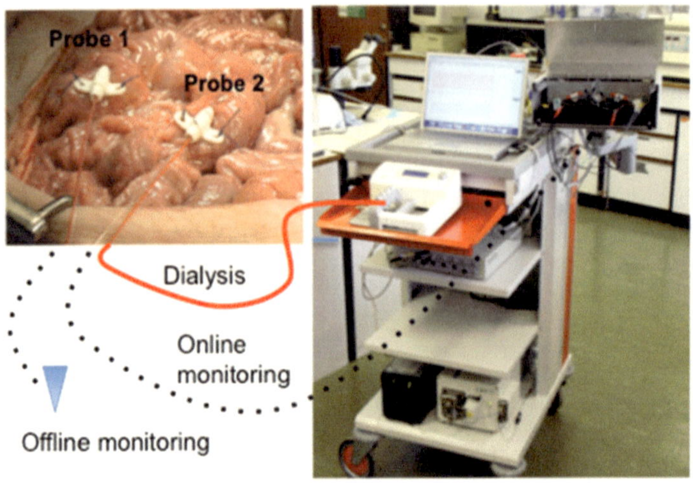

Figure 7. On-line rapid sampling intestinal microdialysis monitoring system. Two probes are implanted in the bowel wall, one as a control (off-line) and one as a test (on-line). The system parts are placed in a laparoscopy trolley allowing the transport of the system from the lab to clinical settings. Reproduced by permission of The Royal Society of Chemistry (157), http://pubs.rsc.org/en/Content/ArticleLanding/2011/AY/c1ay05306j

(158). A preliminary work in animal models was carried out to understand the mechanism of ischemia in compromised bowel, such as that after an anastomosis procedure. Here, the microdialysis was also tunnelled in the seromuscular layer, but in parallel with the site of the anastomosis construction, within a distance of a few millimeters. In this case, glucose and lactate changes occurred almost immediately after the feeding artery transection, which reveals that the tissue cannot rely on the same collateral flow once it has been compromised (by the resection previous to the anastomosis) (157). This has been further illustrated when comparing both data, where a therapeutical window is clearly observed in healthy patients but not in compromised tissue (159) (Figure 8).

The system was recognised as a potential candidate for monitoring early diagnosis of ischemia after AAA repair surgery. A set of data was obtained during the monitoring of aneurysm repair elective surgery patients for up to 2 days in ICU. The probe was implanted in the bowel of seven subjects in the mesenteric border of the sigmoid colon just at the junction of the mesentery with the colon. Although changes in plasma values were observed, dialysate levels for both glucose and lactate were steady. This confirms the fact that microdialysis levels are a good indicator of local changes, but it does not reflect systemic conditions. The lactate/glucose ratio was observed to be constant for all patients for up to 2 days after probe implantation, which strongly indicates the lack of acute ischemic events. Some episodes of transient metabolic ischemia were observed due to a compromised blood supply, which allows for pattern recognition during further studies (160).

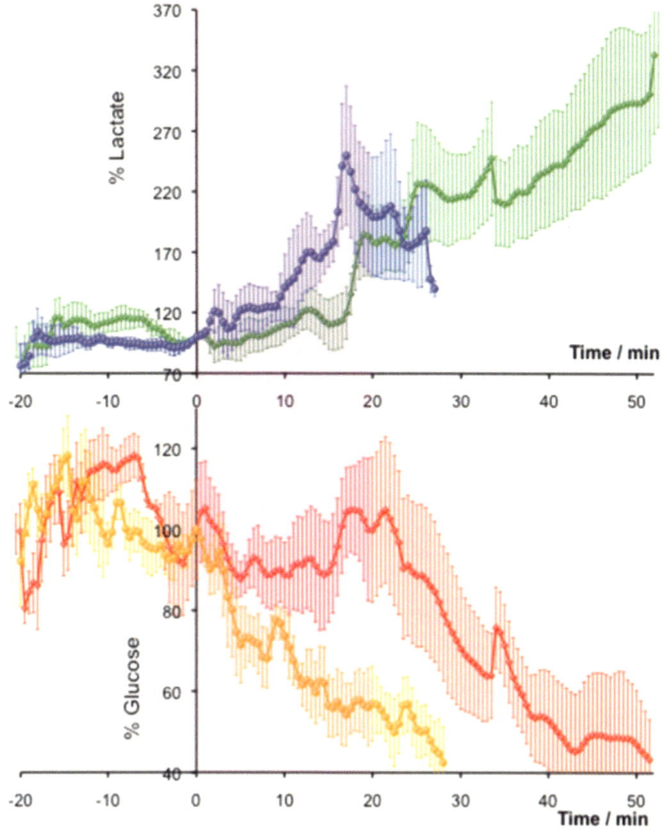

Figure 8. Microdialysis monitoring of healthy tissue in patients versus compromised anastomotic porcine tissue. Percentage of metabolites levels (mean ± sem) monitored during colorectal surgery in patients (red & green traces) and in the anastomosis site of porcine bowel wall models (orange & blue traces). Glucose traces drop from baseline values, while lactate traces rise. Alignment at the transection of main feeding artery (t=0). Reprinted with kind permission from Springer Science & Business Media (159).

6. Conclusion and future trends

Mesenteric ischemia has been known to increase intestinal cell membrane permeability, provoking bacterial translocation and ultimately leading to sepsis and multiple organ failure. An adequate splanchnic perfusion and evaluation of intestinal permeability are crucial to improve outcome rates following surgical procedures. However, current techniques for the diagnosis of leaks are unreliable due to the subjectivity, lack of precision and the delayed manifestation of the symptoms.

Microdialysis has been used to monitor biomarkers in a range of tissues and organs. Clinical studies using intestinal microdialysis have agreed on the advantages of the technique as an early indication of intraoperative and postoperative complications compared with common monitoring of splanchnic circulation. However, off-line detection carries a limitation for the early diagnosis of ischemic insults, since metabolic events are rapid. On-line rapid microdialysis technology takes advantage of the synergetic combination of microdialysis and biosensors, which plays an important role in both point-of-care testing and home care.

Microdialysis has recently been evaluated as a tool to assess the metabolic changes during liver resection, stomach ischemia and for the diagnosis of novel biomarkers of the pancreas that are undetectable in plasma. Preliminary work has been done with microdialysis to monitor key metabolites during and after organ transplantation. Although still in early stage, this presents the potential of monitoring the organ's condition during the transportation. This will allow not only the determination of the suitability of the organ for transplantation, but will also decrease the possibility of occurrence of an ischemic insult by perfusing the organ when it reaches a certain predetermined threshold.

Among some limitations of microdialysis is the trauma caused by the implantation of the probe, which causes an inflammatory response and compromises the results of the investigation. A common solution has been to establish equilibration periods after probe implantation and to develop miniature probes. Since smaller sized probes present high back-pressure, a droplet microdialysis probe has been designed to overcome this issue (161). Alternatively, flat microdialysis geometries can be envisioned, for those tissues where tunnelling of the probe is not necessary. Temporal resolution also limits microdialysis use, hence microfluidic and lab-on-chip devices have been investigated to directly connect the microdialysis with biosensors (162-164). As the microfabrication technology advances, more chips and miniaturised devices will be seen such as micropumps to be implanted in line with the microdialysis inlet and wireless detection systems embedded in the probe design, reducing in this way bulky instrumentation, otherwise required. One of the paramount targets of biomedical research is to be able to create close-loop systems that combine sensing devices with drug delivery systems. Microdialysis probes are currently used for drug delivery and fluid sampling for diagnosis. Hence, it can be envisioned a device where microdialysis is coupled with biosensors for diagnosis and depending on the levels recorded, the mechanism switches to a reverse mode delivering the drug required.

Most microdialysis publications focus on the monitoring of neurochemicals, however, general reviews and book chapters are helpful to understand the fundamentals of the technique and learn how to handle the probes and perform calibration experiments (165-167). Originally, microdialysis probes were fabricated from dialysis fibres connected to an inlet and outlet tubing. With the expansion of microdialysis, few major trades are handling the commercialisation of microdialysis products, producing CE approved sterile probes for human use (141) and for in vitro and animal studies (168, 169).

Author details

Radha Swathe Priya M. and Emma P. Córcoles
Faculty of Health Science and Biomedical Engineering, Universiti Teknologi Malaysia, Skudai, Malaysia

Acknowledgement

The authors would like to acknowledge Universiti Teknologi Malaysia, UTM and Minister of Higher Education of Malaysia, MOHE for the funding for the publication of this chapter.

7. References

[1] Brandt LJ, Boley SJ. AGA Technical Review on Intestinal Ischemia. Gastroenterology. 2000;118(5):954-68.
[2] Loganathan A, Linley JE, Rajput I, Hunter M, Lodge JPA, Sandle GI. Basolateral potassium (IKCa) channel inhibition prevents increased colonic permeability induced by chemical hypoxia. American Journal of Physiology - Gastrointestinal and Liver Physiology. 2011;300(1):G146-G53.
[3] Alexander C, Rietschel ET. Bacterial lipopolysaccharides and innate immunity. J Endotoxin Res. 2001;7(3):167-202.
[4] Davidson MT, Deitch EA, Lu Q, Osband A, Feketeova E, Nemeth ZH, et al. A study of the biologic activity of trauma-hemorrhagic shock mesenteric lymph over time and the relative role of cytokines. Surgery. 2004;136(1):32-41.
[5] Deitch EA, Forsythe R, Anjaria D, Livingston DH, Lu Q, Xu DZ, et al. The Role of Lymph Factors in Lung Injury, Bone Marrow Suppression, and Endothelial Cell Dysfunction in a Primate Model of Trauma-Hemorrhagic Shock. Shock. 2004;22(3):221-8.
[6] Sugi K, Musch MW, Di A, Nelson DJ, Chang EB. Oxidants Potentiate C^2^+- and cAMP-Stimulated Cl^- Secretion in Intestinal Epithelial T84 Cells. Gastroenterol. 2001;120(1):89-98.
[7] Thanou M, Verhoef JC, Marbach P, Junginger HE. Intestinal Absorption of Octreotide: N-Trimethyl Chitosan Chloride (TMC) Ameliorates the Permeability and Absorption Properties of the Somatostatin Analogue In Vitro and In Vivo. J Pharm Sci. 2000;89(7):951-7.
[8] Wiest R, Rath HC. Gastrointestinal disorders of the critically ill. Bacterial translocation in the gut. Best Pract Res Clin Gastroenterol. 2003;17(3):397-425.
[9] Chang JX, Chen S, Ma LP, Jiang LY, Chen JW, chang RM, et al. Functional and morphological changes of the gut barrier during the restitution process after hemorrhagic shock. World J Gastroentero. 2005 Numb 35;11:5485-91.
[10] Ackland G, Grocott MP, Mythen MG. Understanding gastrointestinal perfusion in critical care: so near, and yet so far. Crit Care. 2000;4(5):269-81.
[11] Kanwar S, Windsor AC, Welsh F, Barclay GR, Guillou PJ, Reynolds JV. Lack of Correlation Between Failure of Gut Barrier Function and Septic Complications After Major Upper Gastrointestinal Surgery. Annals Surg. 2000;231(1):88-95.
[12] Alexander JW, Boyce ST, Babcock GF, Gianotti L, Pack MD, Dunn DL. The process of microbial translocation. Ann Surg. 1990;212:496-510.
[13] Berg RD. Bacterial trasnlocation from the gastrointestinal tract. Trends Microbiol. 1995;3(4):149-54.

[14] Tsokos M. Pathology of Sepsis Essentials of Autopsy Practice. 2006:39-85.

[15] Freter R, Abrams GD. Function of Various Intestinal Bacteria in Converting Germfree fice to the Normal State. Infect Immun. 1972;6(2):119-26.

[16] Teshima C, Meddings J. The measurement and clinical significance of intestinal permeability. Current Gastroenterology Reports. 2008;10(5):443-9.

[17] MacFie J, O'Boyle C, Mitchell CJ, Buckley PM, Johnstone D, Sudworth P. Gut origin of sepsis: a prospective study investigating associations between bacterial translocation, gastric microflora, and septic morbidity. Gut. 1999;45(2):223-8.

[18] Porras M, Martín MT, Yang PC, Jury J, Perdue MH, Vergara P. Correlation between cyclical epithelial barrier dysfunction and bacterial translocation in the relapses of intestinal inflammation. Inflammatory Bowel Diseases. 2006;12(9):843-52.

[19] Clayburgh DR, Shen L, Turner JR. A porous defense: The leaky epithelial barrier in intestinal disease. Laboratory Investigation. 2004;84(3):282-91.

[20] Liu Z, Li N, Neu J. Tight junctions, leaky intestines, and pediatric diseases. Acta Paediatr. 2005 Numb 4;94:386-93.

[21] Swidsinski A, Ladhoff A, Pernthaler A, Swidsinski S, Loening-Baucke V, Ortner M, et al. Mucosal flora in inflammatory bowel disease. Gastroenterology. [doi: 10.1053/gast.2002.30294]. 2002;122(1):44-54.

[22] Swank GM, Deitch EA. Role of the Gut in Multiple Organ Failure: Bacterial Translocation and Permeability Changes. World J Surg. 1996;20(4):411-7.

[23] Caplan MS, Kely A, Hsueh W. Endotoxin and hypoxia-induced intestinal necrosis in rats: the role of platelets activating factor. Pediatr Res. 1992;31:428.

[24] Kubes P, Arfors KE, Granger DN. Platelet-activating factor-induced mucosal dysfunction: role of oxidant and granulocytes. Am J Physiol. 1991;260:G965.

[25] Kubes P, Suzuki M, Granger DN. Modulation of PAF-induced leukocyte adherence and increased microvascular permeability. Am J Physiol. 1990;259:G859.

[26] Redl H. Cytokines in severe sepsis and septic shock: Birkhäuser Basel; 1999.

[27] Adams RB, Planchon SM, Roche JK. IFN-gamma Modulation of Epithelial Barrier Function: Time Course, Reversibility, and Site of Cytokine Binding. J Immunology. 1993;150(6):2356.

[28] De-Souza DA, Greene LJ. Intestinal permeability and systemic infections in critically ill patients: Effect of glutamine *. Critical Care Medicine. 2005;33(5):1125-35 10.097/01.CCM.0000162680.52397.97.

[29] Ceppa EP, Fuh KC, Bulkley GB. Mesenteric hemodynamic response to circulatory shock. Curr Opin Crit Care. 2003;9(2):127-32.

[30] Andriantsitohaina R, Suprenant A. Acetylcholine release from guine-pig submucosal neurones dilate arterioles by releasing nitric oxide from endothelium. J Physiol. 1992;453:493.

[31] Falcone JC, Bohlen HG. EDRF from rat intestine and skeletal muscle venules causes dilation of arterioles. Am J Physiol. 1990;258:h1515.

[32] Boughton-Smith NK, Deakin AM, Whittle BJR. Actions of nitric oxide on the acute gastrointestinal damaged induced by PAF in the cat. Agents Actions. 1992;Specs No:C3-9.
[33] Deitch EA. Multiple Organ Failure: Pathophysiology and Potential Future Therapy. Ann Surg. 1992;216(2):117-34.
[34] Kubes P. Nitric oxide modulates epithelial permeability in the feline small intestine. Am J Physiol. 1992;262:G1138.
[35] Kubes P, Granger DN. Nitric oxide modulates microvascular permeability. Am J Physiol. 1992;262(H611).
[36] MacHiedo GW, Zaets SB, Berezina TL, Xu DZ, Feketova E, Spolarics Z, et al. Trauma-hemorrhagic shock-induced red blood cell damage leads to decreased microcirculatory blood flow. Critical Care Medicine. 2009;37(3):1000-10.
[37] Landry D, Oliver J. The ATP-sensitive K^+ channels mediates hypotension in endotoxemia and hypoxic lactic acidosis in dog. J Clin Invest. 1992;89:2071.
[38] Green BT, Tendler DA. Ischemic Colitis: A Clinical Review. South Med J. 2005 Numb 2;98:217-22.
[39] Perry RJ, Martin MJ, Eckert MJ, Sohn VY, Steele SR. Colonic ischemia complicating open vs endovascular abdominal aortic aneurysm repair. J Vasc Surg. 2008;48(2):272-7.
[40] Bauer EP, Redaelli C, Von Segesser LK, Turina MI. Ruptured abdominal aortic aneurysms: Predictors for early complications and death. Surgery. 1993;114(1):31.
[41] Kaplan GG, McCarthy EP, Ayanian JZ, Korzenik J, Hodin R, Sands BE. Impact of Hospital Volume on Postoperative Morbidity and Mortality Following a Colectomy for Ulcerative Colitis. Gastroenterology. [doi: 10.1053/j.gastro.2008.01.004]. 2008;134(3):680-7.e1.
[42] Meissner MH, Johanson KH. Colon infarction after ruptured abdominal aortic aneurysm. Arch Surg. 1992;127:979.
[43] Tollefson DF, Ernst CB. Colon ischemia following aortic reconstruction. Ann Vasc Surg. 1991;5:485.
[44] Karanjia ND, Corder AP, Bearn P, Heald RI. Leakage from stapled low anastomosis after total mesorectal excision for carcinoma of the rectum. Brit J Surg. 1994;81(8):1224.
[45] Alves A, Panis Y, Trancart D, Regimbeau JM, Pocard M, Valleur P. Factors Associated with Clinically Significant Anastomotic Leakage after Large Bowel Resection: Multivariate Analysis of 707 Patients. World J Surg. 2002;26(4):499-502.
[46] Bruce J, Krukowski ZH, Al-Khairy G, Russell EM, Park KGM. Systematic review of the definition and measurement of anastomotic leak after gastrointestinal surgery. Brit J Surg. 2001;88(9):1157-68.
[47] Law WI, Chu KW, Ho JW, Chan CW. Risk factors for anastomotic leakage after low anterior resection with total mesorectal excision. Am J Surg. 2000;179(2):92-6.
[48] Ascione R, Talpahewa S, Rajakaruna C, Reeves BC, Lovell AT, Cohen A, et al. Splanchnic Organ Injury During Coronary Surgery With or Without Cardiopulmonary Bypass: A Randomized, Controlled Trial. The Annals of Thoracic Surgery. [doi: 10.1016/j.athoracsur.2005.06.038]. 2006;81(1):97-103.

[49] Pinsky MR. Both Perfusion Pressure and Flow are Essential for Adequate Resuscitation. Sepsis. 2001;4(2):143-6.

[50] Cancio LC, Kuwa T, Matsui K, Drew GA, Galvez E, Sandoval LL, et al. Intestinal and gastric tonometry during experimental burn shock. Burns. 2007;33(7):879-84.

[51] Cerny V, Cvachovec K. Gastric tonometry and intramucosal pH - theoretical principles and clinical application. Physiol Res. 2000;49(3):289-98.

[52] Marshall AP, West SH. Gastric tonometry and monitoring gastrointestinal perfusion: using research to support nursing practice. Nursing in Critical Care. 2004;9(3):123-33.

[53] Oltean M, Aneman A, Dindelegan G, x00F, lne J, Olausson M, et al. Monitoring of the Intestinal Mucosal Perfusion Using Laser Doppler Flowmetry After Multivisceral Transplantation. Transplantation Proceedings. 2005;37(8):3323-4.

[54] Boyle NH, Manifold D, Jordan MH, Mason RC. Intraoperative assessment of colonic perfusion using scanning laser doppler flowmetry during colonic resection. Journal of the American College of Surgeons. [doi: 10.1016/S1072-7515(00)00709-2]. 2000; 191(5):504-10.

[55] Ramirez FC, Padda S, Medlin S, Tarbell H, Leung FW. Reflectance Spectrophotometry in the Gastrointestinal Tract: Limitations and New Applications. Am J Gastroenterol. 2002;97(11):2780-4.

[56] Hirano Y, Omura K, Yoshiba H, Ohta N, Hiranuma C, Nitta K, et al. Near-Infrared Spectroscopy for Assessment of Tissue Oxygen Saturation of Transplanted Jejunal Autografts in Cervical Esophageal Reconstruction. Surg Today. 2005 Numb 1;35:67-72.

[57] Cautero N, Gelmini R, Villa E, Bagni A, Merighi A, Masetti M, et al. Orthogonal polarization spectral imaging: a new tool in morphologic surveillance in intestinal transplant recipients. Transplantation Proceedings. 2002;34(3):922-3.

[58] Turek Z, Cerny V, Parizkova R. Noninvasive in vivo assessment of the skeletal muscle and small intestine serous surface microcirculation in rat: sidestream dark-field (SDF) imaging. Physiol Res. 2008;57(3):365-72.

[59] Behrendt FF, Tolba RH, Overhaus M, Hirner A, Minor T, Kalff JC. Indocyanine Green Fluorescence Measurement of Intestinal Transit and Gut Perfusion after Intestinal Manipulation. Eur Surg Res. 2004;36(4):210-8.

[60] Assadian A, Assadian O, Senekowitsch C, Rotter R, Bahrami S, Furst W, et al. Plasma d-Lactate as a Potential Early Marker for Colon Ischaemia After Open Aortic Reconstruction. Eur J Vasc Endovasc. 2006;31(5):470-4.

[61] van Haren FMP, Sleigh JW, Pickkers P, van der Hoeven JG. Gastrointestinal perfusion in septic shock. Anaesth Intensive Care. 2007 Numb 5;35:679-94.

[62] Heinonen PO, Jousela IT, Blomqvist KA, Olkkola KT, Takkunen OS. Validation of air tonometric measurement of gastric regional concentrations of CO2 in critically ill septic patients. Intensive Care Medicine. 1997;23(5):524-9.

[63] Salzman AL, Strong KE, Wang H, Wollert PS, Vandermeer TJ, Fink MP. Intraluminal "balloonless" air tonometry: a new method for determination of gastrointestinal mucosal carbon dioxide tension. Critical Care Medicine. 1994;22(1):126-34.

[64] Rombeau JL, Takala J. Summary of round table conference: gut dysfunction in critical illness. Intensive Care Med. 1997;23(4):476-9.

[65] Ballard JL, Stone WM, Hallett JW, Pairolero PC. A Critical Analysis of Adjuvant Techniques Used To Assess Bowel Viability in Acute Mesenteric Ischemia. Am Surg. 1993;59(5):309.

[66] Gaginella TS, editor. Regulatory Mechanisms in Gastrointestinal Function. Florida: CRC Press, Inc; 1995.

[67] Knichwitz G, Brussel T, Reinhold P, Schaumann F, Richter KD, Van Aken H. Early Onset of Regional Intestinal Ischemia Can Be Detected with Carbon Dioxide Tension Measurement Inside the Peritoneal Cavity. Anesth Analg. 2000;91(5):1182-7.

[68] Tenhunen JJ, Uusaro A, Karja V, Oksala N, Jakob SM, Ruokonen E. Apparent Heterogeneity of Regional Blood Flow and Metabolic Changes Within Splanchnic Tissues During Experimental Endotoxin Shock. Anesth Analg. 2003;97(2):555-63.

[69] Hiltebrand LB, Krejci V, tenHoevel ME, Banic A, Sigurdsson GH. Redistribution of Microcirculatory Blood Flow within the Intestinal Wall during Sepsis and General Anesthesia. Anesthesiology. 2003;98(3):658-69.

[70] Krejci V, Hiltebrand L, Banic A, Erni D, Wheatley AM, Sigurdsson GH. Continuous measurements of microcirculatory blood flow in gastrointestinal organs during acute haemorrhage. Brit J Anaesth. 2000;84(4):468-75.

[71] Hiltebrand LB, Krejci V, Banic A, Erni D, Wheatley AM, Sigurdsson GH. Dynamic study of the distribution of microcirculatory blood flow in multiple splanchnic organs in septic shock. Crit Care Med. 2000;28(9):3233-41.

[72] Krejci V, Hiltebrand L, Buchi C, Ali SZ, Contaldo C, Takala J, et al. Decreasing gut wall glucose as an early marker of impaired intestinal perfusion. Crit Care Med. 2006 Numb 9;34:2406-14.

[73] Tugtekin IF, Radermacher P, Theisen M, Matejovic M, Stehr A, Ploner F, et al. Increased ileal-mucosal-arterial PCO~2 gap is associated with impaired villus microcirculation in endotoxic pigs. Intensive Care Med. 2001;27(4):757-66.

[74] Uusaro A, Russell JA, Walley KR, Takala J. Gastric-Arterial PCO~2 Gradient Does Not Reflect Systemic and Splanchnic Hemodynamics or Oxygen Transport After Cardiac Surgery. Shock. 2000;14(1):13-7.

[75] VanderMeer TJ, Wang H, Fink MP. Endotoxemia causes ileal mucosal acidosis in the absence of mucosal hypoxia in a normodynamic porcine model of septic shock. Crit Care Med. 1995;23(7):1217.

[76] Trager K, Radermacher P, Rieger KM, Grover R, Vlatten A, Iber T, et al. Norepinephrine and N^G-monomethyl-L-arginine in hyperdynamic septic shock in pigs: Effects on intestinal oxygen exchange and energy balance. Crit Care Med. 2000;28(6):2007-14.

[77] Liao XP, She YX, Shi CR, Li M. Changes in Body Fluid Markers in Intestinal Ischemia. J Pediatr Surg. 1995;30(10):1412.

[78] Sommer T, Larsen JF. Validation of intramural intestinal microdialysis as a detector of intestinal ischaemia. Scandinavian Journal of Gastroenterology. 2004;39(5):493-9.

[79] Baldini F, Falai A, De Gaudio AR, Landi D, Lueger A, Mencaglia A, et al. Continuous monitoring of gastric carbon dioxide with optical fibres. Sensors and Actuators B: Chemical. [doi: 10.1016/S0925-4005(03)00042-X]. 2003;90(1–3):132-8.

[80] Bours MJL, Swennen ELR, Di Virgilio F, Cronstein BN, Dagnelie PC. Adenosine 5'-triphosphate and adenosine as endogenous signaling molecules in immunity and inflammation. Pharmacology & Therapeutics. [doi: 10.1016/j.pharmthera.2005.04.013]. 2006;112(2):358-404.

[81] Burnstock G. The journey to establish purinergic signalling in the gut. Neurogastroenterology and Motility. 2008;20(SUPPL. 1):8-19.

[82] Christofi FL, Kim M, Wunderlich JE, Xue J, Suntres Z, Cardounel A, et al. Endogenous adenosine differentially modulates 5-hydroxytryptamine release from a human enterochromaffin cell model. Gastroenterology. 2004;127(1):188-202.

[83] Cooke HJ, Wunderlich J, Christofi FL. "The force be with you": ATP in gut mechanosensory transduction. News in Physiological Sciences. 2003;18(2):43-9.

[84] Patel BA, Rogers M, Wieder T, O'Hare D, Boutelle MG. ATP microelectrode biosensor for stable long-term in vitro monitoring from gastrointestinal tissue. Biosensors and Bioelectronics. [doi: 10.1016/j.bios.2010.11.033]. 2011;26(6):2890-6.

[85] Hansberry DR. A Quantum Dot -- Based Diagnostic Immunoassay for Biomarker Detection in Gastrointestinal Inflammatory Diseases: Drexel University; 2011.

[86] Kumari A, Pasini P, Deo Sapna K, Flomenhoft D, Shashidhar H, Daunert S. Biosensors for Quorum Chemical Signaling Molecules: Implications of Bacterial Communication in Gastrointestinal Disorders. Microbial Surfaces: American Chemical Society; 2008. p. 13-27.

[87] Ryou M, Nemiroski A, Azagury D, Shaikh SN, Ryan MB, Westervelt RM, et al. An implantable wireless biosensor for the immediate detection of upper GI bleeding: a new fluorescein-based tool for diagnosis and surveillance (with video). Gastrointestinal Endoscopy. [doi: 10.1016/j.gie.2011.03.1182]. 2011;74(1):189-94.e1.

[88] Frost M, Meyerhoff ME. In vivo chemical sensors: Tackling biocompatibility. Analytical Chemistry. 2006;78(21):7370-7.

[89] Vadgama P. Sensor biocompatibility: Final frontier in bioanalytical measurement. Analyst. 2007;132(6):495-9.

[90] Wisniewski N, Reichert M. Methods for reducing biosensor membrane biofouling. Colloids and Surfaces B: Biointerfaces. 2000;18(3-4):197-219.

[91] Ungerstedt U, Pycock C. Functional correlates of dopamine neurotransmission. Bull Schweiz Akad Med Wiss. 1974 Jul;30(1-3):44-55.

[92] Benveniste H. Brain microdialysis. J Neurochem. 1989 Jun;52(6):1667-79.

[93] Klaus S, Heringlake M, Bahlmann L. Bench-to-bedside review: Microdialysis in intensive care medicine. Crit Care. 2004;8(5):363-8.

[94] Hahn H, Kammerer B, DiMauro A, Salt AN, Plontke SK. Cochlear microdialysis for quantification of dexamethasone and fluorescein entry into scala tympani during round window administration. Hearing Research. [doi: 10.1016/j.heares.2005.12.001]. 2006;212(1–2):236-44.

[95] Jones DA, Parkin MC, Langemann H, Landolt H, Hopwood SE, Strong AJ, et al. On-line monitoring in neurointensive care - Enzyme-based electrochemical assay for simultaneous, continuous monitoring of glucose and lactate from critical care patients. J Electroanal Chem. 2002 DEC 13;538:243-52.

[96] Parkin MC, Hopwood SE, Strong AJ, Boutelle MG. Resolving dynamic changes in brain metabolism using biosensors and on-line microdialysis. Trends Anal Chem. 2003 SEP;22(9):487-97.

[97] Battezzati A, Bertoli S. Methods of measuring metabolism during surgery in humans: focus on the liver-brain relationship. Curr Opin Clin Nutr Metab Care. 2004 Sep;7(5):523-30.

[98] Kennergren C, Mantovani V, Lonnroth P, Nystrom B, Berglin E, Hamberger A. Extracellular amino acids as markers of myocardial ischemia during cardioplegic heart arrest. Cardiology. 1999;91(1):31-40.

[99] Henriksson J. Microdialysis of skeletal muscle at rest. Proceedings- Nutrition Society of London. 1999;58(4):919-23.

[100] Dawson LA. Capillary electrophoresis and microdialysis: current technology and applications. Journal of Chromatography B: Biomedical Sciences and Applications. [doi: 10.1016/S0378-4347(96)00533-6]. 1997;697(1–2):89-99.

[101] Binnert C, Tappy L. Microdialysis in the intensive care unit: a novel tool for clinical investigation or monitoring? Curr Opin Clin Nutr Metab Care. 2002 Numb 2;5:185-8.

[102] Plock N, Kloft C. Microdialysis—theoretical background and recent implementation in applied life-sciences. European Journal of Pharmaceutical Sciences. [doi: 10.1016/j.ejps.2005.01.017]. 2005;25(1):1-24.

[103] Nandi P, Lunte SM. Recent trends in microdialysis sampling integrated with conventional and microanalytical systems for monitoring biological events: A review. Analytica Chimica Acta. [doi: 10.1016/j.aca.2009.07.064]. 2009;651(1):1-14.

[104] Ericsson P, Håkanson R, Rehfeld JF, Norlén P. Gastrin release: Antrum microdialysis reveals a complex neural control. Regulatory Peptides. [doi: 10.1016/j.regpep.2010.01.004]. 2010;161(1–3):22-32.

[105] Cibicek N, Zivna H, Vrublova E, Cibicek J, Cermakova E, Palicka V. Gastric submucosal Microdialysis in the detection of rat stomach ischemia-a comparison of the3H2O efflux technique with metabolic monitoring. Physiological Measurement. 2010;31(10):1355-68.

[106] Bernsand M, Håkanson R, Norlén P. Tachyphylaxis of the ECL-cell response to PACAP: Receptor desensitization and/or depletion of secretory products. British Journal of Pharmacology. 2007;152(2):240-8.

[107] Ericsson P, Norlén P, Bernsand M, Alm P, Höglund P, Håkanson R. ECL cell histamine mobilization studied by gastric submucosal microdialysis in awake rats: Methodological considerations. Pharmacology and Toxicology. 2003;93(2):57-65.

[108] Fykse V, Solligård E, Bendheim MØ, Chen D, Grønbech JE, Sandvik AK, et al. ECL cell histamine mobilization and parietal cell stimulation in the rat stomach studied by microdialysis and electron microscopy. Acta Physiologica. 2006;186(1):37-43.

[109] Kitano M, Bernsand M, Kishimoto Y, Norlén P, Håkanson R, Haenuki Y, et al. Ischemia of rat stomach mobilizes ECL cell histamine. American Journal of Physiology - Gastrointestinal and Liver Physiology. 2005;288(5 51-5):G1084-G90.

[110] Kitano M, Norlén P, Håkanson R. Gastric submucosal microdialysis: a method to study gastrin- and food-evoked mobilization of ECL-cell histamine in conscious rats. Regulatory Peptides. 2000;86(1-3):113-23.

[111] Woo KL, Lunte CE. The development of multiple probe microdialysis sampling in the stomach. Journal of Pharmaceutical and Biomedical Analysis. [doi: 10.1016/j.jpba.2008.04.019]. 2008;48(1):20-6.

[112] Woo KL, Lunte CE. The direct comparison of health and ulcerated stomach tissue: A multiple probe microdialysis sampling approach. Journal of Pharmaceutical and Biomedical Analysis. [doi: 10.1016/j.jpba.2008.05.014]. 2008;48(1):85-91.

[113] Sorensen H. Free Jejunal Flaps Can Be Monitored by Use of Microdialysis. J Reconstr Microsurg. 2008;24(6):443-8.

[114] Takahashi A, Ishimaru H, Ikarashi Y, Kishi E, Maruyama Y. Effects of hepatic nerve stimulation on blood glucose and glycogenolysis in rat liver: Studies with in vivo microdialysis. Journal of the Autonomic Nervous System. [doi: 10.1016/S0165-1838(96)00082-3]. 1996;61(2):181-5.

[115] Nowak G, Ungerstedt J, Wernerman J, Ungerstedt U, Ericzon B-G. Metabolic changes in the liver graft monitored continuously with microdialysis during liver transplantation in a pig model. Liver Transplantation. 2002;8(5):424-32.

[116] Nowak G, Ungerstedt J, Wernerman J, Ungerstedt U, Ericzon BG. Clinical experience in continuous graft monitoring with microdialysis early after liver transplantation. British Journal of Surgery. 2002;89(9):1169-75.

[117] Björnsson B, Winbladh A, Bojmar L, Trulsson LM, Olsson H, Sundqvist T, et al. Remote or Conventional Ischemic Preconditioning –Local Liver Metabolism in Rats Studied with Microdialysis. Journal of Surgical Research. [doi: 10.1016/j.jss.2011.07.038]. (0).

[118] Isaksson B, D'Souza MA, Jersenius U, Ungerstedt J, Lundell L, Permert J, et al. Continuous assessment of intrahepatic metabolism by microdialysis during and after portal triad clamping. Journal of Surgical Research. 2011;169(2):214-9.

[119] Wu Y-S, Tsai T-H, Wu T-F, Cheng F-C. Determination of pyruvate and lactate in primary liver cell culture medium during hypoxia by on-line microdialysis–liquid chromatography. Journal of Chromatography A. [doi: 10.1016/S0021-9673(00)01265-6]. 2001;913(1–2):341-7.

[120] Sun L, Stenken JA, Yang AY, Zhao JJ, Musson DG. An in vitro microdialysis methodology to study 11β-hydroxysteroid dehydrogenase type 1 enzyme activity in liver microsomes. Analytical Biochemistry. [doi: 10.1016/j.ab.2007.06.038]. 2007;370(1):26-37.

[121] Gunaratna C, Kissinger PT. Application of microdialysis to study the in vitro metabolism of drugs in liver microsomes. Journal of Pharmaceutical and Biomedical Analysis. [doi: 10.1016/S0731-7085(97)00042-3]. 1997;16(2):239-48.

[122] Beier H, Kaiser K, Langhans M, Malmendier K, Sluijsmans I, Weiher J. Peritoneal microdialysis in freely moving rodents: An alternative to blood sampling for pharmacokinetic studies in the rat and the mouse. European Journal of Pharmaceutical Sciences. [doi: 10.1016/j.ejps.2006.10.005]. 2007;30(1):75-83.

[123] Saito K, Kanazawa M, Fukudo S. Colorectal distention induces hippocampal noradrenaline release in rats: an in vivo microdialysis study. Brain Research. [doi: 10.1016/S0006-8993(02)03007-X]. 2002;947(1):146-9.

[124] Zhou Q, Gallo JM. In vivo microdialysis for PK and PD studies of anticancer drugs. AAPS Journal. 2005;7(3):E659-E67.

[125] Solligård E, Juel IS, Bakkelund K, Johnsen H, Saether OD, Gronbech JE, et al. Gut barrier dysfunction as detected by intestinal luminal microdialysis. Intensive Care Med. 2004 Jun;30(6):1188-94.

[126] Sommer T, Larsen JF. Intraperitoneal and intraluminal microdialysis in the detection of experimental regional intestinal ischaemia. Br J Surg. 2004 Jul;91(7):855-61.

[127] Jansson K, Ungerstedt J, Jonsson T, Redler B, Andersson M, Ungerstedt U, et al. Human intraperitoneal microdialysis: increased lactate/pyruvate ratio suggests early visceral ischaemia. A pilot study. Scand J Gastroenter. 2003 Sep;38(9):1007-11.

[128] Klaus S, Heringlake M, Gliemroth J, Bruch H-P, Bahlmann L. Intraperitoneal microdialysis for detection of splanchnic metabolic disorders. Langenbeck's Archives of Surgery. 2002;387(7):276-80.

[129] Ungerstedt J, Nowak G, Ericzon BG, Ungerstedt U. Intraperitoneal microdialysis (IPM): a new technique for monitoring intestinal ischemia studied in a porcine model. Shock. 2003 Jul;20(1):91-6.

[130] Sommer T, Larsen JF. Detection of intestinal ischemia using a microdialysis technique in an animal model. World J Surg. 2003 Apr;27(4):416-20.

[131] Kitano M, Sakamoto H, Das K, Komaki T, Kudo M. EUS-guided in vivo microdialysis of the pancreas: a novel technique with potential diagnostic and therapeutic application. Gastrointestinal Endoscopy. [doi: 10.1016/j.gie.2009.05.040]. 2010;71(1):176-9.

[132] Tenhunen JJ, Kosunen H, Alhava E, Tuomisto L, Takala JA. Intestinal Luminal Microdialysis: A New Approach to Assess Gut Mucosal Ischemia. Anaesthesiology. 1999;91(6):1807-15.

[133] Tenhunen JJ, Jakob SM, Takala JA. Gut luminal lactate release during gradual intestinal ischemia. Intensive Care Med. 2001;27(12):1916-22.

[134] Högberg N, Carlsson PO, Hillered L, Meurling S, Stenbäck A. Intestinal ischemia measured by intraluminal microdialysis. Scandinavian Journal of Clinical and Laboratory Investigation. 2012;72(1):59-66.

[135] Solligård E, Juel IS, Spigset O, Romundstad P, Grønbech JE, Aadahl P. Gut luminal lactate measured by microdialysis mirrors permeability of the intestinal mucosa after ischemia. Shock. 2008;29(2):245-51.

[136] Solligård E, Wahba A, Skogvoll E, Stenseth R, Grønbech JE, Aadahl P. Rectal lactate levels in endoluminal microdialysate during routine coronary surgery. Anaesthesia. 2007;62(3):250-8.

[137] Douglas A, Udy AA, Wallis SC, Jarrett P, Stuart J, Lassig-Smith M, et al. Plasma and tissue pharmacokinetics of cefazolin in patients undergoing elective and semielective abdominal aortic aneurysm open repair surgery. Antimicrobial Agents and Chemotherapy. 2011;55(11):5238-42.

[138] Pedersen ME, Dahl M, Qvist N. Intraperitoneal microdialysis in the postoperative surveillance after surgery for necrotizing enterocolitis: A preliminary report. Journal of Pediatric Surgery. 2011;46(2):352-6.

[139] Matthiessen P, Hallbook O, Rutegard J, Simert G, Sjodahl R. Defunctioning Stoma Reduces Symptomatic Anastomotic Leakage After Low Anterior Resection of the Rectum for Cancer: A Randomized Multicenter Trial. Ann Surg. 2007 Numb 2;246:207-14.

[140] Matthiessen P, Strand I, Jansson K, TÃ¶rnquist C, Andersson M, RutegÃ¥rd Jr, et al. Is Early Detection of Anastomotic Leakage Possible by Intraperitoneal Microdialysis and Intraperitoneal Cytokines After Anterior Resection of the Rectum for Cancer? Dis Colon Rectum. 2007;50(11):1918-27.

[141] CMA-Microdialysis. [Feb 2012]; Available from: www.microdialysis.se/.

[142] Seo JH, Leow PL, Cho SH, Lim HW, Kim JY, Patel BA, et al. Development of inlaid electrodes for whole column electrochemical detection in HPLC. Lab on a Chip - Miniaturisation for Chemistry and Biology. 2009;9(15):2238-44.

[143] Wang M, Roman GT, Perry ML, Kennedy RT. Microfluidic chip for high efficiency electrophoretic analysis of segmented flow from a microdialysis probe and in vivo chemical monitoring. Analytical Chemistry. 2009;81(21):9072-8.

[144] Wang M, Slaney T, Mabrouk O, Kennedy RT. Collection of nanoliter microdialysate fractions in plugs for off-line in vivo chemical monitoring with up to 2s temporal resolution. Journal of Neuroscience Methods. 2010;190(1):39-48.

[145] Chaurasia C, Müller M, Bashaw E, Benfeldt E, Bolinder J, Bullock R, et al. AAPS-FDA workshop white paper: Microdialysis principles, application, and regulatory perspectives report from the Joint AAPS-FDA Workshop, November 4–5, 2005, Nashville, TN. The AAPS Journal. 2007;9(1):E48-E59.

[146] Müller M. Microdialysis. British Medical Journal. 2002; 324:588–91.

[147] Baldini F. Microdialysis-based sensing in clinical applications. Analytical and Bioanalytical Chemistry. 2010;397(3):909-16.

[148] Blazkiewicz P, Blazkiewicz K, Verhaege A, Anissimov YG, Roberts MS, Zvyagin AV. Dialysis-assited fiber optic spectroscopy for in situ biomedical sensing. Journal of Biomedical Optics. 2006;11(1).

[149] Pasic A, Koehler H, Klimant I, Schaupp L. Miniaturized fiber-optic hybrid sensor for continuous glucose monitoring in subcutaneous tissue. Sensors and Actuators, B: Chemical. 2007;122(1):60-8.

[150] Zahn JD, Trebotich D, Liepmann D. Microdialysis microneedles for continuous medical monitoring. Biomedical Microdevices. 2005;7(1):59-69.

[151] Böhm S, Olthuis W, Bergveld P. Micromachined double lumen microdialysis probe connector with incorporated sensor for on-line sampling. Sensors and Actuators, B: Chemical. 2000;63(3):201-8.

[152] Pasic A, Koehler H, Schaupp L, Pieber TR, Klimant I. Fiber-optic flow-through sensor for online monitoring of glucose. Analytical and Bioanalytical Chemistry. 2006;386(5):1293-302.

[153] Ricci F, Caprio F, Poscia A, Valgimigli F, Messeri D, Lepori E, et al. Toward continuous glucose monitoring with planar modified biosensors and microdialysis: Study of temperature, oxygen dependence and in vivo experiment. Biosensors and Bioelectronics. 2007;22(9–10):2032-9.

[154] Gramsbergen JB, Cumming P. Serotonin mediates rapid changes of striatal glucose and lactate metabolism after systemic 3,4-methylenedioxymethamphetamine (MDMA, "Ecstasy") administration in awake rats. Neurochemistry International. 2007;51(1):8-15.

[155] Yao T, Okano G. Simultaneous determination of L-glutamate, acetylcholine and dopamine in rat brain by a flow-injection biosensor system with microdialysis sampling. Analytical Sciences. 2008;24(11):1469-73.

[156] Rhemrev-Boom RM, Tiessen RG, Jonker AA, Venema K, Vadgama P, Korf J. A lightweight measuring device for the continuous in vivo monitoring of glucose by means of ultraslow microdialysis in combination with a miniaturised flow-through biosensor. Clinica Chimica Acta. [doi: 10.1016/S0009-8981(01)00574-5]. 2002;316(1–2):1-10.

[157] Córcoles EP, Deeba S, Hanna GB, Paraskeva P, Boutelle MG, Darzi A. Use of online rapid sampling microdialysis electrochemical biosensor for bowel anastomosis monitoring in swine model. Analytical Methods. 2011;3(9):2010-6.

[158] Deeba S, Corcoles EP, Hanna BG, Pareskevas P, Aziz O, Boutelle MG, et al. Use of rapid sampling microdialysis for intraoperative monitoring of bowel ischemia. Diseases of the Colon and Rectum. 2008;51(9):1408-13.

[159] Córcoles EP, Deeba S, Hanna GB, Paraskeva P, Boutelle MG, Darzi A, editors. Bowel ischemia monitoring using rapid sampling microdialysis biosensor system2011.

[160] Corcoles EP, Deeba S, Damji S, Hanna GB, Boutelle MG, Cheshire N, et al. Rapid sampling microdialysis monitorign of post aortic repair intestinal ischemia. J Gastroenterol Hepatol. [Meeting Abstract]. 2011 Oct;26:192-3.

[161] Chen Cf, Drew KL. Droplet-based microdialysis-Concept, theory, and design considerations. Journal of Chromatography A. 2008;1209(1-2):29-36.

[162] Tseng YT, Yang CS, Tseng FG. A perfusion-based micro opto-fluidic system (PMOFS) for continuously in-situ immune sensing. Lab on a Chip - Miniaturisation for Chemistry and Biology. 2009;9(18):2673-82.

[163] Malecha K, Pijanowska DG, Golonka LJ, Kurek P. Low temperature co-fired ceramic (LTCC)-based biosensor for continuous glucose monitoring. Sensors and Actuators, B: Chemical. 2011;155(2):923-9.

[164] Rogers M, Leong C, Niu X, De Mello A, Parker KH, Boutelle MG. Optimisation of a microfluidic analysis chamber for the placement of microelectrodes. Physical Chemistry Chemical Physics. 2011;13(12):5298-303.

[165] Nordström CH. Lessons we have learnt from microdialysis in animals and humans Anaesthesia, Pain, Intensive Care and Emergency Medicine — A.P.I.C.E. 2005:125-38.

[166] Nordström CH, Ungerstedt U. Microdialysis: principles and techniques Anaesthesia, Pain, Intensive Care and Emergency A.P.I.C.E. 2006:61-77.

[167] Ungerstedt U. Continuous Monitoring of Organ Chemistry — a Paradigm Shift in Management of Intensive Care Anaesthesia, Pain, Intensive Care and Emergency A.P.I.C.E. 2008:29-44.

[168] Microbiotech. [Feb 2012]; Available from: www.microbiotech.se/.

[169] Brainlink. [cited Feb 2012]; Available from: www.brainlink.nl

Chapter 11

Challenges in the Diagnosis of Sepsis of the Neonate

Bernhard Resch, Nora Hofer and Wilhelm Müller

Additional information is available at the end of the chapter

http://dx.doi.org/10.5772/50184

1. Introduction

Despite the advances in neonatal care early onset neonatal sepsis remains a serious and potentially life-threatening disease with a mortality rate ranging from 1.5% in term to almost 40% in very low birth weight infants. [1,2] The signs and symptoms of neonatal sepsis may be subtle and nonspecific being clinically indistinguishable from various noninfectious conditions such as respiratory distress syndrome or maladaptation. The current practice of starting empirical antibiotic therapy in all neonates showing infection-like symptoms results in their exposure to adverse drug effects, nosocomial complications, and in the emergence of resistant strains. [3] Accurate and quick diagnosis is therefore essential for both protecting the infant from the consequences of the bacterial invasion and preventing damages deriving from the unnecessary use of antibiotics.

During the last decades efforts have been made to improve the laboratory diagnosis of neonatal sepsis by studying a large variety of inflammatory markers with diverse success. Some, like procalcitonin (PCT) and interleukins, especially interleukin-6 (IL-6), have demonstrated their benefit in clinical practice and are more and more implemented in neonatal wards and neonatal intensive care units. Others, like cell surface markers, show promising results in the research setting but in the clinical everyday practice their use is hindered by the need for sophisticated equipment, trained laboratory staff, and for rapid sample processing that cannot be delayed.

In this review we aim to give a comprehensive overview on laboratory parameters and microbiological techniques for the diagnosis of sepsis in the neonate.

2. Clinical signs of bacterial infection in the neonate

One of the most recent studies on clinical signs associated with neonatal sepsis was published by Modi et al. [4] in 2009 utilizing data from 26 UK neonatal units. The population prevalence of 12 predefined clinical signs of infection captured daily for 28 days including the acute onset of increased oxygen requirement or ventilatory support, increase in apnoea/bradycardia, hypotension, glucose intolerance, impaired peripheral perfusion (capillary refill time >3 s/ pallor/ mottling/ core-peripheral temperature gap >2°C), lethargy/ irritability/ poor handling, temperature instability, ileus/ onset of feed intolerance, increase in serum bilirubin, fall in urine output, metabolic acidosis/base deficit <−10 mmol/l, and anticonvulsant therapy was evaluated. Three or more clinical signs had the best predictive accuracy for a positive blood culture with 76.2% specificity, and 61.5%, 46.9% and 78.2% sensitivity for all positive cultures, cultures yielding coagulase-negative staphylococci, or a recognised pathogen, respectively.

A more simplified but nevertheless widely used approach is to focus on the presence of three or more of the following categories of clinical signs [5]: apnoea/tachypnoea (>60/ min)/nasal flaring/retractions/cyanosis/respiratory distress; bradycardia (<100/ min) or tachycardia (>180/min); hypotonia or seizures; poor skin colour or capillary refilling time >2 seconds; irritability or lethargy. Together with historical factors associated with increased risk for infection including premature rupture of the membranes (PROM) (in term infants >18 hours), maternal fever during labour, and intraamniotic infection/ chorioamnionitis and two or more abnormal values of the so-called sepsis screen (white blood cell count, absolute neutrophil count, immature to total neutrophil – IT – ratio and CRP) findings are supportive of a diagnosis of bacterial infection of the neonate.

A recent review of criteria used for the classification of neonatal sepsis found a high disparity with exact specification in only a quarter of studies [6]. This inconsistency makes comparisons difficult and meta-analysis hardly possible. In 2002 the International Pediatric Sepsis Consensus Conference was held with the aim to create clear definitions for the systemic inflammatory response syndrome (SIRS) and different stages of sepsis for children adaptable for different age groups, ranging from term neonates to adolescents. The definitions should help researchers by creating standardized entry criteria for clinical trials and, thus, making studies comparable [7] following the successful and quickly applied definitions for adults from the American College of Chest Physicians/Society of Critical Care Medicine published in 1992. [8,9] SIRS was diagnosed when at least two of the following four criteria were positive (a or b obligatory): a) core temperature >38.5 °C or <36.0 °C; b) white blood cell count elevated or depressed [10], or >10% immature neutrophils; c) tachycardia >180/min or bradycardia <100/min over a >0.5 hour period without external stimulus or drug therapy; d) tachypnea >60/min or mechanical ventilation for an acute process. Sepsis was defined as SIRS in the presence of or as a result of proven or suspected infection.

The definitions of SIRS and sepsis correlated insufficiently with the diagnosis of culture proven early-onset sepsis, especially in term newborns, in a retrospective cohort study including all newborns with hospitalization within the first 72 hours of life and infants with episodes of suspected late-onset sepsis at our centre between 2004 and 2008. [11] In this age group the criteria showed low sensitivity and low predictive value. Postnatal rather than gestational age seemed to positively influence the correlation with culture proven infections demonstrating a good correlation with late-onset sepsis independent on the gestational age at onset.

In 32 neonates with blood culture proven early-onset bacterial infection using the definition of SIRS two thirds of term newborns and one third of preterm newborns would have been missed in the diagnosis of culture proven bacterial infection. [11] Sensitivity, specificity, positive and negative predictive value of either culture or clinical positive sepsis is shown in table 1. [11,12]

	Weeks Gestational Age				
	Total	**<28**	**28-32**	**33-37**	**>37**
Culture proven early-onset bacterial infection					
Sensitivity	50 (32-68)	67 (30-93)	67 (22-96)	50 (7-93)	31 (9-61)
Specificity	80 (76-84)	66 (46-82)	68 (60-76)	84 (77-89)	90 (84-94)
PPV	15 (9-23)	38 (15-65)	9 (2-20)	7 (1-24)	20 (6-44)
NPV	96 (94-98)	86 (65-97)	98 (93-100)	98 (95-100)	94 (89-97)
Culture proven and clinical early-onset bacterial infection					
Sensitivity	66 (59-74)	77 (56-91)	85 (71-94)	63 (46-78)	48 (34-62)
Specificity	80 (76-84)	66 (46-82)	68 (60-76)	84 (77-89)	90 (84-94)
PPV	54 (47-61)	67 (47-83)	48 (36-59)	49 (34-64)	62 (46-76)
NPV	87 (84-90)	76 (55-91)	93 (86-97)	90 (84-95)	84 (77-89)

Abbreviations: SIRS, systemic inflammatory response syndrome; PPV, positive predictive value; NPV, negative predictive value

Table 1. Sensitivity, specificity, positive and negative predictive value (95% confidence interval) of the definitions of SIRS in the diagnosis of culture proven and clinical early-onset bacterial infection according to different gestational ages (11,12).

In a retrospective cohort study set in our level III neonatal intensive care unit, we aimed to evaluate the role of fever, hypothermia, and temperature instability in term and preterm newborns during the first three days of life and to identify risk factors for early onset sepsis among newborns presenting with these temperature symptoms. [13] Between 2004 and 2007 we included 851 newborns of whom 127 (15%) presented with temperature symptoms during the first three days of life. Sixty-nine (8% of the total cohort) of them had fever (rectal temperature >38.5 °C), 69 (8%) had hypothermia (rectal temperature <36.0 °C), and 55 (6%) had temperature instability, defined as an increase or decrease of rectal temperature of >1.5 °C within three hours. Fourteen of the 127 newborns presenting with temperature symptoms had culture proven early-onset sepsis/pneumonia (33% of all 42 newborns with culture proven sepsis/pneumonia), 67 had clinical sepsis (30% of all 209 newborns with clinical sepsis) and 46 were diagnosed as being sepsis negative (8% of all 600 sepsis negatives). Factors associated with culture proven sepsis/pneumonia in newborns presenting with temperature symptoms were maternal fever (p=.009), chorioamnionitis (p<.001), antibiotic therapy of the mother (p=.04), poor skin colour (p=.001) and syndrome of persistent fetal circulation (p=.01). Thus, every seventh newborn hospitalized at our neonatal intensive care unit developed fever, hypothermia and/or temperature instability during the first three days of life. Two thirds of them had culture proven or clinical sepsis. Despite low sensitivity temperature symptoms were highly specific for bacterial infection in preterm and term newborns.

3. Gold standard blood culture

The isolation of an organism confers many advantages, including the optimal choice and duration of antibiotic treatment. [14] Blood cultures are still the gold standard in the diagnosis of neonatal sepsis. However, obtaining cultures from neonates can be difficult as sample volumes are small and a substantial number of cultures turn out to be contaminated or negative. [15] The minimum volume required for a reliable culture result has been estimated as 1.0 ml. [14] In clinical practice samples often contain less; in a prospective study of 298 sets of blood cultures from critically ill neonates 55% of aerobic culture vessels contained not as much as 0.5 ml of blood. [14] False negative results may arise from insufficient or missing living bacteria in the sample resulting from low specimen volume, only transient bacteremia, or administration of antibiotics prior to sampling including administration of intrapartum antibiotics to the mother. The microbiological results are not available until 24 to 48 hours after sampling and thus have no influence on the initial choice on whether to initiate or withhold antibiotic therapy. Furthermore, obtaining adequate samples from premature infants can be challenging in view of the concerns about blood volume depletion in these infants. Therefore, we are challenged to think beyond the current paradigm of basing sepsis diagnosis in neonates entirely on blood culture results.

4. Polymerase chain reaction and hybridization methods in the detection of bacterial genomes

More recently, an increasing number of reports on the use of molecular methods including polymerase chain reaction (PCR) and hybridization methods in the detection of bacterial genomes in blood samples have appeared. Molecular assays have the advantage of direct pathogen detection in a more rapid turnover time compared to blood cultures with results being available within a few hours. The sensitivity of molecular methods in the diagnosis of sepsis may be higher compared to blood cultures and ranges from 41 to 100% with the majority of studies reporting values between 90 and 100%, with a specificity ranging from 78 to 100%. [16] Molecular assays might eventually replace blood cultures, but will continue as a supplement to blood cultures until they are adequately evaluated. [16] Microarray hybridization and next-generation sequencing techniques can lead not only to rapid identification of organisms, but also to evaluation of organism characteristics such as virulence and antibiotic susceptibility. Another exciting prospect is the ability to quantify bacterial loads (analogous to viral loads), which can then be followed during therapy to assess response. [16]

5. White blood cell count

In a recent paper Murphy and Weiner [17] reported on 100% sensitivity and 100% negative predictive value of two normal white blood cell counts (WBC) within 8 to 12 hours and a negative blood culture at 24 hours for ruling out early-onset sepsis in the neonate. A normal WBC was defined as values between 6.000 and 30.000 per μL, and an IT-ratio as less than

0.2. The strength of the study was the high number of 3213 patients included that retrospectively was identified by an electronic database over a 10 years time period. Data revealed an overall low culture proven sepsis rate of 0.73%. Nevertheless, we would argue not to solely rely on these negative results besides the neonate is asymptomatic.

By means of a retrospective cohort analysis of preterm and term neonates admitted to our NICU between 2004 and 2007, including 737 of a total of 1301 neonates who had at least one WBC count determination during the first 72 hours of life, we sought to proof the usefulness of leukocyte counts in the evaluation of early-onset sepsis. [18] WBC counts were done in 1 to 9 times per case (mean 1.65). Median gestational age was 34 weeks and median birth weight 2137 grams, and preterm to term born ratio was 236 (32%) to 501 (68%). Culture proven EOS was diagnosed in 39 neonates (5.3%), and pathogens yielded Group B streptococci in 51%, Ureaplasma urealyticum in 26%, Escherichia coli in 10%, Staphylococcus aureus in 5%, and single cases with Enterococci (3%), Chlamydia (3%), and Klebsiella (3%) infection. Defining normal WBC counts between 9.000 and 34.000 per µl revealed 39% of cases with culture proven EOS having abnormal values. By a second approach defining normal WBC counts between 8.500 and 21.500 per µl calculated using the Youden index (0.29 for optimal cut-off values, sensitivity 64% and specificity 66%) data revealed 59% of cases having abnormal values. Sensitivity of WBC counts decreased from 0 - 24 hours to 48 - 72 hours of age. The IT-ratio showed sensitivity, specificity, positive predictive and negative predictive value (95% confidence interval) of 14 (5-29), 97 (95-99), 36 (13-65), and 92 (89-94) percent, respectively.

Measurement of immature neutrophil granulocytes has been considered to be a helpful early indicator of various infectious conditions [19,20] and has a long clinical tradition in the diagnosis of bacterial sepsis in neonates. [21] The detection of immature granulocytes (IGs) by microscopic count necessitates experienced laboratory staff; furthermore morphological classification of IGs are subject to a considerable reader bias and interpretative errors; especially in neonates, when leucocytosis occurs frequently during the first days of life, this method seems to provide only limited reproducibility. [22,23] Contrariwise in performing a standard 100-cell manual differential small numbers of IG can often be overlooked in samples of leukopenic patients. Hence, automated measurement of IG counts could represent a reliable and utile method in the prediction of bacterial infection in neonates. Automated hematology analyzers enable a fast, accurate and less-labor intensive method for the detection of IGs and could improve screening and monitoring for neonatal septicemia. [24-26] The detection limit of IGs has been described to be 0.1% which is considerably lower than in a manual smear. The assessment of a complete blood count with white blood cell differential is usually performed as a routine method to evaluate newborns at risk; the automated simultaneous enumeration of IGs provides additional information without the need of further costs and blood sampling, which might be of special importance in preterm babies.

The Sysmex XE-2100 [27] - a multiparameter automated hematology analyzer - offers the possibility to detect IGs including metamyelocytes, myelocytes, and promyelocytes by the measurement of white blood cell differential counts by flow cytometry in the DIFF-channel. In a separate channel, called the IMI-channel not only IGs, but also bands, blasts, and hematopoietic progenitor cells are detected. The reaction principle is based on differences in membrane composition between mature and immature cells. The superiority of the flow cytometric IG count performed by the Sysmex XE-2100 compared to the manual morphology count as a reference method for IG counting has been demonstrated in several studies. [25,28]

To determine the predictive value of the immature granulocyte number and the immature myeloid information in neonatal early-onset sepsis we examined 133 blood samples of patients admitted to our neonatal intensive care unit. [29] The number of immature granulocytes and the immature myeloid information were significantly elevated in 21 neonates with early-onset sepsis compared to 112 controls (median 0.28 vs. 0.05 x 109/L, $p=0.049$ and 639 vs. 89, $p<0.0001$, respectively).

6. C-reactive protein

CRP is one of the most widely available; most studied, and most used laboratory tests for neonatal bacterial infection. It is well known that it provides limited sensitivity when determined during the early phases of the disease, especially at the initial presentation, but provides very high negative predictive values and is thus useful for identifying infants unlikely to be infected or monitoring the response to treatment. [30-33] However, the current literature provides a growing body of evidence suggesting the so far reported characteristics of CRP may not be as suitable for the use in preterm as in term newborns. [34-36] Furthermore, the use of CRP in neonatal sepsis is complicated by a nonspecific rise that starts shortly after birth. [37,38]

Any elevation of serum CRP in the neonate always represents endogenous synthesis, since it passes the placenta in exceedingly low quantities. [39] De novo hepatic synthesis starts very rapidly after a single stimulus with serum concentrations rising above 5 mg/l by about 6 hours and peaking around 48 hours. [40]

For the diagnosis of early onset sepsis in clinical practice the sensitivity is more important compared to the specificity, as the consequences of unnecessarily treating an uninfected infant bear fewer complications than not treating an infected child. Up to date the most used cut-off value is 10 mg/l irrespective of the gestational and postnatal age of the neonate. In view of the physiologic dynamics of CRP during the first days after birth and the influence of gestational age on its response to infection, it appears reasonable to reconsider this static cut-off value and evaluate the possible advantages of the introduction of dynamic reference values. [41] However, the current literature lacks sufficient evidence to make recommendations for the use in clinical practice. CRP reaches the best diagnostic accuracy when combined to another infection marker that compensates for its diagnostic weakness and provides reliable sensitivity during the early phases of sepsis. Suitable markers include but are not limited to PCT, IL-6, and IL-8. Many further parameters may provide similar good results but are not yet sufficiently examined to be applied to clinical practice. CRP is particularly useful for monitoring the response to treatment and for ruling out an infection: A repeated determination of CRP 24 to 48 hours after the initiation of antibiotic therapy has been reported to carry a 99% negative predictive value in accurately identifying uninfected neonates though nothing replaces the clinical impression. CRP values undergo a physiological 3-day-rise after birth. [37,38] This physiologic dynamics as well as certain maternal and perinatal factors may affect interpretation of what constitutes "normal" CRP values in healthy neonates. Furthermore, some reports suggest non-infectious confounders such as meconium aspiration syndrome and perinatal maternal risk conditions may significantly elevate CRP values in symptomatic or at risk neonates and thus confound interpretation of CRP values in the diagnosis of sepsis. [34]

7. Inflammatory cytokines and other inflammatory indices

Sepsis is a pathogen initiated but a cytokine-mediated condition in which immune, inflammatory, and coagulation homeostasis is disturbed. [42] After contact to bacterial antigens inflammatory cytokines and growth factors, and their secondary mediators, which include nitric oxide, thromboxanes, leukotrienes, platelet-activating factor, prostaglandins, and complement, cause activation of the coagulation cascade, the complement cascade, as well as the production of acute-phase reactants. The amount of mediators involved in the inflammatory response to bacterial invasion represents additional opportunity for further improving the diagnosis of sepsis, provided that the right parameter is determined by the right technique at the right time. In fact, each parameter, e.g. acute phase reactants, chemokines and cytokines, has distinct characteristics and a different set of indications and restrictions when applied to different types of infections or even different phases of the infective process.

In 2003 a systematic review of modern diagnostic tests for neonatal sepsis [43] highlighted the following problems by use or recommendation of certain parameters: 1) the cut-off laboratory values that were chosen to distinguish between the presence and absence of infection appear to be unique to each study making any comparisons difficult, 2) the range of test sensitivity and specificity, both calculated and reported, was large, and sensitivities ranged from 57% to 100%, specificities from 43% to 100%, and, similarly, positive likelihood ratios from 1.5 to ∞, 3) the authors also assessed the accuracy of combinations of tests (evaluated in 3 studies) and none of these test combinations had a positive likelihood ratio of more than 10.

Focussing on the early detection of neonatal early-onset sepsis we studied the reliability of procalcitonin (PCT) and interleukin-6 (IL-6) compared with CRP and IT-ratio - used as routine parameter for the diagnosis of bacterial infection - at the age of the first 12 hours of life. [5] In this age-group PCT showed the highest sensitivity followed by CRP, IL-6, and IT-ratio when using ROC analysis with the Youden´s index for optimal cut-off values. The combination of the diagnostic tests revealed the best results for the prediction of bacterial infection within 12 hours of age. The combination of PCT and IL-6 yielded a sensitivity of 89%, a specificity of 91%, a positive predictive value of 94% and a negative predictive value of 84%, the combination of CRP and IT-ratio a sensitivity of 82%, a specificity of 96%, a positive predictive value of 97% and a negative predictive value of 78%. Differences were not significant. The single test results are shown in figure 1 – 4, and the ROC-analysis of all four inflammatory indices is shown in figure 5.

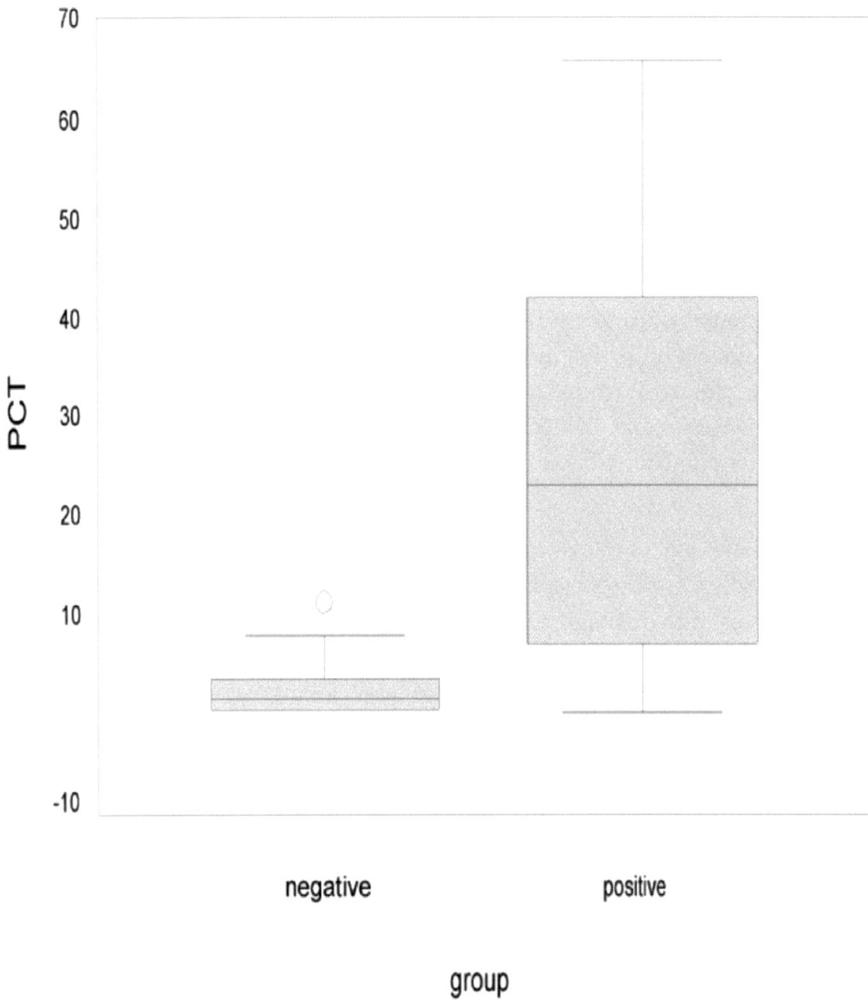

Figure 1. Procalcitonin values (ng/L) of 41 neonates with blood culture positive and clinical early-onset sepsis compared with 27 neonates without sepsis within 12 hours of life (p<0,001).

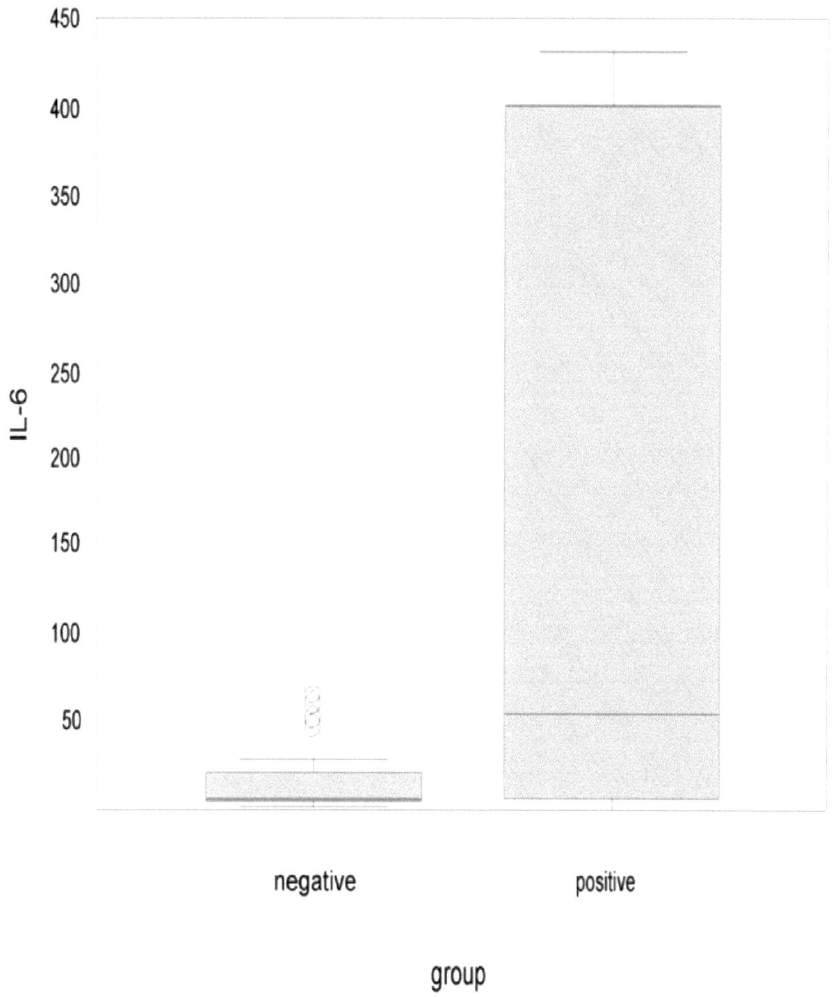

Figure 2. Interleukin-6 values (pg/L) of 41 neonates with blood culture positive and clinical early-onset sepsis compared with 27 neonates without sepsis within 12 hours of life (p<0,001). (5)

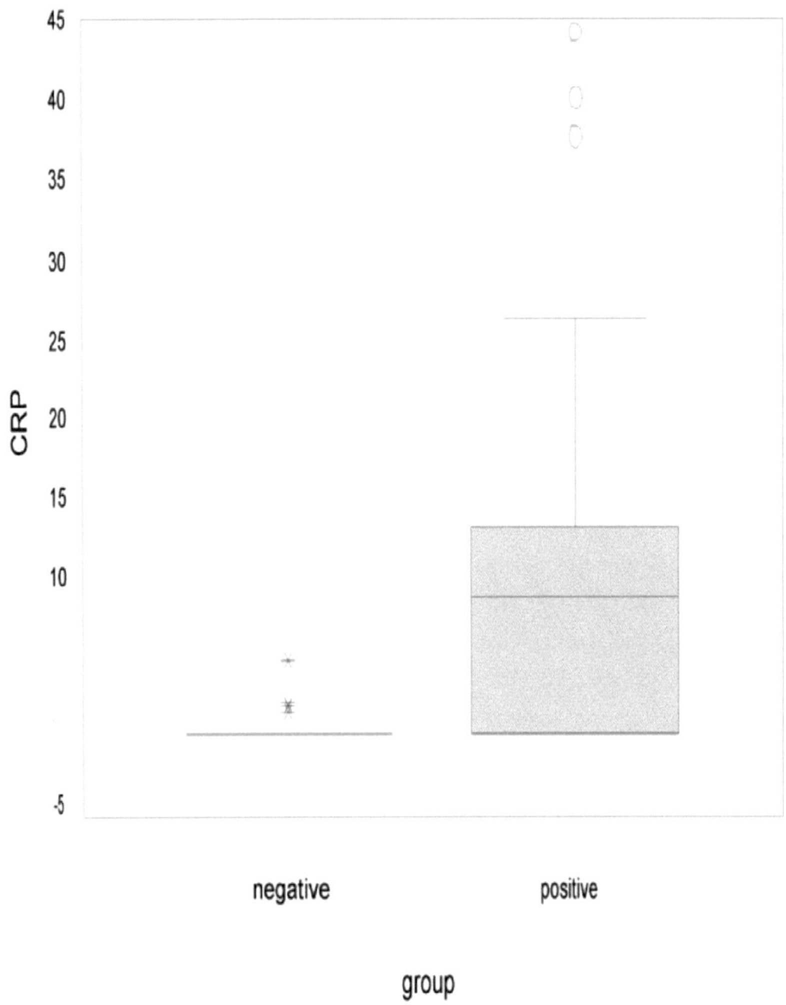

Figure 3. C-reactive protein values (mg/L) of 41 neonates with blood culture positive and clinical early-onset sepsis compared with 27 neonates without sepsis within 12 hours of life (p<0,001). (5)

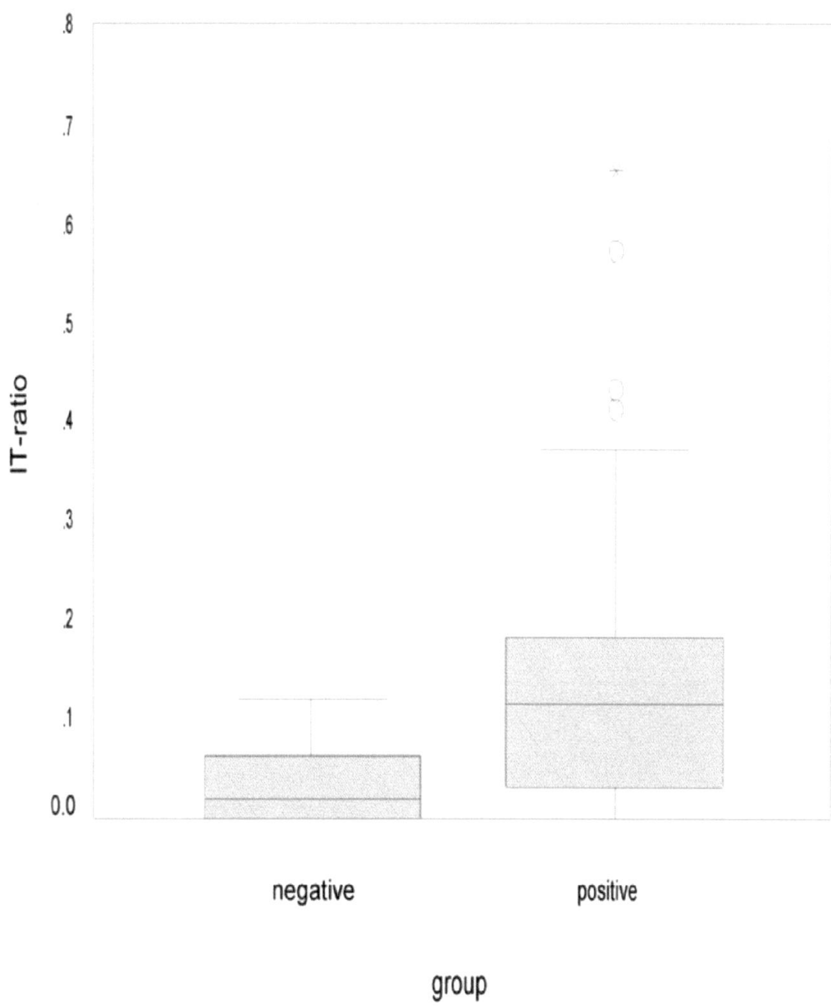

Figure 4. Immature-to-total neutrophil ratio values of 41 neonates with blood culture positive and clinical early-onset sepsis compared with 27 neonates without sepsis within 12 hours of life (p<0,001). (5)

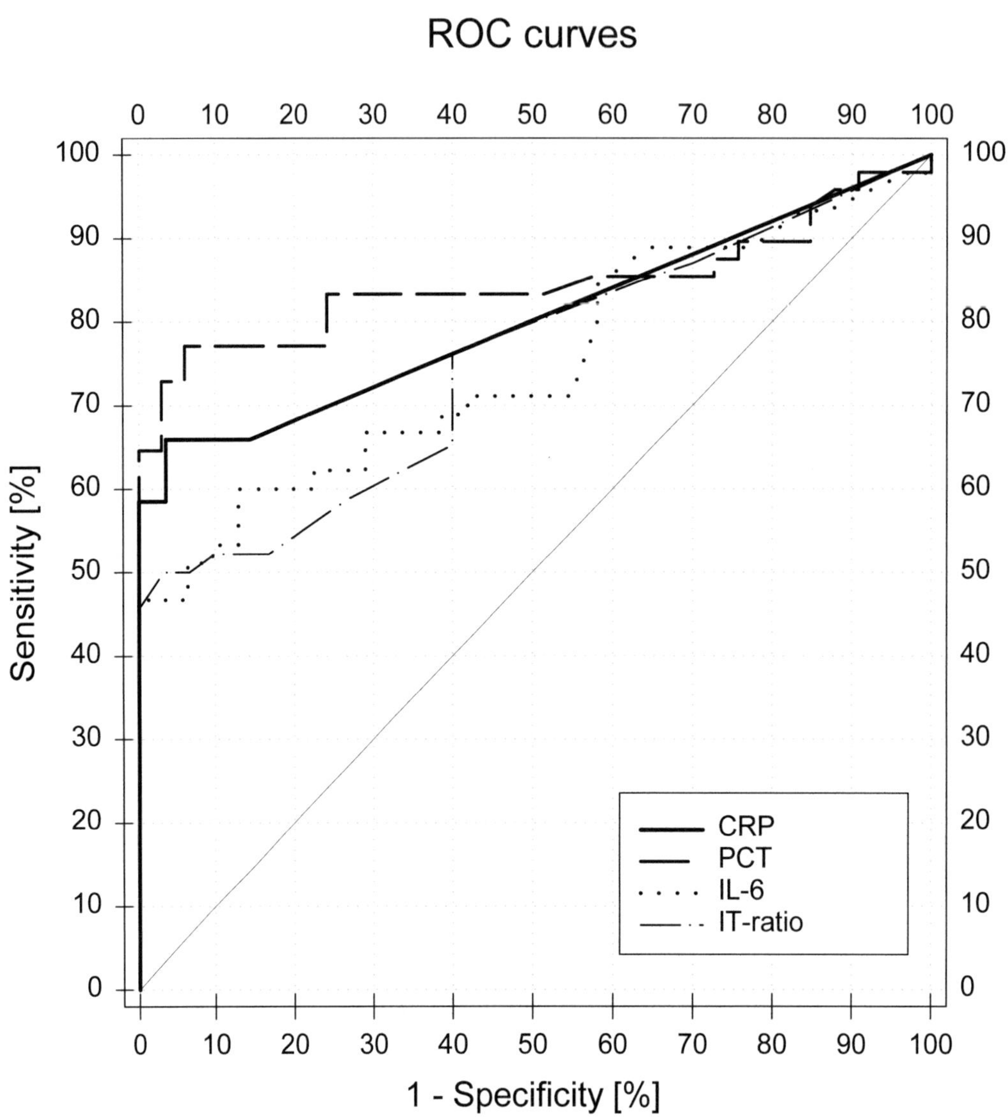

CRP = C-reactive protein, PCT = procalcitonin, IL-6 = interleukin-6, IT-ratio = immature- to-total neutrophil ratio

Figure 5. Receiver operating characteristic curves for values of Procalcitonin, Interleukin-6, CRP, and IT-ratio in 76 neonates within 12 hours of life. Area under the curve was 0,845 (CI 95% 0,741 – 0,949) for PCT; 0,763 (CI 95% 0,641 – 0,884) for IL-6; 0,812 (CI 95% 0,702 – 0,922) for CRP; and 0,770 (CI 95% 0,651 – 0,890) for IT-ratio. Differences were not significant. (5)

Vouloumanou et al. [44] recently analyzed 16 studies (involving 1,959 neonates and including our above mentioned study) that evaluated PCT in neonates with culture proven or clinically diagnosed sepsis in comparison with ill neonates with other conditions. The pooled (95% confidence interval) sensitivity and specificity were 81% (74–87%) and 79% (69–87%), respectively. The area under the ROC curve (AUC) was 0.87. The diagnostic accuracy of PCT seemed higher for neonates with late-onset sepsis (>72 h of life) than for those with early onset sepsis; the AUC for these analyses was 0.95 and 0.78, respectively. However, fewer data were available for late-onset sepsis. High statistical heterogeneity was observed for all analyses. In view of the marked observed statistical heterogeneity, along with the lack of a uniform definition for neonatal sepsis, the authors stated that interpretation of these findings should be done with appropriate caution.

8. Conclusions

At the moment none of the described current diagnostic markers are sensitive and specific enough to influence the judgment whether or not to withhold antimicrobial treatment independent of the clinical findings. Efforts were done to improve diagnostic accuracy by combining multiple markers in order to further enhance the diagnostic accuracy of these mediators in identifying infected neonates. Due to many physiologic changes of inflammatory parameters in the neonatal period and considering the differences between preterm and term infants diagnosis of bacterial infection might better be based on dynamic than static cut-off values during the first 48 to 72 hours of age.

Author details

Bernhard Resch* and Nora Hofer
Research Unit for Neonatal Infectious Diseases and Epidemiology,
Medical University of Graz, Austria

Bernhard Resch and Wilhelm Müller
Division of Neonatology, Department of Pediatric, Medical University of Graz, Austria

9. References

[1] Weston EJ, Pondo T, Lewis MM, Martell-Cleary P, Morin C, Jewell B, Daily P, Apostol M, Petit S, Farley M, Lynfield R, Reingold A, Hansen NI, Stoll BJ, Shane AJ, Zell E, Schrag SJ (2011) The Burden of Invasive Early-onset Neonatal Sepsis in the United States, 2005-2008. Pediatr. Infect. Dis. J. 30:937–941.

[2] Fanaroff AA, Stoll BJ, Wright LL, Carlo WA, Ehrenkranz RA, Stark AR, Bauer CR, Donovan EF, Korones SB, Laptook AR, Lemons JA, Oh W, Papile LA, Shankaran S, Stevenson DK, Tyson JE, Poole WK; NICHD Neonatal Research Network (2007 Trends

* Corresponding Author

in neonatal morbidity and mortality for very low birthweight infants. Am. J. Obstet. Gynecol. 196:147.e1–8.

[3] Murray BE (1994) Can antibiotic resistance be controlled? N. Engl. J. Med. 330:1229–1230.

[4] Modi N, Doré CJ, Saraswatula A, Richards M, Bamford KB, Coello R, Holmes A (2009) A case definition for national and international neonatal bloodstream infection surveillance. Arch. Dis. Child. Fetal Neonatal Ed. 94:F8-12.

[5] Resch B, Gusenleitner W, Müller WD (2003) Procalcitonin and interleukin-6 in the diagnosis of early-onset sepsis of the neonate. Acta Paediatr. 92:243-245.

[6] Reyna-Figueroa J, Yuri-Toala E, Ortiz-Ibarra FJ, Rodríguez-Ramírez E, Limón-Rojas AE (2006) Disparity in the criteria for including patients with neonatal sepsis in scientific medical studies. Are we swimming in a sea without limits? An. Pediatr. (Barc) 65:536-540.

[7] Goldstein B, Giroir B, Randolph A (2005) International pediatric sepsis consensus conference: definitions for sepsis and organ dysfunction in pediatrics. Pediatr. Crit. Care Med. 6:2-8.

[8] American College of Chest Physicians/Society of Critical Care Medicine Consensus Conference: definitions for sepsis and organ failure and guidelines for the use of innovative therapies in sepsis (1992) Crit. Care Med. 20: 864-874.

[9] Trzeciak S, Zanotti-Cavazzoni S, Parrillo JE, Dellinger RP (2005) Inclusion criteria for clinical trials in sepsis: did the American College of Chest Physicians/Society of Critical Care Medicine consensus conference definitions of sepsis have an impact? Chest. 127:242-245

[10] Letsky EA (1999) Haematological values in the newborn. In: Rennie JM, Roberton NRC. Textbook of Neonatology (Third edition). Edinburgh: Churchill Livingstone, p. 1399

[11] Hofer N, Müller W, Resch B (2010) Systemic inflammatory response syndrome (SIRS) definition and correlation with early-onset bacterial infection of the newborn. Arch. Dis. Child. Fetal Neonatal Ed. 95: F151.

[12] Hofer N, Müller W, Resch B (2012) Definitions of SIRS and sepsis in correlation with early and late onset neonatal sepsis. Journal of Pediatric Intensive Care. 1: in press.

[13] Hofer N, Müller W, Resch B (2012) The neonate presenting with temperature symptoms: Role in the diagnosis of early onset sepsis. Pediatr. Int. doi: 10.1111/j.1442-200X.2012.03570.x. [epub ahead]

[14] Neal PR, Kleiman MB, Reynolds JK, Allen SD, Lemons JA, Yu PL (1986) Volume of blood submitted for culture from neonates. J. Clin. Microbiol. 24:353–356.

[15] Escobar GJ (2005) What have we learned from observational studies on neonatal sepsis? Pediatr. Crit. Care Med. 6 (3 Suppl):S138–145.

[16] Venkatesh M, Flores A, Luna RA, Versalovic J (2010) Molecular microbiological methods in the diagnosis of neonatal sepsis. Expert Rev. Anti. Infect. Ther. 8:1037–1048.

[17] Murphy K, Weiner J (2012) Use of leukocyte counts in evaluation of early-onset neonatal sepsis. Pediatr. Infect. Dis. J. 31:1-4

[18] Resch B, Edlinger S, Müller W (2012) White blood cell counts in neonatal early-onset sepsis. Pediatr. Infect. Dis. J. 2012, in press.

[19] Rodwell RL, Leslie AL, Tudehope DI (1988) Early diagnosis of neonatal sepsis using a hematologic scoring system. J. Pediatr. 112:761-767.
[20] Buttarello M, Plebani M (2008) Automated blood cell counts: state of the art. Am. J. Clin. Pathol. 130:104-116.
[21] Akenzua GI, Hui YT, Milner R, Zipursky A (1974) Neutrophil and band counts in the diagnosis of neonatal infections. Pediatrics. 54:38-42.
[22] Chiesa C, Panero A, Osborn JF, Simonetti AF, Pacifico L (2004) Diagnosis of neonatal sepsis: a clinical and laboratory challenge. Clin Chem. 50:279-287.
[23] Schelonka RL, Yoder BA, Hall RB, Trippett TM, Louder DS, Hickman JR, Guerra CG (1995) Differentiation of segmented and band neutrophils during the early newborn period. J Pediatr. 127:298-300.
[24] Briggs C, Harrison P, Grant D, Staves J, MacHin SJ (2000) New quantitative parameters on a recently introduced automated blood cell counter--the XE 2100. Clin Lab Haematol. 22:345-50.
[25] Fernandes B, Hamaguchi Y (2007) Automated Enumeration of Immature Granulocytes. Am. J. Clin. Pathol. 128:454-463.
[26] Nigro KG, O'Riordan M, Molloy EJ, Walsh MC, Sandhaus LM (2005) Performance of an automated immature granulocyte count as a predictor of neonatal sepsis. Am. J. Clin. Pathol. 123:618-624.
[27] Sysmex Corporation (2005) Operators Manual Sysmex XE-2100.
[28] Ansari-Lari MA, Kickler TS, Borowitz MJ (2003) Immature Granulocyte Measurement Using the Sysmex XE-2100 Relationship to Infection and Sepsis. Am. J. Clin. Pathol. 120:795-799.
[29] Cimenti C, Erwa W, Kurt R. Herkner KR, Kasper DC, Müller W, Resch B (2012) The predictive value of immature granulocytes and immature myeloid information in the diagnosis of neonatal sepsis. Clin. Chem. Lab. Med. 2012, in press.
[30] Jaye DL, Waites KB (1997) Clinical applications of C-reactive protein in pediatrics. Pediatr. Infect. Dis. J. 16:735–746
[31] Hengst JM (2003) The role of C-reactive protein in the evaluation and management of infants with suspected sepsis. Adv. Neonatal Care. 3:3–13.
[32] Benitz WE, Han MY, Madan A, Ramachandra P (1998) Serial serum C-reactive protein levels in the diagnosis of neonatal infection. Pediatrics. 102:E41.
[33] Pourcyrous M, Bada HS, Korones SB, Baselski V, Wong SP (1993) Significance of serial C-reactive protein responses in neonatal infection and other disorders. Pediatrics. 92:431–435.
[34] Hofer N, Müller W, Resch B (2011) Non-infectious conditions and gestational age influence C-reactive protein values in newborns during the first 3 days of life. Clin. Chem. Lab. Med. 49:297–302.
[35] Turner MA, Power S, Emmerson AJB (2004) Gestational age and the C reactive protein response. Arch. Dis. Child. Fetal. Neonatal Ed. 89:F272–273.
[36] Doellner H, Arntzen KJ, Haereid PE, Aag S, Austgulen R (1998) Interleukin-6 concentrations in neonates evaluated for sepsis. J. Pediatr. 132:295–299.

[37] Chiesa C, Natale F, Pascone R, Osborn JF, Pacifico L, Bonci E, De Curtis M (2011) C reactive protein and procalcitonin: reference intervals for preterm and term newborns during the early neonatal period. Clin. Chim. Acta. 412:1053–1059.

[38] Chiesa C, Signore F, Assumma M, Buffone E, Tramontozzi P, Osborn JF, Pacifico L (2001) Serial measurements of C-reactive protein and interleukin-6 in the immediate postnatal period: reference intervals and analysis of maternal and perinatal confounders. Clin. Chem. 47:1016–1022.

[39] Kääpä P, Koistinen E (1993) Maternal and neonatal C-reactive protein after interventions during delivery. Acta Obstet. Gynecol. Scand. 72:543-546.

[40] Pepys MB, Hirschfield GM (2003) C-reactive protein: a critical update. J. Clin. Invest. 111:1805-1812.

[41] Hofer N, Zacharias E, Müller W, Resch B (2012) An update on the use of C-reactive protein in early-onset neonatal sepsis: current insights and new tasks. Neonatology. DOI: 10.1159/000336629, in press.

[42] Russell JA (2006) Management of sepsis. N. Engl. J. Med. 355:1699–713.

[43] Malik A, Hui CP, Pennie RA, Kirpalani H (2003) Beyond the complete blood cell count and C-reactive protein: a systematic review of modern diagnostic tests for neonatal sepsis. Arch. Pediatr. Adolesc. Med. 157:511-516.

[44] Vouloumanou EK, Plessa E, Karageorgopoulos DE, Mantadakis E, Falagas ME (2011) Serum procalcitonin as a diagnostic marker for neonatal sepsis: a systematic review and meta-analysis. Intensive Care Med. 37:747–762

Relevance of Procalcitonin for the Diagnosis of Early and Late-Onset Sepsis in Newborns

C. Savagner, B. Leboucher, G. Gascoin-Lachambre and C. Gras-Leguen

Additional information is available at the end of the chapter

http://dx.doi.org/10.5772/50168

1. Introduction

In hospital neonatology, bacterial infections represent significant mortality and morbidity [1-2]. Early diagnosis of bacterial infection in neonatal resuscitation is difficult but essential. Any delay in the initiation of antibiotic therapy is deleterious for prognosis. The lack of specific clinical signs, the elevation of deferred C-reactive protein (CRP) and the time necessary to obtain bacteriological results often delay the establishment of diagnosis. It is usually confirmed by bacteriological analysis of central samples, in particular by exploring blood culture. Recently, new markers of infection status have been proposed for their sensitivity and specificity [3-5]. CRP is currently the most frequent marker used for diagnosis and monitoring of infections in neonates. This is the marker presenting low sensitivity and specificity for initial diagnosis of NS. It rises about 24 hours after the infectious stimulus. Procalcitonin (PCT) is the prohormonal peptide of calcitonin, consisting of 116 amino acids. To date, the site of synthesis and the action of this new biomarker are still unknown. It takes place into extrathyroïdal tissue and its secretion is induced by bacterial endotoxins, with an important role in liver parenchyma [6]. Its increase serum level when bacterial infections have been demonstrated in 1992. These data were confirmed by a prospective pediatric study in 1993 and applied to neonatal monitoring since 1998 [7-12]. In neonatology, studies on the usefulness of PCT are controversial.

For adults, it is shown that in emergencies and general medicine, the PCT may allow a reduction of ABT prescriptions [13-16]. The PCT also helps reduce the indications complementary examinations [17] and durations of ATB in the ICU [18].

2. Diagnosis and management of neonatal sepsis

Bacterial infections can be a devastating complication for newborns and continue to be a significant cause of mortality and long-term morbidity for hospitalized newborns and premature infants [2, 19]. In the United States, the estimated annual incidence of severe sepsis in newborns is 0.3 per 100 live births. The estimated mortality for neonates with severe sepsis is 10.3%, with most deaths occurring within the first 48 hours of infection. Mortality rates vary by causative organisms. Data from the National Institute of Child Health and Human Development Neonatal Research Network reported mortality rates with gram-negative infections at 36% and 32% with fungal infections. Infected infants had significantly longer hospital stays, ongoing neurodevelopmental impairment, and higher mortality rates than very low birth weight infants who did not have late-onset sepsis. The diagnosis of neonatal sepsis is difficult to establish and remains a challenge for neonatal health care providers. Early signs and symptoms of neonatal sepsis are often nonspecific and easily confused with conditions that are expected in this population. The fear of missing a case of neonatal infection with its serious outcomes has led to overuse of antibiotics in the neonatal intensive care environment and the emergence of resistant organisms. Neonatal care providers have evaluated numerous tests searching for one that would be helpful for the diagnosis of NS with a rapid confirmation. Despite extensive investigation over the past decades, there is still no single test to be ideal for the early diagnosis of sepsis in newborns. In usual practice and research, investigations include blood culture and bacteriologic samples, hematological examinations, acute phase reactants (proteins CRP and PCT) and polymerase chain reaction [1]. In this article, we mainly study acute phase proteins, with a special interest for PCT. A recent study demonstrates that level of umbilical cord blood PCT is considered as a risk factor for mortality in very premature infants [20].

3. Early-Onset Neonatal Sepsis (EONS)

Bacterial maternofetal infection is one of the most common cause of neonatal morbidity and mortality. Early diagnosis and treatment are vital to improve outcome. Bacteriological results are not relevant. In the absence of reliable infection markers during the first hours of life, pediatricians often start early antibiotic treatment in newborn infants with risk factors for infection, exposing a considerable number of patients to unnecessary treatment. PCT has been implicated as a sensitive and specific marker of bacterial infection. However, it is well established that PCT concentrations in the neonate show a physiological increase during the first two days of life, which complicates the interpretation of results during this period; CHIESA present the results of work on the kinetics postnatal of the PCT with distribution of PCT values obtained for uninfected and EONS patients between birth and 48 hours of age [9]. Turner [21] study PCT concentration of uninfected and EONS preterm infants between birth and 96 hours of age, with 2 groups to 24-30 and 31—36 weeks gestation; results of these two groups are different.

Serum PCT in cord blood seems to be a useful and early marker of antenatal infection and EONS. In a previous study [22], PCT and CRP concentrations in umbilical cord blood of 197 neonates were measured to evaluate their values as markers for infection. Sixteen of the neonates were infected. The sensitivity, specificity, and negative and positive predictive values were respectively 87.5%, 98.7%, 87.5%, and 98.7% for PCT and 50%, 97%, 67%, and 94% for CRP. Serum PCT in cord blood seems to be a useful and early marker of antenatal infection. PCT measurement in umbilical cord blood appears to be a sensitive and specific marker of antenatal infection, with high positive and negative predictive values. It also presents good positive and negative likelihood ratios, and appears to be more reliable than CRP. Focusing on PCT concentrations in umbilical cord blood before the physiological increase or eventual respiratory or hemodynamic failure makes interpretation for the diagnostic value of PCT concentration easier. On the other hand, the limitation of such an early PCT measurement is that it does not allow the detection of ''late'' maternofetal infection related to perpartum or postnatal contamination.

The detection of infected neonates and its good negative predictive value should result in the reduction number of patients unnecessarily treated. In particular, PCT measurement should allow the clinician to distinguish infections from simple colonizations.

Interestingly, PCT seems to be present in full term and preterm neonates. This reduction in antibiotic prescriptions would represent a direct advantage for neonates, because of the potential toxicity for antibiotics, and an indirect ecological advantage by reducing antibiotic selection pressure. Although the specificity and negative predictive value for PCT in this study were precisely evaluated with a confidence interval of 1%, the number of infected patients was too small to provide definitive sensitivity and positive predictive value. Although these rapid tests look promising for PCT as a useful tool for diagnosing sepsis in newborn infants, our results on a relatively small number of neonates should be confirmed by a properly designed trial.

Two others important studies demonstrate interest for PCT in the diagnosis of NS at 24 hours of age, and in the decision of antibiotic therapy duration [23-24]. Stocker [24], with multicenter study and with large number of subjects and correct methodology, show that Procalcitonin determinations allowed to shorten the duration of antibiotic therapy in newborns with suspected EONS.

4. Late-Onset Neonatal Sepsis (LONS)

Our study [25] has evaluated the contribution of PCT assay to Central catheter during a prolonged hospitalization. Using the quantitative KRYPTOR1-PCT method, we determined the sensitivity (Se) and the specificity (Sp) for PCT and C-reactive protein (CRP). Newborns with a suspicion of BNI were included. They were divided into two groups: not infected (group 0), infected (group 1). Comparing the two groups, we established a threshold value for PCT and CRP using the ROC curves. We also highlighted Se, Sp, positive (VPP) and negative predictive values (VPN) for PCT and CRP.

Forty premature newborns of 28.3 weeks gestational age average were included during a 17 months period. The distribution was as follows: 26 patients in group 0 and 14 patients in the group 1. The threshold value was 0.8 ng/ml for PCT, 6 mg/l for CRP. The Se, Sp, VPP and VPN values were 79, 96, 92 and 89% for PCT, 50, 88, 70 and 77% for CRP. From the ROC curves, the surface under curve was 0.94 for PCT, 0.68 for CRP ($p < 0.05$). In conclusion, this study confirms the interest of PCT assay in the diagnosis of BNI in premature newborns.

There are several biases in our study: the difficulties of sampling in children premature unstable represent a major obstacle to get adequate blood volume in our study. Some infants with nosocomial infection could therefore not be included in this study period, but their number is small (<5) and our sample is probably representative Moreover, Group 0 uninfected children is not a group of healthy children, since they had a clinical suspicion of infection. As a result, the reference values calculated for the PCT from the population in group 0 are not those of children "completely healthy" but children free from infection. Finally, unlike other case-control studies, we have not studied as controls. This mode of recruitment does not allow us to establish normal values really, but seems close to daily practice. Indeed, the difficulty of establishing a diagnosis of infection in neonatal intensive care and neonatology in a population largely consisting of premature is the lack of specificity of clinical signs of appeal that may also be revealing a multitude of other diseases that would be particularly associated with preterm children. Another possible bias in selection: non-homogeneous population, with two children with a digestive surgery. We kept them in the study, this corresponds to the actual recruitment service during the study period.

through grading, defined by the difficulty of defining the bni, is probably one of the main problems of our study. in the absence of gold standard defined, we chose the bacteriological results for reference, but we know that the blood culture may result in false negatives by insufficient sampling or contamination by false positives, this being related to the number blood cultures, the amount of blood and the realization of the sample. we included children with clinical features suggestive of initial infection. we have not included other bni definitions, based on other predictors or proposed for the older child. we have not studied the value of pct and crp markers for confirmation of diagnosis and decision for the continuation or discontinuation of the antibiotic.

The sensitivity of the PCT (nearly 80%) clarifies that the PCT is an interesting marker for the diagnosis of BNI in this study. These results are limited, this corresponds to small numbers, with very wide confidence intervals. The number of studies in the literature on the subject is important enough, but the methodologies are different (Type of study, measurement method, study population, definition of infection. . .) and the results are variable [26-36]. Kuhn et al. [28] found a sensitivity and specificity less important that in our study (Se: 76.5 versus 78.6%; Sp: 82.7 versus 96.2%) in case of nosocomial infection. In contrast, Chiesa et al. [32] with excellent results since the sensitivity and specificity of 100% are obtained. It is Similarly Enguix et al. [33], but it is case- witnesses. Van Rossum et al. [31] indicate that studies give results of sensitivity and specificity vary because of different methodologies or children's associations with early infections (maternofetal) and late (nosocomial). The study Vazzalwar et al. [27] is a cohort study a population of premature infants, finding results satisfactory and in line of great interest to the PCT. The measurement method is the Lumitest1-PCT, in addition, two blood cultures are performed before the initiation antibiotic treatment (one in our study). Other authors found different results: Lopez Sastre et al. [34] and Perez Solis et al. [35] conclude moderate interest in the PCT, but do not compare to the CRP, the result of the Youden index in the study Lopez Sastre et al. is lower than in our study (0.62 versus 0.75). Turner et al. [21] found a similar interest of PCT and CRP, but this study with a methodology and a population different from ours. Isidor et al. [36], with a semi-quantitative method, found values close to our study (likelihood ratio 14.9 and 0.09 versus 20.7 and 0.2). It is important to note that the dosages quantitative PCT in other studies were performed by quantitative technique to immunoluminometric using the PCT-Lumitest1 of Brahms.

A priori, the results obtained with the Kryptor1-PCT and PCT-Lumitest1 well correlated. In our study, from the ROC curve, we determine a threshold value of PCT to 0.8 ng / ml for the diagnosis of BNI. It is relatively comparable to that obtained during the study by Kuhn et al. [3] which includes 38 patients aged three to 61 days of life (16 infected and 22 non-infected) and evaluates the threshold of the PCT to 0.6 ng/ml. Vazzalwar et al. [27] found a threshold value 0.5 ng / ml. This is not what the study authors found following, but it is case-control studies. Chiesa et al. carry out a study [32] in a population composed of 23 infected newborns matched to 92 neonates not infected, aged three to 30 days of life. All newborns PCT infected have a greater than 2 ng / ml and all control children have a PCT less than 1 ng / ml. Enguix et al. [33] also obtained excellent results during a prospective study of 20 newborns infected and 26 infants free of any infection, aged three to 30 days of life, with a threshold value of 6.1 ng / ml. Comparison with other parameters biological, CRP is the marker most commonly used. The sensitivity of the CRP, 50% in our study was 72% in the study Vazzalwar et al. [27] studies similar to ours in terms of methodology and the target population. Cytokines can also assayed in a timely manner to clinical use, but are not yet used in routine. Kuhn et al. [3, 28] compared the value of the assay the PCT, interleukin 6 and interleukin 8 in the early diagnosis of nosocomial infection. The interleukin 6 appears to be the most interesting of the three. In addition, the diagnostic performance of these three markers are greatly increased when combined with dosing

CRP. Using meta-analysis [29, 30], PCT is a valuable additional tool for the diagnosis of NS, but methodologies of studies, and age of patients are different. This sensitive analysis shows that differences in PCT assay producer, gestational age and severity of sepsis in the population studied may partially explain the between-studies heterogeneity.

In conclusion in our study of very premature bearing a central line, with a new quantitative method, the PCT has better sensitivity and specificity than CRP for early diagnosis of nosocomial infection. The dosage of the PCT is useful and applicable in neonatology current in the detection of BNI.

The PCT is an early marker of bacterial infection in NICU. Bacteriological results are also not relevant. In our study using a new quantitative method, the PCT has better sensitivity and specificity than CRP for early diagnosis of nosocomial infection for very premature infants bearing a central line.

However, it is necessary to confirm these results by including more patients.

Larger multicenter trials, in respect with CONSORT statement, are required to validate the routine use of PCT as a marker of LONS in NICU [37].

This could improve the outcome of neonatal infection by initiating early treatment but above all by limiting duration of unnecessary antibiotic treatments.

5. Conclusion

Accurate diagnosis of NS is difficult on account of the imperfect diagnostic sensitivity of laboratory tests. All predisposing factors to infection such as prenatal history, clinical presentation of the newborn, and laboratory results must be considered to treat all those who have infections, and yet minimize the use of antibiotics in those without infection.

A better understanding of the neonatal inflammatory response to infection has led to the identification of multiple diagnostic markers of sepsis. At present, The PCT is an early marker of NS, but none of the current diagnostic markers are sensitive or specific enough to influence with certainty the decision to start antibiotic therapy. These diagnostic markers are promising for the early diagnosis for EONS and LONS, and for discontinuation of antibiotic treatment with suspected sepsis. Further evidence from large multicenter trials is needed to evaluate the newer diagnostic markers prospectively for their incremental diagnostic value before they can be considered reliable for diagnosing early infections and be included as part of a routine sepsis evaluation for neonates. Therefore, the neonatal care provider remains dependent on a thorough history and physical assessment in combination with available laboratory tests to guide treatment for presumptive sepsis while awaiting culture results.

Author details

C. Savagner, B. Leboucher, G. Gascoin-Lachambre
Neonatal Intensive Care Unit, CHU ANGERS, France

C. Gras-Leguen
Neonatal Intensive Care Unit, CHU NANTES, France

Appendix

Abbreviations : CRP, C reactive protein; PCT, Procalcitonin; EONS, Early-onset neonatal sepsis; LONS, Late-onset neonatal sepsis; NS, Neonatal sepsis; BNI, Bacterial nosocomial infection; NICU, Neonatal Intensive Care Unit; ICU, Intensive care unit; ABT, Antibiotherapy.

6. References

[1] Raimondi F, Ferrara T, Maffucci R, Milite P, Del Buono D, Santoro P, Grimaldi LC. Neonatal sepsis: a difficult diagnostic challenge. Clin Biochem. 2011 May;44(7):463-4.

[2] Popowski T, Goffinet F, Batteux F, Maillard F, Kayem G. Prediction of maternofetal infection in preterm premature rupture of membranes: serum maternal markers. Gynecol Obstet Fertil. 2011 May;39(5):302-8.

[3] Kuhn P, Astruc D, Donato L, et al. Quel(s) marqueur(s) inflammatoire(s) pour le diagnostic précoce des infections nosocomiales ? In: G. Moriette, editor. 37e Journées nationales de néonatologie, SFN. Progrès en Néonatologie 2007;27:p. 79-96.

[4] Alt R, Willard D, Messer J, Metais P, Goester C, Mark JJ. Value of C-reactive protein in neonatal bacterial infections. Arch Fr Pediatr. 1982;39:811-3.

[5] Ferrière F. Intérêt de la procalcitonine, nouveau marqueur de l'infection bactérienne. Ann Biol Clin (Paris). 2000;58:49-59.

[6] Hausfater P. Procalcitonin measurement in adult clinical practice. Rev Med Interne. 2007;28:296-305.

[7] Nylen ES, O'Neill W, Jordan MH, Snider RH, Moore CF, Lewis M et al. Serum procalcitonin as an index of inhalation injury in burns. Horm Metab Res. 1992;24:439-42.

[8] Assicot M, Gendrel D, Carsin H, Raymond J, Guilbaud J, Bohuon C. High serum procalcitonin concentrations in patients with sepsis and infection. Lancet. 1993;341:515-8.

[9] Chiesa C, Panero A, Rossi N, Stegagno M, De Giusti M, Osborn JF et al. Reliability of procalcitonin concentrations for the diagnosis of sepsis in critically ill neonates. Clin Infect Dis. 1998;26:664-72.

[10] Maire F, Héraud MC, Loriette Y, Normand B, Bègue RJ, Labbé A. Intérêt de la procalcitonine dans les infections néonatales. Arch Fr Pediatr. 1999;6:503-9.
[11] Lapillonne A, Basson E, Monneret G, Bienvenu J, Salle BL. Lack of specificity of procalcitonin for sepsis diagnostis in premature infants. Lancet. 1998;351: 1211-2.
[12] Ng PC. Diagnostic markers of infection in neonates. Arch Dis Child Fetal Neonatal Ed. 2004 May;89(3):F229-35.
[13] Schuetz P, Christ-Crain M, Thomann R, Falconnier C, Wolbers M, Widmer I et al. Effect of procalcitonin-based guidelines vs standard guidelines on antibiotic use in lower respiratory tract infections: the ProHOSP randomized controlled trial. JAMA. 2009 Sep 9;302(10):1059-66.
[14] Christ-Crain M, Jaccard-Stolz D, Bingisser R, Gencay MM, Huber PR, Tamm M et al. Effect of procalcitonin-guided treatment on antibiotic use and outcome in lower respiratory tract infections: cluster-randomised, single-blinded intervention trial. Lancet. 2004 Feb 21;363(9409):600-7.
[15] Christ-Crain M, Stolz D, Bingisser R, Müller C, Miedinger D, Huber PR, et al. Procalcitonin guidance of antibiotic therapy in community-acquired pneumonia: a randomized trial. Am J Respir Crit Care Med. 2006 Jul 1;174(1):84-93.
[16] Briel M, Schuetz P, Mueller B, Young J, Schild U, Nusbaumer C et al. Procalcitonin-guided antibiotic use vs a standard approach for acute respiratory tract infections in primary care. Arch Intern Med. 2008 Oct 13;168(18):2000-7; discussion 2007-8.
[17] Müller F, Christ-Crain M, Bregenzer T, Krause M, Zimmerli W, Mueller B, ProHOSP Study Group. Procalcitonin levels predict bacteremia in patients with community-acquired pneumonia: a prospective cohort trial. Chest. 2010 Jul;138(1): 121-9.
[18] Bouadma L, Luyt CE, Tubach F, Cracco C, Alvarez A, Schwebel C et al. Use of procalcitonin to reduce patients' exposure to antibiotics in intensive care units (PRORATA trial): a multicentre randomised controlled trial. Lancet. 2010 Feb 6;375(9713):463-74.
[19] Storey I, Bedford Russell A. Perinatal and neonatal mortality in the advent of the neonatal network. Br J Hosp Med (Lond). 2010 Apr;71(4):190-4.
[20] Lautridou A, Ancel PY, Launay E, Denizot S, Orsonneau JL, Roze JC, Gras-Le Guen C. Umbilical cord blood procalcitonin as a risk factor for mortality in very premature infants. Eur J Clin Microbiol Infect Dis. 2012 Mar 1.
[21] Turner D, Hammerman C, Rudensky B, Schlesinger Y, Goia C, Schimmel MS. Procalcitonin in preterm infants during the first few days of life: introducing an age related nomogram. Arch Dis Child Fetal. 2006;91(4):F283-6.
[22] Joram N, Muller JB, Denizot S, Orsonneau JL, Caillon J, Rozé JC and al. Umbilical cord blood procalcitonin and CRP concentrations as markers for early diagnosis of very early onset neonatal infection. Arch. Dis. Child. Fetal Neonatal Ed. 2006;91; 65-66.

[23] Altunhan H, Annagür A, Örs R, Mehmetoğlu I. Procalcitonin measurement at 24 hours of age may be helpful in the prompt diagnosis of early-onset neonatal sepsis. Int J Infect Dis. 2011 Dec;15(12):e854-8.

[24] Stocker M, Hop WC, van Rossum AM. Neonatal Procalcitonin Intervention Study (NeoPInS): Effect of Procalcitonin-guided decision making on duration of antibiotic therapy in suspected neonatal early-onset sepsis: A multi-centre randomized superiority and non-inferiority Intervention Study. BMC Pediatr. 2010 Dec 8; 10:89.

[25] Savagner C, Hoppe A, Montcho Y, Leboucher B, Le Bouedec S, Lemarie C et al. Interest of procalcitonin for diagnosis bacterial nosocomial infections in neonatology: retrospective study of 40 children. Journal of paediatrics and child care (2008) 21, 292-298.

[26] López Sastre JB, Solís DP, Serradilla VR, Colomer BF, Cotallo GD; Grupo de Hospitales Castrillo. Evaluation of procalcitonin for diagnosis of neonatal sepsis of vertical transmission. BMC Pediatr. 2007 Feb 26;7:9.

[27] Vazzalwar R, Pina-Rodrigues E, Puppala BL, Angst DB, Schweig L. Procalcitonin as a screening test for late-onset sepsis in preterm very low birth weight infants. J Perinatol. 2005 Jun;25(6):397-402.

[28] Kuhn P, Escande D, Rivera S, Langlet C, Messer J. Procalcitonine et infection néonatale. Arch Pediatr. 2004;6:585-6.

[29] Vouloumanou EK, Plessa E, Karageorgopoulos DE, Mantadakis E, Falagas ME. Serum procalcitonin as a diagnostic marker for neonatal sepsis: a systematic review and meta-analysis. Intensive Care Med. 2011 May;37(5):747-62.

[30] Yu Z, Liu J, Sun Q, Qiu Y, Han S, Guo X. The accuracy of the procalcitonin test for the diagnosis of neonatal sepsis: a meta-analysis. Scand J Infect Dis. 2010 Oct;42(10):723-33.

[31] Van Rossum AM, Wulkan RW, Oudesluys-Murphy AM. Procalcitonin as an early marker of infection in neonates and children.Lancet Infect Dis. 2004;10:620-30.

[32] Chiesa C, Pacifico L, Rossi N, Panero A, Matrunola M, Mancuso G. Procalcitonin as a marker of nosocomial infections in the neonatal intensive care unit. Intensive Care Med. 2000;26(suppl 2):S175-7.

[33] Enguix A, Rey C, Concha A, Medina A, Coto D, Diéguez MA. Comparaison of procalcitonin with C-réactive protein and serum amyloid for diagnosis of bacterial sepsis in critically ill neonates and children. Intensive Care Med. 2001;27:211-5.

[34] López Sastre JB, Pérez Solís D, Roqués Serradilla V, Fernández Colomer B, Coto Cotallo GD, Krauel Vidal X, et al. Procalcitonin is not sufficiently reliable to be the sole marker of neonatal sepsis of nosocomial origin. BMC Pediatr. 2006;6:16.

[35] Pérez Solís D, López Sastre JB, Coto Cotallo GD, Diéguez Junquera MA, Deschamps Mosquera EM, Crespo Hernández M. Procalcitonin for the diagnosis of nosocomial neonatal sepsis. Ann Pediatr (Barc). 2006;64:349-53.

[36] Isidor B, Caillaux G, Gilquin V, Loubersac V, Caillon J, Roze JC et al. The use of procalcitonin in the diagnosis of late-onset infection in neonatal intensive care unit patients. Scan J Infect dis. 2007;39:1063—6.

[37] Boutron I, Moher D, Altman DG, Schulz KF, Ravaud P; CONSORT Group. Extending the CONSORT statement to randomized trials of nonpharmacologic treatment: explanation and elaboration. Ann Intern Med. 2008 Feb 19;148(4):295-309.

Section 4

Microbiology and Antimicrobial Therapy in Sepsis

Chapter 13

Catheter-Related Bloodstream Infections in Critical Care

Efraín Riveros Pérez

Additional information is available at the end of the chapter

http://dx.doi.org/10.5772/49988

1. Introduction

1.1. High-yield facts

- Central line insertion is a very common procedure in critical care settings, and is associated with infectious complications such as local colonisation and bloodstream infection which leads to bacteremia and sepsis.
- Causative microorganisms are commonly missed on blood cultures, so that empiric therapy must be started in absence of a known pathogen.
- Diagnosis is based on clinical suspicion and microbiological confirmation by means of local and blood cultures (quantitative or semiquantiative).
- The mainstay of treatment is a combination of early antibiotic treatment and catheter removal with insertion at a new site.
- Prevention is the cornerstone of catheter-related infections.
- Multimodular programs (education, surveillance and quality management) and the sophistication of catheter-associated devices have shown benefit on CRBSI rate reduction.
- Strategies must be grouped into bundles.
- CRBSI reduction plans are part of the general ICU quality improvement plan.
- Team work is crucial to the construction and follow-up of the strategies aimed at reducing the infection rate in critically-ill patients.

2. Epidemiology of catheter related bloodstream infections

Central lines are inserted on a routine basis in critical care settings, for IV fluid administration, vasoactive medication infusions and monitoring purposes. As there has been worldwide expansion of intensive care facilities in the last few decades, the insertion of central catheters has increased exponentially. Unfortunately, this procedure carries a risk of morbidity that includes local and bloodstream infections, which translates into higher healthcare costs and eventually into mortality[1-3].

The incidence of catheter-related bloodstream infections (CRBSI) varies widely among different healthcare institutions, ranging between 2,1 per 1.000 catheter-days for peripherally inserted central catheters (PICCs) to 2,7 per 1.000 catheter-days for non-tunneled central lines[4-6]. In the US, it has been estimated that approximately 31.000 deaths per year are attributable to bloodstream infections[7], representing an expenditure of about $18.000 per CRBSI[8]. In Spain the rate of CRBSI has been estimated in the range of 2,1 to 3,4 per 1.000 hospitalized patients[9]. Tacconelli et al. showed that the incidence of CRBSI varies widely among four european countries (France, Germany, Italy and the UK), from 1,12 to 4,2 per 1.000 catheter days[10]. Finally in Latin America and Africa incidence of CRBSI is unknown.

3. Pathogenesis

CRBSI might occur as a result of the entry of pathogenic microorganisms to the bloodstream via four different routes[11]: local insertion site colonisation, catheter hub contamination, hematogenous seeding and infusión of contaminated fluids. Attention has been focused on the two first routes[12-14]. The spread of infection from the insertion site has been widely recognized as the main cause of CRBSI, and the risk factors related to its development have been matter of research during the last two decades. However, hub contamination is relevant for long-term tunneled catheters[15]. CRBSI co-morbidity risk factors identified are insertion technique, insertion site, type and frequency of dressing, frequency of manipulation, duration of catheterization, number of catheter lumens, local and systemic antibiotic use, type of antiseptic solution use and experience of the person in charge of catheter care[16-19]. On the other hand, the presence of renal failure and hemodialysis are independent risk factors for CRBSI[20-21].

Several studies have shown that the causative agent of CRBSI sometimes is difficult to isolate. However, some series have reported that the most common organisms responsible of infection are: *coagulase-negative Staphilococcus, Enterococci, gram negative bacteria (Klebsiella Pneumoniae and E. Coli) and Candida Albicans*[22-24]. Healthcare personnel and patient skin colonization with Staphylococci is common, and is related to CRBSI, whereas *C. Albicans* and *C. Parapsilosis* may be responsable of infusate contamination.

The causative microorganisms of CRBSI are able to produce an exopolysaccaride-rich layer that adheres to the catheter. This layer supports the formation of a microbial biofilm, that allows bacteria to grow on the surface of foreign bodies in contact with bloodflow. This situation confers the causative agent some resistance to antibiotic, making necessary catheter removal in order to erradicate infection. Soon after catheter insertion, a thrombin sheath is formed on the outer and inner surfaces of the device, facilitating adherence of pathogens. This sheath is rich in proteins such as fibronectin, fibrinogen, thrombospondin, laminin and adhesin[25-29]. This last protein is an endogenous protein attractive to coagulase negative

Staphylococci. Once bacteria are attached to adhesin, biofilm covers the microorganisms from the action of immune system and antibiotic action.

Unfortunately, information regarding the causative agent in a particular case is sometimes useless, due to the low rate of positive blood cultures in an ICU population receiving antibiotics for diferent reasons[30,31]. The isolation of a pathogen in blood cultures is a negative prognostic factor[32], whereas it is useful to verify the appropriateness of empiric therapy, which is related to morbidity and mortaity[33,34]. On the other hand, positive cultures at the insertion site do not predict reliably positive blood cultures[35]. Furthermore, false positive cultures may lead to unnecessary anibiotic treatment, prolonged hospital stay[36] and emergence of resistant species[37,38].

4. Diagnosis

It has been found that reliability of clinical findings in CRBSI are not enough to diagnose the disease due to their por performance as diagnostic tests. Fever, one of the most common symptoms, has low specificity, whereas local insertion site inflammatory signs have por sensitivity. Remission of systemic inflammatory response after catheter removal is suggestive but not diagnostic of CRBSI[12,37-39].

The non-uniformity in definition of criteria to diagnose CRBSI has made difficult to compare studies and to issue accurate recommendations regarding diagnosis[12,23]. However, with surveillance purposes, the Centers for Disease Control (CDC) have established the definition of "laboratory confirmed bloodstream infection" (LCBI)[40], consisting in meeting at least one of the following criteria:

- Patient has a recognized pathogen cultured from one or more blood cultures and the pathogen is not related to an infection at another site.
- Patient has fever, chills and/or hypotension as well as positive laboratory cultures from two or more blood samples drawn on separate occasions which are not related to infection at another site and do not reflect contamonation.
- Patient < 1 year of age has at least one of the following signs or symptoms: fever, hypothermia, apnea, or bradicardia (in addition to the above criteria).

It is adequate to process only the catheter tip for culture[23]. Quantitative (positive $>10^2$ cfu) and semiquantitative (positive $>10^5$ cfu) culture techniques are recommended over qualitative cultures[41-45]. It is recommended to culture every catheter removed due to suspicion of infection, but it is not a good practice to send every catheter removed to culture. Secretion draining from the insertion site must be cultured[23].

According to the IDSA guidelines for the diagnosis and management of catheter related infection[23], it is recommended that as long as possible, blood cultures should be drawn prior to antibiotic administration. When dealing with blood cultures, contamination is an issue that must be taken into consideration. Contamination is significant when blood cultures are drawn from a catheter in use, as compared to an adequately obtained sample from a peripheral vein[46-50]. On the other hand, diagnostic accuracy is optimal when quantitative paired blood cultures (concomitant catheter and peripheral) are drawn[51,52]. In summary, an accurate diagnosis of CRBSI can be achieved when clinical signs and symptoms are associated with positive local and paired blood cultures that match in microbiological terms.

5. Management

Empiric antibiotic treatment is a common practice when dealing with CRBSI. The choice of the antimicrobial agent depends on the severity of the systemic illness, the comorbidities, the most likely microorganisms and the local resistance profile. The combination of catheter removal and early antibiotic treatment have shown to be effective (negative blood cultures) in 88% of the cases[53]. Since methicilin-resistant *Staphylococcus Epidermidis* is the most common pathogen, it is reasonable to use Vancomycin as the first choice. In case of MIC ≥ 2 µg/mL, alternatives such as daptomycin are valuable. On the other hand, gram negative microorganisms (including *Pseudomonas Aeruginosa*) should be covered in neutropenic or severely-ill patients. It is not recommended to use linezolid as empiric treatment[23]. Regarding treatment duration, there is no strong evidence in favor of any recommendation. Our experience at Clinica de los Andes (unpublished results) have shown that five days from the first negative blood cultures is associated with no relapse and favorable outcomes. Femoral vein catheters are more prone to develop CRBSI due to the anatomical area of insertion. Furthermore, fungi growth is a common occurrence. This situation warrants antifungal empiric therapy in this subset of patients.

Catheter removal is a mainstay of treatment. However, when an ICU patient with moderate disease has fever, the recommendation is to draw blood samples from the device and from a peripheral vein before making the decision of removal. Most catheters from suspected cases of CRBSI end up being sterile[53-54]. If there is no other possible source of infection, or the patient is severely ill, catheter removal and insertion at a new site are recommended.

The antibiotic regimen must be "de-escalated" depending on blood and local site culture results in order to limit the probability of emergence of resistant species. At our institution we decide to continue the initial antibiotic depending on clinical response over the antibiogram. If the patient is not improving, then the sensitivity tests are taken into account to chang the antimicrobial agent.

6. Prevention: strategies and bundles

Significant efforts have been made at different levels in order to reduce the incidence of CRBSI in intensive care units[55-61]. Most of the initiatives have focused on preventive aspects[62-65], as evidence has shown that educational programs as well as multifactorial model implementation are effective[62-72].

During the last decade, several studies have investigated different strategies aimed at reducing CRBSI by means of prevention[73]. Most of the studies demonstrate benefit derived from multimodule programs including education, surveillance and quality management, and from the development of devices (such as catheter biomaterial and locks, dressings and antiseptic solutions).

The catheter insertion conditions are critical for the development of infections derived from the device. The current recommendation includes the use of a long sleeve gown, surgical cap, face mask, sterile gloves and large sterile sheets that completely cover the patient[74]. Hand hygiene should be the standard practice, but compliance by health care professionals is still poor. In an attempt to enhance compliance, hand rubbing with an alcoholic solution might be as good as hand washing[75]. Chlorhexidine, for example, has shown a better antiseptic performance as compared to regular povidone iodine solutions[76]. However, povidone iodine is preferred in some ICUs, especially in the developing world, due to its low cost and because of the low bacterial and fungal resistance development[77]. In this case, the povidone iodine solution must remain in contact with the skin for at least one minute in order to be effective[76].

The site of insertion of the catheter also influences the infection rate. In general terms, we can say that internal jugular approach is associated with a higher risk of CRBSI but a lower risk of mechanical complications such as pneumothorax. Conversely subclavian insertion requires more expertise but has a significant lower association with infection[2]. A higher infection rate is seen in the femoral approach. Thus, the subclavian approach must be preferred, especially for catheters expected to remain in place for more than 7 days[78]. Femoral catheters must be avoided unless the mechanical complication risks of the subclavian and jugular approaches are prohibitive [79].

Numerous studies have shown that catheter replacement on a scheduled basis does not reduce CRBSI in ICU[80-82]. In fact, the 2011 CDC guidelines argue against this practice[83]. However, guidewire exchange to prevent CRBSI is not recommended[84-86]. Nonetheless, Riveros recently showed that in a medical ICU, with a high average length of stay, the central catheter exchange scheduled on the eighth day was superior to the a change guided by signs of infection[87]. In that study, 315 catheters (163 patients), were analyzed. Significant catheter colonization rates (RR=0,4 CI 95%: 0,1-0,9 $p<0{,}01$) and catheter-related sepsis were significantly lower in the scheduled change group (RR=0,4 CI 95%: 0,1-0,97 $p=0{,}05$). Those findings allow for possibility of scheduled catheter change in selected long-term medical ICU patients. However, further research is needed before clear-cut recommendations may be issued.

Transparent and gauze dressings are supposed to be part of ICU general protocols, but their use is not systematically adopted in routine practice[88]. A randomized controlled trial reported a reduction from 1,3 to 0,4 catheter-days (hazard rate 0,24 95% CI 0,09-0,65) in CRBSI with the use of chlorhexidine-impregnated dressings[89]. Impregnated catheters have been extensively studied but have not been universally used. Despite the theoretical advantage of antibiotic-coated catheters, in a meta-analysis, Walder demonstrated that anti-infective effectiveness of chlorhexidine-sulfadiazine coatings is time-dependent, showing good anti-microbial activity for the first week only[90]. However, the Evidence-based Practice in Infection Control (EPIC) in the UK, recommends the use of impregnated catheters in adults who require the device for one to three weeks[91].

As stated above, the approach to CRBSI is multimodal. Recently, a lot of information has emerged from studies worldwide, regarding changing practices in ICU. These studies use the concept of the "bundle", which includes a definition of objectives such as training[92-94], insertion and catheter care. Simulation training, in addition to improving technical skills in catheter insertion, allows the resident and physician to easily comply with guidelines and checklists[95]. This technique has shown a significant decrease in CRBSI ranging from 71% to 84%[96,97].

Most bundle initiatives have followed to the Michigan bundle proposed by Provonoust[98-105]. The Michigan bundle includes hand hygiene, use of chlorexidine for skin preparation, use of barrier precautions during insertion, a preference for subclavian vein and the removal of unnecessary central lines. The bundle was implemented for the Institute for Health Improvement in the US as part of the 5 million lives campaign[106] and is considered a standard of care. The bundls *per se* is not capable of controlling CRBSI, so that observation and follow-up are mandatory for a prevention strategy to be successful. Riveros et al showed that the implementation of the bundles must be accompanied by a strong ICU quality management program, which ought to have solid foundations in terms of goal definition, follow-up, information system, education and improvement plans[107]. The institution of these plan at different health care centers has produced reports of experiences with impressive results[66]. Finally, the educational programs must be sustained over time, and in order to do so, involvement of ICU staff in the construction and follow-up stages of the process is crucial and has been able to keep CRBSI low[107].

Additional measures to prevent CRBSI include administration sets replacement, including secondary sets and add-on devices, between 96 hours and 7 days[108-112], use of central venous catheters coated with chlorhexidine and silver sulfadiazine to reduce device colonization[113,114], and heparin locks impregnated with antibiotics[115-117].

In conclusion, CRBSI has become more challenging in light of the exponential growth of the critical care patient population worldwide. In order to cope with these changes, ICU healthcare and administrative personnel must work as a team to achieve the goals of a quality plan focused on infection control. The different strategies evidence-based strategies must be part of a bundle, and must be followed on a routine basis as part of improvement plans.

Author details

Efraín Riveros Pérez
Universidad de Boyaca, Clinica de los Andes, Colombia

7. References

[1] Kim JS, Holtom P, Vigen C. Reduction of catheter-related bloodstream infections through the use of a central venous line bundle: Epidemiologic and economic consequences. Am J Infect Control 2011;39:640-6.

[2] Mermel LA. Prevention of intravascular catheter-related infections. Ann Intern Med 2000;132:391-402.
[3] Burke JP. Infection control — a problem for patient safety. N Engl J Med 2003; 348:651-6.
[4] Zingg W, Walder B, Pittet D. Prevention of catheter-related infection: toward zero risk? Current Opinion in Infectious Diseases 2011, 24:377–384.
[5] Maki DG, Kluger DM, Crnich CJ. The risk of bloodstream infection in adults with different intravascular devices: a systematic review of 200 published prospective studies. Mayo Clin Proc 2006; 81:1159–1171.
[6] Lorente L, Henry C, Martin MM, Jimenez A, Mora ML. Central venous catheter-related infection in a prospective and observational study of 2595 catheters. Crit Care 2005; 9: R631-R635.
[7] Klevens RM, Edwards JR, Richards C, Jr., Horan TC, Gaynes RP, et al. (2007) Estimating Health Care-Associated Infections and Deaths in U.S. Hospitals, 2002. Public Health Reports 22: 160–6.
[8] Perencevich EN, Stone PW, Wright SB, Carmeli Y, Fisman DN, et al. (2007) Raising standards while watching the bottom line: making a business case for infection control. Infect Control Hosp Epidemiol 28: 1121–33.
[9] Vaqué J, Roselló J. Prevalencia de infecciones nosocomiales en hospitales espan oles: estudio EPINE [accessed 2011 Sep 4]. Available in: http://www.vhebron.net/preventiva/epine/informe epine 2009 espana.pdf.
[10] Tacconelli E, Smith G, Hieke K, Lafuma A, Bastide P. Epidemiology, medical outcomes and costs of catheter-related bloodstream infections in intensive care units of four European countries: literatura and registry-based estimates. J Hosp Infect. 2009;72:97-103.
[11] Bong JJ, Kite P, Wilco MH, McMahon MJ. Prevention of catheter related bloodstream infection by silver iontophoretic central venous catheters: a randomised controlled trial. J Clin Pathol. 2003 October; 56(10): 731–735.
[12] Maki DG. Infections caused by intravascular devices used for infusion therapy: pathogenesis, prevention, and management of infections due to intravascular therapy. In: Bisno AL, Waldvogel FA, eds. Infections associated with indwelling medical devices, 2nd ed. Washington DC: American Society for Microbiology, 1994:151–212.
[13] Raad I, Darouiche R. Prevention of infections associated with intravascular devices. Curr Opin Crit Care 1996;2:361.
[14] Sitges-Serra A, Girvent M. Catheter-related bloodstream infections. World J Surg 1999;23:589–95.
[15] Mayhall CG. Diagnosis and manage- ment of infections of implantable devices used for prolonged venous access. Curr Clin Top Infect Dis. 1992;12:83-110.
[16] Hosoglu S, Akalin S, Kidir V, Suner A, Kayabas H, Geyik MF. Prospective surveillance study for risk factors of central venous catheter–related bloodstream infections. Am J Infect Control 2004;32:131-4.
[17] Gowardman JR, Montgomery C, Thirlwell S, Shewan J, Idema A, Larsen PD, et al. Central venous catheter-related bloodstream infections: an analysis of incidence and risk factors in a cohort of 400 patients. Intensive Care Med 1998;24:1034-9.

[18] Fraenkel DJ, Rickard C, Lipman J. Can we achieve consensus on central venous catheter-related infections? Anaesth Intensive Care 2000;28:475-90.
[19] Oncu S, Ozsut H, Yildirim A, Ay P, Cakar N, Eraksoy H, et al. Central venous catheter related infections: risk factors and the effect of glycopeptide antibiotics. Ann Clin Microbiol Antimicrobiol 2003;2:3.
[20] AbdulrahmanI S, Al-Mueilo SH, Bokhary HA, Ladipo GOA, Al-Rubaish A. A prospective study of hemodialysis access-related bacterial infections. J Infect Chemother 2002;8:242-6.
[21] Blake PG, Huraib S, VIdall PR. The use of the dual lumen jugular venous catheters as definitive long term access for hemodialysis. Int Artif Organs 1990;13:26-31.
[22] Patil HV, Patil VC, RamteerkarthMN, Kulkarni RD. Central venous catheter-related bloodstream infections in the intensive care unit. Indian J Crit Care Med. 2011 Oct-Dec; 15(4): 213–223.
[23] Mermel LA, Allon M, Bouza E, Craven DE, Flynn P, O'Grady NP, et al. Clinical practice guidelines for the diagnosis and management of intravascular catheter-related infection: 2009 Update by the Infectious Diseases Society of America. Clin Infect Dis. 2009;49:1.
[24] Safdar N, Maki DG. The pathogenesis of catheter-related bloodstream infection with noncuffed short-term central venous catheters. Intensive Care Med (2004) 30:62–67.
[25] Lopes JD, dos Reis M, Brentani RR. Presence of laminin receptors in Staphylo- coccus aureus. Science. 1985;229:275-277.
[26] Herrmann M, Suchard SJ, Boxer LA, et al. Thrombospondin binds to Staphylo- coccus aureus and promotes staphylococcal adherence to surfaces. Infect Immun. 1991;59:279-288.
[27] Herrmann M,Vaudaux PE, Pittet D, et al. Fibronectin, fibrinogen, and laminin act as mediators of adherence of clinical staphy- lococcal isolates to foreign material. J Infect Dis. 1988;158:693-701.
[28] Vaudaux P, Pittet D, Haeberli A, et al. Fibronectin is more active than fibrin or fib-rinogen in promoting Staphylococcus aureus adherence to inserted intravascular catheters. J Infect Dis. 1993;167:633-641.
[29] Nilsson M, Frykberg L, Flock JI, et al. A fibrinogen-binding protein of Staphylo- coccus epidermidis. Infect Immun. 1998; 66:2666-2673.
[30] Previsdomini M, Gini M, Cerutti B, Dolina M, Perren A. Predictors of positive blood cultures in critically ill patients: a retrospective evaluation. Croat Med J. 2012 February; 53(1): 30–39.
[31] McKenzie R, Reimer LG. Effect of antimicrobials on blood cultures in endocarditis. Diagn Microbiol Infect Dis. 1987;8:165–72.
[32] Pazin GJ, Saul S, Thompson ME. Blood culture positivity: suppression by outpatient antibiotic therapy in patients with bacterial endocarditis. Arch Intern Med. 1982;142:263–8.
[33] Pittet D, Tarara D, Wenzel RP. Nosocomial bloodstream infection in critically ill patients: excess length of stay, extra costs, and attributable mortality. JAMA. 1994;271:1598–601.

[34] Schwenzer KJ, Gist A, Durbin CG. Can bacteremia be predicted in surgical intensive care unit patients? Intensive Care Med. 1994;20:425–30.
[35] Bates DW, Goldman L, Lee TH. Contaminant blood cultures and resource utilization. The true consequences of false-positive results. JAMA. 1991;265:365–9.
[36] Ortega M, Marco F, Soriano A, Almela M, Martínez JA, Munoz A, et al. Analysis of 4758 Escherichia coli bacteraemia episodes: predictive factors for isolation of an antibiotic-resistant strain and their impact on the outcome. J Antimicrob Chemother. 2009;63:568–74.
[37] Zarrilli R, Crispino M, Bagattini M, Barretta E, Di Popolo A, Triassi M, et al. Molecular epidemiology of sequential outbreaks of Acinetobacter baumannii in an intensive care unit shows the emergence of carbapenem resistance. J Clin Microbiol. 2004;42:946–53.
[38] Safdar N, Maki DG. Inflammation at the insertion site is not predictive of catheter-related bloodstream infection with short-term, noncuffed central venous catheters. Crit Care Med 2002; 30:2632–5.
[39] Shukrallah B, Hanna H, Hachem R, Ghannam D, Chatzinikolaou I, Raad I. Correlation between early clinical response after catheter removal and diagnosis of catheter-related bloodstream infection. Diagn Microbiol Infect Dis 2007;58:453–7.
[40] Pearson ML. Guideline for prevention of intravascular device-related infections. Hospital Infection Control Practices Advisory Committee. Infect Control Hosp Epidemiol 1996;17:438–73.
[41] Horan TC, Andrus M, Dudeck MA. CDC/NHSN surveillance definition of health care-associated infection and criteria for specific types of infections in the acute care setting. Am J Infect Control 2008; 36:309.
[42] Brun-Buisson C, Abrouk F, Legrand P, Huet Y, Larabi S, Rapin M. Diagnosis of central venous catheter-related sepsis: critical level of quantitative tip cultures. Arch Intern Med 1987; 147:873–7.
[43] Maki DG, Weise CE, Sarafin HW. A semiquantitative culture method for identifying intravenous-catheter–related infection. N Engl J Med 1977; 296:1305–9.
[44] Cleri DJ, Corrado ML, Seligman SJ. Quantitative culture of intra- venous catheters and other intravascular inserts. J Infect Dis 1980; 141:781–6.
[45] Sherertz RJ, Raad, II, Belani A, et al. Three-year experience with sonicated vascular catheter cultures in a clinical microbiology labo- ratory. J Clin Microbiol 1990;28:76–82.
[46] Sherertz RJ, Heard SO, Raad II. Diagnosis of triple-lumen catheter infection: comparison of roll plate, sonication, and flushing meth- odologies. J Clin Microbiol 1997;35:641–6.
[47] Ramsook C, Childers K, Cron SG, Nirken M. Comparison of blood- culture contamination rates in a pediatric emergency room: newly inserted intravenous catheters versus venipuncture. Infect Control Hosp Epidemiol 2000;21:649–51.
[48] Norberg A, Christopher NC, Ramundo ML, Bower JR, Berman SA. Contamination rates of blood cultures obtained by dedicated phlebotomy vs intravenous catheter. JAMA 2003;289:726–9.
[49] Everts RJ, Vinson EN, Adholla PO, Reller LB. Contamination of catheter-drawn blood cultures. J Clin Microbiol 2001; 39:3393–4.

[50] DesJardin JA, Falagas ME, Ruthazer R, et al. Clinical utility of blood cultures drawn from indwelling central venous catheters in hospitalized patients with cancer. Ann Intern Med 1999; 131:641–7.

[51] Martinez JA, Des Jardin JA, Aronoff M, Supran S, Nasraway SA, Snydman DR. Clinical utility of blood cultures drawn from central venous or arterial catheters in critically ill surgical patients. Crit Care Med 2002; 30:7–13.

[52] Safdar M, Fine JP, Maki DG. Meta-analysys: Methods for diagnosing intravascular device-related bloodstream infection. Ann Intern Med. 2005;142:451-466.

[53] Wilcox MH, Tack KJ, Bouza E, et al. Complicated skin and skin- structure infections and catheter-related bloodstream infections: non- inferiority of linezolid in a phase 3 study. Clin Infect Dis 2009;48: 203–12.

[54] Rello J, Coll P, Prats G. Evaluation of culture techniques for diagnosis of catheter-related sepsis in critically ill patients. Eur J Clin Microbiol Infect Dis 1992;11:1192–3.

[55] Cohran J, Larson E, Roach H, Blane C, Pierce P. Effect of intravascular surveillance and education program on rates of nosocomial bloodstream infections. Heart Lung 1996;25:161-4.

[56] Berenholtz SM, Pronovost PJ, Lipsett PA, et al. Eliminating catheter-related bloodstream infections in the intensive care unit. Crit Care Med 2004;32:2014-20.

[57] Warren DK, Cosgrove SE, Deikema DJ, et al. A multicenter intervention to prevent catheter-associated bloodstream infections. Infect Control Hosp Epidemiol 2006;27:662-9.

[58] Reduction in central line-associated bloodstream infections among patients in intensive care units — Pennsylvania, April 2001–March 2005. MMWR Morb Mortal Wkly Rep 2005;54:1013-6.

[59] Monitoring hospital-acquired infections to promote patient safety — United States, 1990–1999. MMWR Morb Mortal Wkly Rep 2000;49:149-53.

[60] Sherertz RJ, Ely EW, Westbrook DM, et al. Education of physicians-in-training can decrease the risk for vascular catheter infection. Ann Intern Med 2000;132:641-8.

[61] Eggimann P, Harbarth S, Constantin MN, Touveneau S, Chevrolet JC, Pittet D. Impact of a prevention strategy targeted at vascular-access care on incidence of infections acquired in intensive care. Lancet 2000;355:1864-8.

[62] Warren DK, Zack JE, Mayfield JL, et al. The effect of an education program on the incidence of central venous catheter-associated bloodstream infection in a medical ICU. Chest 2004;126:1612-8.

[63] Pronovost P, Berenholtz S, Dorman T, Lipsett PA, Simmonds T, Haraden C. Improving communication in the ICU using daily goals. J Crit Care 2003;18:71-5.

[64] Berenholtz SM, Milanovich S, Faircloth A, et al. Improving care for the ventilated patient. Jt Comm J Qual Saf 2004;30:195-204.

[65] Pronovost P, Weast B, Rosenstein B, et al. Implementing and validating a comprehensive unit-based safety program. J Patient Saf 2005;1:33-40.

[66] Pronovost P, Needham D, Berenholtz S, Sinopoli D, Chu H, Cosgrove S, Sexton B, Hyzy R, Welsh R, Roth G, Bander J, Kepros J, Goeschel C. An Intervention to Decrease Catheter-Related Bloodstream Infections in the ICU. N Engl J Med. 2006;355:2725-2732.

[67] O´Grady NP, Alexander M. Dellinger EP. Guidelines for the prevention of intravascular catheter-related infections. Centers for Disease Control and Prevention. Morb Mortal Wkly Rep. 2002;51(RR-10):1-29.

[68] National Nosocomial Infection Surveillance (NNIS) System Report. Data Summary from January 1992 through June 2004, issued October 2004. Am J Infect Control. 2004;32:470-485.

[69] Eggimann P. Diagnosis of intravascular catheter infection. Curr Opin Infect Dis. 2007;20:353-359.

[70] Eggimann P, Pittet D. Infection control in the ICU. Chest. 2001;120:2059-2093.

[71] Wenzel RP, Edmond MB. Team-based prevention of catheter-related infections. 2006;355:2781-2783.

[72] Eggimann P. Prevention of intravascular catheter infection. Curr Opin Infect Dis. 2007;20:360-369.

[73] Timsit JF. Diagnosis and prevention of catheter-related infections. Curr Opin Crit Care. 2007;13:563-571.

[74] Raad II, Hohn DC, Gilbreath BJ, et al. Prevention of central venous catheterrelated infections by using maximal sterile barrier precautions during insertion. Infect Control Hosp Epidemiol 1994; 15 (4 Pt 1):231–238.

[75] Parienti JJ, Thibon P, Heller R, et al. Hand-rubbing with an aqueous alcoholic solution vs. traditional surgical hand-scrubbing and 30-day surgical site infection rates: a randomized equivalence study. JAMA 2002; 288:722–727.

[76] Chaiyakunapruk N, Veenstra DL, Lipsky BA, Saint S. Chlorhexidine compared with povidone-iodine solution for vascular catheter-site care: a meta-analysis. Ann Intern Med 2002; 136:792–801.

[77] Parienti JJ, Du Cheyron D, Ramakers M, et al. Alcoholic povidone-iodine to prevent central venous catheter colonization: a randomized unit-crossover study. Crit Care Med 2004; 32:708–713.

[78] Ruesch S, Walder B, Tramer MR. Complications of central venous catheters: internal jugular versus subclavian access – a systematic review. Crit Care Med 2002; 30:454–460.

[79] Goetz AM, Wagener MM, Miller JM, Muder RR. Risk of infection due to central venous catheters: Effect of site of placement and catheter type. Infect Control Hosp Epidemiol. 1198;19:842-845.

[80] Timsit JF. Scheduled replacement of central venous catheters is not necessary. Infect Control Hosp Epidemiol. 2000 Jun;21(6):371-4.

[81] Eyer S, Brummitt C, Crossley K, Siegel R, Cerra F. Catheter-related sepsis: prospective, randomized study of three methods of long-term catheter maintenance. Crit Care Med 1990; 18:1073–9.

[82] Uldall PR, Merchant N, Woods F, Yarworski U, Vas S. Changing subclavian haemodialysis cannulas to reduce infection. Lancet 1981; 1:1373.

[83] Guidelines for the prevention of intravascular catheter-related infections, Centers for Disease Control and Prevention. 2011.

[84] Cook D, Randolph A, Kernerman P. Central venous catheter replacement strategies: A systematic review of the literatura. Crit Care Med 1997; 25:1417–24.

[85] Mermel LA, McCormick RD, Springman SR, DG. The pathogenesis and epidemiology of catheter-related infection with pulmonary artery Swan-Ganz catheters: a prospective study utilizing molecular subtyping. Am J Med. 1991; 91:197S-205.
[86] Cobb DK, High KP, Sawyer RG. A controlled trial of scheduled replacement of central venous and pulmonary-artery catheters. New Engl J Med. 1992;327:1062-1068.
[87] Riveros E. Cambio de catéter central programado al octavo día es superior al cambio guiado por signos de infección en pacientes críticamente enfermos. Rev Col Anest. 2010;38:445-455.
[88] Trick WE, Vernon MO, Welbel SF, et al. Unnecessary use of central venous catheters: the need to look outside the intensive care unit. Infect Control Hosp Epidemiol 2004; 25:266–268.
[89] Timsit JF, Schwebel C, Bouadma L, et al. Chlorhexidine-impregnated sponges and less frequent dressing changes for prevention of catheter-related infections in critically ill adults: a randomized controlled trial. JAMA 2009; 301:1231–1241.
[90] Walder B, Pittet D, Tramer MR. Prevention of bloodstream infections with central venous catheters treated with antiinfective agents depends on catheter type and insertion time: evidence from a meta-analysis. Infect Control Hosp Epidemiol 2002; 23:748–756.
[91] Pratt RJ, Pellowe CM, Wilson JA, et al. EPIC2: National evidence-based guidelines for preventing healthcare-associated infections in NHS hospitals in England. J Hosp Infect 2007; 65:S1–S64.
[92] Barsuk JH, Cohen ER, McGaghie WC, Wayne DB. Long-term retention of central venous catheter insertion skills after simulation-based mastery learning. Acad Med 2010; 85:S9–S12.
[93] Barsuk JH, McGaghie WC, Cohen ER, et al. Simulation-based mastery learning reduces complications during central venous catheter insertion in a medical intensive care unit. Crit Care Med 2009; 37:2697–2701.
[94] Evans LV, Dodge KL, Shah TD, et al. Simulation training in central venous catheter insertion: improved performance in clinical practice. Acad Med 2010; 85:1462–1469.
[95] Evans LV, Dodge KL. Simulation and patient safety: evaluative checklists for central venous catheter insertion. Qual Saf Healthcare 2010; 19:i42–i46.
[96] Barsuk JH, Cohen ER, Feinglass J, et al. Use of simulation-based education to reduce catheter-related bloodstream infections. Arch Intern Med 2009; 169:1420–1423.
[97] Khouli H, Jahnes K, Shapiro J, et al. Performance of medical residents in sterile techniques during central vein catheterization: randomized trial of efficacy of simulation-based training. Chest 2011; 139:80–87.
[98] Marra AR, Cal RG, Durao MS, et al. Impact of a program to prevent central line-associated bloodstream infection in the zero tolerance era. Am J Infect Control 2010; 38:434–439.
[99] Weber DJ, Brown VM, Sickbert-Bennett EE, Rutala WA. Sustained and prolonged reduction in central line-associated bloodstream infections as a result of multiple interventions. Infect Control Hosp Epidemiol 2010; 31:875–877.

[100] Zingg W, Imhof A, Maggiorini M, et al. Impact of a prevention strategy targeting hand hygiene and catheter care on the incidence of catheter-related bloodstream infections. Crit Care Med 2009; 37:2167–2173.

[101] Apisarnthanarak A, Thongphubeth K, Yuekyen C, et al. Effectiveness of a catheter-associated bloodstream infection bundle in a Thai tertiary care center: a 3-year study. Am J Infect Control 2010; 38:449–455.

[102] DePalo VA, McNicoll L, Cornell M, et al. The Rhode Island ICU collaborative: a model for reducing central line-associated bloodstream infection and ventilator- associated pneumonia statewide. Qual Saf Healthcare 2010; 19:555– 561.

[103] Peredo R, Sabatier C, Villagra A, et al. Reduction in catheter-related bloodstream infections in critically ill patients through a multiple system intervention. Eur J Clin Microbiol Infect Dis 2010; 29:1173–1177.

[104] Pronovost PJ, Goeschel CA, Colantuoni E, et al. Sustaining reductions in catheter related bloodstream infections in Michigan intensive care units: observational study. BMJ 2010; 340:c309.

[105] Venkatram S, Rachmale S, Kanna B. Study of device use adjusted rates in healthcare-associated infections after implementation of 'bundles' in a closedmodel medical intensive care unit. J Crit Care 2010; 25:e11–e18.

[106] Institute for Healthcare Improvement. www.ihi.org [accessed 23 November 2011].

[107] Riveros E, Cendales S. Modelos de calidad y mejoramiento continuo en cuidado intensivo: una mirada a Norte America y Europa. Aplicación en Colombia. Acta Colombiana de Cuidado Intensivo. 2011;11:199-206.

[108] Gillies D, Wallen MM, Morrison AL, Rankin K, Nagy SA, O'Riordan E. Optimal timing for intravenous administration set replacement. Cochrane Database of Systematic Reviews 2005; Issue 4. Art. No.: CD003588. DOI: 10.1002/14651858.CD003588.pub2.

[109] Sitges-Serra A, Linares J, Perez JL, Jaurrieta E, Lorente. A randomized trial on the effect of tubing changes on hub contamination and catheter sepsis during parenteral nutrition. JPEN J Parenter Enteral Nutr. 1985 May-Jun;9(3):322-5.

[110] Snydman DR, Donnelly-Reidy M, Perry LK, Martin WJ. Intravenous tubing containing burettes can be safely changed at 72 hour intervals. Infect Control. 1987 Mar;8(3):113-6.

[111] Maki DG, Botticelli JT, LeRoy ML, Thielke TS. Prospective study of replacing administration sets for intravenous therapy at 48- vs 72-hour intervals. 72 hours is safe and cost-effective. JAMA 1987; 258:1777–81.

[112] Josephson A, Gombert ME, Sierra MF, Karanfil LV, Tansino GF. The relationship between intravenous fluid contamination and the frequency of tubing replacement. Infect Control 1985; 6:367–70.

[113] Carrasco MN, Bueno A, de las Cuevas C, Jimenez S, Salinas I, Sartorius A, Recio T, Generelo M, Ruiz-Ocaña F. Evaluation of a triple-lumen central venous heparin-coated catheter versus a catheter coated with chlorhexidine and silver sulfadiazine in critically ill patients. Intensive Care Med. 2004 Apr;30(4):633-8.

[114] Ostendorf T, Meinhold A, Harter C, Salwender H, Egerer G, Geiss HK, Ho AD, Golschmidt H. Chlorhexidine and silver-sulfadiazine coated central venous catheters in

haematologial patients-A double blind randomised, prospective controlled trial. Support Care Cancer. 2005;13:993-1000.

[115] Garland JS, Alex CP, Henrickson KJ, McAuliffe TL, Maki DG. A vancomycin-heparin lock solution for prevention of nosocomial bloodstream infection in critically ill neonates with peripherally inserted central venous catheters: a prospective, randomized trial. Pediatrics. 2005 Aug;116(2):e198-205.

[116] Filippi L, Pezzati M, Di Amario S, Poggi C, Pecile P. Fusidic acid and heparin lock solution for the prevention of catheter-related bloodstream infections in critically ill neonates: a retrospective study and a prospective, randomized trial. Pediatr Crit Care Med. 2007 Nov;8(6):556-62.

[117] Snaterse M, Rüger W, Scholte op Reimer WJM, Lucas C. Antibiotic-based catheter lock solutions for prevention of catheter-related bloodstream infection: a systematic review of randomised controlled trials. J Hosp Infect. 2010;75:1-11.

Chapter 14

Beware of Unusual Organisms Masquerading as Skin Contaminants

Marilynn R. Fairfax and Hossein Salimnia

Additional information is available at the end of the chapter

http://dx.doi.org/10.5772/50300

1. Introduction

Sepsis or bacterial blood stream infection is diagnosed by culturing blood to see what organisms grow. However, the growth of an organism in a blood culture does not always mean it is the cause of a disease. Some of blood cultures become positive because the needle that punctures the skin becomes contaminated with organisms from the patient's skin. skin and transfers them into the blood culture bottles where they grow. This gives an erroneous impression that the organisms were in the blood, causing disease, rather than on or in the skin.

These false-positive blood cultures, also known as contaminated blood cultures, represent a serious health care problem. The misperception that a patient is bacteremic may prolong hospitalization, increase cost, and lead to serious side effects including drug toxicity and *Clostridium difficile* infection. Use of antibiotics also contributes to the selection for antibiotic resistance. The presence of multi-drug resistant (MDR) bacteria may impact other patients by increasing the chance of hospital-acquired infections. To avoid these undesirable outcomes, the Clinical Laboratory Standards Institute (CLSI; Wayne, Pennsylvania) has promulgated guidelines for the identification and quantification of "contaminated cultures." A single blood culture growing one of the following skin organisms is presumed to be contaminated: coagulase-negative staphylococci (CNS), *Corynebacterium species, Bacillus species* (not *anthrasis*), *Micrococcus species, Streptococcus viridans* (alpha hemolytic streptococci), and *Proprionibacterium acnes*. These are normal skin flora and may be in adenexa below the surface of the skin and thus not subject to removal, even by careful skin preparation. Thus some contaminated cultures are inevitable. Scrupulous attention to cleaning the venipuncture site and barrier protection may contribute to reduced rates of contamination. The nature of the cleaning agent and the time of skin contact are believed to be important. Whether the personnel who draw blood cultures are trained phlebotomists as opposed to nurses or medical residents has been shown to make several percentage points of difference in the percentage of contaminated cultures. It is generally accepted that the target percentage of contaminated blood cultures should be less than 3%. However, many facilities, particularly busy emergency departments (EDs) do not achieve this goal, while other sites have a contamination rate closer to 1%. In many situations, the percentage of positive cultures that are interpreted as contaminants ranges from 25 to 50% of the total number of positive cultures. Further complicating the situation is that in very busy EDs, a second blood culture may not be drawn, and, even if the organism is not a contaminant, it would be classified as such because it could only grow in the single blood culture set. In addition, with the increase in immune-compromised patients, true infections with skin organisms have markedly increased. Both of these observations have lead to increased emphasis on the importance of drawing two blood cultures sets per episode of blood culture collection.

Modern blood culture instrumentation functions optimally with 10 ml of blood per culture bottle, or 20 ml of blood per culture set. This volume should contribute to the detection of low level bacteremias, but it is often difficult to obtain as well, because chronically ill persons, such as renal dialysis, cancer chemotherapy or bone marrow transplant patients may have compromised veins rendering difficult to impossible the collection of two culture sets, each containing an adequate volume of blood [1]. This may lead to false negativity of blood cultures. For a more complete evaluation and extensive references, see the excellent review articles by Hall and Lyman, [2]. and by Weinstein [3].

The Microbiology Division of Detroit Medical Center (DMC) University Laboratories serves the nine hospitals of the DMC (approximately 2000 beds), including two large general hospitals and others specializing in pediatrics, cancer (with a large bone marrow transplant center), acute trauma, rehabilitation, tertiary care, and surgery. In addition, microbiology receives about 50 percent of its specimens from physicians' offices and outpatient clinics, including large adult and pediatric HIV clinics, and serves as the primary or reference laboratory for two specialty hospitals. We receive approximately 80,000 blood culture sets annually. Our combined contaminated culture rate is approximately 3.7% overall. Thus we deal with over 3000 contaminated cultures per year. Not included in this number are those cultures that, although initially apparently filling the criteria for a contaminated culture, have a similar organism appearing in another blood culture within a 7-day period; these are recategorized as true infections.

To avoid working up contaminating organisms, we have established the following guidelines: for organisms that grow in a single blood culture set within seven days, and that appear, based on spot testing, as shown in Table 1, to be *Corynebacteria*, CNS, or alpha (not *Streptococcus pneumoniae* or *S. bovis*) or non-hemolytic streptococci: we do not perform either a complete identification or susceptibility testing. Due to the way we routinely process *Micrococcus sp.*, *Bacillus sp.* not *cereus* or *anthracis*, *Propionibacterium acnes*, and *Clostridium sp.* not *tetani*, they are not subjected to special limited workup as potential "contaminated cultures."

Organism Group	Tests to Identify as Potential Contaminants
Coagulase Negative Staphylococcus	Non-hemolytic, Gram positive cocci in clusters, catalase +, slide and tube coagulase -, pyrrolidinyl arylamidase -, bile esculin -
Streptococcus viridans group	Gram negative cocci in pairs and chains, alpha hemolytic, catalase -, not bile soluble
Streptococcus species, no further identification	Non-hemolytic, Gram + cocci in pairs and chains, catalase -, pyrrolidinyl arylamidase -
Corynebacterium species	Gram positive bacilli of correct morphology, catalase +, non-motile, non-hemolytic

Table 1. Spot tests used to identify potential blood culture contaminants in our laboratory if present in only one blood culture set per 7-day period

We call the Gram stain results of positive blood cultures on each patient to the clinician. If a physician follows up on the culture and finds that the laboratory regards an organism that he considers to be the etiologic agent of disease to be a presumptive contaminant, a call to the laboratory will lead to definitive identification and susceptibility testing. Or if a similar organism grows within 7 days of the original isolate, our laboratory automatically identifies and antibiotic susceptibility tests both organisms. Our clinicians are accustomed to this practice, which has been in place for more than 20 years, and are quick to call the laboratory if they feel that a full workup is warranted.

Our laboratory has detected a number of organisms that at first appeared to be typical contaminants. On further investigation, stimulated by physician request, or subsequent isolation of the same organism, they have proven to be unusual isolates. This chapter describes four of these cases, three of which have been previously published [4, 5, 6]. It describes the methodologies we used to arrive at a definitive identification, and indicates how we came to realize that they were not "typical skin contaminants." This chapter does not highlight the detection of the usual skin flora that appear to be true etiologic agents of disease, although these are far more common. We use the unusual isolates to illustrate laboratory and clinical procedures that are important when the laboratory limits workup of presumed contaminated cultures.

2. Methods

Blood for the detection of infecting organisms is cultured in aerobic and anaerobic bottles of the BACTEC 9240 blood culture system (Becton Dickinson, Deerfield, IL, USA), according to the manufacturer's instructions. When the instrument flags a blood culture bottle as positive, a Gram stain is done and the fluid is subcultured to aerobic and anaerobic agar plates. We use PNA-FISH (AdvanDx, Woburn, Massachusetts) to identify fully within one hour those blood culture organisms that exhibit Gram stain morphology compatible with *Staphylococcus aureus,* or with *Enterococcus species*. Our laboratory uses the MicroScan WalkAway 9600 (WalkAway; Siemans, Deerfield, Illinois) for the organism identification and susceptibility testing reported here. When indicated, we use the RapID Str (Remel, Lenexa, KS), and the API Coryne Strip (bioMerieux, Durham, North Carolina), for organism identification. We also utilize E strips (AB Biodisk, Solna, Sweden) for susceptibility testing as needed. We follow CLSI recommendations for susceptibility testing and result interpretation when recommendations are available (Clinical and Laboratory Standards Institute. Performance Standards for Antimicrobial Susceptibility Testing; Twentieth Information Supplement. CLSI document M100-S20(ISBN 1-56238-716-2). Clinical and Laboratory Standards Institute, 940 W. Valley Rd., Suite 1400, Wayne, Pennsylvania 19087-1898 USA, and Clinical Laboratory Standards Institute. Methods for Antimicrobial Dilution and Disk SusceptibilityTesting of Infrequently Isolated or Fastidious Bacteria; Approved Guideline. CLSI document M45-A [ISBN 1-56238-607-7].Wayne, Pennsylvania.). Ancillary tests whose use is reported in this chapter include leucine amino peptidase (LAP; LAP Disk, Remel), pyrrolidinyl arylamidase (PYR; Identicult-AE-PYR; PML Microbiologicals, Tualatin, Oregon), and the Staphyloslide latex agglutination test (BBL, Lawrence, Kansas). Organism identification by molecular techniques involved amplification and sequencing of 16S rDNA using the MicroSEQ Microbial Identification System as instructed by the manufacturer (Applied Biosystems, Carlsbad, California). Sequence data were analyzed using BLAST at the NCBI web site or the MicroSEQ ID 16S rRNA 500 v2.2 Library.

2.1. Case 1: Organism masquerading as a viridans streptococcus [4]

Case Report: On day 23 after an autologous hemopoietic stem cell transplant for acute lymphocytic leukemia, a 34 y/o man was admitted through the emergency department (ED) with fevers, neutropenia and graft failure. A single blood culture was drawn, and he was begun on empiric vancomycin (VAN) and aztreonam for neutropenic fever. Both the aerobic and anaerobic bottles from that blood culture turned positive on hospital day 3. The organism was initially thought to be a viridans streptococcus. Due to the failure of the recent, apparently successful stem cell transplant, the clinician felt that the patient had a *bone fide* infection. At his request, the organism was tested by MicroScan (PC-20 panel), which showed the organism to be VAN resistant. E-test (AB Biodisc, Solna, SW) revealed Daptomycin (DAP) susceptibility and patient was switched to DAP. Blood cultures drawn on hospital day 3 turned positive on hospital day 6 for the organism, and also for *Escherichia coli* and *Enterococcus faecalis*. Imipenem was added and the patient improved rapidly. After a second bone marrow transplant, he did well.

Laboratory investigation. Both the aerobic and anaerobic blood culture bottles of the single blood culture drawn in the ED, grew gram positive cocci/coccobacilli in pairs and chains at 12 and 24 hours respectively. The bottles were subcultured to standard aerobic and anaerobic media. After 2 days, pinpoint, α-hemolytic colonies grew both aerobically and anaerobically. The organism was catalase negative and was initially thought to be a viridans streptococcus. The next day susceptibility testing (MS PC-20 panel) performed at physician request showed the organism to be VAN R but gave no identification. The patient was switched to DAP, as described above.

The organism was tested on the RapID™ Str panel which identified it as *Streptococcus intermedius, Listeria monocytogenes* or *Pediococcus pentosaceus*, depending on what assumptions were made about ambiguous biochemicals. MicroSeq sequencing and BLAST analysis of the first 500 bases of the 16S rDNA gene revealed the highest identity between our isolate and *Weissella confusa* and *W. cibaria*. We next sequenced the entire 16S rDNA gene. The 1493 base-long sequence showed 100% identity to the sequence of *W. confusa* strain Inje LM S-338 (1492/1493; DQ321751.1).

Approximately 6 months later, a similar VAN-R organism with a slightly different susceptibility profile was isolated from multiple blood cultures of a patient in the burn unit at another of our component hospitals. An alert technologist recognized the biochemical profile from the MicroScan, and sent it for rDNA sequencing to confirm its identity as *W. confusa*. *W. confusa* has been found in fermented foods and has also been reported as a cause of sepsis in 5 other patients [7, 8, 9]. These human cases, like ours, were VAN-R.

Commentary: The MicroScan does not have *W. confusa* in its data base, and thus could not be expected to identify the organism. However, the biochemical reactions were clear cut and allowed recognition of the subsequent patient's isolate. In contrast, the RapID Str panel, which has *W. confusa* in its data base, provided several erroneous identifications, all at high probability, depending on what assumptions were made about ambiguous biochemical reactions. Fortunately our experienced laboratorians realized that the α-hemolysis, the Gram stain morphology, and the VAN resistance rendered each of these identifications unlikely. Molecular identification was definitive.

2.2. Case 2: Organism masquerading as a coagulase-negative Staphylococcus

Case Report: A 45 year old female with congestive heart failure and a long history of end stage renal failure, on dialysis, was admitted through the ED for chest pain and back pain. She was afebrile. A myocardial infarction was ruled out. On hospital day 2 she developed a fever to 102F and two blood cultures were drawn. The initial culture bottle turned positive within 24 hr and the fluid was positive for Gram positive cocci in clusters. PNA-FISH analysis suggested that it was not *S. aureus*. On culture, it first appeared to be a CNS, and thus a presumed skin contaminant. However the second culture turned positive later that day and grew a similar organism, leading to a full workup. Despite negative PNA-FISH and coagulase tests, MicroScan identified the organism as a methicillin-sensitive *S. aureus*. VAN was administered after her dialysis, and her fever resolved within 24 hr. Follow up blood cultures were negative.

Laboratory investigation: The isolate grew in both the aerobic and anaerobic bottles of the both blood culture sets within 24-36 hrs. Staining revealed Gram-positive cocci in clusters. PNA-FISH analyses, performed on the fluid withdrawn from the culture bottles, were negative for *S. aureus*. Both the tube and slide coagulase tests were negative, suggesting coagulase-negative *Staphylococcus species*. However, when the organism was inoculated into the MicroScan panel, it was identified as *S. aureus*. Further, the Staphyloslide latex agglutination test, which detects both clumping factor (the cause of positive slide coagulase tests) and staphylococcal protein A, was positive as would be expected with *S. aureus*. We presume the Staphyloslide detected protein A, since the slide coagulase was negative. The organism utilized mannitol in the presence of salt, again suggesting *S. aureus*. Isolates from all 4 bottles had identical colony morphologies and identical MICs (in μg/ml) including:

Oxicillin 0.5, VAN 1, Erythromycin >4 (Resistant) and Clindamycin resistant by the D test for inducible resistance. 16S rDNA sequencing and BLAST analysis identified the organism as *S. pseudolugdenensis/pettenkorferi.*

Commentary: This isolate was identified with >90% confidence as S. aureus by the MicroScan, and its positive reactions on mannitol salt and on Staphyloslide latex agglutination appeared to confirm its identity as S. aureus. However, the organism's failure to react with the PNA-FISH S. aureus probe and its lack of slide and tube coagulase activity were strongly opposed to this diagnosis. As stated above, we presume that the Staphyloslide latex agglutination test reacted with staphylococcal protein A, which is supposed to be adequate to identify S. aureus. 16S rRNA sequencing and BLAST analysis identified the organism as S. pseudolugdenensis/pettenkorpheri, each of which has been reported to be the etiologic agent of sepsis in some cases, and a presumed skin contaminant in others [10, 11]. The organism seems more likely to represent S. *pettenkorferi*, as S. pseudolugdenensis is reported to by pyrrolidolyl arylamidase positive and our organism was not. Had we not performed the PNA-FISH analysis on this organism, we might have called it a very rare S. aureus that was negative for both slide and tube coagulase. Because of the general susceptibility of the organism, this would not have affected the antibiotic susceptibility result interpretation; but such may not always be the case as CLSI recommends different susceptibility breakpoints for S. aureus and CNS. They further recommend that the S. aureus susceptibility interpretations be used for S. lugdenensis. Whether this should apply to some of the other CNS, and if so to which ones, remain to be determined. Fortunately the patient responded rapidly to VAN therapy. The identity of the organism was not known until after she had been discharged. We had not previously seen such an organism, but over the last several years, other patients, not all of them on dialysis, were found to have infections by similar organisms.

2.3. Case 3: Organism masquerading as a Corynebacterium [5]

Case Report: A 20-year-old female with relapsed T precursor cell leukemia received an allogeneic peripheral blood stem cell transplant from an unmatched male donor (C and DQ mismatch). She engrafted on post-transplant day (PTD) 9, and her maximum neutrophil count was 3.0 x 10^9/L. Transplant complications included hyperacute graft-versus-host disease (GVHD) of the skin, chemotherapy-related mucositis, and neutropenic fever. Therapy included tacrolimus, methylprednisolone, and mycophenolate mofetil.

On PTD 61, she developed abdominal cramping, nausea, vomiting, and diarrhea. Colonoscopy showed diffuse erythema and extensive colitis with numerous erosions. Biopsy confirmed Stage III GVHD. She received intravenous (IV) piperacillin/tazobactam for 14 days for a febrile episode that developed after the endoscopy; blood cultures showed no growth. After 3 days of IV antibiotic therapy, another febrile episode occurred, associated with a blood culture positive for coagulase-negative staphylococcus and *P. acnes*. Therapy with IV vancomycin was added. Within 48 h, after the antibiotics were discontinued, she developed a low-grade fever, and her absolute neutrophil count (ANC) decreased markedly. Therapy with mycophenolate mofetil was discontinued, and filgrastim treatment was begun to raise her ANC.

Two blood cultures drawn over several days were positive for a Gram positive rod which appeared to be a Corynebacterium species. VAN was restarted. One negative blood culture was followed by several more that were positive for the same organism. One of the blood cultures was also positive for Candida glabrata. Therapy with IV micafungin was added. The Hickman catheter, suspected to be the source of the bacteremia/fungemia was removed and the catheter tip grew the bacterium. Because it initially grew in two blood cultures, the presumptive Corynebacterium was identified and susceptibility tested. Based on the susceptibility results, VAN was discontinued, and IV ampicillin, 2 g every 6 hr was administered. The patient became afebrile within 24 hr, and her ANC stabilized at 2 x 10^9/L.

Laboratory Investigation: The organism from the first positive blood culture grew as small, grey, non-hemolytic colonies that were catalase positive, leading to a presumptive identification of *Corynebacterium sp.* Another culture, drawn before the initiation of VAN therapy, was also positive with the same organism. The growth of the organism in multiple blood cultures, and a call to the laboratory by the clinician requesting that the initial isolate be worked up due to the decrease in the patient's ANC, lead to organism identification and susceptibility testing. API Coryne Strips identified all isolates as *Listeria grayi*. Susceptibility testing suggested that it was resistant to VAN (MIC: ≥32 μg/ml) by E Test, but susceptible to ampicilllin (MIC 0.5 mg/ml). After the presumptive source of infection was removed and ampicillin was started, she rapidly became afebrile.

Commentary. *L. grayi* is one of the presumed "non-pathogenic" *Listeria*, although it has been reported as the cause of bacteremia in other immune-compromised hosts [12, 13]. It lacks the beta hemolysin that is a presumed factor in the pathogenesis of the more virulent *L. monocytogenes*. Susceptibility of *L. grayi* to VAN has not been investigated. Although no interpretive criteria for MICs for this rare organism exist, a VAN MIC of ≥32 μg/ml is interpreted as resistant for all organisms which do have such criteria. The ampicillin MIC would be interpreted as susceptible for such organisms. Both interpretations were presumed to apply to this organism, and the assumption were apparently validated by the patient's response to therapy.

2.4. Case 4: Organism masquerading as a Corynebacterium [6]

Case Report: A 39-year-old African-American male, known to be HIV positive, with a recent CD-4 count of 33 cells/mm^3, presented to the ED complaining of epigastric and left upper quadrant pain. He reported allergy to trimethoprim sulfamethoxazole (TMS) and to most beta-lactam antibiotics, although not to cefotetan, which he had received successfully before. He had previously been treated for *Cryptococcus neoformans* meningoencephalitis and for *Toxoplasma gondii* infections of the central nervous system. He reported compliance with the dapsone prescribed for *Pneumocystis* prophylaxis, but only occasionally took his antiretroviral therapy. His temperature was 104.4F and heart rate was 129 beats/min. His neutrophil count was 8600 cells/ $mm^{3.}$ No biochemical abnormalities were detected. Two blood cultures were drawn, and cefotetan and gentamycin were started for a presumed intra-abdominal abscess. Chest roentgenograms were unremarkable. CT scan of the abdomen showed hepatomegaly and calcification of the pancreas. Both adrenal glands were enlarged with heterogeneous attenuation, consistent with abscesses. The kidneys were enlarged with a 2.5 x 3 cm area of attenuation in the right kidney. On hospital day 2, a CT-guided aspiration of an adrenal abscess yielded 15 cc of purulent fluid. Stain of the fluid was interpreted as showing Gram-positive cocci in chains. Antibiotics were continued.

On hospital day 4, growth was detected in the both aerobic bottles of the blood cultures drawn on day 1. Gram stain revealed positive rods. At this time the patient developed electrolyte abnormalities suggesting adrenal insufficiency and a cosyntropin stimulation test showed a blunted response with aldosterone levels < 1 ng/ml.

On hospital day 5 the patient developed hypotension, hypoglycemia, and hyperkalemia: hydrocortisone and fludrocortisone were administered. On hospital day 6, antibiotic susceptibility results of the blood isolate became available. Because of the reported allergy to TMS, doxycycline was added. By the next day (hospital day 7), the patient was afebrile, and felt well. For this reason, even when told that the organism was likely a *Nocardia*, the clinicians elected to continue doxycycline.

On hospital day 22 (day 16 of doxycycline) fever and abdominal pain recurred and the patient reported a headache. Ataxia and grand mal seizures occurred. Blood cultures were drawn. An MRI of the patient's brain revealed numerous small lesions that had not been there a year previously. After questioning about the history of his TMS allergy, which was vague, the patient was started on TMS, imipenem, amikacin, and ciprofloxacin. Other antibiotics were discontinued. Within days, the patient's fever, abdominal pain, and neurologic abnormalities had resolved. He was alive and well 18 months later.

Laboratory Investigation: On hospital day 5, the blood and chocolate agar plates inoculated on day 4 from the positive blood culture bottles grew tiny, beige, non-hemolytic, catalase-positive colonies, suggestive of *Corynebacterium sp.*. These were used to inoculate a MicroScan panel and an API Coryne strip. The next day, the MicroScan panel and the Coryne strip gave no identification but MicroScan MICs were available. Using the CLSI interpretations for Gram positive organisms other than *Streptococcus pneumoniae*, the organism was resistant to ampicillin and gentamicin and susceptible to TMS and to tetracycline (≤ 2 μg/ml). On hospital day 7, the adrenal culture became positive with numerous beige, catalase positive colonies growing on the blood agar plate. When staining revealed Gram positive rods, the original Gram stain was reviewed. The organisms previously thought to be Gram-positive cocci in chains were recognized as beaded, Gram positive rods, a classic finding on Gram stains of *Nocardia*. Examination of the now two-day-old plates from the positive blood cultures revealed that the colonies were larger, irregular and darker with a strong odor of wet dirt, also characteristic of *Nocardia*. The organisms were partially but not fully acid fast. The clinicians were notified that the organism was likely a *Nocardia species*. Biochemical testing was begun and the genus was confirmed based on lysozyme resistance and urease positivity.

On hospital day 8, the MicroScan MIC from the adrenal isolate yielded an MIC for tetracycline of 8 μg/ml, the implications of which were unclear. *Nocardia* generally grow too slowly for MIC determinations, and the technique has not been validated for these organisms. No Nocardia grew on his respiratory culture.

Blood cultures drawn when the patient's fever recurred and he developed seizures also grew beige, catalase-positive colonies with a wet dirt odor, and the Gram stain was positive for beaded Gram positive rods. At the request of the clinicians, it was tested for tetracycline susceptibility and the tetracycline MIC was ≥ 128 μl.

The organism was identified as a member of the *Nocardia asteroides* complex based on its inability to hydrolyze xanthine, tyrosine, or casein within 21 days. 16S rDNA sequencing revealed that the organism was *N. farcinica.*

Commentary: This patient with advanced HIV disease had a complicated course of infection with *N. farcinica,* a virulent member of the *N. asteroides* complex. His therapy was complicated by the initial misinterpretation of the Gram stain morphology, a recurrent problem with *Nocardia* which is frequently beaded, and by the subsequent impression that this rapidly growing organism was a *Corynebacterium*: it grew so rapidly that the possibility of its being *Nocardia* was not considered initially. The hypothesis that the blood isolate should be classified as a skin contaminant that might not be worked up was eliminated when we called the Gram stain result from the first positive blood culture to the clinician who was emphatic about the need to work up the organism, but realization of the genus of the organism and of the fact that the isolates from the adrenals and the blood were identical took several more days.

Unlike our patient's isolates, *Nocardia* usually grow too slowly to be susceptibility tested by MIC, even by accident. The cumbersome agar dilution technique, rather than determination of MICs, is the standard for susceptibility testing of *Nocardia,* so most infections are treated empirically. Before the organism was identified but after the MIC to tetracycline was determined to be very low, this patient was treated with doxycycline and responded dramatically.. Although the initial isolate appeared susceptible, the tetracycline MIC of the organism that appeared after relapse was determined at clinician request: it had increased dramatically into a range that would routinely be interpreted as resistant in other organisms.

Nocardia is still a common cause of death in AIDS patients, but in the U. S. its incidence was low, even prior to the era of highly active antiretroviral therapy, probably since TMS, given to many patients with advanced HIV disease for *Pneumocystis* prophylaxis, is also active against *Nocardia* [14]. Because of his presumed allergy to TMS, this patient received dapsone prophylaxis which does not affect *Nocardia.* Most common infections with *Nocardia* are respiratory, but infections at other body sites in the absence of pulmonary infection are known [14]. The brain is probably the most common extrapulmonary site of infection, with single and multiple abscesses reported. Our patient represents the first case of bilateral adrenal abscesses with adrenal insufficiency which is thought to require more than 90% destruction of the adrenal tissue. Renal abscess is also unusual. Our patient also had positive blood cultures, which are very rare although hematogenous spread of the organism from the lung to extrapulmonary sites is the postulated route of dissemination. Two cases of *Nocardia* bacteremia prior to our patient did have pulmonary disease [15, 16]. However our patient did not, so the source for his initial bacteremia is unclear. Our patient's disease symptoms paralleled the presence, resolution and recurrence of his bacteremia.

3. Discussion

Each year, our laboratory receives approximately 80,000 blood culture sets. On average, about 3.7%, or approximately 3000 of these meet the criteria for contaminated cultures. Some isolates, such as the ones described here meet the initial criteria, but, because of growth in multiple cultures, they are removed from the list and are not represented above. Others are worked up at physician request, and are removed from the list if the organism identification changes. Appropriate classification of and reduced work up of contaminated blood cultures is very important: it saves technologist time, and avoids unnecessary laboratory expenses. It prevents providing a report to the treating physician that could lead to the use of unnecessary antibiotics, and ultimately to harm to the patient due to drug side effects or to the development of antibiotic-associated *Clostridium difficile* infections. It may result in a patient being discharged from the hospital sooner since a diagnosis of sepsis is avoided. It helps retard the selection for drug-resistant bacteria. However, it is important to realize that while some organisms at first appear to be contaminants, they are actually etiologic agents of disease. Most such bacteria are actually skin organisms, often infecting immune-compromised hosts. This chapter highlights the isolation of four unusual organisms that also appeared at first to be contaminants but later proved to be unusual and significant etiologic agents of disease. Three of the four reports have been published previously [4, 5, 6]. However, it has a number of other messages as well.

Our data emphasizes the importance of drawing two blood culture sets at the outset of a new episode of presumed sepsis. Failure to draw the second culture could lead to the failure to work up an organism that is actually the etiologic agent of disease, but appears to be a contaminant found in only one culture.

A related issue is that the organisms discussed here are Gram-positive and most are VAN-resistant. All the isolates on the list of usual skin contaminants are Gram positive, so this is not surprising. The inclusion of VAN in many empiric regimens for presumed sepsis may predispose the at risk patient to subsequent infections with VAN-resistant organisms. .It is clear that VAN cannot be assumed to be the drug of choice for treatment of all Gram positive organisms. In one of the cases presented here, those in the laboratory recognized the importance of the infective organism because it was VAN resistant. Only one blood culture was drawn in the ED, and VAN was part of the empiric antibiotic cocktail started for febrile neutropenia or presumed sepsis. The treatment failure caused by the organism's resistance to VAN lead to the collection of additional cultures, and the same organism grew again. Full work up of the organism was begun, and it was soon recognized that the organism was an unusual isolate, and not the skin organism suggested by the spot testing. Infections with organisms that were susceptible to VAN might have resolved and been missed in this scenario.

Our results also stress the importance of close interactions between the clinicians and laboratory personnel. Workup of several of the organisms reported here was begun at clinician request in the absence of a second blood culture set, or before the second blood culture set had turned positive, because the clinicians were convinced that the patient was septic. They did not want a delay in the proper identification and susceptibility testing of the infecting organism, regardless of the presumptive identification. Such interactions result in good, cost-effective patient care.

It should be noted that such procedures can be a double-edged sword. Clinicians need to be aware that the laboratory limits the work-up of presumed contaminants and intervene quickly as needed. Microbiology laboratory professionals need to be alert to the fact that since the number of immune-compromised patients has increased, the potential for actual infections by normal skin flora is also increased. Furthermore, although in the majority of cases it is good medical practice to not work up the contaminated blood cultures, the clinical microbiologist must keep a high index of suspicion for unusual, low-prevalence pathogens that can resemble routine causes of contaminated blood cultures.

Identification of most of the organisms discussed here was accomplished or confirmed by molecular techniques. At one time organism identification by polymerase chain reaction and DNA sequencing (using 16S rDNA as a target, for example) was regarded as esoteric and prohibitively expensive. Now such testing is offered by many major hospital systems and reference laboratories. Compared to the expense of having laboratory personnel expend significant time and supplies in identifying atypical organisms, molecular identification, whether performed in house or by a reference laboratory, is often more rapid and financially prudent [17].

Author details

Marilynn R. Fairfax and Hossein Salimnia
Department of Pathology, Wayne State University School of Medicine, and Detroit Medical Center University Laboratories, Detroit, Michigan, USA

4. References

[1] Donnino, MW, Goyal N., Terlecki TM., Donnino KF, Miller JB, Otero RM, Howell MD. 2007. Inadequate Blood Volume Collected for Culture: A Survey of Health Care Professionals. Mayo Clin Proc 82: 1069-1072.
[2] Hall KK, Lyman JA. 2006. Updated review of blood culture contamination. Clin Microbiol Rev. 19:788-802.
[3] Weinstein, MP. 2003. Blood culture contamination: persisting problems and partial progress. J. Clin. Microbiol.. 41: 2275-2278.
[4] Salimnia H , Alangaden GJ , Bharadwaj R, Painter TM, Chandraskar PH, Fairfax MR. 2011. Weissella confusa: an unexpected cause of vancomycin-resistant bacteremia in immunocompromised hosts. Transpl. Inf. Dis. 13:294-8.

[5] Salimnia H, Patel D, Lephart PR, Fairfax MR, Chandrasekar PH. 2010. Listeria grayi: vancomycin-resistant, gram-postivive rod causing bacteremia in a stem cell transplant recipient. Transpl. Infect. Dis. 12: 526-528.

[6] Arabi Y, Fairfax MR, Szuba MJ, Crane L, Schuman P. 1996. Adrenal insufficiency, recurrent bacteremia, and disseminated abscesses caused by *Nocardia asteroides* in a patient with acquired immunodeficiency syndrome. Diagn. Microbiol. Infect. Dis. 24:47-51.

[7] Green M, Wadowsky RM, Barbadora K. 1990. Recovery of vancomycin-resistant gram positive cocci from children. J. Clin. Microbiol. 28: 484-488.

[8] Olano A, Chua J, Schroeder S, LaSalvia M, Hall G. 2001. Weissella confusa (basonym: Lactobacillus confusus) bacteremia: a case report. J. Clin. Microbiol 39: 1604-1607.

[9] Flaherty JD, Levett PN, Dewhirst FE, Troe TE, Warren JR, Johnson S. 2003. Fatal case of endocarditis due to Weissella confusa. J. Clin Microbiol. 41: 2237-2239.

[10] Trulzsch K, Grabein B, Schumann A, Mellman A, Antonenka U, Heesemann J, Becker K. 2007. Staphylococcus pettenkoferi sp. nov., a novel coagulase-negative staphylococcal species isolated from human clinical specimens. International Journal of Systematic and Evolutionary Microbiology. 57, 1543–1548.

[11] Tang YW, Han J, McCormac MA, Li H, Stratton CW. 2008. Staphylococcus pseudolugdenensis sp. nov., a pyrrolidonyl arylamidase/ornithine decarboxylase-positive bacterium isolated from blood cultures. Diagn Microbiol Infect Dis. 60:351-359.

[12] Todeschini G, Friso L, Lombardi S, Casaril M, Fontana R, Corrocher R. 1998. A case of Listeria murrayi/grayi bacteremia in a patient with advanced Hodgkin's disease. Eur J Clin Microbiol Infect Dis. 17: 808-810.

[13] Rapose A, Lick SD, Ismail N. 2008. Listeria grayi bacteremia in a heart transplant. Recipient Transpl. Infect. Dis. 10: 434-436.

[14] Uttamchandani RB, Daikos GI, Reyes RR, Fischl MA, Dickenson GM. Yamaguchi E, Kramer MR. 1994. Nocardiosis in patients with advanced human immunodeficiency virus infection: clinical features and outcome. Clin Infect Dis 18: 348-353.

[15] Javaly K, Horowitz, HW, Wormser GP. 1992. Nocardiosis in patients with human immunodeficiency virus infection: report of 2 cases and review of literature. Medicine (Baltimore) 71: 128-138.

[16] Kim J, Minamoto GY, Grieco MH. 1991. Nocardial infection as a complication of AIDS. Report of six cases and review of the literature. Rev Inf Dis 13: 624-629.

[17] Bharadwaj R, Swaminathan S, Salimnia H, Fairfax M, Frey A, Chandrasekar PH. 2012. Clinical impact of the use of 16S rRNA sequencing method for the identification of "difficult-to-identify" bacteria in immunocompromised hosts. Transpl Infect Dis. 14:206–212.

Chapter 15

Blood Culture Systems: From Patient to Result

Andries William Dreyer

Additional information is available at the end of the chapter

http://dx.doi.org/10.5772/50139

1. Introduction

Bacteraemia and sepsis is associated with a high mortality and an increased incidence of hospital stay and associated costs (1, 2). A recent multicentre retrospective evaluation has shown that more than 80% of bacteraemias and fungaemias occur within the hospital or other heathcare settings, with indwelling catheters being the most common source (3).

Blood cultures are still considered to be the 'gold standard' for the detection of microbial pathogens related to bacteraemia and sepsis despite newer molecular techniques (4, 5). This method allows for microbial identification and susceptibility testing to be performed which is a critical component to managing sepsis, however the lack of rapid results and decreased sensitivity for fastidious pathogens has led to the development of improved systems and adjunctive molecular or proteomic testing.

Clinicians need to utilize their respective laboratories' culturing systems optimally by adhering to the correct way of submitting blood culture specimens, understanding the principle of the testing method and making informed decisions regarding the results obtained.

This chapter will focus on the use of blood culture systems in the era of modern technology and aim to highlight the best practice from collection to interpretation of results.

2. The blood culture

The term blood culture refers to a single venipuncture, either from a peripheral site or central or arterial line, with blood inoculated into one or more blood culture bottles. One bottle is considered a blood culture where two or more are considered a set. Multiple sets are from multiple venipunctures and are associated with different sites.

Bacteraemia is defined as the presence of microorganisms in the blood, compared to sepsis which is defined as bacteraemia in the presence of clinical symptoms and signs such as fever, tachycardia, tachypnea and hypotension.

The sensitivity and specificity of the test are influenced by the clinicians' ability to predict bacteraemia or sepsis prior to collection. The clinical indication will guide the timing and the numbers of cultures being send. The person taking the sample will also influence the results by adhering to aseptic technique and inoculating the correct volume.

Blood cultures are taken to establish microbial invasion of the vascular system. Common mechanisms include dissemination from a primary site after inadequate control by host defense mechanisms, intravascular device mediated or infection of the vascular system e.g. infective endocarditis. Transient bacteraemia occur due to translocation of bacteria e.g. during chewing with rapid clearance by immune mechanisms compared to intermittent bacteraemia where bacteria are periodically released into the blood from e.g. an abscess while continuous bacteraemia points to an intravascular infection.

Blood cultures should always be obtained to investigate the possibility of a bacteraemia. Various indications will lead to obtaining these samples (Table 1). Clinical parameters e.g. fever, raised inflammatory markers and suggestive imaging as well as a clinical suspicion of specific disease entities e.g. meningitis, pneumonia, osteomyelitis and pyelonephritis will prompt clinicians to investigate for bacteraemia. Part of the diagnostic criteria for infective endocarditis include obtaining positive blood cultures (6, 7). Blood cultures are taken to confirm or exclude central line associated bloodstream infection (CLABSI) as well as to follow up the response to therapy in certain conditions e.g. fungaemia and infective endocarditis.

Acute bacterial sepsis	Meningitis
	Pneumonia
	Osteomyelitis
	Pyelonephritis
Vascular	Infective endocarditis
Closed space infections	Intra-abdominal abscesses
Catheter related bacteraemia	
Follow up cultures	Fungaemia, infective endocarditis

Table 1. Indications for taking blood cultures

The yield of blood cultures will depend on the site of infection. Up to 99% of blood cultures can be positive with acute suppurative thrombophlebitis, up to 50% with acute bacterial meningitis and only 2% with acute cellulites.

3. Principles of blood culture collection

Collection of blood cultures is a critical component and can either positively affect the patient outcome by providing an accurate diagnosis or adversely affect the outcome by prolonging antimicrobial therapy and the length of hospital stay with the isolation of a contaminant.

3.1. Timing

In general, clinicians will collect blood cultures around the time of temperature elevation to increase the chance of detecting bacteraemia, however this practice can become complicated especially in patients that are hypothermic or unable to mount a temperature response with clinical sepsis. Fever can also be related to non-infectious causes e.g. drug reaction or malignancy. A multiceneter study showed no significant enhanced detection of bacteraemia when taking cultures around elevated temperatures (8).

The general rule of sending two to three blood culture sets from different sites in a period of 24 hours has also been challenged. For continuous bacteraemia e.g. infective endocarditis the first culture are likely to be positive in contrast to patients with intermittent bacteraemia where 3 or more cultures over a period of time may necessary to detect the pathogen. A study showed no difference in taking cultures simultaneously or serially at spaced intervals (9).

Current recommendation with regard to timing and interval include obtaining two sets within minutes apart from two distinct sites at the onset of the 24 hour period with two subsequent sets being taking at different time intervals over the 24 hour period if the clinical condition deteriorates (10).

Blood cultures taken while on antimicrobial therapy will prevent detection of some bacteraemias, therefore sampling should precede administration of antibiotics at all costs. If patients are on antimicrobial therapy, specific resin containing bottles must be used to neutralize antimicrobials and enhance pathogen detection. Antimicrobial therapy should however never be withheld to obtain subsequent cultures at different intervals.

Key points!

1. Blood cultures must be taken on suspicion of bacteraemia and not only around fever spikes.
2. Two sets must be taken at the onset of a 24 hour period within minutes apart.
3. Two more sets can be obtained during the 24 hour period if the clinical condition deteriorates.
4. Blood cultures must be obtained before administration of antimicrobial agents.

3.2. Site

The recommended practice is to obtain a blood culture from a peripheral venipuncture, however patients who are critically ill and where venous access is a problem will have a central venous catheter (CVC) or an arterial line from which sampling can be performed. This practice has been discouraged due to the concerns of possible contamination (11, 12). Other studies have shown the benefit of using sampling from CVCs to detect bacteraemia (13, 14). A recent study by Beutz et al in 2003 evaluated the clinical utility of using blood cultures taken through central venous catheters and peripheral venipunctures in critically ill medical patients and found an overall good negative predictive value, however they warned that in a setting with a high incidence of true bacteraemia the use of taking cultures either through CVCs or peripheral venipunctures should be interpreted with caution, as many critically ill patients who are receiving antimicrobials through their central lines can have negative cultures despite true bacteraemia. They recommend that in patients with a CVC, blood cultures from both the CVC and peripheral venipuncture should be obtained to increase sensitivity but that additional samples may be necessary to trouble shoot discordant results (15). A recent meta-analysis also showed better sensitivity and negative predictive value with cultures taken from an intravascular site and therefore recommends that at least one culture should be from the CVC (16).

The practice of using the two needle technique, removing the needle after drawing the blood and attaching another sterile needle to inoculate the blood into the bottle, is currently discouraged due to the risk of acquiring needlestick injuries although a meta-analysis showed a slight reduction in contamination rates (17).

Key points!

1. Peripheral venipuncture is preferred.
2. If an invasive line is present, do both and correlate.
3. Keep in mind that the culture from the CVC may be negative if antimicrobials are administered through the line, despite true bacteraemia.
4. Although the negative predictive value of one culture is good, the sensitivity of taking a culture either peripherally or through a CVC is not adequate.

3.3. Skin antisepsis

Blood culture contamination can lead to significant increase in healthcare related costs (12). Skin antisepsis therefore plays a critical role in reducing these contaminants.

Various antisepsis agents are commercially available and these agents differ by onset of action, mechanism of action and cost. A comparison between povidine – iodine, 70% isopropyl – alcohol, tincture of iodine and povidine – iodine with 70% alcohol detected no significant difference with regard to blood culture contamination rates (18).

Current infection control bundles for insertion of central line catheters and best practice guidelines for taking of blood cultures recommend using 2% chlorhexidine – gluconate in 70% isopropyl – alcohol as skin antisepsis due to the enhanced activity compared to other formulations (19).

In addition to alcohol containing antiseptics, the use of a prepackage antiseptic may play a role in reducing contamination rates (20). ChloraPrep (Enturia Limited) is a commercial antisepsis system that uses a plastic applicator to release 2% chlorhexidine – gluconate and 70% isopropyl – alcohol into a sponge thereby reducing cross contamination from the care givers' hands. A study by Tepus et al has shown a reduction in culture contamination rates (21) whereas another showed no significant decrease compared to 70% alcohol impregnated wipes (22).

Key points!

1. Various skin antisepsis agents are commercially available.
2. These agents are equally effective in reducing blood culture contamination rates.
3. The current recommended agent for skin antisepsis when performing venipuncture is 2% chlorhexidine – gluconate in 70% isopropyl – alcohol.

3.4. Volume and number of cultures

Adequate sample volume remains a critical factor to detect bacteraemia and have been evaluated extensively over last few years. Clinical and Laboratory Standards Institute (CLSI) recommend four 10 ml bottles to detect 90 – 95% of bacteraemias (23). In order to detect up to 99% of organisms a total of 60 ml of blood will need to be cultured (11).

In the early 1980s Washington proposed that culturing of a higher volume will result in a higher detection rate of blood stream infections (24, 25, 26), however the question arose whether this dictum still holds true for the newer continuous monitoring blood culture systems. Weinstein answered the question by comparing the speed and yield of detection of microorganisms from aerobic bottles inoculated with both 5 ml and 10 ml using a continuous monitoring blood culture system by showing the overall recovery of microorganisms to be higher with the 10 ml inoculated bottles ($P < 0.001$) (27).

An interesting study found that the higher the age of the patient and the severity of the underlying condition significantly influenced the collection and subsequent culturing of lower volumes of blood. The study also demonstrated that in critically ill patients, the higher the volume cultured, the more bacteraemias were detected and the yield of microorganism recovery increased by 3.5% per additional milliliter of blood cultured (28).

Current recommendations include collecting at least two sets of, each 20 ml of blood distributed equally between an aerobic and an anaerobic bottle from two distinct sites (10, 29). Lee et al reported that in order to detect 90% of true bacteraemias, 2 blood culture sets should be taken in a 24 hour period, however to detect > 99% up to 4 blood culture sets may be necessary (30).

Single blood cultures should be discouraged due their lack of sensitivity and difficult interpretation e.g. isolating coagulase negative *staphylococci* (CoNS) from a single blood culture may represent contamination or true bacteraemia (29).

A recent study reported yields from consecutive cultures from patients without infective endocarditis to be 65.1% after the first blood culture, 80.4% after the second blood culture and 95.7% after third blood culture. They also observed a high positivity from the first culture in patients with infective endocarditis which supports the observation of a continuous bacteraemia and fungaemia in this patient group (10).

Although paediatric bottles have been adapted to accommodate much smaller volumes of blood the optimal amount remains unknown. It is common practice to culture not more than

1 – 2 ml of blood in neonates. One study suggests that failure to detect bacteraemia was more likely when culturing < 1 ml of blood (31).

Human blood contains various factors or substances that can interfere with the detection of micro-organisms e.g. host serum factors and also antimicrobial agents. Therefore inoculated blood must be diluted to a point where these substances will have a minimal inhibitory effect. The required dilutional factor has been evaluated before and up to 10 times dilution has been recommended (32, 33), however the blood – broth ratio required for various systems will differ according to manufactures' instruction. The VersaTREK (TREK Diagnostic Systems, Cleveland, Ohio) is adapted to accommodate smaller volumes from as little as 0.1 ml – 10 ml, however the manufacture still recommends using 10 ml to achieve a 1:9 blood – broth ratio in the 80 ml bottle. Inoculating at dilutions higher than 1:10 may be associated with a lower yield due to the decreased overall volume cultured (29).

Key points!

1. The higher the volume, the higher the yield.
2. Up to 4 blood culture sets in a 24 hour period may be necessary to detect > 99% of microorganisms.
3. As least 1 ml must be cultured in neonates.
4. Adequate blood – broth ratio of 1:10 must be achieved to dilute the effects of inhibitory substances and antimicrobials present in the blood.

3.5. Training

Education and training of staff responsible for collection of blood cultures is critical. Studies have shown a decrease in contamination rates associated with combining different measures with training (34, 35) with the one study reporting contamination rates from phlebotomist vs. non-phlebotomists to be 0.8% and 4.7% respectively (35).

Key points!

1. Lower contamination rates are possible with dedicated phlebotomists.

3.6. Clinical information and labeling

Although all positive blood cultures are regarded as significant, false positive results can occur and interpretation becomes critical. Clinical information can aid the laboratory to decide whether an isolate is more likely to be significant or a contaminant (See section on Blood culture contamination).

Labeling of each bottle especially indicating the site through which the sample was taken is of critical importance to the laboratory. Sets taken through catheter lines are more likely to be contaminated and therefore correct labeling can aid interpretation.

Avoid applying the label over the barcode or the bottom of the bottle, this practice cover the sensor that is critical for detection and can result in false positive signals.

Key points!

1. Label bottle with the site where the sample was obtained from.
2. Covering the sensor at the bottom of the bottle can result in false positive signals.

3.7. Blood culture collection kits

This new strategy to decrease blood culture contamination has been implemented in some centers. The kit contains a pre-packaged antiseptic e.g. ChloraPrep sponge, a blood collection set (needle, syringe, safety lock etc), bottles and an instruction leaflet. A study evaluating the impact of these blood culture collection kits showed a reduction in blood culture contamination rates from 9.2% – 3.8%, however introduction of the kit was associated with an unintended yet sustained decrease in the amount of blood cultures collected which may have resulted in an unwanted reduction in the amount of true Gram negative bacteraemias (34). The authors recommend using the kit with ongoing training and ensuring that availability and accessibility are not compromised. Weightman et al also reported a decrease in contamination rates observed at their centre after the introduction of blood culture collection kits from 6% - 2.7% without compromising the amount of investigations performed (35).

Key points!

1. Blood culture collection kits can decrease blood culture contamination rates.

4. Selection of the correct blood culture bottle

Blood culture sets generally consist of and aerobic an anaerobic bottle. Various different bottles are available depending on the continuous monitoring system used. These bottles are specifically designed to optimize recovery of both aerobic and anaerobic organisms. This section will highlight the principles of these bottles by discussing a few examples, more detail with regard to specific bottles not mentioned should be obtained from the manufacturer.

Despite a decrease in the amount of anaerobic organisms isolated, the use of the anaerobic bottle as part of the routine blood culture set continuous. Various authors have questioned this practice (36, 37). Morris et al suggested that an approach of using two aerobic bottles with selective anaerobic culturing could enhance isolation with up to 6% (36), however this approach has not been adapted. Tamayose et al argued strongly to discontinue anaerobic culturing as routine practice and place attention on enhancing fungal isolation. (37). The anaerobic bottle however adds value in the fact that it allows growth of facultative organisms and thus adding to the total volume cultured and thus the sensitivity for organism recovery.

Various culturing media within one system differ with regard to constituents and performance and the choice relies heavily on controlled clinical evaluation. The BacT/ALERT FN medium (bioMérieux, Durham, N.C.) recently replaced the BacT/Alert anerobic FAN medium. They differ in composition with the amount of activated charcoal and broth constituents where the FN bottle contains a higher concentration of activated charcoal as well as trypticase soy broth compared to brain heart infusion. BacT/ALERT also has a standard anaerobic bottle SN which does not contain activated charcoal. Mirret el al compared all three anaerobic bottles with the standard aerobic bottle, the BacT/ALERT FA medium and found better recovery of micro-organisms and a faster time to positivity (TTP) with the FN bottle (38).

Often the culturing media may differ in the structural format e.g. the BacT/ALERT 3D system (bioMérieux, Durham, N.C.) uses plastic bottles compared to the Bactec9240 system (BD Microbiology, Cockeysville,MD) that uses glass bottles. The VersaTREK system (Trek Diagnostic Systems, Cleveland, OH) offers media in two forms for both aerobic and anaerobic isolation, the 40 ml direct draw format which can accommodate 5 ml and an 80 ml format which can accommodate 10 ml. With the direct draw format the blood – broth ratio achieved is 1:8. Samuel et al compared the two media types with simulated blood cultures with clinically relevant microorganisms and found no negative impact on TTP with the smaller volume bottles (39). Caution should be applied in not compromising the total volume cultured when using small volume bottles as the recommended volume to be cultured still remains 30 ml of blood (See section on Principles of blood culture collection).

Some blood culture bottles contain the anticoagulant sodium polyanetholsulphonate (SPS) that can inactivate some of the host serum factors but also have a toxic effect on some organisms. An overall balance is achieved with the correct blood – broth ratio. The blood – broth ratio required and achieved will be different between systems (See section on Principles of blood culture collection). Bottles also differ in terms of the antibiotic binding resins used to limit the effect of inhibitory substances. A study compared the Bactec Plus media and TREK Redox media and found the former to be more efficient in recovering organisms in the presence of antimicrobial substances (40).

Paediatric bottles are specifically adapted to accommodate smaller volumes and often contain additional growth factors and binding resins to enhance organism recovery. A common misconception is that standard bottles cannot be used on paediatric patients and vice versa, however the choice of bottle will be dictated by the volume obtained. Although paediatric bottles are designed to maximize growth from smaller volumes the sensitivity to detect bacteraemia will increase with the volume of blood cultured. In neonates and infants it is assumed that you sample a much smaller pool and therefore the volume necessary to detect bacteraemia must be smaller, however as highlighted before the total volume required is not known and due to restriction in obtaining high volumes from this patient population this answer will keep eluding us. One study however has shown that the chance to fail to detect bacteraemia will increase when culturing < 1 ml in neonates (31).

Some systems provide additional culturing media optimized to detect fungal or mycobacterial pathogens more efficiently, however these will not be addressed in this chapter.

5. From collection to incubation

Over the years blood cultures has been regarded as one of the most import specimen types and microbiology laboratories take great care to process these as rapidly as possible. Blood cultures that have been collected must reach the laboratory as soon as possible and generally receive high attention for immediate incubation to allow optimal growth of organisms and rapid recovery without compromising the specimen.

Although in principle, the bottles must be inserted within the continuous monitoring blood culture systems as soon as possible, various factors can affect the time to insertion (TTI). Some laboratories do not operate a full 24 hours and bottles will then be incubated at 35^{0}C and can only be inserted the following day. Other factors include a delay in reaching the laboratory due to logistics. A study by Saito et al evaluated the effect of delayed insertion of blood culture bottles into continuously monitoring blood culture systems and found that although delayed insertion did not affect the sensitivity for organism recovery the mean TTP for all isolates was significantly shorter if inserted on the same day that the culture was obtained (41).

Time to removal (TTR) is defined as the time elapsed from when the system emits a positive signal until the bottle is removed for subsequent subculturing for organism recovery. A delay in removal of the bottles could be due to closure of the laboratory at night and this can result in obtaining false negative results especially when isolating more fastidious organisms. In our study when evaluating the VersaTREK system against the Bactec9240 system we found that the time to removal (TTR) for some isolates were up to 8 hours and this could have explained some false negative results where the system failed to detect *S. pneumonia* isolates (42). We know that this organism is prone to activate autolysin under stress conditions which may result in poor recovery from blood culture bottles. This phenomena has been observed with the BacT/ALERT 3D system in our laboratory where positive signals were obtained with subsequent no growth, however confirmed after positive agglutination from the bottle sediment (data not shown).

The duration of incubation is calculated from the time of insertion until the time of removal. Bottles will be removed, thus considered negative, when no positive signal is obtained after a certain amount of incubation time has elapsed. This time before removal will depend on the blood culture system used. For manual broth – based systems, 7 days are the recommended incubation time (43) in comparison to various studies that support shorter incubation times of 4 to 5 days with the continuous monitoring blood culture systems (44,45,46).

Extended incubation (up to 14 to 21 days) is still recommended to detect more fastidious organisms specifically the HACEK organisms (*Haemophilus, Actinobacillus, Cardiobacterium, Eikenella,* and *Kingella* species) that are involved in endocarditis (7). Recent reports have shown that the method of detection and not the time of incubation is critical to detect these organisms. Baron et al in 2005 reported evidence that the Bactec9240 system can detect the HACEK organisms within 5 days (47). Alternative methods e.g. a lysis centrifugation system for dimorphic fungi and molecular methods for *Bartonella henselae* may be of more value than prolonged incubation (47, 48). In a multicentre evaluation of 15 826 positive blood cultures only 0.1% of HACEK organisms were detected across all centers with a mean time to detection of 3.4 days. They recommend based on their findings that extended incubation for HACEK organisms is unnecessary (49).

6. The choice of blood culture system

Various commercial blood culture systems are available. The choice of blood culture system will depend on various factors (Table 2). It is the responsibility of the laboratory director to liaise with clinicians on the selection of the best system to achieve the best results for their specific patient population and workload.

The various blood culture systems compete with regard to sensitivity for organism recovery, TTP, workload capacity, user interface and associated costs. Not one system is perfect and able to detect all possible micro-organisms.

These systems all require inoculation of blood into a media bottle. The media are in principle similar, however controlled clinical trials have shown some media to be superior for certain organisms (See section Selection of the correct blood culture bottle).

Sensitivity for organism recovery is the most import parameter when selecting a blood culture system. Studies have shown that the lysis centrifugation systems are more sensitive for the detection of fastidious organisms and dimorphic fungi (25). The continuous monitoring systems have shown superiority with regard to TTP compared to manual systems (50, 51, 52, 53) and are the current preferred systems. TTP has been shown to be a good predictor of clinical outcome in staphylococcal sepsis (54, 55, 56).

Sensitivity for organism recovery
Time to positivity
Workload capacity
User interface
Costs

Table 2. Factors that affect the choice of blood culture system

The workload capacity is important as many laboratories differ in the amount of blood culture they will process. The continuous monitoring systems have the capacity to be expanded to accommodate the workload. The interface must be user friendly e.g. some technologists will review the growth index of the bottle to troubleshoot possible false positive signals. Cost of implementation and maintenance may play a role as well.

6.1. Various commercial blood culture systems – Advantages and disadvantages

There are currently a wide variety of blood culture systems available. Although the continuous monitoring blood culture systems have become the preferred platform, manual systems are still available and used in some settings and will be discussed briefly.

6.1.1. Manual blood culture systems

The conventional manual method entails inoculating a commercially provided blood culture bottle, incubating the bottle at the required temperature and atmosphere with daily inspection of the bottle for macroscopic evidence of growth e.g. turbidity, haemolysis or colonies. Once growth is observed, a sample can be obtained for Gram staining and subculture for further identification. Bottles are incubated for 7 days and terminal subculture is mandatory.

Variations to the conventional manual method is combining agar in the form of paddles to the broth. These systems allow for more frequent subculturing by inverting the bottles to bring the broth into contact with the agar. These bottles can be inspected for growth and Gram staining with presumptive identification to be performed from the agar.

The Septi-Chek (BD Diagnostics) blood culture system is a biphasic-agar slide system that uses a standard blood culture bottle containing brain heart infusion or trypticase soy broth connected to a second plastic chamber with a trisurface panel consisting of chocolate, Mackonkey and malt agar. The slide chamber is screwed onto the bottle after inoculation and incubated at 35°C for 4 – 6 hours. The bottle is then inverted for the first subculture and can be inverted at various intervals thereafter to optimize isolation.

The Oxoid Signal System (Oxoid Unipath, Basingstoke,England) is unique in the sense that it is a one bottle system. After inoculation of a standard blood culture bottle a second chamber is attached with a long needle that extends below the surface of the blood – broth mixture. This closed space system uses CO_2 production to detect growth. Any gas produced will increase the pressure in the headspace and allow some of the blood – broth mixture to enter into the chamber from where sampling, Gram staining and subculturing can be performed. This system thus signals the laboratory towards possible growth without using an automated system. The advantages and disadvantages of these systems are presented in Table 3.

Advantages	Disadvantages
Evaluated favourably in detecting growth	More false positives
Cost effective	Lower yield of anaerobes
Useful in small laboratories with small workload	Labour intensive, need to visibly inspect for growth

Table 3. Advantages and disadvantages of manual blood culture systems

6.1.2. Lysis centrifugation systems

The principle of this test is explained in its name. The Wampole Isostat/ Isolater Microbial System (Inverness Medical) is a single tube test that uses saponin for lyses of erythrocytes and neutrophils, followed by centrifugation and subsequent inoculation of solid agar media for isolation. The system is useful for the recovery of slow growing and fastidious organisms including filamentous moulds, dimorphic fungi and *Bartonella henselae* (29). This method also allows quantification to be performed, however limitations include a higher rate of contamination, excessive hands on time and toxic effects of the saponin that can inhibit growth.

6.1.3. Continuous monitoring blood culture systems

These systems are considered an advance in clinical microbiology and are the current preferred platform for blood culture testing worldwide. With the introduction of these systems in the 1970s they have evolved over time e.g. the Bactec series started with radiometric systems which was later replaced with non – radiometric systems. Today we face automated and computerized continuous monitoring blood culture systems.

The three main commercially available systems are the BacT/ALERT blood culture system (bioMérieux, Durham, N.C), Bactec 9000 series (BD Microbiology, Cockeysville,MD) and the VersaTREK system (Trek Diagnostic Systems, Cleveland, Ohio). All three systems have expandable detection units with self-contained incubation chambers and minimal bottle manipulation as agitation is achieved via rocking or vortexing. The principle of detection of these systems is based on the release of CO_2 in the presence of micro-organism metabolism.

The Bact/ALERT and Bactec systems both depend on a pH change due to the production of CO_2 to detect growth. The Bactec9240 systems' bottles have a sensor at the bottom that emits a fluorescent light as the CO_2 concentration increases, that will pass via an emission filter to a light sensitive diode. The system measures the voltage every 10 minutes and compares the new value with the previous value and emits a positive signal as soon as the threshold value is reached. The BacT/ALERT 3D system uses a CO_2 sensitive chemical sensor that is separated from the blood – broth mixture via a unidirectional membrane. Once the CO_2 concentration increases, the colour will change from green to yellow, this is measured with a photosensitive detector.

The VersaTREK system monitors changes in the bottle headspace every 24 minutes. Both gas consumption and production are monitored. As a result other gasses e.g. O_2 and H_2 are also detected. The system differs from the other systems in that the aerobic bottles are vortexed with a magnetic stir bar to increase oxygenation.

All three systems have been compared for both sensitivity for organism recovery and TTP. Mirret et al compared the VersaTREK system with the BacT/Alert system and found no significant difference for the detection of bacteraemia or fungaemia in clinical isolates (57). Our group compared the VersaTREK system against the Bactec9240 system and found both systems comparable to detect bacteraemia in patients with suspected sepsis however we observed a higher rate of false positive results and postulated that the threshold setting to emit a positive signal might be too low (42). Comparison of the BacT/ALERT system with the Bactec9240 systems showed slight better detection with the former (58). Advantages and disadvantages of these systems are shown in table 4.

Advantages	Disadvantages
Higher sensitivity for organism recovery	High implementation cost
Faster TTP	Equipment must be maintained
Fully automated and computerized	Need continuous power supply
Easy loading and unloading of bottles	
Expandable to accommodate larger or smaller volumes	

Table 4. Advantages and disadvantages of continuous monitoring systems

6.2. Time to positivity

Time to positivity (TTP) is a parameter provided by the automated blood culture system and is calculated from the time of incubation until a positive signal is detected. TTP can be influenced by various factors e.g. the bacterial load, the growth rate of the micro-organism, the presence of antibacterial substances in the blood as well as source of infection and clinical features.

Differential TTP has been used to diagnose CLABSI (59, 60, 61). Two sets of blood cultures are taken at the same time, one through the inserted catheter and the other peripherally. A CLABSI should be suspected if both sets yield the same micro-organisms and the set taken through the line becomes positive (TTP) 120 minutes or earlier than the peripheral set (62).

Short TTP in *S. aureus* bacteraemia can possibly predict the source of infection, specifically an endovascular source and also correlate with the attributable mortality (54).

Combining the TTP with the initial Gram stain result could predict the micro-organism as well as the source of bacteraemia, e.g. patients not on antimicrobial agents with Gram positive cocci in cluster within 14 hours was predictive of *S. aureus*, however the clinical impact of using this approach needs to be evaluated further (63).

7. Interpretation of results

Interpretation of positive blood culture results are challenging to both clinicians and microbiologists. With the background of blood culture contamination rates of up to half of all positive cultures and previously considered contaminants now more frequently implicated in disease the need for tools to assist in distinguishing contaminants from pathogens becomes eminent.

Consensus have been reached with regard to clinical and laboratory parameters that must be taken into consideration to assess positive cultures for significance or contamination. These include fever, leucocytosis, positive imaging, the identity of the organism recovered, the number of sets positive out of the number received, the number of bottles positive within a given set and the TTP (64) (Table 5).

Clinical	Laboratory
Fever	Identity of the microorganism
Leucocytosis	Number of positive sets
Positive imaging	Number of positive bottles (within set)
	Time to positivity

Table 5. Parameters as tools to distinguish contaminants from pathogens in positive blood cultures

The identity of the microorganism can aid interpretation of results (11, 65). According to an evaluation by Weinstein et al in 1997 there are organisms that will be pathogens in > 90% of cases and these include *Staphylococcus aureus, Streptococcus pneumoniae, Escherichia coli,* other *Enterobacteriaceae, Pseudomonas aeruginosa* and *Candida albicans* (66). Despite adequate data from large studies there are other organisms that also presents as true pathogens most of the time e.g. *Streptococcus pyogenes, Streptococcus agalactiae, Listeria monocytogenes, Neisseria meningitidis, Neisseria gonorrhoeae, Haemophilus influenzae, Bacteroides fragilis* group, *Candida* species other than *C. albicans* and *Cryptococcus neoformans* (64). Organisms that represent rarely as pathogens include *Bacillus* species, *Propionibacterium acnes, Corynebacterium* spp other than *C. jeikieum and* Viridans group streptococci (66, 67) (Table 6).

True pathogen	Probable contaminant
Staphylococcus aureus	Coagulase negative staphylococci (CoNS)*
Streptococcus pneumoniae	*Bacillis* species
Escherichia coli	*Propionibacterium acnes*
Other *Enterobacteriaceae*	*Corynebacterium* spp
Pseudomonas aeruginosa	
Candida albicans	

*Contaminant or true pathogen

Table 6. Organism identity to indicate significance or contamination

Other organisms can no longer be judged on their identity with regard to significance, these include CoNS, Viridans group streptococci and *Clostridium* species.

Isolating CoNS from positive blood culture bottles presents a challenge for clinicians in deciding the significance of the finding. Not only are CoNS the most common contaminant isolated but patients who presents with true infection often have mild symptoms which makes the interpretation very difficult (68,69). Various studies are reporting CoNS to be a true pathogen causing blood stream infections especially in patients with indwelling prosthetic devices or central venous catheters (66, 70).

The value of obtaining more than one set of blood cultures not only enhances the yield of detecting bacteraemia, but also aids interpretation when dealing with positive cultures. Contaminants are often obtained from only one set whereas with true bacteraemias multiple blood cultures will grow the same organism (66). Weinstein also reported that if an institution has a baseline contamination rate of about 3%, the chances of recovering the same organism in a two set culture and being a contaminant is less than 1 in a 1000 (64).

Using the TTP as an aid to establish significance have been debated before (64). The principle relies on the assumption that true infection will present with a much larger inoculum vs. contamination and thus result in earlier detection. One of the reasons why TTP can be misleading is the fact that continuous monitoring systems can detect micro-organisms at lower levels much faster than conventional systems.

Using the criteria that if one bottle is positive within a given set relates to contamination should be discouraged. For CoNS this has been evaluated and shown to be inadequate to predict clinical outcome (71).

8. Blood culture contamination

Culture contamination represents false positive results and are not uncommon in microbiology laboratories with rates being reported as high as around 50% of all positive cultures (66, 72). An increase in contamination rates despite advances in the field of microbiology has been observed (66) and this phenomenon could be explained by the increasing use of continuously monitoring blood culture systems and the improved culture media provided for the specific systems that may aid the detection of low numbers contaminants. The increased use of intravascular devices and the practice of taking cultures through invasive lines are also important when considering contamination rates. American Society of Microbiologists published standards that state that blood culture contamination rates must not exceed 3% (73), rates however will differ widely between institutions, but commonly exceeds 7% (74, 75).

The cost of blood culture contamination often exceeds the cost of performing the test (76). A retrospective case-control study evaluated 142 false positive blood cultures and found a significant increase in length of hospital stay as well as laboratory and pharmacy costs, they also calculated that the 254 false positives blood cultures in a year period, added 1372 extra hospital days and £1,270,381 in costs per year (77).

Various strategies have been implemented to decrease blood culture contamination rates e.g. training staff with regard to aseptic collection technique, feedback with regard to contamination rates and implementation of blood culture collection kits. Although skin antisepsis can reduce the burden of contamination, 20% of skin organisms are located deep within the dermis and are unaffected by antisepsis (78). The practice of changing needles before bottle inoculation should be abandoned as it increases the risk to acquire needle stick injuries without decreasing contamination rates (79). Also discarding the initial aliquot of blood taken from CVCs does not reduce contamination (80).

9. New technologies used in conjunction with blood culture systems in the diagnosis of sepsis

In hospital settings where resistance profiles of circulating micro-organisms are known, the use of rapid identifying methods to guide empiric antimicrobial usage is critical to improve patient outcomes. Research efforts are focused on developing molecular tests that can be performed without prior culturing with continuous monitoring systems, however these assays are limited to date. Molecular assays performed on positive blood culture bottles has improved sensitivity compared to conventional culturing methods, and has decreased turnaround times compared to routine culture (81). Study by Karahan have shown the use of molecular methods to evaluate false positive signals for identifying microbial DNA of organisms that might have been inhibited by high leucocytes count or antimicrobials (82).

The Lightcycler® SeptiFast (Roche Diagnostics, Manheim, Germany) is a multiplex realtime PCR system that can detect up to 25 common pathogens involved in sepsis from one single blood sample within 6 hours. Various studies have evaluated the use and confirm increased detection of circulating microbial DNA compared with conventional blood culture (83, 84,85). Study by Lucignano et al evaluated the use in the paediatric population with suspected sepsis with sensitivity and specificity reported of 85% and 95% respectively. Significantly higher yields were observed from patients already on antimicrobial therapy (86). Although this method is considered culture – independent, most studies agree that this system does not replace conventional blood culturing and the clinical significance of detecting higher amounts of microbial DNA must be further evaluated.

A new strategy for the detection of blood stream pathogens include PCR/Electrospray ionization and mass spectrometry (PCR/ESI-MS). This technique in short amplifies broadly conserved regions of bacterial and fungal genomes followed by mass spectrometric analysis by weighing the PCR amplicons and comparing the product with known standards. The commercial assay is the Bac Spectrum Assay that runs on the PLEX-ID (Abbott Molecular). A study by Eshoo et al showed good sensitivity and specificity for the detection of *Erlichia* species in the blood from patients with suspected erlichiosis with the identification of additional bacterial pathogens that was determined to be clinically relevant (89). This new method will likely change the future of diagnosis of bloodstream pathogens however clinical relevant studies needs to be performed.

The Prove-it sepsis assay (Mobidiag, Helsinki, Finland) is a DNA-based microarray platform can identify more than 50 Gram positive and Gram negative bacteria that can cause sepsis (87) as well as detect the presence of the *mecA* gene that codes for methicillin resistance in *S. aureus* (88) from positive blood culture bottles. Sensitivity and specificity compared to conventional culture are reported to be 94.7% and 98.8% respectively (81). The study also showed an 18 hour faster turnaround time for identification compared to conventional culture. Due to the multiplexing capabilities this assay can also be expanded to detect pathogens involved in fungaemia.

The Xpert MRSA/SA Blood culture assay (Cepheid) was evaluated favourably for the detection of an the discrimination between methicillin resistant *staphylococcus aureus* (MRSA) and methicillin susceptible *staphylococcus aureus* (MSSA) (90) . Although this method is limited with regard to the range of pathogens it will guide initial empiric therapy towards a better clinical outcome.

Another new approach to enhance earlier specie identification from positive blood culture bottles following Gram staining include the Peptide Nucleic Acid Fluorescence *In situ* Hybridization assay (PNA-FISH). This assay uses probes that target specific conserved bacterial and fungal genomic regions and can distinguish between e.g. *S. aureus* and non – *S. aureus* as well as different *Candida* species (91, 92, 93).

Matrix-assisted Laser Desorption/Ionization–time of flight (MALDI-TOF) mass spectrometry (MS) is currently widely applied on post culture isolates for rapid identification. The system use MS signals created and compare them to standard signal patterns within a database. The use directly from positive blood culture bottles needs further evaluation but the advantage of this technology shows promise for the future.

The various new technologies appears attractive, however implementation will come at great cost and are not cost effective for routine laboratories at present. Certainly the rapidly of results being generated and the ability to detect pathogens unlikely to grew on conventional media comes as a great advantage. The clinical significance of enhanced detection of circulating microbial DNA must be established.

10. Conclusion

The use of blood culture systems still remain the gold standard for the detection of bacteraemia. It is important to understand the process from collection to obtaining a result to aid interpretation and improve the clinical outcome. While the continuous monitoring systems are the preferred platform for testing, various new methods are on the horizon that will aid or even replace these systems, only time will tell.

Author details

Andries William Dreyer*
Department of Medical Microbiology, University of Pretoria and
the National Health Laboratory Services (NHLS) Tshwane Academic Division, South Africa

11. References

[1] Orsi GB, Di Stefano L, Noah N. Hospital-acquired, laboratory-confirmed bloodstream infection: increased hospital stay and direct costs. Infect Control Hosp Epidemiol 2002 Apr;23(4):190-197.

[2] Rello J. Impact of nosocomial infections on outcome: myths and evidence. Infect Control Hosp Epidemiol 1999 Jun;20(6):392-394.

[3] Pien BC, Sundaram P, Raoof N, Costa SF, Mirrett S, Woods CW, et al. The clinical and prognostic importance of positive blood cultures in adults. Am J Med 2010 Sep;123(9):819-828.

* Corresponding Author

[4] Gaibani P, Rossini G, Ambretti S, Gelsomino F, Pierro AM, Varani S, et al. Blood culture systems: rapid detection--how and why? Int J Antimicrob Agents 2009;34 Suppl 4:S13-5.

[5] Mancini N, Carletti S, Ghidoli N, Cichero P, Burioni R, Clementi M. The era of molecular and other non-culture-based methods in diagnosis of sepsis. Clin Microbiol Rev 2010 Jan;23(1):235-251.

[6] Durack DT, Lukes AS, Bright DK. New criteria for diagnosis of infective endocarditis: utilization of specific echocardiographic findings. Duke Endocarditis Service. Am J Med 1994 Mar;96(3):200-209.

[7] Fowler VG Jr, Scheld WM, Bayer AS. Endocarditis and intravascular infections. In: Mandell GL, Bennett JE, Dolin R, eds. Mandell, Douglas and Bennett's principles and practice of infectious diseases, 6th ed. Philadelphia. Elsevier, 2005:975–1022.

[8] Riedel S, Bourbeau P, Swartz B, Brecher S, Carroll KC, Stamper PD, et al. Timing of specimen collection for blood cultures from febrile patients with bacteremia. J Clin Microbiol 2008 Apr;46(4):1381-1385.

[9] Li J, Plorde JJ, Carlson LG. Effects of volume and periodicity on blood cultures. J Clin Microbiol 1994 Nov;32(11):2829-2831.

[10] Cockerill FR,3rd, Wilson JW, Vetter EA, Goodman KM, Torgerson CA, Harmsen WS, et al. Optimal testing parameters for blood cultures. Clin Infect Dis 2004 Jun 15;38(12):1724-1730.

[11] Weinstein MP, Murphy JR, Reller LB, Lichtenstein KA. The clinical significance of positive blood cultures: a comprehensive analysis of 500 episodes of bacteremia and fungemia in adults. II. Clinical observations, with special reference to factors influencing prognosis. Rev Infect Dis 1983 Jan-Feb;5(1):54-70.

[12] Bates DW, Goldman L, Lee TH. Contaminant blood cultures and resource utilization. The true consequences of false-positive results. JAMA 1991 Jan 16;265(3):365-369.

[13] DesJardin JA, Falagas ME, Ruthazer R, Griffith J, Wawrose D, Schenkein D, et al. Clinical utility of blood cultures drawn from indwelling central venous catheters in hospitalized patients with cancer. Ann Intern Med 1999 Nov 2;131(9):641-647.

[14] Martinez JA, DesJardin JA, Aronoff M, Supran S, Nasraway SA, Snydman DR. Clinical utility of blood cultures drawn from central venous or arterial catheters in critically ill surgical patients. Crit Care Med 2002 Jan;30(1):7-13.

[15] Beutz M, Sherman G, Mayfield J, Fraser VJ, Kollef MH. Clinical utility of blood cultures drawn from central vein catheters and peripheral venipuncture in critically ill medical patients. Chest 2003 Mar;123(3):854-861.

[16] Falagas ME, Kazantzi MS, Bliziotis IA. Comparison of utility of blood cultures from intravascular catheters and peripheral veins: a systematic review and decision analysis. J Med Microbiol 2008 Jan;57(Pt 1):1-8.

[17] Spitalnic SJ, Woolard RH, Mermel LA. The significance of changing needles when inoculating blood cultures: a meta-analysis. Clin Infect Dis 1995 Nov;21(5):1103-1106.

[18] Calfee DP, Farr BM. Comparison of four antiseptic preparations for skin in the prevention of contamination of percutaneously drawn blood cultures: a randomized trial. J Clin Microbiol 2002 May;40(5):1660-1665.

[19] Adams D, Quayum M, Worthington T, Lambert P, Elliott T. Evaluation of a 2% chlorhexidine gluconate in 70% isopropyl alcohol skin disinfectant. J Hosp Infect 2005 Dec;61(4):287-290.
[20] Malani A, Trimble K, Parekh V, Chenoweth C, Kaufman S, Saint S. Review of clinical trials of skin antiseptic agents used to reduce blood culture contamination. Infect Control Hosp Epidemiol 2007 Jul;28(7):892-895.
[21] Tepus D, Fleming E, Cox S, Hazelett S, Kropp D. Effectiveness of Chloraprep in reduction of blood culture contamination rates in emergency department. J Nurs Care Qual 2008 Jul-Sep;23(3):272-276.
[22] McLellan E, Townsend R, Parsons HK. Evaluation of ChloraPrep (2% chlorhexidine gluconate in 70% isopropyl alcohol) for skin antisepsis in preparation for blood culture collection. J Infect 2008 Dec;57(6):459-463.
[23] Clinical and Laboratory Standards Institute (CLSI). Principles and Procedures for Blood Cultures; Approved Guideline. CLSI document M47-A. Wayne, PA: Clinical and Laboratory Standards Institute 2007.
[24] Hall MM, Ilstrup DM, Washington JA,2nd. Effect of volume of blood cultured on detection of bacteremia. J Clin Microbiol 1976 Jun;3(6):643-645.
[25] Henry NK, McLimans CA, Wright AJ, Thompson RL, Wilson WR, Washington JA,2nd. Microbiological and clinical evaluation of the isolator lysis-centrifugation blood culture tube. J Clin Microbiol 1983 May;17(5):864-869.
[26] Ilstrup DM, Washington JA,2nd. The importance of volume of blood cultured in the detection of bacteremia and fungemia. Diagn Microbiol Infect Dis 1983 Jun;1(2):107-110.
[27] Weinstein MP, Mirrett S, Wilson ML, Reimer LG, Reller LB. Controlled evaluation of 5 versus 10 milliliters of blood cultured in aerobic BacT/Alert blood culture bottles. J Clin Microbiol 1994 Sep;32(9):2103-2106.
[28] Bouza E, Sousa D, Rodriguez-Creixems M, Lechuz JG, Munoz P. Is the volume of blood cultured still a significant factor in the diagnosis of bloodstream infections? J Clin Microbiol 2007 Sep;45(9):2765-2769.
[29] Weinstein MP. Current blood culture methods and systems: clinical concepts, technology, and interpretation of results. Clin Infect Dis 1996 Jul;23(1):40-46.
[30] Lee A, Mirrett S, Reller LB, Weinstein MP. Detection of bloodstream infections in adults: how many blood cultures are needed? J Clin Microbiol 2007 Nov;45(11):3546-3548.
[31] Szymczak EG, Barr JT, Durbin WA, Goldmann DA. Evaluation of blood culture procedures in a pediatric hospital. J Clin Microbiol 1979 Jan;9(1):88-92.
[32] Auckenthaler R, Ilstrup DM, Washington JA,2nd. Comparison of recovery of organisms from blood cultures diluted 10% (volume/volume) and 20% (volume/volume). J Clin Microbiol 1982 May;15(5):860-864.
[33] Salventi JF, Davies TA, Randall EL, Whitaker S, Waters JR. Effect of blood dilution on recovery of organisms from clinical blood cultures in medium containing sodium polyanethol sulfonate. J Clin Microbiol 1979 Feb;9(2):248-252.

[34] Thomas S, Cheesbrough J, Plumb S, Bolton L, Wilkinson P, Walmsley J, et al. Impact of a blood culture collection kit on the quality of blood culture sampling: fear and the law of unintended consequences. J Hosp Infect 2011 Aug;78(4):256-259.

[35] Weightman NC, Kerr KG. Blood culture contamination: having your cake and eating it. J Hosp Infect 2012 Jan;80(1):101-102.

[36] Morris AJ, Wilson ML, Mirrett S, Reller LB. Rationale for selective use of anaerobic blood cultures. J Clin Microbiol 1993 Aug;31(8):2110-2113.

[37] Tamayose MH, Yamane N, Kisanuki K, Kawai M, Nakasone I. Laboratory-based evaluation of significance to routinely use anaerobic blood culture bottles: analysis of positivity and rapidity to detect positive cultures. Rinsho Byori 2009 Dec;57(12):1145-1150.

[38] Mirrett S, Petti CA, Woods CW, Magadia R, Weinstein MP, Reller LB. Controlled clinical comparison of the BacT/ALERT FN and the standard anaerobic SN blood culture medium. J Clin Microbiol 2004 Oct;42(10):4581-4585.

[39] Samuel LP, Pimentel JD, Tibbetts RJ, Martin R, Hensley R, Meier FA. Comparison of time to positivity of the VersaTREK(R) REDOX 80-mL and the REDOX EZ draw 40-mL blood culture bottles for common bacterial bloodstream pathogens. Diagn Microbiol Infect Dis 2011 Oct;71(2):101-105.

[40] Miller NS, Rogan D, Orr BL, Whitney D. Comparison of BD Bactec Plus blood culture media to VersaTREK Redox blood culture media for detection of bacterial pathogens in simulated adult blood cultures containing therapeutic concentrations of antibiotics. J Clin Microbiol 2011 Apr;49(4):1624-1627.

[41] Saito T, Iinuma Y, Takakura S, Nagao M, Matsushima A, Shirano M, et al. Delayed insertion of blood culture bottles into automated continuously monitoring blood culture systems increases the time from blood sample collection to the detection of microorganisms in bacteremic patients. J Infect Chemother 2009 Feb;15(1):49-53.

[42] Dreyer AW, Ismail NA, Nkosi D, Lindeque K, Matthews M, van Zyl DG, et al. Comparison of the VersaTREK blood culture system against the Bactec9240 system in patients with suspected bloodstream infections. Ann Clin Microbiol Antimicrob 2011 Feb 5;10:4.

[43] Reimer LG, Wilson ML, Weinstein MP. Update on detection of bacteremia and fungemia. Clin Microbiol Rev 1997 Jul;10(3):444-465.

[44] Johnson AS, Touchie C, Haldane DJ, Forward KR. Four-day incubation for detection of bacteremia using the BACTEC 9240. Diagn Microbiol Infect Dis 2000 Dec;38(4):195-199.

[45] Wilson ML, Mirrett S, Reller LB, Weinstein MP, Reimer LG. Recovery of clinically important microorganisms from the BacT/Alert blood culture system does not require testing for seven days. Diagn Microbiol Infect Dis 1993 Jan;16(1):31-34.

[46] Doern GV, Brueggemann AB, Dunne WM, Jenkins SG, Halstead DC, McLaughlin JC. Four-day incubation period for blood culture bottles processed with the Difco ESP blood culture system. J Clin Microbiol 1997 May;35(5):1290-1292.

[47] Baron EJ, Scott JD, Tompkins LS. Prolonged incubation and extensive subculturing do not increase recovery of clinically significant microorganisms from standard automated blood cultures. Clin Infect Dis 2005 Dec 1;41(11):1677-1680.
[48] Weinstein MP. Emerging data indicating that extended incubation of blood cultures has little clinical value. Clin Infect Dis 2005 Dec 1;41(11):1681-1682.
[49] Petti CA, Bhally HS, Weinstein MP, Joho K, Wakefield T, Reller LB, et al. Utility of extended blood culture incubation for isolation of Haemophilus, Actinobacillus, Cardiobacterium, Eikenella, and Kingella organisms: a retrospective multicenter evaluation. J Clin Microbiol 2006 Jan;44(1):257-259.
[50] Nolte FS, Williams JM, Jerris RC, Morello JA, Leitch CD, Matushek S, et al. Multicenter clinical evaluation of a continuous monitoring blood culture system using fluorescent-sensor technology (BACTEC 9240). J Clin Microbiol 1993 Mar;31(3):552-557.
[51] Krisher KK, Whyburn DR, Koepnick FE. Comparison of the BacT/Alert pediatric blood culture system, Pedi-BacT, with conventional culture using the 20-milliliter Becton-Dickinson supplemented peptone broth tube. J Clin Microbiol 1993 Apr;31(4):793-797.
[52] Kirkley BA, Easley KA, Washington JA. Controlled clinical evaluation of Isolator and ESP aerobic blood culture systems for detection of bloodstream infections. J Clin Microbiol 1994 Jun;32(6):1547-1549.
[53] Rohner P, Pepey B, Auckenthaler R. Comparison of BacT/Alert with Signal blood culture system. J Clin Microbiol 1995 Feb;33(2):313-317.
[54] Khatib R, Riederer K, Saeed S, Johnson LB, Fakih MG, Sharma M, et al. Time to positivity in Staphylococcus aureus bacteremia: possible correlation with the source and outcome of infection. Clin Infect Dis 2005 Sep 1;41(5):594-598.
[55] Marra AR, Edmond MB, Forbes BA, Wenzel RP, Bearman GM. Time to blood culture positivity as a predictor of clinical outcome of Staphylococcus aureus bloodstream infection. J Clin Microbiol 2006 Apr;44(4):1342-1346.
[56] Sowden D, Anstey C, Faddy M. Blood culture time to positivity as a predictor of mortality in community acquired methicillin-susceptible Staphylococcus aureus bacteremia. J Infect 2008 Apr;56(4):295-296.
[57] Mirrett S, Hanson KE, Reller LB. Controlled clinical comparison of VersaTREK and BacT/ALERT blood culture systems. J Clin Microbiol 2007 Feb;45(2):299-302.
[58] Jamal W, Tamaray G, Pazhoor A, Rotimi VO. Comparative evaluation of BacT/ALERT 3D and BACTEC systems for the recovery of pathogens causing bloodstream infections. Med Princ Pract 2006;15(3):223-227.
[59] Catton JA, Dobbins BM, Kite P, Wood JM, Eastwood K, Sugden S, et al. In situ diagnosis of intravascular catheter-related bloodstream infection: a comparison of quantitative culture, differential time to positivity, and endoluminal brushing. Crit Care Med 2005 Apr;33(4):787-791.
[60] Blot F, Nitenberg G, Chachaty E, Raynard B, Germann N, Antoun S, et al. Diagnosis of catheter-related bacteraemia: a prospective comparison of the time to positivity of hub-blood versus peripheral-blood cultures. Lancet 1999 Sep 25;354(9184):1071-1077.

[61] Raad I, Hanna HA, Alakech B, Chatzinikolaou I, Johnson MM, Tarrand J. Differential time to positivity: a useful method for diagnosing catheter-related bloodstream infections. Ann Intern Med 2004 Jan 6;140(1):18-25.
[62] Weber DJ, Rutala WA. Central line-associated bloodstream infections: prevention and management. Infect Dis Clin North Am 2011 Mar;25(1):77-102.
[63] Martinez JA, Pozo L, Almela M, Marco F, Soriano A, Lopez F, et al. Microbial and clinical determinants of time-to-positivity in patients with bacteraemia. Clin Microbiol Infect 2007 Jul;13(7):709-716.
[64] Weinstein MP. Blood culture contamination: persisting problems and partial progress. J Clin Microbiol 2003 Jun;41(6):2275-2278.
[65] MacGregor RR, Beaty HN. Evaluation of positive blood cultures. Guidelines for early differentiation of contaminated from valid positive cultures. Arch Intern Med 1972 Jul;130(1):84-87.
[66] Weinstein MP, Towns ML, Quartey SM, Mirrett S, Reimer LG, Parmigiani G, et al. The clinical significance of positive blood cultures in the 1990s: a prospective comprehensive evaluation of the microbiology, epidemiology, and outcome of bacteremia and fungemia in adults. Clin Infect Dis 1997 Apr;24(4):584-602.
[67] Hall KK, Lyman JA. Updated review of blood culture contamination. Clin Microbiol Rev 2006 Oct;19(4):788-802.
[68] von Eiff C, Peters G, Heilmann C. Pathogenesis of infections due to coagulase-negative staphylococci. Lancet Infect Dis 2002 Nov;2(11):677-685.
[69] Rahkonen M, Luttinen S, Koskela M, Hautala T. True bacteremias caused by coagulase negative Staphylococcus are difficult to distinguish from blood culture contaminants. Eur J Clin Microbiol Infect Dis 2012 Mar 31.
[70] Tokars JI. Predictive value of blood cultures positive for coagulase-negative staphylococci: implications for patient care and health care quality assurance. Clin Infect Dis 2004 Aug 1;39(3):333-341.
[71] Mirrett S, Weinstein MP, Reimer LG, Wilson ML, Reller LB. Relevance of the number of positive bottles in determining clinical significance of coagulase-negative staphylococci in blood cultures. J Clin Microbiol 2001 Sep;39(9):3279-3281.
[72] Zwang O, Albert RK. Analysis of strategies to improve cost effectiveness of blood cultures. J Hosp Med 2006 Sep;1(5):272-276.
[73] Washington II JA, Cumitech IA. Blood cultures II. In: Reller LB, Murray PR, MacLowry JO, editors. American Society for Microbiology; 1982.
[74] Gander RM, Byrd L, DeCrescenzo M, Hirany S, Bowen M, Baughman J. Impact of blood cultures drawn by phlebotomy on contamination rates and health care costs in a hospital emergency department. J Clin Microbiol 2009 Apr;47(4):1021-1024.
[75] Schifman RB, Strand CL, Meier FA, Howanitz PJ. Blood culture contamination: a College of American Pathologists Q-Probes study involving 640 institutions and 497134 specimens from adult patients. Arch Pathol Lab Med 1998 Mar;122(3):216-221.
[76] Segal GS, Chamberlain JM. Resource utilization and contaminated blood cultures in children at risk for occult bacteremia. Arch Pediatr Adolesc Med 2000 May;154(5):469-473.

[77] Alahmadi YM, Aldeyab MA, McElnay JC, Scott MG, Darwish Elhajji FW, Magee FA, et al. Clinical and economic impact of contaminated blood cultures within the hospital setting. J Hosp Infect 2011 Mar;77(3):233-236.
[78] Selwyn S, Ellis H. Skin bacteria and skin disinfection reconsidered. Br Med J 1972 Jan 15;1(5793):136-140.
[79] Smart D, Baggoley C, Head J, Noble D, Wetherall B, Gordon DL. Effect of needle changing and intravenous cannula collection on blood culture contamination rates. Ann Emerg Med 1993 Jul;22(7):1164-1168.
[80] Dwivedi S, Bhalla R, Hoover DR, Weinstein MP. Discarding the initial aliquot of blood does not reduce contamination rates in intravenous-catheter-drawn blood cultures. J Clin Microbiol 2009 Sep;47(9):2950-2951.
[81] Tissari P, Zumla A, Tarkka E, Mero S, Savolainen L, Vaara M, et al. Accurate and rapid identification of bacterial species from positive blood cultures with a DNA-based microarray platform: an observational study. Lancet 2010 Jan 16;375(9710):224-230.
[82] Karahan ZC, Mumcuoglu I, Guriz H, Tamer D, Balaban N, Aysev D, et al. PCR evaluation of false-positive signals from two automated blood-culture systems. J Med Microbiol 2006 Jan;55(Pt 1):53-57.
[83] Mancini N, Clerici D, Diotti R et al. Molecular diagnosis of sepsis in neutropenic patients with haematological malignancies. J Med Microbiol 2008; 57: 601–604.
[84] Louie RF, Tang Z, Albertson TE, Cohen S, Tran NK, Kost GJ. Multiplex polymerase chain reaction detection enhancement of bacteremia and fungemia. Crit Care Med 2008; 36: 1487–1492.
[85] Westh H, Lisby G, Breysse F, Boddinghaus B, Chomarat M, Gant V, et al. Multiplex real-time PCR and blood culture for identification of bloodstream pathogens in patients with suspected sepsis. Clin Microbiol Infect 2009 Jun;15(6):544-551.
[86] Lucignano B, Ranno S, Liesenfeld O, Pizzorno B, Putignani L, Bernaschi P, et al. Multiplex PCR allows rapid and accurate diagnosis of bloodstream infections in newborns
[87] Roth SB, Jalava J, Ruuskanen O, Ruohola A, Nikkari S. Use of an oligonucleotide array for laboratory diagnosis of bacteria responsible for acute upper respiratory infections. J Clin Microbiol 2004 Sep;42(9):4268-4274.
[88] Eigner U, Weizenegger M, Fahr AM, Witte W. Evaluation of a rapid direct assay for identification of bacteria and the mec A and van genes from positive-testing blood cultures. J Clin Microbiol 2005 Oct;43(10):5256-5262.
[89] Eshoo MW, Crowder CD, Li H, Matthews HE, Meng S, Sefers SE, et al. Detection and identification of Ehrlichia species in blood by use of PCR and electrospray ionization mass spectrometry. J Clin Microbiol 2010 Feb;48(2):472-478.
[90] Wolk DM, Struelens MJ, Pancholi P, Davis T, Della-Latta P, Fuller D, et al. Rapid detection of Staphylococcus aureus and methicillin-resistant S. aureus (MRSA) in wound specimens and blood cultures: multicenter preclinical evaluation of the Cepheid Xpert MRSA/SA skin and soft tissue and blood culture assays. J Clin Microbiol 2009 Mar;47(3):823-826.

[91] Chapin K, Musgnug M. Evaluation of three rapid methods for the direct identification of *Staphylococcus aureus* from positive blood cultures. *J. Clin. Microbiol.* 41(9), 4324–4327 (2003).

[92] Oliveira K, Brecher SM, Durbin A *et al.* Direct identification of *Staphylococcus aureus* from positive blood culture bottles. *J. Clin. Microbiol.* 41(2), 889–891 (2003).

[93] Shepard JR, Addison RM, Alexander BD *et al.* Multicenter evaluation of the *Candida albicans/Candida glabrata* peptide nucleic acid fluorescent *in situ* hybridization method for simultaneous dual-color identification of *C. albicans* and *C. glabrata* directly from blood culture bottles. *J. Clin. Microbiol.* 46(1), 50–55 (2008).

Chapter 16

Sepsis: Antimicrobial Therapy

Renato Finkelstein and Ilana Oren

Additional information is available at the end of the chapter

http://dx.doi.org/10.5772/51714

1. Introduction

Twenty years ago a consensus committee of experts proposed standardized terminology and definitions for sepsis, organ failure, bacteremia, systemic inflammatory response syndrome (SIRS) and other related clinical conditions (1). Nevertheless, these terms are still a source of confusion and very often used interchangebly in clinical pratice.Whatever will be the accepted definition, sepsis is a clinical syndrome that complicates severe infection. However, in terms of antimicrobial therapy, diagnosing sepsis is not sufficient. The approach to the patient with sepsis includes also a tremendous challenge of establishing the etiologic agent, the anatomical site, the extent of the infectious problem and the possible underlying disease associated with the infection. Approximately 10 percent of patients with sepsis do not receive prompt antibiotic therapy for the implicated pathogen, and the mortality rate is 10 to 15 percent higher for such patients than for those who receive prompt, appropriate antibiotic therapy (2-3). Overall mortality from severe sepsis or septic shock ranges from 30% to 60% despite aggressive medical care (5-6). In the presence of septic shock, each hour delay in achieving administration of effective antibiotics is associated with a measurable increase in mortality (7). Therefore, antimicrobial therapy plays a central role in the management of these patients and the importance of the initial empiric regimen cannot be underestimated. The approach to critically ill patients with a suspected severe infection includes a well-accepted willingness to begin empirical broad-spectrum antibiotic therapy before the microbiological results are obtained. Intravenous antibiotic therapy should be started as early as possible and within the first hour of recognition of severe sepsis or septic shock. Appropriate cultures should be obtained before initiating antibiotic therapy, but should not prevent prompt administration of antimicrobial therapy. These recommendations are also emphasized in the recent guidelines for management of severe sepsis and septic shock (8). Nevertheless, even the broadest antibiotic regimen cannot "blindly" cover all pathogens responsible for sepsis and the choice of the initial antimicrobial therapy in sepsis should be guided by a systematic bedside evaluation, paired with a judicious use of laboratory methods and other medical technologies. This will facilitate to determine the suspected focus of primary infection, one of major determinants in the choice of antibiotics. The antibiotic regimen should be selected taking in consideration the most common pathogens causing infections at these sites. However, even for the same site of infection choices are frequently different depending whether infections are community-acquired or health care-associated. The site of infection (e.g. central nervous system, endocardium) is also important when considering other factors such as pharmacokinetics, dosing and bactericidal properties of antimicrobial drugs. Other important factors such as knowledge of local endemic diseases, microbiological data and patterns of resistance increase the likelihood of prescribing appropriate antimicrobial therapy. Based on these principles, this review will focus on the antimicrobial therapy for the most common causes of sepsis and, in particular, discuss the most appropriate choices to be used until the causative organism and its antibiotic susceptibilities are defined.

2. Common clinical conditions and pathogens associated with sepsis

2.1. Severe community-acquired pneumonia

Several large series of patients with severe sepsis have shown that the lungs are the most commonly identified site of primary infection (9-11).Pneumonia is among the top ten most common causes of death among all age groups in the United States, the sixth leading cause of death in those 65 years or older, and the single most common cause of infection-related mortality (12). Although the majority of patients with community-acquired pneumonia (CAP) are treated as outpatients, approximately 10% of patients with community-acquired pneumonia will develop severe disease, as defined by admission to an intensive care unit (ICU) due to the presence of shock requiring vasopressors or respiratory failure requiring mechanical ventilation (13). This population represents the greatest proportion of pneumonia-related mortality and healthcare expenditure occurs among the patients who are hospitalized. Using a pathophysiological approach to characterize the causes of clinical failure, it was found that severe sepsis and cardiac deterioration are the main causes of clinical failure in hospitalized patients with CAP (14).The Infectious Diseases Society of America/American Thoracic Society (IDSA/ATS) Consensus Guidelines on the Management of Community-Acquired Pneumonia in Adults strongly recommend direct admission to an ICU for patients with septic shock requiring vasopressors or with acute respiratory failure requiring intubation and mechanical ventilation (15).The clinical challenge of treating community-acquired pneumonia is the large number of microbial agents that can cause disease, the difficulty in making a clinical and etiologic diagnosis, and the fact that no single antimicrobial regimen can cover all the possible etiologies. Recommendations for diagnostic testing remain controversial. The most clear-cut indication for extensive diagnostic testing is in the critically ill CAP patient. Such patients should at least have blood drawn for culture and an endotracheal aspirate obtained if they are intubated. Blood cultures are positive in only 4 to 18 of patients hospitalized with community-acquired pneumonia (16); however a positive blood cultures is highly specific, may allow narrowing antibiotic use, and may identify the presence of unusual organisms that would not be adequately covered by routine empirical antibiotic coverage (17). Other difficulties in treating these patients include a long list of bacterial, fungal, viral, and protozoal agents that may cause severe acute CAP and because, by the time of presentation, evaluation rarely results in a specific etiologic diagnosis. Therefore, antibiotic therapy is almost always begun empirically. *S. pneumoniae* and *L. pneumophila* are the organisms most commonly involved in cases of severe pneumonia, however a large number of other microorganisms must be considered. A review of 9 studies that included 890 patients with CAP who were admitted to the ICU demonstrates that the most common pathogens in the ICU population were (in descending order of frequency) *S. pneumoniae, Legionella* species, *H. influenzae,* Enterobacteriaceae species, *S. aureus,* and *Pseudomonas* species (18).In some series, *M. pneumoniae* is involved in up to 11% of patients with community-acquired pneumonia requiring intensive care (19). The following empirical antibiotic treatment is the minimal recommended by the joint IDSA/ATS guidelines for severe CAP, i.e., patients needing hospitalization in ICU (15):

1. β-lactam (cefotaxime, ceftriaxone, or ampicillin-sulbactam) **plus** either azithromycin or a fluoroquinolone (ciprofloxacin). For penicillin-allergic patients, a respiratory fluoroquinolone (levofloxacin, moxifloxacin) and aztreonam are recommended.
2. For *Pseudomonas* infection, it is recommended the use of an antipneumococcal, antipseudomonal β-lactam (piperacillin-tazobactam, cefepime, imipenem, or meropenem) plus either ciprofloxacin or levofloxacin (750-mg dose) or the above β-lactam plus an aminoglycoside (gentamicin, amikacin) and azithromycin or the above β-lactam plus an aminoglycoside and an respiratory fluoroquinolone. For penicillin-allergic patients, substitute aztreonam for the above β-lactam.
3. For community-acquired methicillin-resistant *Staphylococcus aureus* (MRSA) infection, add vancomycin or linezolid.

Infections with the overwhelming majority of CAP pathogens will be adequately treated by use of the recommended empirical regimens. The emergence of methicillin-resistant *S. aureus* as a CAP pathogen and the small but significant incidence of CAP due to *P. aeruginosa* are the exceptions. Once the etiology of CAP has been identified, antimicrobial therapy should be directed at that pathogen; however two major issues are of concern. The first is whether bacteremic pneumococcal pneumonia should be treated with dual therapy. The second is that if the patient has concomitant pneumococcal meningitis, the efficacy of fluoroquinolone monotherapy is uncertain. Therefore, discontinuation of combination therapy after results of cultures are known is most likely safe in non-ICU patients (15).

3. Nosocomial pneumonia

Nosocomial pneumonia (NP), and its most serious form, ventilator-associated pneumonia (VAP), is a major cause of morbidity and mortality in the ICU. NP accounts for up to 25% of all ICU infections and for more than 50% of the antibiotics prescribed (20).In this setting, nearly 90% of episodes of NP occur during mechanical ventilation. Rates of VAP are related to the duration of mechanical ventilation and have been estimated to be 3% per day during the first 5 days and 2% per day thereafter (21). NP and VAP may be caused by a wide spectrum of bacterial pathogens, they may be polymicrobial, and are rarely due to viral or fungal pathogens in immunocompetent hosts (22).Time of onset of pneumonia is an important epidemiologic variable and risk factor for specific pathogens and outcomes in patients with NP and VAP. For patients who experience onset of infection within the first 4 days of hospitalization (early-onset VAP) and who have no risk factor for health care-related pneumonia or multidrug-resistant pathogens, *S. pneumoniae,* methicillin-susceptible *S. aureus, H. influenzae,* and antimicrobial-susceptible enteric gram-negative bacilli (e.g., *Klebsiella pneumoniae* and *Enterobacter* species) are the most common causative pathogens (22). For these patients a limited-spectrum antimicrobial therapy (i.e., ceftriaxone, a fluoroquinolone such levofloxacin or moxafloxacin, ampicillin/sulbactam, or ertapenem) may be appropriate. For patients who develop severe infection later during their hospital stay (late-onset VAP) additional antimicrobial-resistant bacteria (e.g., *P. aeruginosa, Acinetobacter* species, and MRSA) may also be responsible for infection (23) and a broad-spectrum combination antimicrobial therapy should be initiated promptly, with a commitment to de-escalating the treatment on the basis of serial clinical and microbiologic data. The recommended combinations (22) include an antipseudomonal cephalosporin (cefepime, ceftazidime), an antipseudomonal carbapenem(imipenem, meropenem), particularly when an extended-spectrum β-lactamase-positive strain is suspected, or a β-lactam/β-lactamase inhibitor (piperacillin–tazobactam) plus either an antipseudomonal fluoroquinolone (ciprofloxacin or levofloxacin) or an aminoglycoside (amikacin, gentamicin, or tobramycin) plus either vancomycin or linezolid (if MRSA risk factors are present or there is a high incidence locally). If an aminoglycoside is one of the agents used instead of quinolones, a macrolide (e.g. azithromycin) should also be given if *Legionella pneumophila* is suspected. Ultimately, the choice of agent should be based on ICU-specific trends in pathogens and their susceptibility patterns. VAP due to multiple drug-resistant microorganisms is one of the most dreadful complications that occurs in critically ill patients and, in this setting, infections caused by carbapenem-resistant *A. baumannii and K. pneumoniae* are of special concern because very few treatment options exist. If VAP caused by these pathogens are considered, polymyxyns (e.g. colistin) appears to be a safe and effective alternative (24). A recent prospective, randomized trial has demonstrated that fixed-dose of linezolid was more effective than a dose-optimized vancomycin regimen for treatment of methicillin-resistant *Staphylococcus aureus* nosocomial pneumonia, although the 60-day mortality was similar (25). Cases of non-nosocomial health care-associated pneumonia, defined as pneumonia occurring within 48-72 hours of hospitalization in a patient with extensive contact with the health care system (e.g. nursing home residence, hemodialysis dependence, recent hospitalization), are treated with the same regimens recommended for NP.

4. Urinary tract infection

The term *urosepsis* is commonly used to describe the sepsis syndrome caused by urinary tract infection (UTI). In large series of patients with sepsis, the urinary tract was considered to be source of infection in approximately 10% to 22 % of cases (9, 11). Sepsis is much more likely to occur among patients with upper UTI and complicated UTI, the latter defined as infection that occurs in a urinary tract with functionally, metabolically, or anatomically abnormalities (26). Infections occurring in patients with indwelling catheters and calculi, infection in men, pregnant women, children, and in patients who are hospitalized or in health care–associated settings also may be considered complicated (27). However, sepsis may be also a clinical presentation of acute uncomplicated pyelonephritis in young women (26). UTI in some adult patients groups, such as those with spinal cord injury, long-term catheterization, or diabetes, may progress to severe, life threatening pyelonephritis, abscess formation, or septicemia (28). In contrast to other community and nosocomial infections, there have been few new pathogens identified as important causes of UTI. *E. coli* accounts for approximately 80% of uncomplicated UTI (28); however, a broad range of bacteria can cause nosocomial UTI, and many are resistant to multiple antimicrobial agents. *E. coli*, although significantly less prevalent than in uncomplicated UTI, is still the most common cause of nosocomial bacteriuria in medical-surgical ICUs. Other gram-negative bacteria such as *Klebsiella* spp., *Serratia* spp., *Citrobacter* spp., *Enterobacter* spp., *Pseudomonas aeruginosa*, and gram-positive cocci, including coagulase negative staphylococci and *Enterococcus* spp., cause most of the other infections (29, 30). In patients with nosocomial UTI in medical-surgical ICUs reported in the U.S. National Nosocomial Infection Surveillance System from 1992 to 1998, *C. albicans* constituted 15.3% and all fungal isolates 31.2% of all urinary isolates (30). Urosepsis, in general, is easily diagnosed by positive urine and blood cultures with the same pathogens, but until microbiological results are available, empirical treatment should be selected considering the pharmacokinetics of the agent, its spectrum of activity relative to the anticipated pathogens and potential for adverse effects. Therapeutic management for uncomplicated infection has been compromised by increasing antimicrobial resistance, particularly global dissemination of the CTXM-15 extended spectrum β-lactamase (ESBL) producing Escherichia coli ST-131 strain (31).Guidelines developed by the Infectious Diseases Society of America (IDSA) and the European Society for Microbiology and Infectious Diseases (ESCMID) (32) recommends that women with pyelonephritis requiring hospitalization may be initially treated with an intravenous antimicrobial regimen, such as a fluoroquinolone (ciprofloxacin, ofloxacin) when the prevalence of resistance of community uropathogens is not known to exceed 10%. If the prevalence of fluoroquinolone resistance is thought to exceed 10%, an initial intravenous dose of a long-acting parenteral antimicrobial, such as ceftriaxone or a consolidated 24-h dose of an aminoglycoside (gentamicin), with or without ampicillin, an aminoglycoside (gentamicin), with or without ampicillin or an extended-spectrum penicillin (piperacillin, mezlocillin), with or without an aminoglycoside, or a carbapenem (imipenem, meropenem) is recommended. Patients with community-acquired urosepsis may be managed in a similar manner. Among patients with complicated nosocomial UTI the concern of multidrug resistance is much greater and the choice of antibiotic agent for empiric treatment should be based on available information, including the urine Gram-stain results, previous urine culture results, or the antimicrobial sensitivity patterns of urinary pathogens isolated in the patient's hospital or long-term care facility (26, 29). Other potential concerns with these choices include the increasing prevalence of resistance to fluoroquinolones in institutional settings and the frequency of enterococcal infections (29). In patients with nosocomial urosepsis, one should consider a broader-spectrum drug such as piperacillin-tazobactam or a carbapenem for empiric treatment. If the urine Gram stain shows gram-positive cocci (most likely enterococci or staphylococci), treatment with vancomycin is reasonable (33). The antimicrobial regimen should be tailored as appropriate when the infecting strain has been identified and antimicrobial susceptibilities are known.

5. Intraabdominal infections

Intraabdominal infections (IAIs) are one of the most common causes of sepsis (9, 11) and they comprehend a great number of pathological conditions. According to the source, site and extension of the infections, IAIs may be classified in several manners (34); they may be retroperitoneal and intraperitoneal, primary (without an evident source) or secondary, diffuse or localized (peritoneal or visceral abscesses), community acquired or health care–associated. The term complicated intra-abdominal infections is also commonly used and it implies an infections that extend beyond the hollow viscus of origin into the peritoneal space and that is associated either with abscess formation or peritonitis (35). The bacteria that cause intra-abdominal infections are derived from the indigenous flora of the gastrointestinal tract. Anaerobic bacteria are predominant in IAIs because they are the main component of the gastrointestinal tract flora, outnumbering aerobic and facultative bacteria in the ratio of 1,000 to 10,000 to one (36). Most cases of secondary peritonitis are polymicrobial and anaerobes play a major role (37-39).The predominant aerobic are *Escherichia coli, Enterococcus faecalis, Klebsiella* spp., *Enterobacter* spp., and the main anaerobic bacteria are anaerobic Gram-negative bacilli (including *Bacteroides fragilis* group and pigmented *Prevotella* and *Porphyromonas*), *Peptostreptococcus*, and *Clostridium* spp. (40). Recently, an Expert Panel of the Surgical Infection Society and the IDSA prepared guidelines intended for managing patients with IAIs (41). These guidelines make therapeutic recommendations on the basis of the severity of infection, which is defined for these guidelines as a composite of patient age, physiologic derangements, and background medical conditions. Many of these recommendations, intended for patients with severe infection or those considered at risk of complications, are also relevant for patients with IAI and sepsis and they are summarized as follow:

1. Appropriately collected, anaerobic and aerobic cultures should be performed. These include blood cultures and specimen collected from the intra-abdominal focus of infection which are representative of the material associated with the clinical infection.
2. Appropriate source control procedures are essential for nearly all patients with IAIs. These procedures include drainage of infected foci, control of ongoing peritoneal contamination by diversion or resection, and repair of anatomic and physiological function to the extent feasible.

3. The recommended empirical antibiotic treatment of adult patients with severe community-acquired infection and all patients with health care-associated infections are similar and should include antimicrobial regimens with broad-spectrum activity against gram-negative organisms, including an carbapenem (meropenem, imipenem, doripenem), or piperacillin-tazobactam (all with excellent antianaerobic activity), or ceftazidime or cefepime in combination with metronidazole (also excellent antianaerobic activity). Quinolones (ciprofloxacin, levofloxacin) in combination with metronidazole also may be used for empirical treatment if hospital surveys indicate >90% susceptibility of *E. coli* to this class of drugs. Aztreonam plus metronidazole is an alternative, but addition of an agent effective against gram-positive cocci is recommended.
4. The empiric use of agents effective against enterococci, particularly against *Enterococcus faecalis* is also recommended in this situation and includes drugs such as ampicillin, piperacillin, piperacillin-tazobactam, or vancomycin.
5. Empiric use of vancomycin should be provided to patients with health care-associated intra-abdominal infection who are known to be colonized with MRSA or who are at risk of having an infection due to this organism because of prior treatment failure and significant antibiotic exposure.
6. Antifungal therapy is not routinely included in the empiric regimen, unless gram-stains or cultures indicate that these organisms may be involved in the infection. In this case, patients with sepsis should be treated with an echinocandin (caspofungin, micafungin, or anidulafungin)
7. All antimicrobial therapy should be tailored when culture and susceptibility reports become available.

6. Skin and soft tissue infections

The spectrum of manifestations skin and soft tissue infections (SSTI) is wide, varying from otherwise healthy people with severe infection and sepsis to patients with major co-morbidities and relatively minor infection; patients with extensive cellulitis and systemic symptoms who can be managed with antibiotics alone to patients with necrotizing limb-threatening infection that requires life-saving surgery. SSTIs have been classified in several manners, including according to the anatomical site of infection (42), to their microbial etiology or by severity (43), or clinical characteristics (44). SSTIs may be caused by a large number of microorganisms. Therefore, in establishing a diagnosis, it is critical to ask patients about animal exposure, travel history, underlying diseases, recent trauma, bites, burns, and water exposure; and to recognize the signs of different types of infection in an effort to limit the spectrum of causes to a more reasonable differential diagnosis. Eron *et al.* (45) classify these infections according to the severity of local and systemic signs, thereby developing a system that guides the clinical management and treatment decisions for patients with SSTIs. Accordingly, class 4 in this classification includes sepsis syndrome and life-threatening infection (e.g. necrotizing fasciitis), the most serious presentations of complicated SSTI. A discussion on all causes of SSTIs is beyond the scope of this chapter. Instead, we will focus our discussion only on necrotizing fasciitis (NF), probably the most important clinical presentation of complicated SSTI associated with sepsis. NF (44, 46), is a relatively rare but often life-threatening necrotizing infection of subcutaneous tissue and fascia. About 20% of patients have no visible skin lesion. In others, the initial presentation may be a trivial lesion or that of cellulitis, which can advance very rapidly. Clinical signs that the process involves the deeper tissue planes include failure to respond to initial antibiotic therapy, a hard, wooden feel of the subcutaneous tissue, altered mental status, bullous lesions and skin necrosis or ecchymoses. According to the microbiological characteristics, NF has two major types. In type I, the polymicrobial form (most originating from the bowel flora), up to 15 different anaerobic (e.g. *Clostridium, Bacteroides, Prevotella, and Peptostreptococcus*) and aerobic organisms (*E. coli, Klebsiella, Proteus*) may be cultured. Four major clinical settings of Type I NF are recognized: (1) surgical procedures involving the bowel or penetrating abdominal trauma, (2) decubitus ulcer or a perianal abscess, (3) at the site of injection in injection drug users, and (4) spread from a Bartholin abscess or a minor vulvovaginal infection. Nevertheless, some cases are caused by a single pathogen, particularly anaerobic *Streptococcus* species. Type II NF is monomicrobial and classically has been caused by Group A Streptococcus (GAS) (*Streptococcus pyogenes*). Most cases of NF caused by GAS (also known as hemolytic streptococcal gangrene, "flesh-eating disease") are community acquired and present in the limbs. An underlying cause (e.g. diabetes, peripheral vascular disease) is common. Cases of NF that arise after varicella or trivial injuries are almost always due to *S. pyogenes*. The mortality in this group is high, approaching 50%–70% in patients with hypotension and organ failure (44).Other causes of NF are: *V. vulnificus, A. hydrophila*, anaerobic streptococci (i.e., *Peptostreptococcus* species), and community-acquired MRSA (47). A definitive bacteriologic diagnosis is best established by culture of tissue specimens obtained during operation or by positive blood culture results. Aggressive surgical intervention is the major therapeutic modality in cases of necrotizing fasciitis. Antimicrobial therapy must be directed at the pathogens and several antibiotic choices for treating NF (44) are summarized as follow:

1. Treatment of polymicrobial NF must include agents effective against both aerobes and anaerobes. Choices include: a) ampicillin which may cover susceptible enteric aerobic organisms (e.g. *E. coli*) and gram-positive organisms, such as *Peptostreptococcus* species, group B, C, or G streptococci, and some anaerobes; b) clindamycin which is useful for coverage of anaerobes and aerobic gram-positive cocci, including most *S. aureus* serogroups; c) metronidazole which has the greatest anaerobic spectrum against the enteric gram-negative anaerobes (but it is less effective against the gram-positive anaerobic cocci); d) gentamicin or a fluorquinolone (ciprofloxacin), ticarcillin-clavulanate, or piperacillin-tazobactam, which may cover resistant gram-negative rods. The practice guidelines of the Infectious Diseases Society of America for treating NF consider a combination of ampicillin-sulbactam plus clindamycin plus ciprofloxacin as the best choice of antibiotics for community-acquired mixed infections (44).
2. Necrotizing fasciitis caused by group A streptococci should be treated with clindamycin and penicillin.

3. A history of water exposure or fish injury or handling in a patient with NF is typical of infections caused by *A. hydrophila*, and, in particular, V. *vulnificus*, the most common recognized marine pathogen of SSTIs. A combination therapy with cefotaxime or ceftazidime (which are also recommended for treating infections due to Aeromonas infection) and minocycline is suggested for treating adult patients with bacteremia and severe soft-tissue infection caused by *V. vulnificus* (48).
4. *S. aureus*, particularly MRSA, is the most common Gram-positive aerobe cause of complicated SSTIs. The increased prevalence of hospital-acquired MRSA has been noted worldwide and more recently also in the community setting (CA-MRSA) (46). In the Unites States, the predominant CA-MRSA clone is USA300 which has caused several numerous outbreaks including prison innmates, professional football players and others populations (46). Therefore, the IDSA guidelines for the management of patients with MRSA infections (49), recommend that empirical therapy for MRSA should be considered pending culture data in adult hospitalized patients with complicated SSTI (deeper soft-tissue infections, surgical/traumatic wound infection, major abscesses, cellulitis, and infected ulcers and burns). In addition to surgical debridement and broad-spectrum antibiotics these recommendations include the following options: intravenous vancomycin, oral or intravenous linezolid 600 mg twice daily, daptomycin 4 mg/kg/dose IV once daily, telavancin 10 mg/kg/dose IV once daily, and clindamycin 600 mg IV or PO 3 times a day. A β-lactam antibiotic (e.g. cefazolin) may be considered in hospitalized patients with nonpurulent cellulitis with modification to MRSA-active therapy if there is no clinical response. Seven to 14 days of therapy is recommended but should be individualized on the basis of the patient's clinical response. Obviously, the oral route is not recommended for septic patients.

7. Neutropenic fever

Fever occurs frequently during chemotherapy-induced neutropenia: about 30% of patients with solid tumors and > 80% of those with hematological malignancies will develop fever during at least one of the chemotherapy cycles associated with neutropenia (50). Mortality rate of sepsis in neutropenic patients is extremely high. Bacteremia occurs in 10-15% of all patients, with most episodes occurring in the setting of prolonged and profound neutropenia (absolute neutrophil count < 100) (51-53). Substantial fluctuations in the epidemiologic spectrum of bloodstream infections have occurred over the past 40 years. Early in the development of cytotoxic chemotherapy, during the 1960s and 1970s, gram-negative pathogens, particularly *E. coli, Klebsiella* spp., *Enterobacter* spp., *Pseudomonas aeruginosa* and *Stenotrophomonas* spp., predominated. In the 1980s and 1990s, gram-positive organisms became more common, because of the increasing use of indwelling intravenous catheters (53-58). Nowadays, there is again a trend toward a predominance of infections caused by gram-negative pathogens and in particular those due to multidrug-resistant (MDR) bacteria. Extended spectrum beta-lactamase (ESBL) producing gram-negative rods, especially *Klebsiella* and *Enterobacter* species, are sometimes susceptible only to carbapenems (59-60). Carbapenemase-producing *Klebsiella* and *Pseudomonas* species emerged recently and cause infections that are resistant to carbapenems (61). However, severe infections caused by gram-positive resistant pathogens such as MRSA and vancomycin-resistant *Enterococcus* (VRE), or penicillin resistant *pneumococci* and *viridans streptococci* are still prevalent in certain centers (62-64). An update which is intended as guidelines for the use of antimicrobial agents in managing patients with cancer who experience chemotherapy-induced fever and neutropenia was recently published by the IDSA (65). Accordingly, patients presenting with fever and neutropenia should receive empirical antibiotic therapy immediately after the initial clinical evaluation and after appropriate cultures are obtained. The initial empiric antibiotic treatment recommended for high risk patients with neutropenia, is monotherapy with an antipseudomonal beta-lactam agent, such as cephalosporin (cefepime), or a carbapenem (imipenem, meropenem), or a penicillin drug (piperacillin/tazobactam). Addition of an aminoglycoside (gentamicin, amikacin) as a combination therapy has not been proven beneficial in a meta-analysis of numerous trials (66). Modifications in the above regimens should be considered according to local epidemiological data and patient's specific risk factors. For instance, vancomycin, linezolid or daptomycin should be considered in the initial management of patients known to be colonized or previously infected with MRSA or VRE; for patients previously infected or colonized with ESBL-producing gram-negative rods, one should consider the early use of a carbapenem; colonization with carbapenem-resistant Enterobacteriacea (CRE) may justify the addition of drugs such as colistin or tigecycline. Empirical antibiotics are considered vital in febrile neutropenic patients. Although up to 23% of these episodes are associated with bacteremia (67), treatment should be continued even if blood cultures remain negative. Finally, high risk patients who have received intensive cytotoxic chemotherapy are at risk for invasive fungal infection. Yeasts which cause bloodstream infections (primarily *Candida* species), and molds which cause sino-pulmonary infections (primarily *Aspergillus species*) typically cause infections which are manifested by persistent or recurrent fever in patients with prolonged neutropenia, rather than causing initial fever in the course of neutropenia (68). Empirical antifungal coverage should be considered in high-risk patients after 4-7 days of a broad-spectrum antibacterial regimen and no identified fever source. For over 3 decades, amphotericin B was the drug used for empiric antifungal treatment, based on a study of Pizzo *et al* (69) which showed decrease mortality associated with this practice. In the last decade, a number of trials have identified roles for other antifungal agents with anti-yeast and anti-mold activity, like lipid formulations of amphotericin B, or echinocandins (caspofungin) and broad spectrum azoles (voriconazole), based on their lower toxicity compared to traditional amphotericin B (70-74).

8. Catheter related bloodstream infections (CRBSI)

Approximately 80,000 CRBSIs occur in ICUs every year (75). CRBSI is defined when bacteremia or fungemia occurs in a patient who has an intravascular device and a positive blood culture obtained from a peripheral vein, clinical manifestation of infection, and no apparent source for bloodstream infection other than the catheter. A positive result of semiquantitative catheter tip culture (>15 cfu) with the same pathogen, or of simultaneous quantitative blood cultures obtained from catheter and peripheral blood (ratio of >3:1 cfu/ml of blood, respectively) or differential time to positivity (≥ 2 hours) between catheter and peripheral vein blood culture are also required for this the definition (76). Gram staining routine culture with additional culture for fungi and acid-fast organisms as indicated, obtained from any exudate at the insertion site of the catheter, are important diagnostic tools, particularly when assessing immunocompromised patients. Several characteristics are associated with an increased risk of CRBSI with the most important being the type of the intravascular device (short-term central venous catheters are at the highest risk) (77), the intended use of the catheter (e.g. for total parenteral therapy nutrition use), the insertion site (femoral site at highest risk), the frequency with which the catheter is accessed, the characteristics of the patient, the experience of the individual who installs the catheter and the use of proven infection control measures (78-79). The pathogens that most commonly cause CRBSI differ a little according to the catheter type. In order of prevalence, the 4 groups of microbes that most commonly cause CRBSI associated with percutaneously inserted, noncuffed catheters are as follows: coagulase-negative staphylococci, *S. aureus, Candida* species, and enteric gram-negative bacilli. For surgically implanted catheters and peripherally inserted CVCs, they are coagulase-negative staphylococci, enteric gram-negative bacilli, *S. aureus*, and *P. aeruginosa* (79). The following discussion includes current recommendations for the management of CRBSI as updated by the IDSA in 2009 and emphasizes the most important aspects relevant to patients with CRBSI and sepsis (76). Most situations involving patients with CRBSI and sepsis require the removal of the catheter. Exceptions for this rule are patients with limited access sites and uncomplicated CRBSI involving long-term catheters (e.g., patients undergoing hemodialysis) due to pathogens other than *S. aureus, P. aeruginosa, Bacillus* species, *Micrococcus* species, Propionibacteria, fungi, or mycobacteria. In these patients treatment may be attempted without catheter removal, with the use of both systemic and antimicrobial lock therapy if there is a prompt response to antibiotic therapy (80, 81). The antibiotic lock should be changed every 24-48 hours. The concentration of the antibiotic in the lock solution should be at least 1000 times higher than the MIC of the microorganism treated (82). Although a declining incidence, MRSA represents approximately 7.5% of all reported ICU central line-associated bloodstream infections (83). In addition, coagulase-negative staphylococci are the most common cause of catheter-related infection. Most of these pathogens exhibit methicillin resistance, and this should be considered when choosing empirical therapy for catheter-related infection (84-85). Consequently, vancomycin should be recommended for the initial empiric antibiotic regimen of patients with CRBSI and sepsis. This regimen should include coverage for gram-negative bacilli using a fourth-generation cephalosporin (cefepime), or a carbapenem (imipenem, meropenem), or a beta-lactam/beta-lactamase inhibitor combinations (piperacillin/tazobactam), with or without an aminoglycoside (gentamicin, tobramicin, amikacin). Based on local antimicrobial epidemiologic and susceptibility data, empirical coverage for multidrug resistant gram-negative bacilli with additional drugs (e.g. colistin) may also be considered. A fungal etiology, mainly invasive *Candida* infection, should be suspected in septic patients with any of the following risk factors: TPN administration, prolonged use of broad-spectrum antibiotics, hematologic malignancy, femoral catheterization, or colonization with candida species in multiple sites (86, 87). An echinocandin (caspofungin, anidulafungin) is the recommended empirical treatment for patients with recent azole exposure, patients with moderately severe to severe illness, or patients who are at high risk of infection due to *C. glabrata* or *C. krusei* (88). Therefore, this class of drugs should be preferred for the empirical treatment when sepsis is present. Transition to fluconazole is recommended for patients who have isolates susceptible to fluconazole (e.g.,*Candida albicans*) and who are clinically stable. Duration of treatment depends on the pathogen involved. CRBSI caused by coagulase-negative staphylococci should be treated for 5-7 days if the catheter is removed, and for 10-14 days in combination with antibiotic lock therapy, if the catheter is retained. *S. aureus* CRBSI should be generally treated for 4-6 weeks. A short duration of treatment (minimum of 14 days) can be considered in the absence of following conditions: a) diabetes mellitus; b) immunosuppression; c) prosthetic intravascular devices or grafts; d) endocarditis or suppurative thrombophlebitis; e) metastatic infection. The same approach may be adopted if fever and bacteremia resolved after 72 hours of treatment or if the infected catheter was removed.

9. Conclusion

Sepsis is a clinical syndrome that complicates severe infection and is associated with high mortality rates despite aggressive medical care. Antimicrobial therapy plays a central role in the management of these patients. Early institution of empirical but appropriate antibiotic treatment can influence the outcome and this is optimally done through a systematic bedside clinical evaluation, paired with a judicious use of laboratory methods and other medical technologies until the causative organism and its antibiotic susceptibilities are defined.

Author details

Renato Finkelstein
Infectious Diseases Unit, Rambam Medical Center,
The Bruce Rapport Faculty of Medicine, Technion-Israel Institute of Technology, Haifa, Israel

Ilana Oren
The Bruce Rapport Faculty of Medicine, Technion-Israel Institute of Technology, Haifa, Israel

10. References

[1] Bone RC, Balk RA, Cerra, Dellinger RP, Fein AM, Knaus WA, ScheinRM, Sibbald WJ. Definitions for sepsis and organ failure and guidelines for the use of innovative

therapies in sepsis.The ACCP/SCMM Consensus Conference Committee.American College of Chest Physicians/Society of Critical Care Medicine.Chest 1992; 20:864-874.

[2] Pittet D, Thievent B, Wenzel RP, Li N, Auckenthaler R, Sutter PM. Bedside prediction of mortality from bacteremic sepsis: a dynamic analysis of ICU patients. Am J RespirCrit Care Med 1996;153:684-693.

[3] Opal SM, Fisher CJ Jr, Dhainaut JFA, Brase R, Lowry SF, Sadoff JC, Slotman GJ, Levy H, Balk RA, Shelly MP, Pribble JP, LaBrecque JF, Lookabaugh J, Donovan H, Dubin H, Baughman R, Norman J, DeMaria E, Matzel K, Abraham E, Seneff M. Confirmatory interleukin-1 receptor antagonist trial in severe sepsis: a phase III, randomized, double-blind, placebo-controlled, multicenter trial. The Interleukin-1 Receptor Antagonist Sepsis Investigator Group.Crit Care Med. 1997;25(7):1115-24.

[4] Angus DC,Linde-Zwirble WT.; LidickerJC, GillesC, JosephPMR. Epidemiology of severe sepsis in the United States: Analysis of incidence, outcome, and associated costs of care. Critical Care Medicine. 29(7):1303-1310.

[5] SasseKC, NauenbergE, LongA, AntonB; TuckerHJ, HuTW. Long-term survival after intensive care unit admission with sepsis. Critical Care Medicine 1995; 23 (6):1040-1047.

[6] Annane D, Aegerter P, Jars-Guincestre MC, Guidet B. Current Epidemiology of Septic Shock. The CUB-Réa Network.Am J Respir Crit Care Med. 2003;168: 165-172.

[7] Kumar A, Roberts D, Wood KE, Light B, Parrillo JE, Sharma S, Suppes R, Feinstein D, Zanotti S, Taiberg, L, Gurka D, Kumar A, Cheang M. Duration of hypotension before initiation of effective antimicrobial therapy is the critical determinant of survival in human septic shock. Critical Care Medicine 2006;34: 1589-1596.

[8] Dellinger RP, Levy MM, Carlet JM, Bion J, Parker MM, Jaeschke R, Reinhart K, Angus DC, Brun-Buisson C, Beale R, Calandra T, Dhainaut JF, Gerlach H, Harvey M, Marini JJ, Marshall J, Ranieri M, Ramsay G, Sevransky J, Thompson BT, Townsend S, Vender JS, Zimmerman JL, Vincent JL; International Surviving Sepsis Campaign Guidelines Committee. Surviving Sepsis Campaign: International guidelines for management of severe sepsis and septic shock: 2008. Crit Care Med. 2008;36(1):296-327.

[9] Angus DC, Birmingham MC, Balk RA, ScannonPJ, Collins D, Kruse JA, Graham DR, Dehidia HV, Homann SH, MacIntyre N. E5 murine monoclonal antiendotoxin antibody in gram-negative sepsis—A randomized controlled trial.*JAMA* 2000; 283:1723-1730.

[10] Rivers E, Nguyen B, Havstad S, Ressler J, Muzzin A, Knoblich B, Peterson E, Tomlanovich M. Early goal-directed therapy in the treatment of severe sepsis and septic shock. N Engl J Med. 2001;345(19):1368-1377.

[11] Bernard GR, Wheeler AP, Russell JA, Schein R, Summer WR, Steinberg KP, Fulkerson WJ, Wright PE, Christman BW, Dupont WR, Higgins SB, Swindell BB. The effects of

ibuprofen on the physiology and survival of patients with sepsis. N Engl J Med 1997; 336:912-918.

[12] Minino A, Heron AP, Smith BL.Death, preliminary data for 2004.*National Vital Statistics Report* 2006; 54(19):1-52.

[13] Pachon J, Prados D, Capote F, et al: Severe community-acquired pneumonia: Etiology, prognosis, treatment. *Am Rev Respir Dis* 1990; 142:369-373.

[14] Aliberti S, Amir A, Peyrani P, Peyrani P, Allen M, Moffet BK, Myers J, Shaib F, Cirini M, Bordon J, Blasi F, Ramirez JA. Zilberberg MD, Shorr AF, Micek ST, Mody SH, Kollef H. Incidence, etiology, timing, and risk factors for clinical failure in hospitalized patients with community-acquired pneumonia. *Chest* 2008; 134:955–962.

[15] Mandell LA, Wunderinck RG, Anzueto A, Barlett JG, Campbell GD, Dean NC, Dowell SF, File Jr. TM, Musher DM, Niederman MS, Torres A, Whitney CG.Infectious Diseases Society of America/American Thoracic Society Consensus Guidelines on the Management of Community-Acquired Pneumonia in Adults. Clin Infec Dis 2007; 44, Supplement 2: S27-S72

[16] Metersky ML, Ma A, Bratzler DW, Houck PM. Predicting bacteremia in patients with community-acquired pneumonia. Am J Respir Crit Care Med 2004; 169:342-347

[17] Craven D: Blood cultures for community-acquired pneumonia - piecing together a mosaic for doing less. Am J Respir Crit Care Med 2004; 169:327-335.

[18] FileTM. Community-acquired pneumonia. Lancet *2003;362:1991-2001.*

[19] Donowitz GR. Acute pneumonia. In: Mandell GL, Bennett JE, Dolin R (Eds). Principles and practice of infectious diseases (7th edition), Elsevier. 2010; pp:891-916.

[20] Richards MJ, Edwards JR, CulverDH, GaynesRP. Nosocomial infections in medical intensive care units in the United States. Crit Care Med 1999; 27:887-892.

[21] Cook DJ, Walter SD, Cook RJ, Griffith LE,Guyatt GH, Leasa D, Jaeschke RZ, Brun-Buisson C. Incidence of and risk Factors for ventilator-associated pneumonia in critically Ill Patients. Ann Intern Med 1998 129:433-440.

[22] Guidelines for the Management of Adults with Hospital-acquired, Ventilator-associated, and Healthcare-associated Pneumonia. Am. J. Respir. Crit. Care Med 2005; 171:388-416.

[23] Niederman MS. Use of Broad-Spectrum Antimicrobials for the Treatment of Pneumonia in Seriously Ill Patients: Maximizing Clinical Outcomes and Minimizing Selection of Resistant Organisms. Clin Infect Dis2006;42:S72-S81.

[24] Garnacho-Montero J, Ortiz-Leyba C, Jiménez-Jiménez FJ, Barrero-Almodóvar AR, García-Garmendia JL, Bernabeu-Wittell M, Gallego-Lara SL, Madrazo-Osuna J. Treatment of multidrug-resistant *Acinetobacter baumannii* ventilator-associated pneumonia (VAP) with intravenous colistin: a comparison with imipenem-susceptible VAP. Clin Infect Dis 2003; 36:1111-1118.

[25] Wunderink RG, Niederman MS, Kollef MH, Shorr AF, Kunkel MJ, Baruch A, McGee WT, Reisman A, Chastre J. Linezolid in methicillin-resistant *Staphylococcus aureus*

nosocomial pneumonia: a randomized, controlled study. Clin Infect Dis 2012; 54:621-629.

[26] Stamm WE, Hooton TM. Management of urinary tract infections in adults. N Engl J Med 1993;329:1328-1334.

[27] Sobel JD, Kaye D. Urinary tract infections. In: Mandell GL, Bennett JE, Dolin R (Eds). Principles and practice of infectious diseases (7th edition), Elsevier. 2010; pp:957-985.

[28] Stamm WE. Scientific and clinical challenges in the management of urinary tract infections. Am J Med 2002; 113:S1-S4.

[29] Nicolle LE. Catheter-related urinary tract infection. Drugs Aging 2005; 22:627-639.

[30] Richards MJ, Edwards JR, Culver DH, et al: Nosocomial infections in combined medical-surgical intensive care units in the United States. Infect Control Hosp Epidemiol 2000; 21:510-515.

[31] Nicolle LE. Update in adult urinary tract infection. Curr Infect Dis Rep 2011; 13:552-560.

[32] Gupta K, Hooton TM, Naber KG, Wullt B, Colgan R, Miller LG, Moran GJ, Nicolle LE, Raz R, Schaeffer AJ, Soper DE. International clinical practice guidelines for the treatment of acute uncomplicated cystitis and pyelonephritis in women: a 2010 update by the Infectious Diseases Society of America and the European Society for Microbiology and Infectious Diseases. Clin Infect Dis 2011 (52): e103-e120.

[33] Hooton TM. Nosocomial urinary tract infections. In: Mandell GL, Bennett JE, Dolin R (Eds). Principles and practice of infectious diseases (7th edition), Elsevier. 2010; pp:3725-3737.

[34] Levinson ME, Bush LM. Peritonitis and intraperitoneal abscesses. In: Mandell GL, Bennett JE, Dolin R (Eds). Principles and practice of infectious diseases (7th edition), Elsevier. 2010; pp:1011-1034.

[35] Solomkin JS, Mazuski JE, Baron EJ, Sawyer RG, Nathens AB, DiPiro JT, Buchman T, Dellinger EP, Jernigan J, Gorbach S, Chow AW, Bartlett J. Guidelines for the selection of anti-infective agents for complicated intra-abdominal infections. Clin Infect Dis.2003; 37:997-1005.

[36] Hao WL, Lee YK.Microflora of the gastrointestinal tract: a review. Methods Mol Biol 2004; 268:491–502

[37] Finegold SM: Abdominal and perineal infections. In: Finegold SM, ed. Anaerobic Bacteria in Human Disease, New York: Academic Press; 1977:257-313.

[38] Gorbach SL, Thadepalli H, Norsen J: Anaerobic microorganisms in intra-abdominal infections. In: Balows A, de Haan RM, Dowell Jr VR, Guze LB. Anaerobic Bacteria: Role in Disease, Springfield, IL: Charles C Thomas; 1974:399-407.

[39] Lorber B, Swenson RM: The bacteriology of intra-abdominal infections. Surg Clin North Am 1975; 55:1349-1354.

[40] Brook I. Microbiology and management of abdominal Infections. Dig Dis Sci 2008; 53:2585-2591.

[41] Solomkin JS, Mazuski JE, Radley JS, Rodvold KA, Goldstein EJC, Baron EJ, O'Neill PJ, Chow AW, Dellinger EP, Eachempati SR, Gorbach S, Hilfiker M, May AK, Nathens AB, Sawyer RG, Bartlett JG. Diagnosis and Management of complicated intra-abdominal infection in adults and children: guidelines by the Surgical Infection Society and the Infectious Diseases Society of America. Clin Infect Dis. 2010;50:133-164.

[42] Dryden MS. Complicated skin and soft tissue infection. J Antimicrob Chemother 2010; 65 Suppl 3: iii35–44.

[43] Di Nubile MJ, Lipsky BA. Complicated infections of the skin and skin structures: when the infection is more than skin deep. J Antimicrob Chemother 2004; 53 Suppl 2: ii37–50.

[44] Stevens DL, Bisno AL, Chambers HF, Everett ED, Dellinger P, Gorbach SL, Hirshmann JV, Kaplan EL, Montoya JG, Wade JC. Practice Guidelines for the Diagnosis and Management of Skin and Soft-Tissue Infections. Clin Infect Dis 2005; 41: 1373-1406.

[45] Eron LJ, Lipsky BA, Low DE, Nathwani D, Tice AD, Volturo GA. Managing skin and soft tissue infections: expert panel recommendations on key decision points. J Antimicrob Chemother 2003; 52 Suppl 1: i3–17.

[46] Stevens DL. Treatment for skin and soft tissue and surgical site infections due to MDR gram-positive bacteria. J Infect 2010; 59:S32-S39.

[47] Miller LG, Perdreau-Remington F, Rieg G, Mehdi S, Perlroth J, Bayer AS. Necrotizing fasciitis caused by community-associated methicillin-resistant *Staphylococcus aureus* in Los Angeles. N Engl J Med 2005:352:1445-1453

[48] Finkelstein R, Oren I. Soft tissue infections caused by marine bacterial pathogens: epidemiology, diagnosis, and management. Cur Infect Dis Rep Dis 2011; 13:470-477.

[49] Liu C, Bayer A, Cosgrove SE, Daum RS, Fridkin SK, Gorwitz RJ, Kaplan SL, Karshmer AW, Levine DP, Murray BE, Rybak MJ, Talan DA, Chambers HF. Clinical practice guidelines by the Infectious Diseases Society of America for the treatment of methicillin-resistant *Staphylococcus aureus* infections in adults and children. Clin Infect Dis 2011; 52:1-38.

[50] Klastersky J.Management of fever in neutropenic patients with different risks of complications. Clin Infect Dis. 2004; 39 Suppl 1:S32-7.

[51] Bodey GP, Buckley M, Sathe YS, Freireich EJ. Quantitative relationships between circulating leukocytes and infection in patients with acute leukemia. Ann Intern Med. 1966; 64(2):328-40.

[52] Rosenberg PS, Alter BP, Bolyard AA, Bonilla MA, Boxer LA, Cham B, Fier C, Freedman M, Kannourakis G, Kinsey S, Schwinzer B, Zeidler C, Welte K, Dale DC; Severe Chronic Neutropenia International Registry. The incidence of leukemia and mortality from

sepsis in patients with severe congenital neutropenia receiving long-term G-CSF therapy. Blood. 2006; 107(12):4628-35.

[53] Ramphal R. Changes in the etiology of bacteremia in febrile neutropenic patients and the susceptibilities of the currently isolated pathogens. Clin Infect Dis. 2004; 39 Suppl 1:S25-31.

[54] Zinner SH. Changing epidemiology of infections in patients with neutropenia and cancer: emphasis on gram-positive and resistant bacteria. Clin Infect Dis. 1999; 29(3):490-4.

[55] Wisplinghoff H, Seifert H, Wenzel RP, Edmond MB. Current trends in the epidemiology of nosocomial bloodstream infections in patients with hematological malignancies and solid neoplasms in hospitals in the United States. Clin Infect Dis 2003; 36(9):1103-10.

[56] Cattaneo C, Quaresmini G, Casari S, Capucci MA, Micheletti M, Borlenghi E, Signorini L, Re A, Carosi G, Rossi G. Recent changes in bacterial epidemiology and the emergence of fluoroquinolone-resistant *Escherichia coli* among patients with haematological malignancies: results of a prospective study on 823 patients at a single institution. J Antimicrob Chemother. 2008 Mar; 61(3):721-8.

[57] Oliveira AL, de Souza M, Carvalho-Dias VM, Ruiz MA, Silla L, Tanaka PY, Simões BP, Trabasso P, Seber A, Lotfi CJ, Zanichelli MA, Araujo VR, Godoy C, Maiolino A, Urakawa P, Cunha CA, de Souza CA, Pasquini R, Nucci M. Epidemiology of bacteremia and factors associated with multi-drug-resistant gram-negative bacteremia in hematopoietic stem cell transplant recipients. Bone Marrow Transplant. 2007; 39(12):775-81.

[58] Chen CY, Tang JL, Hsueh PR, Yao M, Huang SY, Chen YC, Chen YC, Shen MC, Wang CH, Tsai W, Chang SC, Tien HF, Luh KT. Trends and antimicrobial resistance of pathogens causing bloodstream infections among febrile neutropenic adults with hematological malignancy. J Formos Med Assoc. 2004; 103(7):526-32.

[59] Johnson MP, Ramphal R. Beta-lactam-resistant *Enterobacter* bacteremia in febrile neutropenic patients receiving monotherapy.J Infect Dis 1990; 62(4):981-3.

[60] Johnson PR, Liu Yin JA, Tooth JAA randomized trial of high-dose ciprofloxacin versus azlocillin and netilmicin in the empirical therapy of febrile neutropenic patients.J Antimicrob Chemother 1992; 30(2):203-14.

[61] Aubron C, Poirel L, Fortineau N, Nicolas P, Collet L, Nordmann P. Nosocomial spread of Pseudomonas aeruginosa isolates expressing the metallo-beta-lactamase VIM-2 in a hematology unit of a French hospital. Microb Drug Resist 2005;11(3):254-9.

[62] Morris PG, Hassan T, McNamara M, Hassan A, Wiig R, Grogan L, Breathnach OS, Smyth E, Humphreys H. Emergence of MRSA in positive blood cultures from patients with febrile neutropenia-a cause for concern. Support Care Cancer. 2008; 16(9):1085-8.

[63] Weinstock DM, Conlon M, Iovino C, Aubrey T, Gudiol C, Riedel E, Young JW, Kiehn TE, Zuccotti G. Colonization, bloodstream infection, and mortality caused by

vancomycin-resistant enterococcus early after allogeneic hematopoietic stem cell transplant. Biol Blood Marrow Transplant. 2007; 13(5):615-21.

[64] Carratalà J, Rosón B, Fernández-Sevilla A, Alcaide F, Gudiol F. Bacteremic pneumonia in neutropenic patients with cancer: causes, empirical antibiotic therapy, and outcome. Arch Intern Med. 1998; 158(8):868-72.

[65] Freifeld AG, Bow EJ, Sepkowitz KA, Boeckh MJ, Ito JI, Mullen CA, Raad II, Rolston KV, Young JA, Wingard JR.Executive summary: clinical practice guideline for the use of antimicrobial agents in neutropenic patients with cancer: 2010 Update by the Infectious Diseases Society of America. Clin Infect Dis. 2011; 52(4):427-31.

[66] Paul M, Soares-Weiser K, Grozinsky S, Leibovici L. Beta-lactam versus beta-lactam-aminoglycoside combination therapy in cancer patients with neutropaenia. Cochrane Database Syst Rev.2003;(3):CD003038.

[67] Klastersky J, Ameye L, Maertens J, Georgala A, Muanza F, Aoun M, Ferrant A, Rapoport B, Rolston K, Paesmans M. Bacteraemia in febrile neutropenic cancer patients. Int J Antimicrob Agents. 2007; 30 Suppl 1:S51-9.

[68] Rüping MJ, Vehreschild JJ, Cornely OA. Patients at high risk of invasive fungal infections: when and how to treat. Drugs. 2008;68(14):1941-62.

[69] Pizzo PA, Robichaud KJ, Gill FA, Witebsky FG. Empiric antibiotic and antifungal therapy for cancer patients with prolonged fever and granulocytopenia. Am J Med 1982;72:101–11.

[70] Walsh TJ, Finberg RW, Arndt C, Hiemenz J, Schwartz C, Bodensteiner D, Pappas P, Seibel N, Greenberg RN, Dummer S, Schuster M, Holcenberg JS. Liposomal amphotericin B for empirical therapy in patients with persistent fever and neutropenia. National Institute of Allergy and Infectious Diseases Mycoses Study Group. N Engl J Med 1999; 340(10):764-71.

[71] Walsh TJ, Teppler H, Donowitz GR, Maertens JA, Baden LR, Dmoszynska A, Cornely OA, Bourque MR, Lupinacci RJ, Sable CA, dePauw BE. Caspofungin versus liposomal amphotericin B for empirical antifungal therapy in patients with persistent fever and neutropenia. N Engl J Med. 2004; 351(14):1391-402.

[72] Wingard JR, White MH, Anaissie E, Raffalli J, Goodman J, Arrieta AL Amph/ABLC Collaborative Study Group. A randomized, double-blind comparative trial evaluating the safety of liposomal amphotericin B versus amphotericin B lipid complex in the empirical treatment of febrile neutropenia. Clin Infect Dis. 2000; 31(5):1155-63.

[73] Fleming RV, Kantarjian HM, Husni R, Rolston K, Lim J, Raad I, Pierce S, Cortes J, Estey E. Comparison of amphotericin B lipid complex (ABLC) vs. ambisome in the treatment of suspected or documented fungal infections in patients with leukemia. Leuk Lymphoma. 2001 Feb; 40(5-6):511-20.

[74] Boogaerts M, Winston DJ, Bow EJ, Garber G, Reboli AC, Schwarer AP, Novitzky N, Boehme A, Chwetzoff E, De Beule K. Itraconazole Neutropenia Study Group. Intravenous and oral itraconazole versus intravenous amphotericin B deoxycholate as

empirical antifungal therapy for persistent fever in neutropenic patients with cancer who are receiving broad-spectrum antibacterial therapy. A randomized, controlled trial. Ann Intern Med. 2001;135(6):412-22.

[75] Mermel LA. Prevention of intravascular catheter-related infections. Ann Intern Med 2000; 132(5):391-402.

[76] Mermel LA, Allon M, Bouza E, Craven DE, Flynn P, O'Grady NP, Raad II, Rijnders BJ, Sherertz RJ, Warren DK. Clinical practice guidelines for the diagnosis and management of intravascular catheter-related infection: 2009 update by the Infectious Diseases Society of America. Clin Infect Dis. 2009; 49(1):1-45.

[77] Maki DG, Kluger DM, Crnich CJ. The risk of bloodstream infection in adultswith different intravascular devices: a systematic review of 200 published prospective studies. Mayo Clin Proc 2006; 81(9):1159-71.

[78] O'Grady NP, Alexander M, Dellinger EP, Gerberding JL, Heard SO, Maki DG, Masur H, McCormick RD, Mermel LA, Pearson ML, Raad II, Randolph A, Weinstein RA. Guidelines for the prevention of intravascular catheter-related infections. Centers for Disease Control and Prevention. MMWR Recomm Rep. 2002; 51(RR-10):1-29.

[79] Safdar N, Mermel LA, Maki DG. The epidemiology of catheter-related infection in the critically ill. In: O'Grady N, Pittet D, eds. Catheter related infections in the critically ill. New York, NY: Kluwet, 2004: 1-23.

[80] Fernandez-Hidalgo N, Almirante B, Calleja R, Ruiz I, Planes AM, Rodriguez D, Pigrau C, Pahissa A. Antibiotic-lock therapy for long-term intravascular catheter-related bacteraemia: results of an open, non-comparative study.J Antimicrob Chemother. 2006; 57(6):1172-80.

[81] Fortún J, Grill F, Martín-Dávila P, Blázquez J, Tato M, Sánchez-Corral J, García-San Miguel L, Moreno S. Treatment of long-term intravascular catheter-related bacteraemia with antibiotic-lock therapy. J Antimicrob Chemother. 2006; 58(4):816-21.

[82] Kropec A, Huebner J, Wursthorn M, Daschner FD. In vitro activity of vancomycin and teicoplanin against *Staphylococcus aureus* and *Staphylococcus epidermidis* colonizing catheters. Eur J ClinMicrobiol Infect Dis. 1993; 12(7):545-8.

[83] Burton D, Edwards JR, Horan TC, Jernigan JA, Fridkin SK. Methicillin-Resistant *Staphylococcus aureus* Central Line–Associated Bloodstream Infections in US Intensive Care Units, 1997-2007 JAMA 2009;301:727-736.

[84] Miragaia M, Couto I, Pereira SF, Kristinsson KG, Westh H, Jarløv JO, Carriço J, Almeida J, Santos-Sanches I, Lencastre H. Molecular characterization of methicillin-resistant *Staphylococcus epidermidis* clones: evidence of geographic dissemination. *J Clin Microbiol* 2002; 40:430-8.

[85] Pottumarthy S, Fritsche TR, Jones RN. Evaluation of alternative disk diffusion methods for detecting mecA-mediated oxacillin resistance in an international collection of staphylococci: validation report from the SENTRY Antimicrobial Surveillance Program. Diagn Microbiol Infect Dis 2005 ;51:57-62.

[86] Lorente L, Jiménez A, Santana M, Iribarren JL, Jiménez JJ, Martín MM, Mora ML. Microorganisms responsible for intravascular catheter-related bloodstream infection according to the catheter site. Crit Care Med 2007; 35(10):2424-7.

[87] Raad I, Hanna H, Boktour M, Girgawy E, Danawi H, Mardani M, Kontoyiannis D, Darouiche R, Hachem R, Bodey GP. Management of central venous catheters in patients with cancer and candidemia. Clin Infect Dis 2004; 38(8):1119-27.

[88] Pappas PG, Kauffman CA, Andes D, Benjamin, Jr. DK, Calandra, TF, Edwards, Jr JE, Filler SG, Fisher JF, Kullberg BJ, Zeichner LO, Reboli AC, Rex JH, Walsh TJ, Sobel JD. Clinical Practice Guidelines for the Management Candidiasis: 2009 Update by the Infectious Diseases Society of America. Clin Infect Dis 2009; 48(5): 503-535.

Section 5

Sepsis in Specific Populations

Chapter 17

Infections in Leukemia

Rekha Chandran, Morgan Hakki and Stephen Spurgeon

Additional information is available at the end of the chapter

http://dx.doi.org/10.5772/50193

1. Introduction

Despite significant advances in supportive care, infectious complications continue to be a significant cause of morbidity and mortality in leukemia patients. The implementation of empiric antibiotic therapy in febrile neutropenia led to dramatic reduction in mortality and was hailed as a turning point in cancer treatment (1). Nonetheless, the development of more effective and dose intensive salvage chemotherapy regimens, incorporation of monoclonal antibodies, use of consolidation and maintenance strategies, and increased use of indwelling venous catheters have increased susceptibility to infections and changed the spectrum of infections in patients with leukemia (1). Specifically, multidrug resistant organisms, as well as those previously considered innocuous have emerged. Even under the optimal circumstances i.e. timely diagnosis and implementation of appropriate therapy, infections in leukemia remain a therapeutic challenge. Furthermore, delayed recognition and/or poor implementation of the appropriate treatment strategy can lead to significant morbidity and mortality while potentially increasing the economic burden associated with the infections seen in this immunocompromised population. Therefore, it is imperative that clinicians caring for this vulnerable group of patients have a thorough understanding of the infectious complications associated with leukemia and leukemia directed therapy.

This chapter includes a discussion of

a. Basic concepts and definitions;
b. Pathogenesis of infections in acute and chronic leukemia;
c. Spectrum of infections, with a focus on new and emerging infections;
d. Risk of certain infections associated with specific chemotherapy medications;
e. Clinical evaluation of suspected infection;
f. Treatment strategies, including empiric therapy and management of documented infection;

g. Role of prophylactic and preventive measures, in patients with acute and chronic leukemia;
h. Economic impact and outcomes.

1.1. Basic concepts and definitions

Fever in a neutropenic patient is usually defined as a single temperature >38.3ºC (101ºF), or a sustained temperature >38ºC (100.4ºF) for more than one hour (2).

Neutropenia is defined as an absolute neutrophil count (ANC) of less than 500cells/ microL whereas ANC less than 100 cells /microL is indicative of profound neutropenia (2).

Innate immunity refers to the body's natural resistance. It provides the first line of defense against a variety of pathogens. Innate immunity is not disease or pathogen specific and is composed of anatomic (skin and mucous membranes), physiologic (body temperature, gastric pH), and chemical (complement system) mediators, lysozyme and toll like receptors, phagocytic, and inflammatory aspects (3).

Adaptive immunity mediated by lymphocytes is a slower but highly specific response to antigen stimulation (3). B and T lymphocytes receive whole or partially processed antigens from antigen presenting cells from lymphoid tissue (lymph nodes and the spleen). These cells multiply at the site of infection to evoke a highly targeted antigenic response. Cytotoxic T (CD8+) lymphocytes spearhead the body's defense against intracellular pathogens. Helper T(CD4+) lymphocytes play a supportive role in providing necessary signals to CD8+ T lymphocytes that help not just in the primary response to infection, but also in the generation of memory CD8+ T cells and recruitment of CD8+ cells at the site of infection (4). B lymphocytes secrete antibodies, process and present antigens and transform into a pool of memory B cells for future defense (4). This capacity to retain immunologic memory is the distinguishing feature of adaptive immunity. Studies in murine models have demonstrated that NK cells, not just B and T lymphocytes possess the capacity to transform into memory cells (5). Immunologists have customarily considered Natural killer (NK) cells as a part of the innate system due to their ability to respond rapidly albeit non- specifically to infection (5). However unlike B and T lymphocytes that can generate responses to an unlimited range of antigen-specific receptors, NK cells can generate antigen specific responses limited to a population but not at an individual level. These cells are thought to represent a developmental transition between the innate and adaptive immune systems (5).

1.2. Pathogenesis of infections in leukemia

The acute leukemias are characterized by the rapid proliferation of immature progenitor cells and include acute myelogenous leukemia (AML) and acute lymphoblastic leukemia (ALL). Chronic leukemias typically run a more indolent course. This group includes chronic myelogenous leukemia (CML), chronic lymphocytic leukemia (CLL) and hairy cell leukemia (HCL). The accumulation and slow proliferation of mature appearing but functionally incompetent leukocytes is the common underlying pathology in chronic leukemias. The clinical presentations of infections are determined by a complex interplay between the pathogen and its virulence and the defense mechanisms of the host and the degree to which this is impaired.

Disease specific factors associated with host immune response

Studies in the early twentieth century led to a gradual shift in our understanding of the pathogenesis of infections. It became apparent that infections were not solely determined by the inherent virulence of the organism but also the susceptibility of the host (6).

In acute leukemia normal hematopoiesis is replaced by abnormal maturation and dysregulated proliferation of leukocytes (7). Coupled with significant bone marrow infiltration, this leads to decreased production of normal granulocytes resulting in neutropenia and impaired granulocyte function. Additionally, the presence of a large number of immature myeloid cells can inhibit antigen specific T cell response (8) Therefore, newly diagnosed leukemia patients often present with concurrent infections (7). Treatment with standard induction regimens results in prolonged neutropenia that can last weeks, rendering the host highly susceptible to bacterial and fungal infections (7). Furthermore, polymorphonuclear leucocyte function may be adversely affected by several chemotherapeutic medications such as high dose glucocorticoids, vincristine, vinblastine, carmustine, cyclophosphamide and 6- mercaptopurine (9). The risk of severe infections is not uniform among these patients and is related to the degree and duration of neutropenia (7) with the risk of developing more serious infections increasing with prolonged neutropenia (10) (11), the use of salvage chemotherapy, and previous antibiotic exposures (12). In acute leukemia patients, the risk of infection does not fully abate after achieving remission as patients can have prolonged defects in humoral immunity (13). This risk increases further with relapse of disease (14).

In addition, chemotherapy-induced mucosal disruption of the oropharynx and gastrointestinal tract enables normal commensals to access the bloodstream and cause invasive disease (15). In the 1980s, the use of central lines became widespread and contributed to the increased incidence of blood stream and systemic infections with skin flora (15).

Patients with CLL have defects in both humoral and cellular immunity as a result of their underlying malignancy, as well as therapy-related immune suppression from chemotherapeutics such as alkylating agents, purine analogues and monoclonal antibodies (16). Although these drugs have dramatically improved CLL outcomes, the predisposition to serious infections can result in significant morbidity - 80% of CLL patients will have a significant infection over the course of their disease, with up to 60% of people dying from infection (17).

B cell defects in patients with CLL can lead to hypogammaglobulinemia in the majority of patients (up to 70% within seven years of diagnosis) (18). Deficiencies can be seen in all three classes of immunoglobulins -IgG, A and M and is worse with advanced disease stage (19, 20). Severity and incidence of infections particularly respiratory infections correlated with low levels of serum IgG (19) as well as IgA (21,22). Decreased levels of opsonizing antibodies typically result in infections due to encapsulated organisms such as Streptococcus pneumoniae, Haemophilus influenza, and Neisseria meningitides (17). These patients also tend to respond poorly to vaccination (23). Impaired function of NK cells (lack of azurophilic granules that are necessary for normal killing activity (24)), neutrophils (reduced chemotaxis and migration) and monocytes and macrophage system have also been noted. T cells show a number of defects including abnormalities in gene expression and CD30 response, decreased CD4 to CD8 ratio (25), impaired Th2 polarization, and reversible acquired CD40 ligand deficiency (26)) all of which prevent T cells from initiating or maintaining and completing an immune response(18). Furthermore, patients can develop disease or therapy related neutropenia. These multiple immune defects predispose patients to bacterial, fungal, and viral infections.

Although the advent of improved diagnostics and more effective therapies have largely obviated the need for splenectomy across a number of hematologic malignancies, it may be performed for diagnostic reasons or in the setting of symptomatic splenomegaly, refractory autoimmune hemolytic anemia or thrombocytopenia (27,28). The spleen is a large mass of lymphoid tissue pivotal in filtering blood borne pathogens. It is also an antibody producing organ (29) and plays a role in the activation of alternative complement pathway which may be abnormal in those with anatomic or functional asplenia (30). Splenectomy therefore further predisposes this already at risk population serious infections including rapidly fatal infections with encapsulated organisms (see above), babesiosis, and capnocytophaga canimorsus (31-34).

HCL is an uncommon adult B-cell lymphoid leukemia that typically runs an indolent course and like CLL, many patients do not require immediate treatment (35). Clinical features include pancytopenia, splenomegaly (which may be complicated by rupture or infarction), and absolute monocytopenia (35). Infections remain a significant problem, presumably due to neutropenia and monocytopenia (36), and have been found to be prognostic. For example, survival at 4 years from diagnosis is markedly lower in individuals who have had infections as opposed to those who have not (49% versus 92%, p=0.0012)(36).

Age and malnutrition

Other factors that have been evaluated in the pathogenesis of infections in patients with leukemia include age and nutritional deficiencies. Fanci and colleagues compared the effect of age on the incidence of nosocomial infections in patients with acute leukemia older than 60 yrs compared to younger patients (37). The authors concluded that the risk of infection was no different in the study groups despite the added decline in immune function with age. However these results needed to be evaluated with caution as they were likely confounded by the fact that elderly patients with relapsed/ refractory disease were generally treated with less aggressive treatment regimens (37) which inherently may be associated with less infectious risk.

Nutritional deficiencies may also adversely affect the ability of normal tissue to withstand toxicity from chemotherapy resulting in need for discontinuation or dose reduction of chemotherapy (38); however, its impact on infections in leukemia is not well defined.

Key points

- In acute leukemia there are quantitative and qualitative defects in leukocyte function.
- The risk of infections in neutropenic fever is determined by the severity and duration of neutropenia.
- Disruption of mucosal lining due to toxic effects of chemotherapeutic drugs and the use of central venous catheters contribute to the risk of infection due to commensal organisms.
- In CLL both humoral and cellular immunity are impaired leading to a predilection to infection with encapsulated and intracellular organisms respectively.
- Patients with HCL are also at increased risk for infections which may be associated with worse outcomes.

1.3. Spectrum of infections in leukemia patients

Febrile neutropenia

The most common bacterial pathogen in the 1960s in neutropenic patients was Staphylococcus aureus (10,39). However, presumably due to the widespread use of methicillin, fatal staphylococcal infection rates dropped from 23.5% in 1954 to 3.1% in 1963 according to a ten year review of National Cancer Institute data (40). This success was dampened in the late 1960s and early 1970s by the emergence of aerobic gram-negative bacilli such as Klebsiella pneumonia, enterobacter , E. coli, Pseudomonas and other enteric organisms such as enterococci and anerobes(39). Cephalothin, a first-generation cephalosporin, led to improved outcomes with these infections. This period marked the emergence of Pseudomonas aeruginosa as a major pathogen associated with high mortality rates in this population (39). Although polymyxin and gentamicin were available as monotherapies to treat Pseudomonas bacteremia, the use of the first anti-pseudomonal carboxy penicillin carbenicillin, in combination with gentamicin, significantly reduced mortality from 60% in the 1960s to 10-30% in the 1980s (39).

In the 1990s, given their oral route of administration, broad spectrum of activity including against gram negatives, good bioavailability, and general low toxicity, prophylactic fluoroquinolone use became widespread. In addition, emerging resistance patterns resulted in an increased reliance on third generation cephalosporins for prophylaxis, empiric therapy for neutropenic fever, or treatment of gram negative infections. These developments, along with the increased use of implantable venous catheters, shifted the spectrum of infections back towards gram positive organisms such as staphylococcus and streptococcus species (41). Use of H2 antagonists and other antacids in conjunction with fluoroquinolones have also been implicated as a potential contributing factor to this shift (41,42).

Bloodstream infections (BSI) are commonly associated with mucositis, cellulitis, pneumonia, neutropenic enterocolitis, invasive fungal disease and central venous catheters (43,44) . The clinical presentations of BSI may vary from bacteremia to fulminant shock. In a survey of 49 hospitals between 1995 and 2001, the frequency of gram positive bloodstream infections increased from 62% in 1995 to 76% in 2001(45). The source of BSI was not identified in 52% of cases in this study. One hospital based study reported the re-emergence of gram negative organisms in primary nosocomial BSI (46). Interestingly, a seasonal increase in the incidence of gram negative BSI, particularly Acinetobacter, and to a lesser degree E.coli has recently been noted, stressing a need for greater vigilance during summer months (47). The epidemiology of BSI is included in Table 1. Coagulase negative staphylococci, Staphylococcus aureus, Viridans streptococci, and gram negatives are the most likely pathogens. Although candida is well known as a cause of catheter related blood stream infection, atypical catheter related infections from mycobacteria, nocardia, and Tsukamurella have been reported (48-52).

It should be emphasized that gram-negative organisms continue to dominate the scene as the most frequent pathogens causing infections in febrile neutropenic patients. Apart from BSI, other sites of infection include the respiratory tract (pneumonia, sinus), skin and soft tissue (mucositis and cellulitis), gastrointestinal (diarrhea , typhlitis, perirectal abscess, and enterocolitis) and genitourinary tract (UTI,) in order of frequency (53-55). Neutropenic enterocolitis, notorious for its morbidity and mortality may be further complicated by polymicrobial BSI due to aerobic gram negative bacilli and anerobes such as Clostridium septicum (56). The gastrointestinal tract (including the oral cavity) is often the site of origin of polymicrobial BSI. Elting and colleagues delineated factors associated with the poor response to treatment in a large study of polymicrobial infections in cancer patients. These included persistent neutropenia (25%), pneumonia (19%), and bloodstream infection caused by multiple gram-negative organisms (49%) (57) .

Clinical syndromes	**Pathogens/ Risk factors**
Upper gastrointestinal -Gingivostomatitis and periodontal lesions	Streptococci, gram negatives, herpes simplex, candida and uncommon bacteria like stomatococcus and aerococcus
Gastrointestinal infections- Typhlitis, neutropenic enterocolitis, perirectal abscess	Gram negatives and anerobes, C-diff.
Lower respiratory tract infections- Pneumonia (64)(65)	Gram negative bacilli, pneumococci, moulds, virus e.g CMV
Blood stream infections (45,66).	Coagulase negative staphylococcus (the most common isolate), S. aureus, E.coli and P.aeruginosa
Polymicrobial infections (67)	Gram-positive, anaerobic, or fungal , often seen with concurrent presence of a gram-negative bacillus.
Skin and soft tissue -cellulitis and folliculitis	Streptococci, staphylococci, anaerobes and gram negatives

Table 1. Sites of infection in neutropenic patients

Clostridium difficile associated diarrhea is common is patients with acute leukemia especially AML (58,59). It accounts for approximately one third of episodes of diarrhea and is more common with older age, number and duration of antibiotics and prolonged neutropenia prior to onset of diarrhea (59). Fluoroquinolone use has been implicated in the increased incidence of resistant Clostridium difficile (C-diff) infections (60). Toxin negative

Clostridium infections which have been described in up to 10% of patients, are particularly problematic, and require endoscopic studies for diagnosis (61). C-Diff therapy consists of metronidazole or, in severe cases, oral vancomycin (62), which has become the initial agent of choice at some institutions (63) due to increasing emergence of metronidazole resistance. Fidaxomicin is a new macrocyclic antibiotic has been shown to have clinical cure rates similar to vancomycin but superior in terms of lower recurrence rates (62). Table 1 summarizes the clinical syndromes, sites of infection and associated pathogens in neutropenic patients.

Resistant bacterial pathogens

Patients with leukemia are predisposed to infections and thus exposed to multiple antibiotics during the course of their therapy. The emergence of resistant organisms in this cohort of patients can be catastrophic.

1. Methicillin resistant Staphylococcus aureus (MRSA): accounts for 20-30% of nosocomial BSI and can lead to metastatic complications such as deep tissue and focal abscesses (e.g epidural, splenic), endocarditis and septic arthritis. MRSA is resistant to penicillin, cephalosporins and quinolones.
2. Vancomycin resistant staphylococci (VRSA): has become a growing concern no doubt due to the widespread use of vancomycin. Although linezolid and daptomycin can be used, these isolates may be less sensitive to these agents as well (68).
3. Vancomycin sensitive and vancomycin resistant enterococci (VRE): Risk factors include neutropenia, fluoroquinolone use, and previous treatment with vancomycin. E. faecium, which is often vancomycin resistant, has now surpassed E. faecealis as the predominant organism and is associated with a two-fold risk of higher mortality-in excess of 70% in the setting of neutropenia. In an attempt to decrease this risk, some centers have begun to isolate immunosuppressed VRE-colonized patients and employ barrier precautions (i.e. gowns, gloves); however, it is not yet clear if this approach impacts the outcomes of VRE infections. Linezolid and daptomycin are reasonable therapeutic options for the treatment of VRE infection. (41,69,70).
4. Multidrug resistant gram negative organisms have become especially problematic presumably due to the widespread use of antibiotics in this population. Extended spectrum beta-lactamase producing bacteria, such as Klebsiella and E coli, are resistant to fluoroquinolones, cephalosporins and penicillins (71). The carbapenams are usually effective in treatment. However in cases of carbapenamase producing Klebsiella, colistin can be used. Multidrug resistant pseudomonas requires colistin or polymixin B therapy (72).

Fungal infections

Invasive fungal infections (IFI) have been implicated as a complication in leukemia since the 1940s (10) and continue to be a major cause of morbidity and mortality in leukemia patients. Autopsy studies identified IFI as a cause of persistent fever and subsequent demise in neutropenic patients unresponsive to broad spectrum antibiotic therapy (10). The use of empiric antifungal therapy led to improved survival; however, it was often difficult to confirm a diagnosis of IFI. This in turn often led to overtreatment with antifungal medications and thereby significant treatment related costs and morbidity (73). Table 2 outlines the spectrum of fungal infections in neutropenic seen in leukemia patients. Although candidiasis and aspergillosis continue to be the predominant pathogens, additional fungi have emerged (Table 2). IFI should be suspected in the setting of persistent fever despite broad spectrum antibiotics.

Fungal Pathogen	Clinical features
Candida spp. (74)	Most common IFI infection. Severe immune suppression, broad spectrum antibiotics and central venous catheters are risk factors. Clinical presentation can range from BSI, gastrointestinal candidiasis and acute disseminated candidiasis.
Trichosporon spp. (75)(76)	Unusual fungal infection more often diagnosed per case reports in AML patients. It presents similar to candidemia and may also be associated with skin, kidney and lung findings if disseminated.
Cryptococcus(76)	Rare in leukemia, likely due to widespread prophylaxis with fluconazole, but if seen, occurs most often in AML, CLL and CML. Underlying severe T cell depletion, diabetes mellitus and use of steroids are added risk factors. Lung and nervous system often affected.
Aspergillus sp(77)(78)(74)(79)	Lungs, sinus and CNS infections often seen. Risk factors include prolonged neutropenia especially AML and steroid use (non neutropenic patients). Lung infections can present as fever, cough, pleuritic chest pain and massive pulmonary hemorrhage. Nodular pneumonia and CT finding of a nodule with a halo sign are characteristic. Serum galactomannan (GM) assay used with variable success in screening and diagnosis. Bronchoalveolar lavage (BAL) galactomannan optical density > 3.0 had 100% positive predictive value and less than 0.5 had high negative predictive value. False positive GM may be seen with concomitant administration of piperacillin/tazobactam, severe gastrointestinal mucosal disruption, and pneumocystis (*PJP*).
Zygomycetes (80-82)	Presents similar to aspergillus infections. Pathogenesis involves vascular invasion and tissue infarction manifesting as pulmonary, rhinocerebral and cutaneous infections. May progress rapidly; mortality in excess of 80% in disseminated disease.
Scedosporium (76)(83)	Can cause skin or pulmonary involvement. Associated with high mortality. Surgical drainage of fluid collections in skin, joint or soft tissue and systemic treatment are the cornerstones of therapy.
Endemic mycoses (84-88)	Reactivation of endemic fungal infections such as histoplasmosis, blastomycosis and coccidiomycosis can occur in the setting of immune suppression and can occur several years after leaving the region of original infection. Histoplasmosis may present in a disseminated fashion.

Table 2. Fungal infections in leukemia

Key points

- In neutropenic patients gram negative organisms remain the most frequent pathogens at sites other than blood stream infections.
- Gram positive organisms particularly oral commensals emerged as the leading cause of bloodstream infections in the 1980s.

- A number of factors such as the increased use of antibiotic prophylaxis and indwelling venous catheters have altered the spectrum of infections in leukemia patients.
- Clostridium Difficile infection has emerged as a major cause of morbidity in leukemia patients.
- Persistent fever after 4-7 days of broad spectrum antibiotics may indicate occult IFI.

Non- neutropenic patients

Among non-neutropenic patients with leukemia, a number of bacterial, viral, fungal and other opportunistic infections have been described. With the introduction of newer immunosuppressive or more aggressive therapies such as purine analogues, multiagent combination chemotherapy, monoclonal antibodies and steroids, the increased frequency of more atypical infections. With the introduction of newer immunsosuppressive or more aggressive therapies more atypical infections, such as CMV, Pneumocystis jirovecci pneumonia (PJP), liseria meningitis, and IFI have been seen highlighting the need for deliberation when selecting the the appropriate treatment regimen. Individuals at greatest risk of infection include those who have active disease, have undergone multiple previous treatment regimens, and longer disease duration (18).

Among the infections in patients with both acute and chronic leukemia, listeriosis is notable for its predilection for the central nervous system (90, 91). Listeria is a gram positive bacillus that gains entry into the blood stream via the gastrointestinal tract (90) . Listeriosis can present with bacteremia or with CNS involvement (meningitis (92), meningoencephalitis or cerebritis). Steroid therapy and nucleoside analogs such as fludarabine, which deplete T cells, are treatment associated risk factors (90). Ampicillin is the drug of choice, although vancomycin, carbapenams, fluoroquinolones and linezolid have good in vitro activity. Among viral infections, herpes virus reactivation is relatively common, with localized Herpes zoster reported more often than (93) disseminated infections (94-96). In addition, Epstein-Barr virus (EBV) reactivation is important and has been implicated in Richter's transformation (97).

Tuberculosis is seen in CLL more frequently than in other hematological malignancies (98). This is especially true for patients treated with fludarabine and the anti-CD52 monoclonal antibody alemtuzumab (as described in section C) (98). Atypical mycobacterial (99) infection in chronic leukemia is linked to a high mortality especially if disseminated (99-101). Clinical sites include skin (102,103), lung and multifocal osteomyelitis (104), but occasionally there may be no signs and symptoms other than fever. Bone marrow culture has a high diagnostic yield.

PJP can rapidly progress from fever and dyspnea to acute respiratory failure in a few hours (16). Parasitic infections such as toxoplasmosis and strongyloidiasis are rare in leukemic patients but have been described. For example, cerebral toxoplasmosis has been linked to patients with fludarabine refractory CLL with profound CD4 lymphopenia (105) and is associated with high mortality.

Key points

- Non-neutropenic patients with leukemia are susceptible to a host of bacterial, viral, IFI and other opportunistic infections.
- Patients with CLL and HCL who have been treated with newer immunosuppressive therapies remain profoundly lymphopenic several months after cessation of therapy and at risk for various opportunistic infections.
- Factors associated with increased risk of infection include duration of disease, T cell depletion, active disease and individuals who have undergone multiple prior therapies.

Other emerging pathogens

Unless the treating physician is aware of the pathogenic potential of bacteria widely believed to be harmless in the immunocompetent host, positive culture results may be dismissed as insignificant or as a contaminant.

- *Fusarium* is a mold that can cause rapidly fatal infections. Skin involvement is common and blood cultures are often positive. High dose liposomal amphotericin is the treatment of choice (106-110).
- *Corynebacterium* (e.g *Corynebacterium pseudodiphtheriticum* , *Corynebacterium jeikeium*) *Corynebacterium* is a gram positive bacillus that may present clinically as catheter related infections, pneumonia, endocarditis, urinary infections, keratitis and sepsis (111). Immunoglobulin deficiency in CLL is a predisposing factor (112). Mortality in the neutropenic host can be as high as 34% (111). *Corynebacterium jeikeium* is resistant to multiple antibiotics and vancomycin is the recommended antibiotic of choice (113).
- *Stenotrophomonas maltophilia* is a gram negative bacillus that normally resides in the oral mucosa. Patients with prolonged neutropenia and T cell defects may present with life threatening syndromes of hemorrhagic pneumonia and *ecthyma gangrenosum. Trimethoprim-sulfamethoxazole and fluoroquinolone-based multidrug combination regimens are used as first line treatment* (114-117).
- *Bacillus cereus*: A gram-positive rod that is typically associated with foodborne illness in the immunocompetent host. Patients can present with pneumonia, necrotizing gastritis, septic shock, multiorgan failure, disseminated intravascular coagulation, brain abscess, critical illness polyneuropathy and myopathy. Leukemia patients, particularly ALL patients, are more vulnerable. Risk factors that predict poor outcomes include severe neutropenia, presence of central venous catheters and CNS symptoms (118-122).
- *Lactobacillus* is a gram positive bacillus that may cause infection in the neutropenic patient. It presents usually as sepsis or pneumonia. Importantly, vancomycin has poor activity against *Lactobacillus,* and treatment with penicillin or related compounds is recommended instead (123).

1.4. Risk of infections due to specific chemotherapy agents

Alkylating agents and Anthracyclines

Anthracyclines (idarubicin, daunorubicin, and doxorubicin) are unique among chemotherapeutic drugs in that they induce apoptosis of hematopoietic cell lines (124) in the

G_0-G_1 phases of the cell cycle. They can deplete the peripheral T-cell pool and cause neutropenia secondary to myelosuppresion.(124) which can result in bacterial infections and IFI. However the incidence of gram negative infections and ≥ grade3 /4 infections (i.e. requiring IV antibiotics) may be reduced by the use of pegylated liposomal doxorubicin possibly due to reduced overall myelotoxicity (125).

Alkylating agents (e.g chlorambucil, cyclophosphamide, melphalan, bendamustine etc) cause DNA damage and prevent DNA repair activity both in normal and leukemic cells (126). Pyogenic infections due to Staphylococcus aureus, Streptococcus pneumoniae, Haemophilus influenza, Klebsiella and E. coli account for the vast majority of infections in patients treated with alkylating agents (17). These frequently involve the respiratory tract; however, infections of the urinary tract, skin and soft tissue can also occur. BSI are more likely to be seen in neutropenic patients. Candidiasis and aspergillosis occur in patients with prolonged neutropenia or who are treated concomitantly with high-dose steroids, prolonged antibiotic therapy, combination chemotherapy. Nocardia, listeria, mycobacteria and *PJP* can occur but are uncommon in CLL patients treated with alkylating agents alone (17).

Purine and Pyrimidine analogues

Purine nucleosides cladribine, fludarabine and pentostatin have been extensively used in CLL, HCL and other indolent B cell lymphoproliferative disorders. The risk of infections with these agents is related to both quantitative and qualitative T cell defects. Their use can result in prolonged suppression of all T cells especially CD4 cells, which can last up to 11-40 months after completion of treatment (127) (17). Consequently, as noted previously, the spectrum of infections broadens to include organisms such as Listeria, Nocardia, and mycobacteria. Disseminated candidiasis and aspergillosis are well recognized offenders. Concurrent treatment with steroids increases the likelihood of pneumocystis infections (93). Viral infections are common, especially varicella zoster virus (VZV) infection, which may be complicated by a high incidence of post-herpetic neuralgia. Reactivation of hepatitis B, adenovirus and cytomegalovirus (CMV) infections have been described (17). Cladribine has been used in CLL and HCL and can also cause prolonged suppression of CD4 cells which may recover at a a median of 40 months after therapy with CD8 cells returning to normal at 3 months (127). Purine nucleosides are stem cell toxic (128) and thus, may induce severe bone marrow suppression. The incidence of severe neutropenia has been reported as varying from 16-42% (129,130) and may persist for many months after completion of therapy. However, documented infections-where a pathogen is identified- are less common at 7-13%(129,130). Clofarabine is a second-generation nucleoside analog approved for the treatment of childhood ALL. It has been studied alone or in combination with cytarabine or idarubcin in adult patients with relapsed and/or refractory acute leukemia (131,132). The risk of myelosuppression and neutropenic fever is very high. In one study, Grade 4 neutropenia (ANC < 500) occurred in all patients and 38% developed a bacterial infection (12).

Of the **pyrimidine analogs**, cytarabine (cytosine arabinoside, Ara-C) is widely used in the treatment of both AML and ALL. Mayer and colleagues presented the results of using low

(100 mg/m^2), intermediate (400 mg/m^2) and high dose cytosine arabinoside (3 gm/m^2) for post remission chemotherapy in adult patients with AML. Myelosuppression resulted in ≥ Grade 3 neutropenic fever -significant to require hospital admission- in 71% (133) of patients in the high dose arm. Treatment-related deaths during remission, attributable to infections occurred in 1, 6 and 5% percent of the patients assigned to the low, intermediate and high dose groups respectively (133).

Corticosteroids

Corticosteroids are synthetic analogs of hormones produced in the adrenal cortex and are frequently used in the management of leukemia patients, particularly those with lymphoid malignancies. Despite their widespread benefits, the risk of infections is well known. Steroids impair T cell and neutrophil function, may camouflage classic signs and symptoms of inflammation, and are an independent risk factor for serious opportunistic infections in patients receiving other immunosuppressive therapy such as induction chemotherapy, alkylating agents and nucleoside analogues (17) (89).

A wide spectrum of bacterial, viral (CMV, HSV, VZV), fungal, tubercular and opportunistic infections have been reported in patients treated with chronic steroids (134,135).

Infections associated with corticosteroids are dependent on the route of administration (parenteral worse risk than oral route), dose, and duration of therapy -daily dose greater than 10 mg per day or a cumulative dose of more than 700 mg- as evidenced by data from 71 clinical trials (135). Unfortunately this analysis excluded trials in which patients were already on antiviral, antibacterial or antifungal prophylaxis, preventative practices common in this group of patients.

Monoclonal antibodies

Monoclonal antibodies have gained popularity for the treatment of various hematological malignancies. They potentially allow for more narrowly directed therapy for these diseases by targeting specific antigens expressed on the cell surface of malignant cells. However, normal hematopoetic cells express the target as well, resulting in off target effects. While a number immune conjugates, which incorporate antibody directed delivery of various toxins, have been developed, the majority of commercially available monoclonal antibodies rely on complement mediated and antibody mediated cytotoxicity against the malignant cells (136) which can disrupt adaptive immunity.

Rituximab is directed against CD20, which is a cell surface antigen expressed on B cells. It has limited use in CLL as monotherapy in part due to the limited expression of CD20 on malignant B cells in CLL (137). However, it has been shown to significantly improve outcomes when added to other agents (138). Neutropenia that can be seen including late onset neutropenia occuring several weeks to months after treatment, is typically self-limited with no clinically significant risk of infections, and appears to be linked to B cell recovery (139). Rituximab has been associated with reactivation of hepatitis B infection, which may be severe enough to require urgent liver transplantation (140), as well as progressive multifocal leukoencephalopathy (PML), which is due to reactivation of JC virus (141,142).

Ofatumumab is a novel fully humanized anti-CD20 monoclonal antibody recently approved for the treatment of CLL refractory to alemtuzumab and fludarabine (148). In the pivotal study, Grade 5 (fatal) infections were seen in 10% (149) of patients with pneumonia being the most frequent cause of infection. In a similar study 8-12% of patients developed grade 3 or 4 infections while receiving ofatumumab treatment (150) although the degree of additional immunosuppression mediated directly by ofatumumab is debatable as these patients were already severely immunosuppressed at the initation of therapy. Similar to rituximab, ofatumumab can cause neutropenia, however, the risk of grade 3 or 4 neutropenia in this heavily pre-treated populations was significantly higher (42% grade 3, 18% grade 4) (151).

Alemtuzumab: Alemtuzumab is a humanized monoclonal antibody directed against CD52, a cell surface glycopeptide expressed on virtually all human lymphocytes, monocytes and macrophages, a small subset of granulocytes, but not on erythrocytes, platelets or bone marrow stem cells (137). Alemtuzumab is used in the treatment of CLL and T cell prolymphocytic leukemia. Given the near ubiquitous expression of CD52 on immune cells, treatment results in the loss of circulating T cells, leading to defective cell mediated immunity and neutropenia in approximately 1/3 of patients. As a result, CMV reactivation occurs in 15 to 25% of patients and is the most commonly observed opportunistic infection (137,143-145). Other infections include herpes simplex, varicella zoster, *PJP*, candidiasis, cryptococcosis, toxoplasmosis and mold infections(aspergillosis and mucormycosis) (17) It is recommended that all patients receiving alemtuzumab receive antiviral prophylaxis (acyclovir, valacyclovir or famciclovir). Although valganciclovir is effective in preventing CMV reactivation (146), it can suppress bone marrow function and current guidelines recommend weekly screening for CMV viremia using PCR, and pre- emptive treatment with ganciclovir or foscarnet when patients are symptomatic or show increase in viremia (144). In a Cancer and Leukemia Group (CALGB) study by Lin et al (147) alemtuzumab was administered to patients who received induction therapy with fludarabine and rituximab. Improved complete response was noted, but event free survival did not improve due to serious infections (including listeria meningitis, CMV reactivation and PCP pneumonia) which occurred up to 7 months after completion of therapy (147).

Tyrosine Kinase inhibitors

Tyrosine kinase inhibitors (TKI) disrupt T-cell receptor mediated T-cell proliferation, activation and selective inhibition of memory CTL responses without interfering with primary T or B cell responses. *Imatinib* is the first agent in this class and has significantly improved the outcomes of CML patients (152). In a study of 250 CML patients treated with imatinib the most frequently seen infections were pneumonia, herpes zoster reactivation and urinary tract infections. The incidence of opportunistic infections was low (153).

Dasatinib is a multikinase inhibitor used for CML and ALL. It acts both as an antineoplastic and immunosuppressive agent at doses 140 mg or above. Grade 3 or 4 infections are more problematic in the accelerated phase compared to the chronic phase of the disease (89% versus 45%) (154) which is likely related to the underlying disease process.

Nilotinib

Nilotinib is an orally bioavailable TKI with increased selectivity for bcr-abl relative to other targets such as Src family or c-kit kinases. This probably accounts for the high efficacy of nilotinib without severe myelosuppression (155). Although all tyrosine kinase inhibitors cause myelosuppression, nilotinib is associated with more garden variety types of infections. In a phase II trial involving 280 patients with CML in chronic phase, grade 3/4 neutropenia (ANC < 1000) was noted in 29% of patients with a median duration of 15 days and need for dose interruptions or modifications in 10% of patients (155).

Key points

- Atypical infections are common in patients with CLL and HCL treated with monoclonal antibodies and purine nucleosides.
- Alemtuzumab is particularly immunosuppressive and its use requires close monitoring for CMV reactivation as well as prophylaxis for *PJP* and fungal infections.
- Concurrent use of steroids significantly increases the risk of infections.
- Risk of severe infections may persist for months after cessation of therapy.
- The risk of infections in patients with CML receiving TKIs is relatively low.

1.5. Initial evaluation and risk stratification

Neutropenic fever is a medical emergency and thus requires prompt evaluation and initiation of empiric therapy. While a variety of noninfectious causes including transfusion of blood products, medications, and the underlying malignancy itself, may cause fever, the presence of fever should always be presumed to be due to an underlying infection until proven otherwise. Initial evaluation of the neutropenic patient should include a complete history, with special attention given to identifying prior chemotherapies, previous infectious complications, and recent or current prophylactic antimicrobial therapies. A thorough physical examination, blood and bodily fluid cultures -based on clinical suspicion-, and appropriate radiographic imaging are integral to the evaluation of these patients. Clinicians should be aware that in the neutropenic host, signs and symptoms of infection may be blunted by a decreased inflammatory response and therefore, a high index of clinical suspicion is essential for expeditious diagnosis and treatment. For example, only 8% of neutropenic patients with pneumonia produce sputum compared to 84% in non neutropenic patients (64).

In order to better stratify which patients require more intensive management, scoring systems and treatment algorithms have been devised. For example, the Multinational Association for Supportive Care in Cancer (MASCC) scoring system is a well validated tool for risk stratification of febrile neutropenic patients based on the burden of illness (mild, moderate or severe), absence of hypotension, absence of chronic obstructive lung disease, absence of dehydration, age less than 60 years, outpatient status at the time of onset of fever and solid tumor or lymphoma with no previous fungal infection (156,157). A cumulative score of 20 or more is predictive of a less than 5% chance of developing serious medical complications. This is a valuable tool to identify low risk patients who may be treated as an outpatient (158). However, it is more common practice to observe the patient in the hospital for at least 24 hours on empiric IV antibiotics to confirm low risk status (159).

Key points

- Patients with neutropenic fever should undergo a rapid and comprehensive evaluation.
- MASCC scoring can be used as a general guide to help risk stratify patients and identify those who would benefit from outpatient treatment noting that most leukemia patients are high risk and warrant a period of hospitalization.

1.6. Treatment of infections

The four basic approaches to infections in leukemia patients include **prophylactic** (prevention of infection in high risk individuals by appropriate medications), **empiric** (initiating treatment on symptomatic individuals before positive cultures), **pre-emptive** (initiating treatment on the basis of positive or rising titers at the onset of clinical or radiological signs(160)) and **traditional** (treatment based on positive cultures).

During the 1950s it was not common practice to initiate antibacterial therapy before a specific pathogen was identified (10). Not surprisingly, this fundamental principle was associated with high mortality rate among neutropenic leukemia patients. Early randomized trials failed to demonstrate improved outcomes with the use of empiric antibiotics in the management of febrile neutropenia (161). However, shortly thereafter, subsequent studies in leukemia patients showed a significant benefit for patients treated with empiric antibiotic therapy prior to bacteriological data becoming available (162,163). This established the paradigm of empiric antibiotic use which is still used to guide the initial approach to managing neutropenic leukemia patients. In the setting of neutropenic fever, treatment of the most likely focus should be initiated and include coverage for the most virulent and prevalent pathogens. In the absence of an obvious focus, broad spectrum empiric therapy covering gram positives and gram negatives should be initiated and be guided by institutional protocols based on local resistance patterns pending results of initial tests. Initial combination therapy should take into consideration any recent antibiotic prophylaxis, prior infections including with resistant organisms, presenting signs and symptoms, exam findings, severity of infection, organ function, and co-morbidities.

The three basic antibiotic regimens include: 1) monotherapy with an antipseudomonal beta-lactam such as cefepime, 2) a beta lactam plus an aminoglycoside or a fluoroquinolone, and 3) a glycopeptide in addition to beta lactam monotherapy. Due to the concern for emergence of resistance, vancomycin is not routinely used in the empiric treatment of neutropenic fever unless any of the following criteria are met: positive blood cultures with smears showing gram positive cocci, critically ill patients, presence of skin or soft tissue infection, suspicion of catheter related infection, or known colonization or prior infection with MRSA (2).

There are several options for the treatment of MRSA infection. Vancomycin has been used traditionally for this indication. Vancomycin dosing should be adjusted based on trough levels, with a goal trough of 15-20 mcg/mL.(164) Toxicities associated with high trough levels include renal injury, ototoxicity, and myelosuppresison. Vancomycin should not be used to treat MRSA infection if the MIC of the MRSA is ≥ 2 μg/ml due to a high rate of treatment failure (164). Daptomycin has become the second-line agent of choice for MRSA infections. Daptomycin can induce eosinophilic pneumonia (165) and has been associated with rhabdomyolysis (package insert). Linezolid has the advantage of good bioavailability after oral administration, but is bacteriostatic against MRSA and therefore, should be used with caution in life-threatening MRSA infections. Myelosuppression, serotonin syndrome when administered concurrently with serotonin uptake inhibitors (SSRI)), and rhabdomyolysis are notable linezolid related toxicities (166,167). Ceftaroline is a new cephalosporin that has activity against MRSA and is approved for use in skin and soft tissue infections (168). Doxycycline, TMP/SMX, and clindamycin all possess activity against most MRSA isolates but are traditionally reserved for the treatment of non-life threatening infections such as uncomplicated skin and soft tissue infections.

Even with the initiation of the appropriate empiric antibiotic, it may take days for fevers to abate in neutropenic patients; however, if fevers persist without an obvious focus or culture result after 4-7days of antibacterial therapy, persistent fever atypical organisms and IFI must be considered. In this case, empiric antifungal therapy may be initiated while further diagnostic tests are done. Prompt removal of catheters is essential if suspected to be the source of infection. Due to the widespread use of fluconazole and posaconazole as antifungal prophylaxis, the possibility of azole resistance should be borne in mind. In the treatment of candidemia, IDSA guidelines recommend fluconazole for the less critically ill who have not been exposed to this drug or echinocandins, such as micafungin or caspofungin (169). Voriconazole or liposomal amphotericin may be used as first line in more critically ill individuals. Voriconazole has emerged as a safe and more efficacious alternative to liposomal amphotericin for the empiric treatment of fungal infections in febrile neutropenia (170) and as the primary therapy of invasive aspergillosis (171) based on two landmark randomized trials. The 2008 IDSA guidelines recommend voriconazole as first line therapy for invasive aspergillosis (2,74). This drug has high bioavailability in both oral and intravenous forms. For patients who fail voriconazole or therapy is limited by toxicity such as hallucinations, hepatotoxicity, or skin rash, conventional amphotericin B or liposomal preparation can be used (74). Both forms of amphotericin have similar success rates but the latter has less toxicity allowing for the use of higher doses. Infusional toxicity (fever, chills, and hypotension), potassium and magnesium wasting and frequent renal toxicity are complications of amphotericin.

The three echinocandins in clinical use are caspofungin, micafungin and anidulafungin. This class of medications inhibits the synthesis of 1,3-β-D-glucan, an essential component of the fungal cell wall (172). All three drugs are fungistatic against Aspergillus spp although the minimal effective concentration for micafungin and anidulafungin are 2- 10 fold lower than caspofungin (172). Caspofungin has been approved for use in refractory aspergillosis or invasive disease where other treatment options cannot be tolerated. It has also been used as a single agent in pulmonary aspergillosis in patients with hematological malignancies (173).

Micafungin has a clinical efficacy that is comparable to caspofungin (174). Unlike, the other echinocandins anidulafungin is unique in that it undergoes elimination by breakdown in the bile rather than via hepatic metabolism (172) and like micafungin has the added advantage of not requiring dose reduction in moderate liver disease (172).

Surgical debridement followed by antifungal treatment for zygomycosis (mucormycosis) with lipid formulations of amphotericin B is the standard of care (74). Posaconazole is recommended as salvage therapy but not as first line (175). Voriconazole is the drug of choice in the treatment of scedosporium (176). The optimal duration of therapy in these infections has not been determined by clinical trials and is largely determined by the treating physician.

Observational studies have indicated increased mortality with delay in starting antifungal therapy (177,178). The dilemma in initiating prompt antifungal therapy is complicated by the fact that fewer than 5% patients who receive empiric therapy go on to develop or demonstrate evidence of IFI in the first 48 hours (179). Therefore, with the increasing availability of newer diagnostic techniques in IFI, there is an interest in active surveillance with non-culture based methods and initiation of treatment before the onset of signs and symptoms. This pre-emptive therapy, although being practiced by clinicians, is still considered experimental (180) and the NCCN (National Comprehensive Cancer Network) does not currently recommend pre- emptive therapy due to lack of sufficient evidence to support routine use (181). However, a number of leukemia centers have adopted prophylactic and empiric treatment strategies which incorporate anti-fungal therapy. Although combination therapy for invasive aspergillosis has shown therapeutic promise in a number of small studies (182,183), this approach has not been validated in large prospective randomized studies and is not currently recommended.

In *PJP* infections, CXR can show bilateral alveolar infiltrates although a normal CXR does not exclude the diagnosis. Gold standard for diagnosis is direct immunofluorescence to detect the organism although recently measurement of 1-3-beta-d- glucan is being studied with interest. So far it has not shown reliable prognostic value and can be elevated in several mycoses making it a very non- specific test (184,185). Trimethoprim/ sulfamethoxazole is the first line of therapy and is the standard prophylactic agent. Other options include pentamidine, trimerexate atovaquone and clindamycin. A high index of suspicion should be maintained especially in patients who have received ongoing steroids or T-cell depleting therapies.

Key points:

- Empiric treatment with broad spectrum coverage in the absence of an obvious focus should follow institutional guidelines according to local resistance patterns.
- Delay in instituting empiric antibiotic and antifungal therapy is associated with worse outcomes.
- One should consider IFI if fever persists > 4-7 days in the setting of appropriate broad spectrum antibiotic therapy and negative cultures.

- If a source of infection is identified, the therapy should be appropriately tailored/ adjusted.
- Preemptive therapy involves active surveillance to detect viral and fungal infections based on rising titers and institution of treatment with onset of symptoms
- A number of antifungal therapies are available for the treatment of fungal infections in leukemia patients and should be selected based on the suspected pathogen, severity of illness, and co-morbidities.
- *PJP* infection should be suspected in patients with unexplained hypoxia, even in the setting of a normal chest xray, especially in patients who have received T-cell depleting therapy.

1.7. Prophylaxis

Due to the high mortality and costs associated with infections, there is a great interest in preventing them. Various approaches have been adopted and this is an area of active research.

Antibiotics: IDSA recommends prophylactic FQ for high risk patients defined as patients with expected durations of prolonged and profound neutropenia(ANC ≤ 100 cells/mm3 for > 7 days)(2) Among the FQ, ciprofloxacin has maximum activity against Pseudomonas whereas levofloxacin has the added advantage of activity against some gram positives and once a day dosing at the expense of less anti- pseudomonal coverage(186). The main concern with the use of FQ has been the emergence of resistant bacteria. However, surprisingly, in the setting of febrile neutropenia, this increase in resistant organisms has not translated into increased infectious mortality. (187).(60)

Antiviral: NCCN recommends acyclovir or valacyclovir for patients with acute leukemia or T cell depleting therapy for HSV seropositive individuals throughout the neutropenic phase and a minimum of 2 months after alemtuzumab therapy or until the circulating CD4 count is more than 0.2×10^9/L (181). Patients who are inactive carriers of hepatitis B virus should receive lamivudine 100 mg daily for 3 months following cessation of chemotherapy (181). Preemptive influenza chemoprophylaxis with oseltamivir, amantadine or rimantidine is recommended after known exposure to a confirmed case during an established outbreak (181).

Antifungals: Outside of bone marrow transplant there is very little evidence to support the routine use of antifungal prophylaxis. IDSA recommends prophylaxis against candida with fluconazole, itraconazole, voriconazole, posaconazole, micafungin, or caspofungin for patients undergoing intensive remission induction or salvage chemotherapy in acute leukemia (2). In this group IDSA also recommends use posaconazole for prophylaxis against aspergillosis (2). In patients with AML or myelodysplastic syndrome undergoing chemotherapy posaconazole prevented IFI compared to fluconazole or itraconazole and was associated with improved overall survival (188). NCCN recommends antifungal prophylaxis only in leukemia patients receiving mucotoxic regimens including cytarabine and anthracycline (181) *PJP* prophylaxis is recommended for patients receiving alemtuzumab (181) however, many centers have adapted widespread use of *PJP* prophylaxis in patients receiving any T-cell depleting therapy.

Colony stimulating factors (CSF): The main benefit of CSF is in hastening time to recovery of neutrophil function and number of hospital days but these have not been shown to affect mortality (189). ASCO guidelines recommend use of CSF in patients at increased risk of complications from prolonged neutropenia such as age > 65 yr, poor performance status, malnutrition, advanced cancer, bone marrow infiltration, active or open wounds, and/or extensive prior treatment (190). Secondary prophylaxis is recommended in individuals who experienced complications due to neutropenia during a prior cycle (190). Given the potential concern for promotion of myeloid stimulation in active AML, myeloid growth factors are typically not given during primary induction therapy. However, they are typically utilized in patients after consolidation therapy.

Intravenous immunoglobulin (IVIG): IVIG is not routinely advised in patients with CLL due to lack of known benefit in preventing life threatening infections. However, it should be considered in those with recurrent sinopulmonary infections or in those with underlying refractory CLL. In a multicenter double-blind study, 84 CLL patients at high risk for infections (history of hypogammaglobulinemia, infections, or both) were randomized to receive IV immunoglobulin G (IVIG) (400 mg/kg) every 3 weeks or placebo. Although moderate bacterial infections were reduced by 50%, there was no subsequent reduction in mortality (191). Another study found that the number of infection related admissions was reduced with IVIG administration (192). However in a cost effective analysis it was determined that IVIG therapy resulted in a 0.8 day per patient per quality adjusted life year at a cost of $6 million per year gained implying a prohibitive cost for minimal benefit (193). This was mainly due to the loss of quality of life due to the need to receive IV infusion every 3 weeks. The authors estimated that even if immune globulin were to be given free of cost, treatment would result in a net savings of only $814 because of lower infection rates and, thus, lower medical costs. At a cost of $50 per treatment, the marginal cost of treatment equals that of no treatment (193).

Active immunization: Annual influenza vaccination is recommended for all cancer patients lifelong (2). Immunization responses in CLL patients are variable but suboptimal. One study found that 73% of stage zero CLL patients had decreased levels of at least one immunoglobulin. Vaccination is most successful if used earlier in the disease, when immunoglobulin levels are better preserved, and if protein or conjugated vaccines are used (194). Response to hemophilus and tetanus vaccines may be enhanced by the use of adjuvant ranitidine but it has no beneficial effect on the response to vaccination with unconjugated polysaccharide antigens (195). Given the immunosuppressive effects of leukemia directed treatment, it is recommended that vaccines not be performed in the peri-chemotherapy period. Live vaccines including polio (oral), typhoid (oral), yellow fever, measles, mumps, rubella, BCG and Herpes zoster should not be administered to patients with CLL (18).

Vaccine based strategies to prevent IFI are hampered by the fact that the population that will most benefit from this approach is able to mount the least immune response..

Torosantucci et al have developed a fungal vaccine consisting of laminarin that was protective against candidiasis and aspergillosis (196). Currently, developing vaccines for this immunosuppressed patient population remains an active area of research (197).

Key points

- Prophylactic antibiotics, antivirals and antifungals should be given to patients at highest risk for these infections.
- The role of IVIG in CLL is controversial and not routinely recommended due to lack of cost effectiveness although moderate reduction in infections have been noted and its use should be considered in patients with hypogammaglobulinemia and recurrent sinopulmonary infections.
- Patients with CLL should be vaccinated earlier in their disease to reap maximum benefit due to decline in antibody response with disease duration.
- Live virus vaccines should be avoided in immunosuppressed patients.
- Growth factors shorten the duration of neutropenia but do not impact mortality.

1.8. Economic burden and outcomes of infections in leukemia

Infections increase the costs of treatment in patients with leukemia and can drastically influence the economic burden of the disease (198). There are no recent direct studies that have addressed the economic burden related to infections in patients with leukemia. However, in 2000, aggregate US hospital costs were 2.1 billion dollars with AML being the most costly leukemia followed by ALL, CML and CLL (198). In patients with CLL, infections have been shown to contribute to higher total cost of care (198). Patients with leukemia who are critically ill have worse outcomes than non- cancer patients. Relapsed/ refractory status of disease and high Sequential Organ Failure Assessment (SOFA) score (a simple and objective score that allows for calculation of both the number and the severity of organ dysfunction in six organ systems -respiratory, coagulation, liver, cardiovascular, renal, and neurologic) (199) have been found to be predictive of high mortality (200). Among ICU survivors 1 year mortality for acute leukemia patients is lower than patients with other malignancies (201). In a study by Thakkar et al evaluating predictors of outcome for patients with acute leukemia admitted to the ICU, respiratory distress was the most frequently observed reason for ICU admission or transfer with the majority requiring ventilator support (202). The two, six, and twelvemonth overall survival was 24 (27%), 16 (18%), and 14 (16%), respectively. Higher APACHE II score (a severity of disease classification system that helps prognostically risk stratify acutely ill patients) (203), use of vasopressors, undergoing bone marrow transplantation preparative regimen, and adverse cytogenetics were predictors of worse outcomes whereas a new diagnosis of leukemia, type of leukemia and age were not significant. (202).

A study by Schapira in 1993 evaluated the economic cost of survival in patients with hematologic malignancies. Factors noted to be significant for survival included: the nadir platelet count and albumin level prior to and during the ICU stay, the BUN, creatinine, and the need for mechanical ventilation. Seventy-eight percent of patients survived less than five months and spent less than two and a half months at home after discharge. Fifty percent of patients expired during their ICU stay. The cost per year of life gained for the entire group of patients was $189,339 per.admission (204). However, this study did not differentiate between relapsed/refractory or de novo disease. Documented infection was noted in 54.7% of individuals who expired in the hospital. Among patients who were discharged from the hospital, documented infections were noted in 29.3% of patients who survived for less than 6 months but in only 16% of patients who survived for more than 6 months. Taken together, these studies highlight the impact of infections in leukemia patients, especially those with relapsed/refractory disease, with a direct correlation to hospital mortality and post discharge survival (204).

Careful patient selection improves outcomes without the burden of futile economic costs. It has been recommended that patients with good performance status, where life prolonging treatment options are available- especially patients with new or recent diagnosis of leukemia, should be given the benefit of intensive care support, while patients with poor prognosis who may benefit from a palliative care approach should not. This is often a difficult choice for the treating provider. A middle of the road approach might be to initiate ICU care unless declined by the patient with a goal to regularly reassess the patients wishes and/or condition (205) and proceed to comfort care if continued aggressive therapies are deemed to be of minimal benefit.

Key points

- Intensive care costs for treatment of patients with leukemia are significant
- Careful selection of patients improves outcomes without adding significantly to economic costs.
- Patients with refractory or relapsed leukemia and poor performance status are unlikely to benefit from ICU stay
- Identifying low risk patients with neutropenia using MASCC scoring can help minimize the costs of treatment of neutropenic fever.

2. Summary

With rapid advances in diagnostic techniques and availability of newer chemotherapeutic and antibiotic medications in the armamentarium against leukemia, the spectrum of infections continues to change. Clinicians face evolving clinical, diagnostic and ethical challenges to select the most cost effective and evidence based care. The cornerstone of therapy should however be an individualized and patient oriented approach in order to achieve the best outcomes.

Author details

Rekha Chandran
Legacy Health System Portland, OR

Morgan Hakki
Division of Infectious Disease Oregon Health and Science University Portland, OR

Stephen Spurgeon
Center for Hematologic Malignancies Oregon Health and Science University Portland, OR

3. References

[1] Viscoli C, Varnier O, Machetti M. Infections in Patients with Febrile Neutropenia: Epidemiology, Microbiology, and Risk Stratification. Clinical Infectious Diseases 2005 April 01;40(Supplement 4):S240-S245.
[2] Freifeld AG, Bow EJ, Sepkowitz KA, Boeckh MJ, Ito JI, Mullen CA, et al. Clinical practice guideline for the use of antimicrobial agents in neutropenic patients with cancer: 2010 Update by the Infectious Diseases Society of America. Clin Infect Dis 2011 Feb 15;52(4):427-431.
[3] Goldsby R. Overview of the immune system. In: Kuby J, editor. Immunology. Fifth ed.; 2003. p. 5-9.
[4] Nakanishi Y, Lu B, Gerard C, Iwasaki A. CD8(+) T lymphocyte mobilization to virus-infected tissue requires CD4(+) T-cell help. Nature 2009 Nov 26;462(7272):510-513.
[5] Sun JC, Lanier LL. Natural killer cells remember: an evolutionary bridge between innate and adaptive immunity? Eur J Immunol 2009 Aug;39(8):2059-2064.
[6] Casadevall A, Pirofski LA. Host-pathogen interactions: redefining the basic concepts of virulence and pathogenicity. Infect Immun 1999 Aug;67(8):3703-3713.
[7] Young L. Management of infections in leukemia and lymphoma. In: Rubin R, Young L, editors. Clinical approach to infection in the compromised host. 4th ed. p. 497-522.
[8] Almand B, Clark JI, Nikitina E, van Beynen J, English NR, Knight SC, et al. Increased Production of Immature Myeloid Cells in Cancer Patients: A Mechanism of Immunosuppression in Cancer. The Journal of Immunology 2001 January 01;166(1):678-689.
[9] Pickering LK, Ericsson CD, Kohl S. Effect of chemotherapeutic agents on metabolic and bactericidal activity of polymorphonuclear leukocytes. Cancer 1978 Oct;42(4):1741-1746.
[10] Bodey GP. Fever and neutropenia: the early years. Journal of Antimicrobial Chemotherapy 2009 May 01;63(suppl 1):i3-i13.
[11] Gil L, Styczynski J, Komarnicki M. Infectious complication in 314 patients after high-dose therapy and autologous hematopoietic stem cell transplantation: risk factors analysis and outcome. Infection 2007 Dec;35(6):421-427.
[12] Tse E, Leung AY, Sim J, Lee HK, Liu HS, Yip SF, et al. Clofarabine and high-dose cytosine arabinoside in the treatment of refractory or relapsed acute myeloid leukaemia. Ann Hematol 2011 Nov;90(11):1277-1281.
[13] Ashman LK, Drew PA, Toogood IR, Juttner CA. Immunological competence of patients in remission from acute leukaemia: apparently normal T cell function but defective pokeweed mitogen-driven immunoglobulin synthesis. Immunol Cell Biol 1987 Apr;65 (Pt 2)(Pt 2):201-210.

[14] BODEY GP, BUCKLEY M, SATHE YS, FREIREICH EJ. Quantitative Relationships Between Circulating Leukocytes and Infection in Patients with Acute Leukemia. Annals of Internal Medicine 1966 February 01;64(2):328-340.
[15] Viscoli C, Castagnola E. Factors predisposing cancer patients to infection. Cancer Treat Res 1995;79:1-30.
[16] Morrison VA. Infectious complications in patients with chronic lymphocytic leukemia: pathogenesis, spectrum of infection, and approaches to prophylaxis. Clin Lymphoma Myeloma 2009 Oct;9(5):365-370.
[17] Wadhwa PD, Morrison VA. Infectious complications of chronic lymphocytic leukemia. Semin Oncol 2006 Apr;33(2):240-249.
[18] Dearden C. Disease-Specific Complications of Chronic Lymphocytic Leukemia. ASH Education Program Book 2008 January 01;2008(1):450-456.
[19] Itala M, Helenius H, Nikoskelainen J, Remes K. Infections and serum IgG levels in patients with chronic lymphocytic leukemia. Eur J Haematol 1992 May;48(5):266-270.
[20] Zhu YD, Xu W, Miao KR, Cao X, Fan L, Liu Q, et al. Abnormality of serum immunoglobulin in peripheral blood of patients with chronic lymphocytic leukemia. Zhongguo Shi Yan Xue Ye Xue Za Zhi 2009 Oct;17(5):1159-1162.
[21] Beard LJ, Ferrante A. IgG4 deficiency in IgA-deficient patients. Pediatr Infect Dis J 1989 Oct;8(10):705-709.
[22] French MA, Harrison G. Serum IgG subclasses in patients with an increased susceptibility to respiratory tract infections. Aust N Z J Med 1987 Aug;17(4):402-406.
[23] Sinisalo M, Aittoniemi J, Kayhty H, Vilpo J. Vaccination against infections in chronic lymphocytic leukemia. Leuk Lymphoma 2003 Apr;44(4):649-652.
[24] Kay NE, Zarling JM. Impaired natural killer activity in patients with chronic lymphocytic leukemia is associated with a deficiency of azurophilic cytoplasmic granules in putative NK cells. Blood 1984 Feb;63(2):305-309.
[25] Gorgun G, Holderried TA, Zahrieh D, Neuberg D, Gribben JG. Chronic lymphocytic leukemia cells induce changes in gene expression of CD4 and CD8 T cells. J Clin Invest 2005 Jul;115(7):1797-1805.
[26] Cantwell M, Hua T, Pappas J, Kipps TJ. Acquired CD40-ligand deficiency in chronic lymphocytic leukemia. Nat Med 1997 Sep;3(9):984-989.
[27] Cusack JC,Jr, Seymour JF, Lerner S, Keating MJ, Pollock RE. Role of splenectomy in chronic lymphocytic leukemia. J Am Coll Surg 1997 Sep;185(3):237-243.
[28] Thiruvengadam R, Piedmonte M, Barcos M, Han T, Henderson ES. Splenectomy in advanced chronic lymphocytic leukemia. Leukemia 1990 Nov;4(11):758-760.
[29] Bohnsack JF, Brown EJ. The role of the spleen in resistance to infection. Annu Rev Med 1986;37:49-59.
[30] Wara DW. Host defense against Streptococcus pneumoniae: the role of the spleen. Rev Infect Dis 1981 Mar-Apr;3(2):299-309.
[31] Ensor CR, Russell SD, Wittstein IS, Conte JV. Capnocytophagia canimorsus sepsis in an asplenic heart transplant candidate with a left ventricular assist system. Prog Transplant 2011 Jun;21(2):121-123.

[32] Lammers AJ, de Porto AP, Florquin S, de Boer OJ, Bootsma HJ, Hermans PW, et al. Enhanced vulnerability for Streptococcus pneumoniae sepsis during asplenia is determined by the bacterial capsule. Immunobiology 2011 Aug;216(8):863-870.

[33] Scheiermann P, Rosch I, Nerlich AG, Huf R, Kunz SN, Janner F, et al. Unusual presentation of Streptococcus pneumoniae-induced septic shock 36 years after splenectomy. Infection 2011 Jun;39(3):283-285.

[34] Wormser GP, Lombardo G, Silverblatt F, El Khoury MY, Prasad A, Yelon JA, et al. Babesiosis as a cause of fever in patients undergoing a splenectomy. Am Surg 2011 Mar;77(3):345-347.

[35] Naik RR, Saven A. My treatment approach to hairy cell leukemia. Mayo Clin Proc 2012 Jan;87(1):67-76.

[36] Golomb HM, Hadad LJ. Infectious complications in 127 patients with hairy cell leukemia. Am J Hematol 1984 May;16(4):393-401.

[37] Fanci R, Leoni F, Longo G. Nosocomial infections in acute leukemia: comparison between younger and elderly patients. New Microbiol 2008 Jan;31(1):89-96.

[38] Alexandre J, Gross-Goupil M, Falissard B, Nguyen M-, Gornet J-, Misset J-, et al. Evaluation of the nutritional and inflammatory status in cancer patients for the risk assessment of severe haematological toxicity following chemotherapy. Annals of Oncology 2003 January 01;14(1):36-41.

[39] Hathorn JW, Rubin M, Pizzo PA. Empirical antibiotic therapy in the febrile neutropenic cancer patient: clinical efficacy and impact of monotherapy. Antimicrob Agents Chemother 1987 Jul;31(7):971-977.

[40] Hersh EM, Bodey GP, Nies BA, Freireich EJ. Causes of Death in Acute Leukemia. JAMA: The Journal of the American Medical Association 1965 July 12;193(2):105-109.

[41] Donowitz GR, Maki DG, Crnich CJ, Pappas PG, Rolston KVI. Infections in the Neutropenic Patient— New Views of an Old Problem. ASH Education Program Book 2001 January 01;2001(1):113-139.

[42] Elting LS, Bodey GP, Keefe BH. Septicemia and shock syndrome due to viridans streptococci: a case-control study of predisposing factors. Clin Infect Dis 1992 Jun;14(6):1201-1207.

[43] Madani TA. Clinical infections and bloodstream isolates associated with fever in patients undergoing chemotherapy for acute myeloid leukemia. Infection 2000 Nov-Dec;28(6):367-373.

[44] Bakhshi S, Padmanjali KS, Arya LS. Infections in childhood acute lymphoblastic leukemia: an analysis of 222 febrile neutropenic episodes. Pediatr Hematol Oncol 2008 Jun;25(5):385-392.

[45] Wisplinghoff H, Seifert H, Wenzel RP, Edmond MB. Current trends in the epidemiology of nosocomial bloodstream infections in patients with hematological malignancies and solid neoplasms in hospitals in the United States. Clin Infect Dis 2003 May 1;36(9):1103-1110.

[46] Albrecht SJ, Fishman NO, Kitchen J, Nachamkin I, Bilker WB, Hoegg C, et al. Reemergence of gram-negative health care-associated bloodstream infections. Arch Intern Med 2006 Jun 26;166(12):1289-1294.
[47] Eber MR, Shardell M, Schweizer ML, Laxminarayan R, Perencevich EN. Seasonal and temperature-associated increases in gram-negative bacterial bloodstream infections among hospitalized patients. PLoS One 2011;6(9):e25298.
[48] Zainal Muttakin AR, Tan AM. Mycobacterium fortuitum catheter-related sepsis in acute leukaemia. Singapore Med J 2006 Jun;47(6):543-545.
[49] Karthaus M, Doellmann T, Klimasch T, Krauter J, Heil G, Ganser A. Central venous catheter infections in patients with acute leukemia. Chemotherapy 2002 Jul;48(3):154-157.
[50] Karunakaran R, Halim HA, Ng KP, Hanifah YA, Chin E, Jaafar FL, et al. Tsukamurella tyrosinosolvens intravascular catheter-related bacteremia in a haematology patient: a case report. Eur Rev Med Pharmacol Sci 2011 Nov;15(11):1343-1346.
[51] Kontoyiannis DP, Jacobson KL, Whimbey EE, Rolston KV, Raad II. Central venous catheter-associated Nocardia bacteremia: an unusual manifestation of nocardiosis. Clin Infect Dis 2000 Aug;31(2):617-618.
[52] Watson ME,Jr, Estabrook MM, Burnham CA. Catheter-associated Nocardia higoensis bacteremia in a child with acute lymphocytic leukemia. J Clin Microbiol 2011 Jan;49(1):469-471.
[53] Jagarlamudi R, Kumar L, Kochupillai V, Kapil A, Banerjee U, Thulkar S. Infections in acute leukemia: an analysis of 240 febrile episodes. Med Oncol 2000 May;17(2):111-116.
[54] Gupta A, Singh M, Singh H, Kumar L, Sharma A, Bakhshi S, et al. Infections in acute myeloid leukemia: an analysis of 382 febrile episodes. Med Oncol 2010 Dec;27(4):1037-1045.
[55] Sharma A, Lokeshwar N. Febrile neutropenia in haematological malignancies. J Postgrad Med 2005;51 Suppl 1:S42-8.
[56] Rolston KVI, Bodey GP, Safdar A. Polymicrobial Infection in Patients with Cancer: An Underappreciated and Underreported Entity. Clinical Infectious Diseases 2007 July 15;45(2):228-233.
[57] Elting LS, Bodey GP, Fainstein V. Polymicrobial septicemia in the cancer patient. Medicine (Baltimore) 1986 Jul;65(4):218-225.
[58] Apostolopoulou E, Raftopoulos V, Terzis K, Elefsiniotis I. Infection Probability Score: a predictor of Clostridium difficile-associated disease onset in patients with haematological malignancy. Eur J Oncol Nurs 2011 Dec;15(5):404-409.
[59] Schalk E, Bohr UR, Konig B, Scheinpflug K, Mohren M. Clostridium difficile-associated diarrhoea, a frequent complication in patients with acute myeloid leukaemia. Ann Hematol 2009 Jun 17.
[60] Leibovici L, Paul M, Cullen M, Bucaneve G, Gafter-Gvili A, Fraser A, et al. Antibiotic prophylaxis in neutropenic patients: new evidence, practical decisions. Cancer 2006 Oct 15;107(8):1743-1751.

[61] Andreyev HJ, Davidson SE, Gillespie C, Allum WH, Swarbrick E, British Society of Gastroenterology, et al. Practice guidance on the management of acute and chronic gastrointestinal problems arising as a result of treatment for cancer. Gut 2012 Feb;61(2):179-192.

[62] Tillotson GS, Tillotson J. Clostridium difficile--a moving target. F1000 Med Rep 2011;3:6.

[63] Zar FA, Bakkanagari SR, Moorthi KM, Davis MB. A comparison of vancomycin and metronidazole for the treatment of Clostridium difficile-associated diarrhea, stratified by disease severity. Clin Infect Dis 2007 Aug 1;45(3):302-307.

[64] Sickles EA, Greene WH, Wiernik PH. Clinical Presentation of Infection in Granulocytopenic Patients. Arch Intern Med 1975 May 1;135(5):715-719.

[65] Lanoix JP, Schmit JL, Douadi Y. Bacterial lung sepsis in patients with febrile neutropenia. Curr Opin Pulm Med 2012 May;18(3):175-180.

[66] Madani TA. Clinical infections and bloodstream isolates associated with fever in patients undergoing chemotherapy for acute myeloid leukemia. Infection 2000 Nov-Dec;28(6):367-373.

[67] Rolston KV, Bodey GP, Safdar A. Polymicrobial infection in patients with cancer: an underappreciated and underreported entity. Clin Infect Dis 2007 Jul 15;45(2):228-233.

[68] Appelbaum PC. Reduced glycopeptide susceptibility in methicillin-resistant *Staphylococcus aureus* (MRSA). Int J Antimicrob Agents 2007 Nov;30(5):398-408.

[69] Linden PK. Treatment options for vancomycin-resistant enterococcal infections. Drugs 2002;62(3):425-441.

[70] Hayakawa K, Marchaim D, Martin ET, Tiwari N, Yousuf A, Sunkara B, et al. Comparison of the clinical characteristics and outcomes associated with vancomycin-resistant Enterococcus faecalis and vancomycin-resistant E. faecium bacteremia. Antimicrob Agents Chemother 2012 Feb 21.

[71] Paterson DL, Bonomo RA. Extended-spectrum beta-lactamases: a clinical update. Clin Microbiol Rev 2005 Oct;18(4):657-686.

[72] Li J, Nation RL, Milne RW, Turnidge JD, Coulthard K. Evaluation of colistin as an agent against multi-resistant Gram-negative bacteria. Int J Antimicrob Agents 2005 Jan;25(1):11-25.

[73] Klastersky J. The changing face of febrile neutropenia-from monotherapy to moulds to mucositis. Why empirical therapy? J Antimicrob Chemother 2009 May;63 Suppl 1:i14-5.

[74] Leventakos K, Lewis RE, Kontoyiannis DP. Fungal Infections in Leukemia Patients: How Do We Prevent and Treat Them? Clinical Infectious Diseases 2010 February 01;50(3):405-415.

[75] Suzuki K, Nakase K, Kyo T, Kohara T, Sugawara Y, Shibazaki T, et al. Fatal Trichosporon fungemia in patients with hematologic malignancies. Eur J Haematol 2010 May;84(5):441-447.

[76] Segal BH, Bow EJ, Menichetti F. Fungal infections in nontransplant patients with hematologic malignancies. Infect Dis Clin North Am 2002 Dec;16(4):935-64, vii.

[77] D'Haese J, Theunissen K, Vermeulen E, Schoemans H, De Vlieger G, Lammertijn L, et al. Detection of galactomannan in bronchoalveolar lavage fluid samples of patients at

risk for invasive pulmonary aspergillosis: analytical and clinical validity. J Clin Microbiol 2012 Apr;50(4):1258-1263.

[78] Nicolle MC, Benet T, Thiebaut A, Bienvenu AL, Voirin N, Duclos A, et al. Invasive aspergillosis in patients with hematologic malignancies: incidence and description of 127 cases enrolled in a single institution prospective survey from 2004 to 2009. Haematologica 2011 Nov;96(11):1685-1691.

[79] Ulusakarya A, Chachaty E, Vantelon JM, Youssef A, Tancrede C, Pico JL, et al. Surveillance of Aspergillus galactomannan antigenemia for invasive aspergillosis by enzyme-linked immunosorbent assay in neutropenic patients treated for hematological malignancies. Hematol J 2000;1(2):111-116.

[80] Bethge WA, Schmalzing M, Stuhler G, Schumacher U, Krober SM, Horger M, et al. Mucormycoses in patients with hematologic malignancies: an emerging fungal infection. Haematologica 2005 Nov;90 Suppl:ECR22.

[81] Pagano L, Caira M, Candoni A, Offidani M, Martino B, Specchia G, et al. Invasive aspergillosis in patients with acute myeloid leukemia: a SEIFEM-2008 registry study. Haematologica 2010 Apr;95(4):644-650.

[82] Pagano L, Offidani M, Fianchi L, Nosari A, Candoni A, Piccardi M, et al. Mucormycosis in hematologic patients. Haematologica 2004 Feb;89(2):207-214.

[83] Cunningham R, Mitchell DC. Amphotericin B responsive Scedosporium apiospermum infection in a patient with acute myeloid leukaemia. J Clin Pathol 1996 Jan;49(1):93-94.

[84] Blair JE, Smilack JD, Caples SM. Coccidioidomycosis in patients with hematologic malignancies. Arch Intern Med 2005 Jan 10;165(1):113-117.

[85] Hombach M, Stulz P, Arnold W, Pfyffer GE. Pulmonary Coccidioides nodule in a Swiss patient with chronic lymphatic leukaemia. J Med Microbiol 2008 Nov;57(Pt 11):1427-1430.

[86] Isotalo PA, Ford JC, Veinot JP. Miliary blastomycosis developing in an immunocompromised host with chronic lymphocytic leukaemia. Pathology 2002 Jun;34(3):293-295.

[87] van Koeveringe MP, Brouwer RE. Histoplasma capsulatum reactivation with haemophagocytic syndrome in a patient with chronic lymphocytic leukaemia. Neth J Med 2010 Dec;68(12):418-421.

[88] Weeks E, Jones CM, Guinee V, Shallenberger R, Sarosi GA, Bunnell PA. Histoplasmosis in hairy cell leukemia: case report and review of the literature. Ann Hematol 1992 Sep;65(3):138-142.

[89] Anaissie EJ, Kontoyiannis DP, O'Brien S, Kantarjian H, Robertson L, Lerner S, et al. Infections in Patients with Chronic Lymphocytic Leukemia Treated with Fludarabine. Annals of Internal Medicine 1998 October 01;129(7):559-566.

[90] Goulet V, Hebert M, Hedberg C, Laurent E, Vaillant V, De Valk H, et al. Incidence of listeriosis and related mortality among groups at risk of acquiring listeriosis. Clin Infect Dis 2012 Mar 1;54(5):652-660.

[91] Ferrand H, Tamburini J, Mouly S, Bouscary D, Bergmann JF. Listeria monocytogenes meningitis following imatinib mesylate-induced monocytopenia in a patient with chronic myeloid leukemia. Clin Infect Dis 2005 Dec 1;41(11):1684-1685.

[92] Levidiotou S, Charalabopoulos K, Vrioni G, Chaidos A, Polysoidis K, Bourantas K, et al. Fatal meningitis due to Listeria monocytogenes in elderly patients with underlying malignancy. Int J Clin Pract 2004 Mar;58(3):292-296.

[93] Morrison VA. Management of Infectious Complications in Patients with Chronic Lymphocytic Leukemia. ASH Education Program Book 2007 January 01;2007(1):332-338.

[94] Grimm W, Korting HC, Stolz W. Disseminated herpes zoster in chronic lymphatic leukemia. Hautarzt 1989 Sep;40(9):582-585.

[95] Rodnan GP, Rake GW. Disseminated herpes zoster complicating chronic lymphatic leukemia; report of case of electron-microscope study of vesicle fluid. N Engl J Med 1956 Mar 8;254(10):472-474.

[96] Zanolli MD, Powell BL, McCalmont T, White WL, Jorizzo JL. Granuloma annulare and disseminated herpes zoster. Int J Dermatol 1992 Jan;31(1):55-57.

[97] Dolcetti R, Carbone A. Epstein-Barr virus infection and chronic lymphocytic leukemia: a possible progression factor? Infect Agent Cancer 2010 Nov 22;5:22.

[98] Silva FA, Matos JO, de Q Mello FC, Nucci M. Risk factors for and attributable mortality from tuberculosis in patients with hematologic malignances. Haematologica 2005 Aug;90(8):1110-1115.

[99] Green L, Coumbe A, Sawicka E, De Lord C. Mycobacterium kansasii in a patient with hairy cell leukaemia. Br J Haematol 2009 Jan;144(1):2.

[100] Goldschmidt N, Nusair S, Gural A, Amir G, Izhar U, Laxer U. Disseminated Mycobacterium kansasii infection with pulmonary alveolar proteinosis in a patient with chronic myelogenous leukemia. Am J Hematol 2003 Nov;74(3):221-223.

[101] Thaker H, Neilly IJ, Saunders PG, Magee JG, Snow MH, Ong EL. Remember mycobacterial disease in hairy cell leukaemia (HCL). J Infect 2001 Apr;42(3):213-214.

[102] Awais A, Tam CS, Kontoyiannis D, Ferrajoli A, Duvic M, Cortes J, et al. Rapid resolution of Mycobacterium marinum chronic skin infection during lenalidomide herapy for chronic lymphocytic leukemia. Clin Infect Dis 2008 Apr 1;46(7):e69-71.

[103] Dungarwalla M, Field-Smith A, Jameson C, Riley U, Chapman A, Bunker CB, et al. Cutaneous Mycobacterium chelonae infection in chronic lymphocytic leukaemia. Haematologica 2007 Jan;92(1):e5-6.

[104] Meyer JJ, Gelman SS. Multifocal osteomyelitis due to Mycobacterium szulgai in a patient with chronic lymphocytic leukemia. J Infect 2008 Feb;56(2):151-154.

[105] Abedalthagafi M, Rushing EJ, Garvin D, Cheson B, Ozdemirli M. Asymptomatic diffuse "encephalitic" cerebral toxoplasmosis in a patient with chronic lymphocytic eukemia: case report and review of the literature. Int J Clin Exp Pathol 2009 Mar 15;3(1):106-109.

[106] Austen B, McCarthy H, Wilkins B, Smith A, Duncombe A. Fatal disseminated fusarium nfection in acute lymphoblastic leukaemia in complete remission. J Clin Pathol 2001 un;54(6):488-490.

[107] Chi CC, Wang SH. Disseminated cutaneous Fusarium moniliforme infections in a eukemic child. Int J Dermatol 2007 May;46(5):487-489.

[108] Gutierrez Paredes EM, Gamez Perez L, Gonzalez Rodriguez AJ, Ramon Quiles D, Monteagudo Castro C, Jorda Cuevas E. Disseminated fusariosis in mmunocompromised patients. Eur J Dermatol 2011 Sep-Oct;21(5):753-755.

[109] Hermansen NE, Ralfkiaer EM, Kjeldsen L. Disseminated fusariosis in a patient with acute lymphoblastic leukaemia. Ugeskr Laeger 2008 Sep 8;170(37):2892.

[110] Jossi M, Ambrosioni J, Macedo-Vinas M, Garbino J. Invasive fusariosis with prolonged ungemia in a patient with acute lymphoblastic leukemia: case report and review of the iterature. Int J Infect Dis 2010 Apr;14(4):e354-6.

[111] van der Lelie H, Leverstein-Van Hall M, Mertens M, van Zaanen HC, van Oers RH, Thomas BL, et al. Corynebacterium CDC group JK (Corynebacterium jeikeium) sepsis n haematological patients: a report of three cases and a systematic literature review. Scand J Infect Dis 1995;27(6):581-584.

[112] Gompelmann D, Kappes J, Heussel CP, Schnabel PA, Herth FJ. Corynebacterium pseudodiphtheriticum causing severe pneumonia in secondary immunoglobulin deficiency. Dtsch Med Wochenschr 2011 Dec;136(48):2503-2506.

[113] Wang CC, Mattson D, Wald A. Corynebacterium jeikeium bacteremia in bone marrow ransplant patients with Hickman catheters. Bone Marrow Transplant 2001 Feb;27(4):445-449.

[114] Araoka H, Fujii T, Izutsu K, Kimura M, Nishida A, Ishiwata K, et al. Rapidly progressive fatal hemorrhagic pneumonia caused by Stenotrophomonas maltophilia in hematologic malignancy. Transpl Infect Dis 2012 Jan 30.

[115] Soga Y, Saito T, Nishimura F, Ishimaru F, Mineshiba J, Mineshiba F, et al. Appearance of multidrug-resistant opportunistic bacteria on the gingiva during leukemia treatment. Periodontol 2008 Jan;79(1):181-186.

[116] Son YM, Na SY, Lee HY, Baek JO, Lee JR, Roh JY. Ecthyma Gangrenosum: A Rare Cutaneous Manifestation Caused by Stenotrophomonas maltophilia in a Leukemic Patient. Ann Dermatol 2009 Nov;21(4):389-392.

[117] Teo WY, Chan MY, Lam CM, Chong CY. Skin manifestation of Stenotrophomonas maltophilia infection--a case report and review article. Ann Acad Med Singapore 2006 Dec;35(12):897-900.

[118] Gurler N, Oksuz L, Muftuoglu M, Sargin F, Besisik S. Bacillus cereus catheter related bloodstream infection in a patient with acute lymphoblastic leukemia. Mediterr J Hematol Infect Dis 2012;4(1):e2012004.

[119] Hirabayashi K, Shiohara M, Suzuki T, Saito S, Tanaka M, Yanagisawa R, et al. Critical llness Polyneuropathy and Myopathy Caused by Bacillus Cereus Sepsis in Acute Lymphoblastic Leukemia. J Pediatr Hematol Oncol 2012 Jan 12.

[120] Inoue D, Nagai Y, Mori M, Nagano S, Takiuchi Y, Arima H, et al. Fulminant sepsis caused by Bacillus cereus in patients with hematologic malignancies: analysis of its prognosis and risk factors. Leuk Lymphoma 2010 May;51(5):860-869.

[121] Le Scanff J, Mohammedi I, Thiebaut A, Martin O, Argaud L, Robert D. Necrotizing gastritis due to Bacillus cereus in an immunocompromised patient. Infection 2006 Apr;34(2):98-99.

[122] Nishikawa T, Okamoto Y, Tanabe T, Kodama Y, Shinkoda Y, Kawano Y. Critical illness polyneuropathy after Bacillus cereus sepsis in acute lymphoblastic leukemia. Intern Med 2009;48(13):1175-1177.

[123] Fruchart C, Salah A, Gray C, Martin E, Stamatoullas A, Bonmarchand G, et al. Lactobacillus species as emerging pathogens in neutropenic patients. Eur J Clin Microbiol Infect Dis 1997 Sep;16(9):681-684.

[124] Ferraro C, Quemeneur L, Prigent A, Taverne C, Revillard J, Bonnefoy-Berard N. Anthracyclines Trigger Apoptosis of Both G0-G1 and Cycling Peripheral Blood Lymphocytes and Induce Massive Deletion of Mature T and B Cells. Cancer Research 2000 April 01;60(7):1901-1907.

[125] Hunault-Berger M, Leguay T, Thomas X, Legrand O, Huguet F, Bonmati C, et al. A randomized study of pegylated liposomal doxorubicin versus continuous-infusion doxorubicin in elderly patients with acute lymphoblastic leukemia: the GRAALL-SA1 study. Haematologica 2011 Feb;96(2):245-252.

[126] Decker BC. Alkylating Agents. In: Kufe DW, Pollock RE, Weichselbaum RR, editors. Holland-Frei Cancer Medicine. 6th edition ed.: Hamilton ON; 2003.

[127] Seymour J, Kurzrock R, Freireich E, Estey E. 2-chlorodeoxyadenosine induces durable remissions and prolonged suppression of CD4+ lymphocyte counts in patients with hairy cell leukemia. Blood 1994 May 15;83(10):2906-2911.

[128] Dimopoulos MA, Gertz MA, Kastritis E, Garcia-Sanz R, Kimby EK, LeBlond V, et al. Update on Treatment Recommendations From the Fourth International Workshop on Waldenström's Macroglobulinemia. Journal of Clinical Oncology January 1, 2009 anuary 1, 2009;27(1):120-126.

[129] Lauria F, Bocchia M, Marotta G, Raspadori D, Zinzani PL, Rondelli D. Weekly administration of 2-chlorodeoxyadenosine in patients with hairy-cell leukemia is effective and reduces infectious complications. Haematologica 1999 Jan;84(1):22-25.

[130] Saven A, Burian C, Adusumalli J, Koziol JA. Filgrastim for cladribine-induced neutropenic fever in patients with hairy cell leukemia. Blood 1999 Apr 15;93(8):2471-2477.

[131] Faderl S, Ferrajoli A, Wierda W, Huang X, Verstovsek S, Ravandi F, et al. Clofarabine combinations as acute myeloid leukemia salvage therapy. Cancer 2008 Oct 15;113(8):2090-2096.

[132] Jeha S, Kantarjian H. Clofarabine for the treatment of acute lymphoblastic leukemia. Expert Rev Anticancer Ther 2007 Feb;7(2):113-118.

[133] Mayer RJ, Davis RB, Schiffer CA, Berg DT, Powell BL, Schulman P, et al. Intensive Postremission Chemotherapy in Adults with Acute Myeloid Leukemia. N Engl J Med 1994 10/06; 2012/04;331(14):896-903.

[134] Klein NC, Go CH, Cunha BA. Infections associated with steroid use. Infect Dis Clin North Am 2001 Jun;15(2):423-32, viii.

[135] Stuck AE, Minder CE, Frey FJ. Risk of infectious complications in patients taking glucocorticosteroids. Rev Infect Dis 1989 Nov-Dec;11(6):954-963.

[136] Laros-van Gorkom BA, Huisman CA, Wijermans PW, Schipperus MR. Experience with alemtuzumab in treatment of chronic lymphocytic leukaemia in the Netherlands. Neth J Med 2007 Oct;65(9):333-338.

[137] Christian BA, Lin TS. Antibody therapy for chronic lymphocytic leukemia. Semin Hematol 2008 Apr;45(2):95-103.

[138] Hallek M, Fischer K, Fingerle-Rowson G, Fink AM, Busch R, Mayer J, et al. Addition of rituximab to fludarabine and cyclophosphamide in patients with chronic lymphocytic eukaemia: a randomised, open-label, phase 3 trial. Lancet 2010 Oct 2;376(9747):1164-1174.

[139] Grant C, Wilson WH, Dunleavy K. Neutropenia associated with rituximab therapy. Curr Opin Hematol 2010 Nov 22.

[140] Coppola N, Tonziello G, Pisaturo M, Messina V, Guastafierro S, Fiore M, et al. Reactivation of overt and occult hepatitis B infection in various immunosuppressive settings. J Med Virol 2011 Nov;83(11):1909-1916.

[141] Chakraborty S, Tarantolo SR, Treves J, Sambol D, Hauke RJ, Batra SK. Progressive Multifocal Leukoencephalopathy in a HIV-Negative Patient with Small Lymphocytic Leukemia following Treatment with Rituximab. Case Rep Oncol 2011 Jan;4(1):136-142.

[142] Herold T, Seiler T, Egensperger R, Trumm C, Bergmann M, Franke D, et al. Progressive multifocal leukoencephalopathy after treatment with rituximab, fludarabine and cyclophosphamide in a patient with chronic lymphocytic leukemia. Leuk Lymphoma 2012 Jan;53(1):169-172.

[143] Skoetz N, Bauer K, Elter T, Monsef I, Roloff V, Hallek M, et al. Alemtuzumab for patients with chronic lymphocytic leukaemia. Cochrane Database Syst Rev 2012 Feb 15;2:CD008078.

[144] Osterborg A, Foa R, Bezares RF, Dearden C, Dyer MJ, Geisler C, et al. Management guidelines for the use of alemtuzumab in chronic lymphocytic leukemia. Leukemia 2009 Nov;23(11):1980-1988.

[145] Montillo M, Ricci F, Miqueleiz S, Tedeschi A, Morra E. Alemtuzumab in the treatment of fludarabine refractory B-cell chronic lymphocytic leukemia (CLL). Biologics 2008 Mar;2(1):41-52.

[146] O'Brien S, Ravandi F, Riehl T, Wierda W, Huang X, Tarrand J, et al. Valganciclovir prevents cytomegalovirus reactivation in patients receiving alemtuzumab-based herapy. Blood 2008 Feb 15;111(4):1816-1819.

[147] Lin TS, Donohue KA, Byrd JC, Lucas MS, Hoke EE, Bengtson EM, et al. Consolidation herapy with subcutaneous alemtuzumab after fludarabine and rituximab induction

herapy for previously untreated chronic lymphocytic leukemia: final analysis of CALGB 10101. J Clin Oncol 2010 Oct 10;28(29):4500-4506.
[148] Veliz M, Pinilla-Ibarz J. Role of ofatumumab in treatment of chronic lymphocytic eukemia. J Blood Med 2011;2:71-77.
[149] Gravanis I, Ersboll J, Skovlund E, Abadie E, Marty M, Pignatti F. The European Medicines Agency review of ofatumumab (Arzerra(R)) for the treatment of chronic ymphocytic leukemia in patients refractory to fludarabine and alemtuzumab: summary of the scientific assessment of the European medicines agency committee for medicinal products for human use. Oncologist 2010;15(12):1335-1343.
[150] Wierda WG, Kipps TJ, Mayer J, Stilgenbauer S, Williams CD, Hellmann A, et al. Ofatumumab As Single-Agent CD20 Immunotherapy in Fludarabine-Refractory Chronic Lymphocytic Leukemia. Journal of Clinical Oncology 2010 April 01;28(10):1749-1755.
[151] Lemery SJ, Zhang J, Rothmann MD, Yang J, Earp J, Zhao H, et al. U.S. Food and Drug Administration Approval: Ofatumumab for the Treatment of Patients with Chronic Lymphocytic Leukemia Refractory to Fludarabine and Alemtuzumab. Clinical Cancer Research 2010 September 01;16(17):4331-4338.
[152] Pinilla-Ibarz J, Flinn I. The expanding options for front-line treatment in patients with newly diagnosed CML. Crit Rev Oncol Hematol 2012 Apr 7.
[153] Breccia M, Girmenia C, Latagliata R, Loglisci G, Santopietro M, Federico V, et al. Low ncidence rate of opportunistic and viral infections during imatinib treatment in chronic myeloid leukemia patients in early and late chronic phase. Mediterr J Hematol Infect Dis 2011;3(1):e2011021.
[154] Talpaz M, Shah NP, Kantarjian H, Donato N, Nicoll J, Paquette R, et al. Dasatinib in matinib-Resistant Philadelphia Chromosome–Positive Leukemias. N Engl J Med 2006 06/15; 2012/04;354(24):2531-2541.
[155] Kantarjian HM, Giles F, Gattermann N, Bhalla K, Alimena G, Palandri F, et al. Nilotinib (formerly AMN107), a highly selective BCR-ABL tyrosine kinase inhibitor, is effective in patients with Philadelphia chromosome–positive chronic myelogenous eukemia in chronic phase following imatinib resistance and intolerance. Blood 2007 November 15;110(10):3540-3546.
[156] de Naurois J, Novitzky-Basso I, Gill MJ, Marti FM, Cullen MH, Roila F, et al. Management of febrile neutropenia: ESMO Clinical Practice Guidelines. Ann Oncol 2010 May;21 Suppl 5:v252-6.
[157] Klastersky J, Paesmans M, Rubenstein EB, Boyer M, Elting L, Feld R, et al. The Multinational Association for Supportive Care in Cancer risk index: A multinational scoring system for identifying low-risk febrile neutropenic cancer patients. J Clin Oncol 2000 Aug;18(16):3038-3051.
[158] Del Prete SA, Ryan SP, Jacobson JS, Erichson RB, Weinstein PL, Grann VR. Safety and costs of treating neutropenic fever in an outpatient setting. Conn Med 1999 Dec;63(12):713-717.

[159] Marti FM, Cullen MH, Roila F, On behalf of the ESMO Guidelines Working Group. Management of febrile neutropenia: ESMO Clinical Recommendations. Annals of Oncology 2009 May 01;20(suppl 4):iv166-iv169.

[160] Herbrecht R, Berceanu A. β-d-Glucan Detection Test: A Step Toward Preemptive Therapy for Fungal Infections in Leukemic Patients? Clinical Infectious Diseases 2008 March 15;46(6):886-889.

[161] BOGGS DR, FREI E, ZIERDT CH. FEVER IN MALIGNANT NEOPLASTIC DISEASE: A CONTROLLED STUDY OF TETRACYCLINE THERAPY*. Annals of Internal Medicine 1960 October 01;53(4):754-764.

[162] CURTIN JA, MARSHALL BD,Jr. Use of antibiotics in cancer and leukemia. J Chronic Dis 1962 Jul;15:713-718.

[163] Schimpff S, Satterlee W, Young VM, Serpick A. Empiric Therapy with Carbenicillin and Gentamicin for Febrile Patients with Cancer and Granulocytopenia. N Engl J Med 1971 05/13; 2012/03;284(19):1061-1065.

[164] Liu C, Bayer A, Cosgrove SE, Daum RS, Fridkin SK, Gorwitz RJ, et al. Clinical Practice Guidelines by the Infectious Diseases Society of America for the Treatment of Methicillin-Resistant Staphylococcus Aureus Infections in Adults and Children. Clinical nfectious Diseases 2011 January 04.

[165] Kalogeropoulos AS, Tsiodras S, Loverdos D, Fanourgiakis P, Skoutelis A. Eosinophilic pneumonia associated with daptomycin: a case report and a review of the literature. J Med Case Reports 2011 Jan 17;5(1):13.

[166] Butterfield JM, Lawrence KR, Reisman A, Huang DB, Thompson CA, Lodise TP. Comparison of serotonin toxicity with concomitant use of either linezolid or comparators and serotonergic agents: an analysis of Phase III and IV randomized clinical trial data. J Antimicrob Chemother 2012 Feb;67(2):494-502.

[167] Carroll MW, Choi H, Min S, Hwang S, Park H, Song T, et al. Rhabdomyolysis in a Patient Treated with Linezolid for Extensively Drug Resistant (XDR) Tuberculosis. Clin nfect Dis 2012 Mar 15.

[168] Duplessis C, Crum-Cianflone NF. Ceftaroline: A New Cephalosporin with Activity against Methicillin-Resistant Staphylococcus aureus (MRSA). Clin Med Rev Ther 2011 Feb 10;3:a2466.

[169] Pagano L, Fianchi L, Fanci R, Candoni A, Caira M, Posteraro B, et al. Caspofungin for he treatment of candidaemia in patients with haematological malignancies. Clin Microbiol Infect 2010 Mar;16(3):298-301.

[170] Walsh TJ, Pappas P, Winston DJ, Lazarus HM, Petersen F, Raffalli J, et al. Voriconazole compared with liposomal amphotericin B for empirical antifungal therapy in patients with neutropenia and persistent fever. N Engl J Med 2002 Jan 24;346(4):225-234.

[171] Herbrecht R, Denning DW, Patterson TF, Bennett JE, Greene RE, Oestmann JW, et al. Voriconazole versus amphotericin B for primary therapy of invasive aspergillosis. N Engl J Med 2002 Aug 8;347(6):408-415.

[172] Chen SC, Slavin MA, Sorrell TC. Echinocandin antifungal drugs in fungal infections: a comparison. Drugs 2011 Jan 1;71(1):11-41.

[173] Candoni A, Mestroni R, Damiani D, Tiribelli M, Michelutti A, Silvestri F, et al. Caspofungin as first line therapy of pulmonary invasive fungal infections in 32 mmunocompromised patients with hematologic malignancies. Eur J Haematol 2005 Sep;75(3):227-233.

[174] Eschenauer G, Depestel DD, Carver PL. Comparison of echinocandin antifungals. Ther Clin Risk Manag 2007 Mar;3(1):71-97.

[175] Spellberg B, Ibrahim AS. Recent advances in the treatment of mucormycosis. Curr nfect Dis Rep 2010 Nov;12(6):423-429.

[176] Chen SC, Blyth CC, Sorrell TC, Slavin MA. Pneumonia and lung infections due to emerging and unusual fungal pathogens. Semin Respir Crit Care Med 2011 Dec;32(6):703-716.

[177] Clancy CJ, Yu VL, Morris AJ, Snydman DR, Nguyen MH. Fluconazole MIC and the Fluconazole Dose/MIC Ratio Correlate with Therapeutic Response among Patients with Candidemia. Antimicrobial Agents and Chemotherapy August 2005 August 2005;49(8):3171-3177.

[178] von Eiff M, Roos N, Schulten R, Hesse M, Zuhlsdorf M, van de Loo J. Pulmonary aspergillosis: early diagnosis improves survival. Respiration 1995;62(6):341-347.

[179] Verweij PE, Maertens J. Moulds: diagnosis and treatment. Journal of Antimicrobial Chemotherapy 2009 May 01;63(suppl 1):i31-i35.

[180] Maertens J, Marchetti O, Herbrecht R, Cornely OA, Fluckiger U, Frere P, et al. European guidelines for antifungal management in leukemia and hematopoietic stem cell transplant recipients: summary of the ECIL 3--2009 update. Bone Marrow Transplant 2011 May;46(5):709-718.

[181] Baden LR. Prevention and treatment of cancer related infections. National comprehensive cancer network guidelines 2011;Version 2.2011.

[182] Caillot D, Thiebaut A, Herbrecht R, de Botton S, Pigneux A, Bernard F, et al. Liposomal amphotericin B in combination with caspofungin for invasive aspergillosis in patients with hematologic malignancies: a randomized pilot study (Combistrat trial). Cancer 2007 Dec 15;110(12):2740-2746.

[183] Rojas R, Molina JR, Jarque I, Montes C, Serrano J, Sanz J, et al. Outcome of Antifungal Combination Therapy for Invasive Mold Infections in Hematological Patients is ndependent of the Chosen Combination. Mediterr J Hematol Infect Dis 2012;4(1):e2012011.

[184] Koo S, Baden LR, Marty FM. Post-diagnostic kinetics of the (1 --> 3)-beta-d-glucan assay in invasive aspergillosis, invasive candidiasis and Pneumocystis jirovecii pneumonia. Clin Microbiol Infect 2012 Jan 23.

[185] Marty FM, Koo S. Role of (1-->3)-beta-D-glucan in the diagnosis of invasive aspergillosis. Med Mycol 2009;47 Suppl 1:S233-40.

[186] Cullen M, Baijal S. Prevention of febrile neutropenia: use of prophylactic antibiotics. Br Cancer 2009 Sep;101 Suppl 1:S11-4.

[187] Bucaneve G, Micozzi A, Menichetti F, Martino P, Dionisi MS, Martinelli G, et al. Levofloxacin to prevent bacterial infection in patients with cancer and neutropenia. N Engl J Med 2005 Sep 8;353(10):977-987.

[188] Cornely OA, Maertens J, Winston DJ, Perfect J, Ullmann AJ, Walsh TJ, et al. Posaconazole vs. Fluconazole or Itraconazole Prophylaxis in Patients with Neutropenia. N Engl J Med 2007 01/25; 2012/04;356(4):348-359.

[189] Gurion R, Belnik-Plitman Y, Gafter-Gvili A, Paul M, Vidal L, Ben-Bassat I, et al. Colony-stimulating factors for prevention and treatment of infectious complications in patients with acute myelogenous leukemia. Cochrane Database Syst Rev 2011 Sep 7;(9)(9):CD008238.

[190] Smith TJ, Khatcheressian J, Lyman GH, Ozer H, Armitage JO, Balducci L, et al. 2006 Update of Recommendations for the use of White Blood Cell Growth Factors: an Evidence-Based Clinical Practice Guideline. J Clin Oncol 2006 Jul 1;24(19):3187-3205.

[191] Unknown a. Intravenous immunoglobulin for the prevention of infection in chronic ymphocytic leukemia. A randomized, controlled clinical trial. Cooperative Group for he Study of Immunoglobulin in Chronic Lymphocytic Leukemia. N Engl J Med 1988 Oct 6;319(14):902-907.

[192] Jurlander J, Geisler CH, Hansen MM. Treatment of hypogammaglobulinaemia in chronic lymphocytic leukaemia by low-dose intravenous gammaglobulin. Eur J Haematol 1994 Aug;53(2):114-118.

[193] Weeks JC, Tierney MR, Weinstein MC. Cost effectiveness of prophylactic intravenous mmune globulin in chronic lymphocytic leukemia. N Engl J Med 1991 Jul 11;325(2):81-86.

[194] Sinisalo M, Vilpo J, Itala M, Vakevainen M, Taurio J, Aittoniemi J. Antibody response o 7-valent conjugated pneumococcal vaccine in patients with chronic lymphocytic eukaemia. Vaccine 2007 Dec 21;26(1):82-87.

[195] Van der Velden AM, Van Velzen-Blad H, Claessen AM, Van der Griend R, Oltmans R, Rijkers GT, et al. The effect of ranitidine on antibody responses to polysaccharide vaccines in patients with B-cell chronic lymphocytic leukaemia. Eur J Haematol 2007 ul;79(1):47-52.

[196] Cassone A, Torosantucci A. Opportunistic fungi and fungal infections: the challenge of a single, general antifungal vaccine. Expert Rev Vaccines 2006 Dec;5(6):859-867.

[197] Spellberg B. Vaccines for invasive fungal infections. F1000 Med Rep 2011;3:13.

[198] Redaelli A, Stephens JM, Laskin BL, Pashos CL, Botteman MF. The burden and outcomes associated with four leukemias: AML, ALL, CLL and CML. Expert Rev Anticancer Ther 2003 Jun;3(3):311-329.

[199] Jones AE, Trzeciak S, Kline JA. The Sequential Organ Failure Assessment score for predicting outcome in patients with severe sepsis and evidence of hypoperfusion at the ime of emergency department presentation. Crit Care Med 2009 May;37(5):1649-1654.

[200] Park HY, Suh GY, Jeon K, Koh WJ, Chung MP, Kim H, et al. Outcome and prognostic actors of patients with acute leukemia admitted to the intensive care unit for septic shock. Leuk Lymphoma 2008 Oct;49(10):1929-1934.

[201] Mokart D, Etienne A, Esterni B, Brun JP, Chow-Chine L, Sannini A, et al. Critically ill cancer patients in the intensive care unit: short-term outcome and 1-year mortality. Acta Anaesthesiol Scand 2012 Feb;56(2):178-189.

[202] Thakkar SG, Fu AZ, Sweetenham JW, Mciver ZA, Mohan SR, Ramsingh G, et al. Survival and predictors of outcome in patients with acute leukemia admitted to the ntensive care unit. Cancer 2008 May 15;112(10):2233-2240.

[203] Knaus WA, Draper EA, Wagner DP, Zimmerman JE. APACHE II: a severity of disease classification system. Crit Care Med 1985 Oct;13(10):818-829.

[204] Schapira D, Studnicki J, Bradham D, Wolff P, Jarrett A, Aziz N. Heroic measures when reating patients with hematologic malignancies - the economic cost of survival. Int J Oncol 1993 Nov;3(5):987-993.

[205] Markou N, Demopoulou E, Myrianthefs P. The critically ill patient with cancer - indications for Intensive Care Unit admission and outcomes. J BUON 2008 Oct-Dec;13(4):469-478.

Section 6

Treatment of Sepsis-Associated Dysfunctions

Chapter 18

Continuous Renal Replacement Therapies in Patients with Severe Sepsis and Septic Shock

F.J. García-Miguel

Additional information is available at the end of the chapter

http://dx.doi.org/10.5772/50254

1. Introduction

Acute renal failure (ARF) that requires replacement therapy is a common problem in critically ill patients. The treatment of ARF is one the aspects that has evolved over the management of critically ill patients in the last 25 years. Conventional Hemodialysis presents problems when used in these patients, often being unable to remove enough fluid, due to hemodynamic instability and hypotension that often results. In 1977, Kramer et al. describe the technique of continuous arteriovenous hemofiltration, which, by eliminating slow and continuous ultrafiltration allows good control of electrolyte balance in patients with ARF and oliguria, with good hemodynamic tolerance in critically ill patients. Later modifications of the technique, continuous venovenous hemodiafiltration and hemofiltration get the plasmatic clearance depends less on the ultrafiltration rate determined by blood pressure, and allow more effective clearance. This coupled with the fact that different forms of continuous hemofiltration allow control of uremic and intravascular volume without restriction of protein intake or liquids and requires no specialized personal in dialysis techniques, has become a technique widely used in intensive care units (1,2).

However, the use of continuous renal replacement techniques therapies (CRRT) in patients with severe sepsis or multiple organ dysfunction syndrome (MODS) to remove inflammatory mediators and, therefore, anticipate or mitigate multiorgan dysfunction is still controversial, since this involves the use of hemofiltration in patients that do not require (or not yet needed) replacement of their kidney function (3-6). The sequence of events leading to septic shock and MODS is initiated by endotoxins or other structural components of microorganisms that cause inappropriate inflammatory response through the cells responsible for immunity, and release of inflammatory mediators such as cytokines, active products of complement, arachidonic acid metabolites, nitric oxide, oxygen reactive substances, proteases, etc.. The consequences are tissue damage and hypotension by myocardial depression and vasodilation (7). Current therapeutic strategies against sepsis are still based on the pharmacology of the immunoinflammatory cascade, however so far very few studies in stage III and IV with these "pro-sepsis" drugs who have achieved favorable results in improving the survival of patients. For this reason the hypothesis that CRRT may modulate this broad and inappropriate tissue inflammation by eliminating inflammatory mediators remains highly attractive (8,9).

2. Principal advantages of CRRT in severe sepsis patients

Theoretically, hemofiltration has several advantages over the pharmacological approach of the sepsis treatment:

- The simultaneous extraction of various mediators should be more effective than selective treatment against a single mediator.
- Hemofiltration only removes plasmatic mediators and thus limits the deleterious systemic effect preserving the local effect (which is considered essential for the elimination of microorganisms and damaged tissue).
- The effect of hemofiltration is more pronounced for those mediators who are in a higher plasma concentration (10).

But although hemofiltration may have some advantages over “prosepsis” drugs, is not a perfect solution, because this treatment also has limitations (2):

1. Hemofiltration can only extract substances present in plasma in unbound form to proteins, but the mediators may be absent because of transient release (TFN and IL-1 for example), being limited effect and release the tissue compartment, and so on. In addition, although they may be inflammatory mediators in the ultrafiltrate of CRRT, has not yet been able to demonstrate that their removal produces a significant decrease in serum levels or there is clinical improvement of the inflammatory response.
2. Most mediators have a molecular weight range (between 600 and 54,000 daltons) and thus can be eliminated by diffusion as this is a process dependent on molecular weight. However, this molecular weight if it is compatible with the extraction convective through high-flux membranes (threshold passage of substances close to 30,000 daltons).
3. Hemofiltration may even be detrimental for all substances indiscriminately remove circulating mediators including beneficial counterregulatory substances, other essential endogenous substances and drugs such as antimicrobials.
4. The use of biocompatible membranes may generate mediators of inflammation.
5. Hemofiltration is an invasive technique that requires the placement of catheters and continuous anticoagulation, and,
6. CRRT are expensive and represent a significant workload (2).

The choice of dialytic technique in severe sepsis patients is dependent upon a variety of factors including availability, the expertise of the clinician, hemodynamic stability, and the degree to which solutes and/or fluid must be removed. In addition, comorbid conditions may affect the decision:

- Abdominal drains and/or new incisions generally preclude peritoneal dialysis.
- Severe peripheral vascular disease or coagulopathy are general contraindications to cannulation of a major artery. Patients at high risk for bleeding during CAVH can be treated with minimal dose heparin or regional citrate anticoagulation (if there is a diffusion component) to prevent clotting in the dialyzer (1).

Although hemodialysis is the standard modality in hemodynamically stable patients with acute renal failure, CRRT is used in selected cases. The determining factors of which modality is chosen include the catabolic state, hemodynamic stability, and whether the primary goal is solute removal (eg, uremia, hyperkalemia), fluid removal, or both (11,12).

CRRTs in patients with acute kidney injury are most often selected when hemodynamic instability precludes the use of standard three to four hour intermittent dialysis. While randomized controlled trials have failed to prove better outcomes with CRRTs when compared to intermittent dialysis, many clinicians prefer them because of their ease of use and the security perceived by slow therapy. Since there is no proven benefit of CRRT versus intermittent dialysis in this setting, the renal replacement modality selection is based on ease of operation and perceived benefit.

Solute removal occurs primarily by diffusion from the plasma into the dialysate during dialysis and, to a much lesser degree, by convection during ultrafiltration as solvent drag carries small and intermediate sized solutes with the water. Smaller solutes (such as urea and electrolytes) are removed in roughly the same concentration as the plasma with hemofiltration; as a result, the rate of solute clearance is equal to the ultrafiltration rate unless there is concurrent diffusive loss. There is also no change in the plasma concentrations of small solutes with hemofiltration alone, unless they are lowered by dilution by the administration of replacement fluid to prevent extracellular volume depletion.

The rate of solute diffusion is determined by a number of factors including:

- The surface area and unit **solute** permeability of the dialysis membrane.
- The blood and dialysate flow rates which, if increased, maintain a maximum concentration gradient between these two compartments.
- The duration of dialysis (only if a favorable concentration gradient persists for continued diffusion).

In comparison, the rate of solute removal by ultrafiltration is influenced by:

- The transmembrane pressure gradient that provides the driving force for ultrafiltration.
- The surface area and unit **water** permeability of the dialysis membrane.
- The duration of hemofiltration.
- The blood flow rate, which acts indirectly by moving nonfiltered plasma proteins away from the inner wall of the dialysis membrane; preventing local protein accumulation maintains water permeability.

These determinants apply to hemodialysis/hemofiltration, but not to peritoneal dialysis.

Hypotension, either at baseline or during the procedure, may be a limiting feature with conventional hemodialysis but should not occur with slow fluid and solute removal in peritoneal dialysis. However, the latter is often not an option in acutely ill patients.

Slow fluid and solute removal can also be achieved with CRRT. In addition to being better tolerated hemodynamically, CRRT is also as efficient in removing solutes over the course of 24 to 48 hours as conventional hemodialysis. Although the clearance rate of small solutes (such as urea) is slower per unit time with CRRT (17 mL/min with CAVHD versus more than 160 mL/min with hemodialysis), the rates are closer at 24 hours and more urea is removed over 48 hours with CRRT than with a single run of hemodialysis (13-18).

Hemodynamic stability: Daily or every other day conventional hemodialysis is the standard dialytic regimen for the hemodynamically stable patient with severe acute renal failure. However, hypotension, due in part to **rapid** fluid and solute removal, is one of the most common complications with this technique, making it less desirable in the patient who is hypotensive or hemodynamically unstable. In contrast, the rate of fluid and solute removal is **slow** and hypotension is less common with the CRRTs, such as continuous arteriovenous hemofiltration or hemodialysis (19-22). A review of the characteristics of the different types of CRRT is available elsewhere.

CRRT has the additional advantage of effectively removing excess fluid in hypotensive patients, while hemodialysis is frequently limited by a further reduction in blood pressure in this setting.

The relative hemodynamic instability associated with hemodialysis is related to several factors:

- The rapid rate of solute removal results in an abrupt fall in plasma osmolality that induces further extracellular volume depletion by promoting osmotic water movement into the cells. The reduction in plasma osmolality itself may contribute to the development of hypotension.
- Hemodialysis may impair the protective sympathetic response to volume depletion.

It must be emphasized, however, that the protection afforded by CRRT is **relative**, not absolute. Hypotension can still occur if too much fluid is removed or if fluid is removed too quickly.

Solute removal: In addition to being better tolerated hemodynamically, CRRT is also as efficient in removing solutes over the course of 24 to 48 hours as conventional hemodialysis. Although the clearance rate of small solutes (such as urea) is slower per unit time with CRRT (17 mL/min with CAVHD versus more than 160 mL/min with hemodialysis), the rates are closer at 24 hours and more urea is removed over 48 hours with CRRT than with a single run of hemodialysis (Table 1) (23).

Removal of immunomodulatory substances in sepsis: The less porous membranes used with conventional hemodialysis are less efficient in removing middle to large molecules with cardiodepressant, vasodilatory, or immunomodulatory properties in septic or highly catabolic patients. Examples of such toxins are endotoxin, interleukin-1, complement anaphylatoxins, platelet activating factor, and tumor necrosis factor (21,24,25).

Technique	Operating conditions	Urea clearance mL/min	L/day	Inulin clearance mL/min	Inulin clearance L/day
CAVH	Postdilution, UFR 8 mL/min	8	11.5	6.4	9.2
CAVH	Postdilution, UFR 14 mL/min	14	20	11	16
CAVH	Predilution, UFR 14 mL/min	16	23.5	11	16
CAVHD	Qd 1 L/h, UFR 3 mL/min	19.7	28	2.4	3.5
CVVH	UFR 17 mL/min	17	24	13.6	19.6
CVVHD	Qd 1 L/h, UFR 12 ml/min Postdilution	29	42	9.6	13.8
CEPD	8 L/day, 1 L ultrafiltration	6.3	9	2	3
HD	4 hours	160	38	6	2

The clearance of small (urea) and intermediate (inulin) sized solutes with the different forms of continuous renal replacement therapy, continuous equilibrium peritoneal dialysis (CEPD), and standard hemodialysis (HD). Although urea clearance is much slower with CRRT than with hemodialysis per unit time, the quantity of urea cleared is almost the same over the course of one or two days because of the continuous therapy. When there is no dialysis (as with CAVH or CVVH), the urea clearance is **equal to the ultrafiltration rate** (UFR) unless there is predilution with replacement fluid. Intermediate sized solutes are cleared to a much greater degree with CRRT, since more permeable membranes are used. The values for inulin clearance assume a sieving coefficient of 0.8.
Qd: dialysate flow rate.

Table 1. Solute clearance continuous renal replacement therapy (23).

Experimental and some clinical evidence suggest that large volume hemofiltration more effectively removes some of these substances, possibly leading to better preservation of cardiovascular function (26-29). One report, for example, evaluated 16 patients with sepsis, multiple organ dysfunction, and acute renal failure (28). Hemofiltration did not induce significant mediator activation and did not lead to cytokine removal. There was, however, increased removal of complement anaphylatoxins. Furthermore, the ultrafiltrate from these patients significantly stimulated peripheral blood mononuclear cells in vitro and enhanced tumor necrosis factor release; on the other hand, it reduced lymphocyte production of IL-2 and IL-6. These effects were not seen with ultrafiltrate from normal volunteers.

The ability of hemofiltration to remove immunomodulatory substances may lead to an improvement in patient outcome among those with sepsis and acute kidney injury. Although not yet studied in large randomized prospective controlled studies, there is some evidence that hemofiltration may provide some benefit in those with sepsis and acute renal failure (30-36):

- In a pilot prospective study, 20 patients with septic shock and acute renal failure were randomly assigned to either high (65 mL/kg per hour) or low volume (35 mL/kg per hour) hemofiltration (36). High volume hemofiltration was associated with decreased mean norepinephrine dose and increased urine output. Survival at 28 days was the same in both groups.

- One retrospective study evaluated the effects of isovolemic hemofiltration on physiological and clinical outcomes in 80 patients with septic shock and oliguric acute kidney injury (31). Prior to 1999, 40 patients had received conventional supportive therapy; subsequently, 40 patients received hemofiltration at 45 mL/kg per hour over the first six hours, which was followed by conventional CVVH. Incorporation of isovolemic hemofiltration into the treatment regimen significantly improved oxygenation and mean arterial pressure. Survival at 28 days was also significantly better (55 versus 28 percent).

Further study in larger better designed studies is required to understand the role of this modality in acute renal failure and sepsis. Furthermore, the early initiation of this intervention (isovolemic hemofiltration) may be very important. However, a randomized prospective study found that early intervention with low volume hemofiltration (25 mL/kg per hour) was deleterious in those with severe sepsis (37).

Effect on mortality: No modality of renal replacement therapy in the critically ill patient with acute renal failure, including intermittent hemodialysis, peritoneal dialysis, and the many forms of CRRT, has been clearly shown to have a survival benefit (1,38).

3. Terminology - Different models of CRRT

There are many variations of CRRT and the remainder of this topic will provide a general overview of the nomenclature that has been developed. The different modalities are categorized according to the access characteristics (blood or peritoneal, venovenous or arteriovenous) (Table 2) (39).

Blood access
Arteriovenous
Continuous arteriovenous hemofiltration
Continuous arteriovenous hemodialysis
Continuous arteriovenous hemodiafiltration
Venovenous
Continuous venovenous hemofiltration
Continuous venovenous hemodialysis
Continuous venovenous hemodiafiltration
Slow continuous ultrafiltration
Slow low efficiency dialysis or dialfiltration
Slow low efficiency daily dialysis
Extended daily dialysis
Peritoneal access
Continuous equilibrium peritoneal dialysis

Table 2. Continuous renal replacement therapies (39)

Arteriovenous or venovenous: Arteriovenous (AV) refers to the use of an arterial catheter that allows blood to flow into the extracorporeal circuit by virtue of the systemic blood pressure. A venous catheter is placed for return. Venovenous (VV) is an alternative modality in which both catheters or one dual lumen catheter are placed in veins. An extracorporeal blood pump is required to circulate blood through the extracorporeal circuit.

The advantage of arteriovenous access is that it is simple to set up and does not require an extracorporeal blood pump. It does, however, require arterial puncture with an attendant risk of arterial embolization. Blood flow may also be unreliable in patients who are hypotensive or have severe peripheral vascular disease.

Venovenous access, on the other hand, does not require arterial access, involves less systemic anticoagulation, uses only one dual lumen catheter, and has faster and more reliable blood flow than with arterial access. The only disadvantage is the requirement for an extracorporeal blood pump (39).

Hemodialysis: Hemodialysis (HD) refers to the transport process by which a solute **passively diffuses down its concentration gradient** from one fluid compartment (either blood or dialysate) into the other. During HD, urea, creatinine, and potassium move from blood to dialysate, while other solutes, such as calcium and bicarbonate, move from dialysate to blood. The dialysate flows countercurrent to blood flow through the dialyzer to maximize the concentration gradient between the compartments and therefore to maximize the rate of solute removal. The net effect is the production of desired changes in the plasma concentrations of these solutes: a reduction in the blood urea nitrogen and plasma creatinine concentration; and an elevation in the plasma calcium and bicarbonate concentrations (39).

Hemofiltration: Hemofiltration (HF) refers to the use of a hydrostatic pressure gradient to induce the filtration (or **convection**) of plasma water across the membrane of the hemofilter. The frictional forces between water and solutes (called **solvent drag**) results in the convective transport of small and middle molecular weight solutes (less than 5000 Daltons) in the same direction as water. Substitution fluid is usually required to prevent excessive fluid removal.

The process of HF itself removes smaller solutes (such as urea and electrolytes) in roughly the **same concentration as the plasma**. There is therefore no change in the plasma concentrations of these solutes by HF, in contrast to those achieved by HD. However, the administration of substitution fluid will lower by dilution the plasma concentrations of those solutes (such as urea and creatinine) not present in the substitution fluid (39).

Hemodiafiltration: Hemodiafiltration (HDF) refers to a combination of dialysis and filtration. Solute loss primarily occurs by diffusion dialysis but 25 percent or more may occur by hemofiltration (39).

Continuous replacement therapies (CRRT): the acronyms that have derived from the above concepts describe continuous therapies with the following general characteristics.

Continuous arteriovenous hemofiltration (CAHV): CAVH uses AV access to remove fluid and solutes by convection. Its per hour efficiency of solute removal is generally quite low, since no diffusion occurs. Thus, 24 hour/day operation or the addition of enhancing techniques is required. Ultrafiltration in CAVH is allowed at a greater degree than required for the restoration of euvolemia to increase solute removal. As a result, replacement fluid is necessary to prevent volume depletion. However, the rate of solute clearance with CAVH is still relatively low even at a high UFR (table 1). One method to increase the removal of urea (and probably other small, lipid-soluble solutes) is to administer the replacement fluid before the filter; this **predilution** lowers the plasma urea concentration, thereby allowing urea to diffuse from within red cells into the plasma water. The increased total extracellular urea entering the filter enhances the urea clearance rate by approximately 15 percent, especially if 200 mmHg of suction is also used (40,41).

As with any hemofiltration procedure, the aim is to keep the filtration fraction at 10 to 20 percent. At 40 percent and above, sludging occurs in the filter, compromising further fluid removal (42).

Continuous venovenous hemofiltration (CVVH): CVVH is similar to CAVH except that an extracorporeal blood pump is required that allows the physician to control the flow rates within the system (43). The blood pump assures a fast and stable Qb that can be set, for example, at approximately 250 mL/min. If the hematocrit is 33 percent, then the plasma flow rate will be 167 mL/min. A filtration fraction of 10 percent in this setting results in a UFR of 16.7 mL/min, which is equal to 1 L/h or 24 L/day (four times greater than that with SCUF). Most of this fluid will need to be replaced; if given before the filter (predilution), the urea clearance will again be enhanced by approximately 15 percent. Water exchanges of 40 to 60 L/day are usually sufficient, but catabolic patients with an increased urea load may require more than 60 L/day (44).

The more predictable blood flow rate and the associated ability to achieve a high ultrafiltration rate make CVVH preferable to CAVH when solute removal is important, as in hypercatabolic patients with a high BUN (table 1).

Slow continuous ultrafiltration (SCUF): SCUF is strictly a dehydrating procedure with no intent to substantially remove solute. Access can be arteriovenous or venovenous. SCUF is similar to CAVH or CVVH except that the ultrafiltration rate is held at a lower rate; thus, SCUF is primarily used when the fluid removal goals are modest.

Slow continuous ultrafiltration (SCUF) is designed to remove up to **6 to 7 L** of fluid per day without requiring replacement fluid other than for hyperalimentation. Solute removal is **minimal** with this technique, being limited by the low ultrafiltration rate and lack of dialysis. As an example, the clearance of urea and other small solutes is equal to the ultrafiltration rate of approximately 4 to 5 mL/min. Thus, SCUF is not useful in patients who are uremic or hyperkalemic.

Either arteriovenous or venovenous access can be used for SCUF. Arteriovenous access, without an extracorporeal pump, is generally sufficient to achieve the desired rate of fluid loss. The low ultrafiltration rate (UFR) of about 5 mL/min does not require a high rate of blood flow (Qb) through the filter. The Qb can be estimated by flushing the extracorporeal circuit with saline and then measuring the time for blood to refill the circuit. The volume of the lines and filter are noted in the manufacture's package literature.

Practical goals are a UFR of 5 mL/min and a Qb of 80 mL/min. If the hematocrit is between 35 and 40 percent, then this Qb represents a plasma flow of approximately 50 mL/min with a filtration fraction of 10 percent. If necessary, the UFR can be increased by raising Qb or by adding suction to the filtrate drainage system (45). The Qb can be raised by increasing the systemic blood pressure or by inserting an extracorporeal blood pump into the circuit. Short catheters with wide internal diameters that have been specifically designed for CAVH should be used for arterial access, since they maximize Qb (46).

In some cases, however, the UFR is too rapid. In this setting, ultrafiltration can be slowed by raising the level of the bag into which the ultrafiltrate drains. Most SCUF is now performed with venovenous access, and UFR is completely controlled by the operating parameters of the automated equipment.

Continuous arteriovenous hemodialysis *(CAVHD or CAVD respectively):* CAVHD or CAVD is similar to CAVH with two exceptions: dialysate is run at a low flow rate countercurrent to the direction of blood flow; and the ultrafiltration rate is not maximized to protect against the development of hypotension. Fluid removal is slower than with CAVH alone, but a greater reduction in solute concentration is achieved.

CAVHD differs from CAVH in that dialysis fluid flows through the filter in a compartment separated from the blood by the dialysis membrane. The efficiency of CAVHD is, as with CAVH, dependent upon Qb. However, the UFR is not as high as that achievable with CAVH alone. Thus, fluid removal with CAVHD is slower, but a greater rate of solute clearance can be achieved (table 1).

Clearance rates with CAVHD are dependent upon both blood and dialysate flow rates, which determine the concentration gradient between these two compartments. At Qb values above 80 mL/min, the dialysate fluid tends to become saturated with small solutes (ie, the concentration in the dialysate approaches that in the plasma, preventing further diffusive loss). In this setting, the main way to increase clearance is to raise the dialysate flow rate (Qd) from 1 up to 2 L/h (47,48). Once the Qd reaches 2 L/h, additional attempts to enhance clearance should be directed at increasing Qb, either by using a blood pump or turning up the pump rate if it is already in use.

A final way to raise solute clearance above that achieved by diffusion is to increase convective clearance. This can be achieved by enhancing ultrafiltration beyond the amount necessary to reestablish euvolemia, with replacement fluid then being given to prevent volume depletion. Thus, the highest solute clearances are achieved in CAVHD with a high Qb, high Qd, high UFR, and high rate of fluid replacement. For all the therapies discussed the highest clearances are in the extracorporeal pumped venovenous therapies.

Continuous venovenous hemodialysis (CVVHD or CVVD): CVVHD or CVVD utilizes venovenous access and a blood pump, but is otherwise similar to CAVHD. CVVHD combines the processes of diffusive and convective clearances; as with CVVH, it utilizes a blood pump to maximize the delivery of blood to the extracorporeal device. The transmembrane pressure generated by the blood pump assures net ultrafiltration unless the dialysate outflow is regulated to ensure that ultrafiltration is retarded. Under routine operating conditions, the blood flow (Qb) varies from 150 to 300 mL/min and the dialysate flow (Qd) from 1 to 2 L/hour.

The equipment required to provide CVVHD can be simple or complex. As an example, components, such as a blood pump, may be combined with separate infusion pumps; by comparison, specialized equipment made by many vendors can be utilized alone to deliver fresh dialysate to the filter and to govern the rate of dialysate exiting the filter.

Some machines also can be utilized for CVVHD. This system uses a proportioning system to generate bicarbonate dialysate from concentrate. The Qd can be adjusted to as high as 6 L/h, thereby providing an enormous clearance potential with continuous therapy. This approach can be applied for as little as eight hours per day (or nocturnally) because the solute clearance is high and the ultrafiltration needs can frequently be realized in this short period (49,59). This hybrid dialytic intervention, named sustained or slow low efficiency dialysis (SLED), or extended daily dialysis (EDD), may soon become the "gold standard" for renal replacement therapy during acute renal failure.

Continuous arteriovenous hemodiafiltration (CAVHDF): CAVHDF is similar to CAVHD except that ultrafiltration is allowed at a rate beyond that necessary to reestablish euvolemia. From the viewpoint of solute removal, CAVHDF combines diffusion to aggressively removal small solutes with convection to remove large solutes. Because the volume of fluid ultrafiltered is so large, replacement fluid must be given to maintain euvolemia.

Continuous venovenous hemodiafiltration *or CVVHDF* is similar to CAVHDF, except that venovenous access is utilized and a blood pump is required.

Continuous equilibrium peritoneal dialysis (CEPD): CEPD is a long-dwell procedure similar to CAPD. A semipermanent peritoneal dialysis catheter is placed. Rapid exchanges are used initially to attain fluid and solute balance (as in acute PD). This is followed by longer dwell times to maintain this balance.

Continuous flow peritoneal dialysis: In this variant of peritoneal dialysis, there are two points of access into the peritoneal cavity, one for continuous inflow of fresh dialysate, the other for efflux of used dialysate. Clearances still primarily depend upon the flow rate of dialysate up to a point in PD, because peritoneal blood flow is limited. However, continuous flow PD clearances exceed those of CEPD (39).

4. Efficacy of CRRT in patients with severe sepsis or septic shock

Continuous renal replacement therapies (CRRTs) involve either dialysis (diffusion-based solute removal) or filtration (convection-based solute and water removal) treatments that operate in a continuous mode (22,51-53). Variations of CRRT might run 12 to 14 hours, especially during daytime periods of full staffing. This regimen has become more prevalent in Europe and has been called "go slow dialysis." The major advantage of continuous therapy is the slower rate of solute or fluid removal per unit of time. Thus, CRRT is generally better tolerated than conventional therapy, since many of the complications of intermittent hemodialysis are related to the rapid rate of solute and fluid loss.

Severe sepsis and septic shock carry a high mortality and account for a large proportion of patients admitted to intensive care units (54-57). It is widely accepted that the release of large amounts of pro- and anti-inflammatory mediators that occurs in severe sepsis contributes to the development of multiple organ dysfunction syndrome (MODS) (8,58-60), including ARF. Theoretically, high-dose CRRT could remove mediators by convection and/or adsorption (44,61) and reduce mortality, even in the absence of ARF (62). However, most current clinical practice guidelines suggest that the traditional doses of CRRT used in ARF, with or without sepsis, are insufficient to remove these mediators and recommend using at least 35 ml/kg/hour of ultrafiltration (10,63).

In order to assess the efficacy of CRRT in patients with severe sepsis or septic shock, we performed a systematic search in Medline, Embase, Web of Knowledge, Cochrane Library and Clinicaltrials.gov and a hand search of the retrieved studies. We included both randomised controlled clinical trials and subgroups of randomised trials that assessed the effect of continuous renal replacement therapies (at traditional or high doses) and reported clinical outcomes in adult patients with severe sepsis or septic shock (effect on mortality, hemodinamic effect, pulmonary function, etc.). Recently, two large randomised clinical trials in patients with ARF (ATN study (64,65) and RENAL study (66,67) have seriously challenged these recommendations. Additionally, four recent meta-analyses about effectiveness of CRRT in critical patients with ARF have described no impact on the mortality or secondary outcomes of these techniques. The uncertainty regarding the effectiveness of CRRT in patients with sepsis without renal failure is even greater.

The results of systematic review about the efficacy in severe septic patients with ARF suggest that the addition of CRRT or its use at high doses does not improve the clinical outcomes of patients with severe sepsis or septic shock with or without ARF and irrespective of the technique used or the definition of ARF. Albeit conventional haemofiltration, haemofiltration using high cut-off filters, high volume haemofiltration and haemodiafiltration are clearly different, the results are consistent and homogeneous, evidencing a lack of effect. With regard to mortality, only one trial (68) reported a significant reduction in mortality. However this was a small study (based on 28 events) (69), which was stopped early by benefit (70-72), which reported an unusual reduction in mortality (risk ratio of 0.31). Therefore, there is a high probability that it was a false positive. After exclusion of this trial, the heterogeneity was greatly reduced and the pooled relative risk was 1.

A specific consideration should be done with respect to three studies comparing conservative treatment versus CVVH or high volume haemo-filtration (37,73), or in patients without ARF (8) respectively. Although it is doubtful whether these studies should be analysed together due to differences in design, a subgroup analysis did not reveal any subgroup effect.

Only one study (64) included different types of renal replacement therapies, specially continuous and intermittent, showed specifically that the schedule of application of renal replacement therapies was not a factor capable to modifying the effect on mortality.

With respect to other outcomes such as improvement in haemodynamic status or pulmonary oxygenation, much of the available evidence comes from animal and non-randomised studies (mainly pre-post studies without external control groups (35,74-76) not included in this review. However, the evidence based on randomised controlled trials is consistent with that of mortality. Only one study with significant methodological limitations reported a reduction in the use of vasopressors in the experimental group (36), and none of the trials reviewed reported an improvement in gas exchange, duration of mechanical ventilation, development of MODS or length of stay. Respect to other outcomes, two recent meta-analyses (77,78) found no effect of high-dose renal replacement therapy on dialysis dependence or length of stay in patients with ARF.

We did not detect any difference of effect of haemofiltration according to the three groups of doses used. However, only two small studies used doses higher than 65 ml/kg/hour. The dose for attaining a sepsis could very likely be different from the dose used for renal support in ARF. Currently there is an ongoing randomised clinical trial (79) addressing this issue. In any case, the results of our review do not support the routine use of doses higher than 35 ml/kg in patients with severe sepsis with or without ARF.

Similarly, this review is limited to studies comparing high-dose haemofiltration-haemodiafiltration or standard haemofiltration-haemodiafiltration versus traditional dosage or no haemofiltration. Thus, the study results cannot be generalised to other haemofiltration techniques with dialysis (e.g. highadsorption filters, filters of high porosity or plasmapheresis).

A further limitation of studies is that six of the 12 studies which met the inclusion criteria were actually not designed to study patients with severe sepsis and septic shock. These studies evaluated patients with ARF and some had very low numbers of septic patients. Furthermore, these groups of septic patients may not have been defined in the same way across studies. Therefore, the external validity of our study is limited by the scarcity of randomised controlled trials addressing specifically clinical outcomes of renal replacement therapies in septic patients. Indeed, almost all the studies that compared high versus low doses were performed in patients with ARF. The effect of high doses in septic patients without acute kidney injury therefore cannot be fully evaluated until well-designed and powered trials are performed.

Finally, the efficacy of haemofiltration in patients with non-infectious systemic inflammatory response syndrome is beyond the scope of this chapter. It is possible that patients with systemic inflammatory response syndrome (post-cardiac arrest syndrome (80), severe trauma (81,82), pancreatitis (83), severe burns (84) experience a massive release of mediators and therefore may benefit from early haemo-filtration. In contrast, patients with sepsis undergo haemofiltration at a later stage in the course of the disease. It can be hypothesised that the haemofiltration in patients with sepsis is performed outside the therapeutic window when organ damage has already occurred. Further research is needed to address this issue.

5. Conclusions

Regarding these theoretical limitations and potential deleterious effects, it is clear that we can not indicate sistematically hemofiltration in sepsis and SMDO according to hypothesis, however attractive they may be. We have to assess the use of these techniques derived from the knowledge of studies with scientific evidence. The systematic review of the Literature gives us the following conclusions:

1. Is not very strong the evidence that ultrafiltrate obtained from the septic patient's employing continuous hemofiltration remove any clinically important mediator. This is not so with respect to the NTF and the IL-1, two proinflammatory cytokines that are believed to play an important role in the pathogenesis of inflammatory syndrome (Evidence Class IIa or evidence for its usefulness or effectiveness) (85-87).
2. Most animal models using endotoxic or bacterial stimulus or suggest that hemofiltration plays a beneficial effect on survival. However, when we use a true model of infection in humans, nobody has been able to show beneficial effects. Clinical studies do not establish, nor excluded, a positive impact on mortality (Evidence Class IIb evidence or less evidence for utility and effectiveness) (88,89).
3. Experimental animal models of hypodynamic sepsis, again with the exception of true infection model, suggest that continuous hemofiltration allows the extraction of cardio depressor mediators, thereby producing a beneficial effect greater the higher filtration rate. Also controlled clinical studies show an attenuation of the hemodynamic response, suggesting a modulation of the inflammation (Evidence Class I or evidence or general agreement beneficial use, useful and effective) (90-94).
4. When analyzing the oxygen transport respiratory parameters they demonstrated a strong evidence of improved oxygenation and peripheral oxygen extraction with the use of continuous hemofiltration (Evidence Class I or evidence or general agreement beneficial use, useful and effective). The mechanism It is not clear. It may be reflect an improvement in blood flow through redistribution to peripheral level in hypoxic cells, or it may be that there are circulating factors that are eliminated by hemofiltration and they are responsible for the inadequate peripheral oxygen extraction (95).
5. Finally, the beneficial effects observed with hemofiltration it may be not necessarily attributed to the removal of inflammatory mediators. Some of these findings may be explained by reduced temperature, handling of the water balance (reducing the water extravascular lung or optimizing the Starling curve of patients) or metabolic changes (as may be the correction of acidosis), which increases the effect of catecholamines (5,6,15,96,97).

In summary, Continuous Renal Replacement Therapy (CRRT) may be required in patients with severe ARF. Although most patients are treated with hemodialysis, an alternative approach is the use of CRRT. A number of possible differences between intermittent hemodialysis and CRRT include hemodynamic stability, solute removal, removal of substances in those with sepsis, and effects on mortality. However, the best evidence available does not support the routine use of CRRT in patients with sepsis. Further research is necessary regarding the efficacy of early high-dose CRRT in patients with severe systemic inflammatory response syndrome of non-infectious origin.

Author details

F.J. García-Miguel
Department of Anaesthesiology and Reanimation, Hospital del Tajo, Aranjuez, Madrid, Spain

6. References

[1] Golper TA. Continuous renal replacement therapy in acute kidney injury (acute renal failure). http://www.uptodate.com. Last updated. Oct 17, 2011.
[2] García Miguel FJ. Mirón Rodríguez MF. Extracorporeal hemofiltration techniques: support treatment in sepsis and multiple-organ dysfunction syndrome. Act Anest Reanim (Madrid) 2008;18:37-40.
[3] Honore PM, Joannes-Boyau O. The French Hemodiafe Trial. Int J Artif Organs 2006;29:1190-2.
[4] Joannes-Boyau O, Honore PM, Boer W. Hemofiltration: the case for removal of sepsis mediators from where they do ham. Crit Care Med 2006;34:2244-6.
[5] Pestaña D, Casanova E, Villagrán MJ, Tormo C, Pérez-Chrzanowska H, Redondo J, et al. Continuous hemofiltration in hyperthermic septic shock patients. J Trauma 2007;63:751-6.
[6] Uchino S, Bellomo R, Morimatsu H, Morgera S, Schetz M, Tan I, et al. Continuous renal replacement therapy: a worldwide practice survey. The beginning and ending supportive therapy for the kidney (B.E.S.T. kidney) investigators. Intensive Care Med 2007;33:1563-70.
[7] Morgera S; Haase M, Rocktäschel J, Vargas-Hein O, Krausch D, et al. Intermittent high-permiability hemofiltration modulates inflammatory response in septic patients with multiorgan failure. Nephron Clin Pract 2003;75-80.
[8] Cole L, Bellomo R, Hart G, Journois D, Davenport P, Tipping P, et al. A phase II randomized, controlled trial of continuous hemofiltration in sepsis. Crit Care Med 2002;30:100-6.
[9] Hörner C, Shuster S, Planchky J, Hofer S, Martin E, Weigand MA. Hemofiltration an immune response in severe sepsis. J Surg Res 2007;142:59-65.
[10] Bouman CS, Oudemans-van Straaten HM, Schultz MJ, Vroom MB. Hemofiltration in sepsis and systemic inflammatory response syndrome: the role of dosing and timing. J Crit care 2007;22:1-12.
[11] Ghani RA, Zainudin S, Ctkong N, Rahman AF, Wafa SR, Mohamed M, et al. serum IL-6 and IL 1-ra with sequential organ failure assessment scores in septic patients receiving high-volume haemofiltration and continuous venovenous haemofiltration. Nephrolgy (Carlton) 2006;11:386-93.
[12] Ronco C, Brendolan A, Lonnemann G, Bellomo R, Piccinni P, Digito A, et al. A pilot study of coupled plasma with adsorption in septic shock. Crit Care Med 2002;30:1250-5.

[13] Morgera S, Slowinski T, Melzer C, Sobottke V, Vargas-Hein O, Volk T, et al. Renal replacement therapy with high-cutoff hemofilters: impact of convection and diffusion on cytokine clearances and protein status. Am J Kidney Dis 2004;43:444-53.
[14] Boereboom FT, Ververs FF, Blankestijin PJ, Savelkoul TJ, van Dijk A. Vancomycin clearance during continuous haemofiltration in critically ill patients. Intensive Care Med 1999;25:1100-4.
[15] Morgera S, Haase M, Kuss T, Vargas-Hein O, Zuckermann-Becker H, Melzer C, et al. Pilot study on the effects of high-cutoff hemofiltration on the need for norepinephrine in septic patients with acute renal failure. Crit Care Med 2006;34:2099-104.
[16] Kline JA, Gordon BE, Williams C, Blumenthal S, Watts JA, Díaz-Buxo J. Large-pore haemodialysis in acute endotoxin shock. Crit Care Med 1999;27:588-96.
[17] Düngen HD, von Heymann C, Ronco C, Kox WJ, Spies CD. Renal replacement therapy: physical properties of hollow fibers influence efficiency. Int J Artif Organs 2001;24:357-66.
[18] Naka T, Egi M, Bellomo R, Cole L, French C, Botha J, et al. Commercial low-citrate anticoagulation haemofiltration in high risk patients with frequent filter clotting. Anaesth Intensive Care 2005;33:601-8.
[19] Golper TA. Indications, technical considerations, and strategies for renal replacement therapy in the intensive care unit. J Intensive Care Med 1992; 7:310-7.
[20] Forni LG, Hilton PJ. Continuous hemofiltration in the treatment of acute renal failure. N Engl J Med 1997; 336:1303-9.
[21] Ronco C. Continuous renal replacement therapies for the treatment of acute renal failure in intensive care patients. Clin Nephrol 1993; 40:187-98.
[22] Manns M, Sigler MH, Teehan BP. Continuous renal replacement therapies: an update. Am J Kidney Dis 1998; 32:185-207.
[23] Golper TA, Cigarran-Guldris S, Jenkins RD, Brier ME, The role of convection during simulated continuous arteriovenous hemodialysis. Contrib Nephrol 1991;93:146-8.
[24] Ziegler EJ, Fisher CJ Jr, Sprung CL, Straube RC, sadoff JC, Foule GE, et al. Treatment of gram-negative bacteremia and septic shock with HA-1A human monoclonal antibody against endotoxin. A randomized, double-blind, placebo-controlled trial. The HA-1A Sepsis Study Group. N Engl J Med 1991; 324:429-36.
[25] Moldawer LL. Interleukin-1, TNF alpha and their naturally occurring antagonists in sepsis. Blood Purif 1993; 11:128-33.
[26] Stein B, Pfenninger E, Grünert A, Deller A. Influence of continuous haemofiltration on haemodynamics and central blood volume in experimental endotoxic shock. Intensive Care Med 1990; 16:494-9.
[27] Gomez A, Wang R, Unruh H, Light RB, Bose D, Chau T, et al. hemofiltration reverses left ventricular dysfunction during sepsis in dogs. Anesthesiology 1990; 73:671-85.
[28] Hoffmann JN, Hartl WH, Deppisch R, Hartl WH, Inthorn D. Hemofiltration in human sepsis: evidence for elimination of immunomodulatory substances. Kidney Int 1995; 48:1563-70.
[29] Barzilay E, Kessler D, Berlot G, Gullo A, Geber D, Ben Zeev I. Use of extracorporeal supportive techniques as additional treatment for septic-induced multiple organ failure patients. Crit Care Med 1989; 17:634-7.

[30] Storck M, Hartl WH, Zimmerer E, Inthorn D. Comparison of pump-driven and spontaneous continuous haemofiltration in postoperative acute renal failure. Lancet 1991; 337:452-5.

[31] Piccinni P, Dan M, Barbacini S, Carraro R, Lieta E, Marafon S. Early isovolaemic haemofiltration in oliguric patients with septic shock. Intensive Care Med 2006; 32:80-6.

[32] Cole L, Bellomo R, Journois D, Davenport P, Baldwing I, Tipping P. High-volume haemofiltration in human septic shock. Intensive Care Med 2001; 27:978-86.

[33] Kvist T, Reit C. Results of endodontic retreatment: a randomized clinical study comparing surgical and nonsurgical procedures. J Endod 1999; 25:814-7.

[34] Cole L, Bellomo R, Silvester W, Reeves JH. A prospective, multicenter study of the epidemiology, management, and outcome of severe acute renal failure in a "closed" ICU system. Am J Respir Crit Care Med 2000; 162:191-6.

[35] Honore PM, Jamez J, Wauthier M, Lee PA, Dugernier T, Pirenne B, et al. Prospective evaluation of short-term, high-volume isovolemic hemofiltration on the hemodynamic course and outcome in patients with intractable circulatory failure resulting from septic shock. Crit Care Med 2000; 28:3581-7.

[36] Boussekey N, Chiche A, Faure K, Devos P, Guery B, d'Escrivan T, et al. A pilot randomized study comparing high and low volume hemofiltration on vasopressor use in septic shock. Intensive Care Med 2008; 34:1646-53.

[37] Payen D, Mateo J, Cavaillon JM, Fraisse F, Floriot C, Vicaut E. Impact of continuous venovenous hemofiltration on organ failure during the early phase of severe sepsis: a randomized controlled trial. Crit Care Med 2009; 37:803-10.

[38] Latour-Pérez J, Palencia-Herrejón E, Gómez-Tello V, Baeza-Román A, García-García MA, Sánchez Artola B. Intensity of continuous renal replacement therapies in patients with severe sepsis and septic shock: a systematic review and meta-analysis. Anaesth Intensive Care 2011;39:373-83.

[39] Golper TA. Continuous renal replacement therapies. Overview. http://www.uptodate.com. Last updated. mar 20, 2012.

[40] Kaplan AA. Predilution versus postdilution for continuous arteriovenous hemofiltration. Trans Am Soc Artif Intern Organs 1985; 31:28-32.

[41] Kaplan AA. Clinical trials with predilution and vacuum suction: enhancing the efficiency of the CAVH treatment. ASAIO Trans 1986; 32:49-51.

[42] Golper TA. Continuous arteriovenous hemofiltration in acute renal failure. Am J Kidney Dis 1985; 6:373-86.

[43] Macias WL, Mueller BA, Scarim SK, Robinson M, Rudy DW. Continuous venovenous hemofiltration: an alternative to continuous arteriovenous hemofiltration and hemodiafiltration in acute renal failure. Am J Kidney Dis 1991; 18:451-8.

[44] Ronco C, Bellomo R, Homel P, Brendolan A, Dan M, Piccini P, et al. Effects of different doses in continuous veno-venous haemofiltration on outcomes of acute renal failure: a prospective randomised trial. Lancet 2000; 356:26-30.

[45] Kaplan AA, Longnecker RE, Folkert VW. Suction-assisted continuous arteriovenous hemofiltration. Trans Am Soc Artif Intern Organs 1983; 29:408-13.

[46] Olbricht CJ, Haubitz M, Häbel U, Frei U, Koch KM. Continuous arteriovenous hemofiltration: in vivo functional characteristics and its dependence on vascular access and filter design. Nephron 1990; 55:49-57.
[47] Sigler MH, Teehan BP. Solute transport in continuous hemodialysis: a new treatment for acute renal failure. Kidney Int 1987; 32:562-71.
[48] van Geelen JA, Vincent HH, Schalekamp MA. Continuous arteriovenous haemofiltration and haemodiafiltration in acute renal failure. Nephrol Dial Transplant 1988; 3:181-6.
[49] Hu, KT, Yeun, JY, Craig, M, et al. Extended daily dialysis: An alternative to continuous venovenous hemofiltration in the intensive care unit. Blood Purif 1999; 17:28.
[50] Marshall MR, Golper TA, Shaver MJ, Alam MG, Chatoth DK. Sustained low-efficiency dialysis for critically ill patients requiring renal replacement therapy. Kidney Int 2001; 60:777-85.
[51] Kanagasundaram NS, Paganini EP. Critical care dialysis--a Gordian knot (but is untying the right approach?). Nephrol Dial Transplant 1999; 14:2590-4.
[52] Ronco C, Bellomo R, Kellum JA. Continuous renal replacement therapy: opinions and evidence. Adv Ren Replace Ther 2002; 9:229-44.
[53] Mehta RL. Continuous renal replacement therapy in the critically ill patient. Kidney Int 2005; 67:781.
[54] Vincent J-L, Sakr Y, Sprung CL, Ranieri VM, Reinhart K, Gerlach H et al. Sepsis in European intensive care units: results of the SOAP study. Crit Care Med 2006; 34:344-53.
[55] Brun-Buisson C, Meshaka P, Pinton P, Vallet B. EPISEPSIS: a reappraisal of the epidemiology and outcome of severe sepsis in French intensive care units. Intensive Care Med 2004; 30:580-8.
[56] Esteban A, Frutos-Vivar F, Ferguson ND, Penuelas O, Lorente JA, Gordo F et al. Sepsis incidence and outcome: contrasting the intensive care unit with the hospital ward. Crit Care Med 2007; 35:1284-9.
[57] Adrie C, Alberti C, Chaix-Couturier C, Azoulay E, De Lassence A, Cohen Y et al. Epidemiology and economic evaluation of severe sepsis in France: age, severity, infection site, and place of acquisition (community, hospital, or intensive care unit) as determinants of workload and cost. J Crit Care 2005; 20:46-58.
[58] Pinsky MR, Vincent JL, Deviere J, Alegre M, Kahn RJ, Dupont E. Serum cytokine levels in human septic shock. Relation to multiple-system organ failure and mortality. Chest 1993; 103:565-75.
[59] Bone RC, Grodzin CJ, Balk RA. Sepsis: a new hypothesis for pathogenesis of the disease process. Chest 1997; 112:235-43.
[60] Koch T. Origin and mediators involved in sepsis and the systemic inflammatory response syndrome. Kidney Int Suppl 1998; 64:S66-9.
[61] Ronco C, Tetta C, Mariano F, Wratten ML, Bonello M, Bordoni V et al. Interpreting the mechanisms of continuous renal replacement therapy in sepsis: the peak concentration hypothesis. Artif Organs 2003; 27:792-801.
[62] Bagshaw SM, George C, Bellomo R. Early acute kidney injury and sepsis: a multicentre evaluation. Crit Care 2008; 12:R47.

[63] Bellomo R, Honore PM, Matson J, Ronco C, Winchester J. Extracorporeal blood treatment (EBT) methods in SIRS/Sepsis. Int J Artif Organs 2005; 28:450-8.
[64] Palevsky PM, Zhang JH, O'Connor TZ, Chertow GM, Crowley ST, Choudhury D et al. Intensity of renal support in critically ill patients with acute kidney injury. N Engl J Med 2008; 359:7-20.
[65] Bonventre JV. Dialysis in acute kidney injury – more is not better. N Engl J Med 2008; 359:82-4.
[66] Bellomo R, Cass A, Cole L, Finfer S, Gallagher M, Lo S et al. Intensity of continuous renal-replacement therapy in critically ill patients. N Engl J Med 2009; 361:1627-38.
[67] Palevsky PM. Renal support in acute kidney injury – how much is enough? N Engl J Med 2009; 361:1699-701.
[68] Saudan P, Niederberger M, De Seigneux S, Romand J, Pugin J, Perneger T et al. Adding a dialysis dose to continuous hemofiltration increases survival in patients with acute renal failure. Kidney Int 2006; 70:1312-7.
[69] Pogue J, Yusuf S. Overcoming the limitations of current meta-analysis of randomised controlled trials. Lancet 1998; 351:47-52.
[70] Higgins J, Altman De. Assessing risk of bias in included studies. In: Higgins J, Green Se, eds. Cochrane Handbook for Systematic Reviews of Interventions Version 501 (updated September 2008). The Cochrane Collaboration 2008.
[71] Montori VM, Devereaux PJ, Adhikari NKJ, Burns KEA, Eggert CH, Briel M et al. Randomized trials stopped early for benefit: a systematic review. JAMA 2005; 294:2203-9.
[72] Bassler D, Briel M, Montori VM, Lane M, Glasziou P, Zhou Q et al. Stopping randomized trials early for benefit and estimation of treatment effects: systematic review and meta-regression analysis. JAMA 2010; 303:1180-7.
[73] Sander A, Armbruster W, Sander B, Daul AE, Lange R, Peters J. Hemofiltration increases IL-6 clearance in early systemic inflammatory response syndrome but does not alter IL-6 and TNF alpha plasma concentrations. Intensive Care Med 1997; 23:878-84.
[74] Lange R, Erhard J, Sander A, Scherer R, Eigler F. Use of continuous veno-venous high volume hemofiltration (CVVHVH) in patients with multiple organ failure. Principle and applications. Zentralbl Chir 1996; 121:535-40.
[75] Klouche K, Cavadore P, Portales P, Clot J, Canaud B, Beraud JJ. Continuous veno-venous hemofiltration improves hemodynamics in septic shock with acute renal failure without modifying TNFalpha and IL6 plasma concentrations. J Nephrol 2002; 15:150-7.
[76] Cornejo R, Downey P, Castro R, Romero C, Regueira T, Vega J et al. High-volume hemofiltration as salvage therapy in severe hyperdynamic septic shock. Intensive Care Med 2006; 32:713-22.
[77] Casey ET, Gupta BP, Erwin PJ, Montori VM, Murad MH. The dose of continuous renal replacement therapy for acute renal failure: a systematic review and meta-analysis. Ren Fail 2010; 32:555-61.
[78] Van Wert R, Friedrich JO, Scales DC, Wald R, Adhikari NKJ. High-dose renal replacement therapy for acute kidney injury: Systematic review and meta-analysis. Crit Care Med 2010; 38:1360-9.

[79] Haemofiltration Study: IVOIRE (High Volume in Intensive Care). From http://www.clinicaltrials.gov/ct2/show/NCT00241228?term=IVOIRE&rank=1 Accessed August 2010.

[80] Laurent I, Adrie C, Vinsonneau C, Cariou A, Chiche J-D, Ohanessian A et al. High-volume hemofiltration after out-of-hospital cardiac arrest: a randomized study. J Am Coll Cardiol 2005; 46:432-7.

[81] Sanchez-Izquierdo JA, Perez Vela JL, Lozano Quintana MJ, Alted Lopez E, Ortuno de Solo B, Ambros Checa A. Cytokines clearance during venovenous hemofiltration in the trauma patient. Am J Kidney Dis 1997; 30:483-8.

[82] Sanchez-Izquierdo RJA, Alted E, Lozano MJ, Perez JL, Ambros A, Caballero R. Influence of continuous hemofiltration on the hemodynamics of trauma patients. Surgery 1997; 122:902-8.

[83] Jiang H-L, Xue W-J, Li D-Q, Yin A-P, Xin X, Li C-M, Gao J-L. Influence of continuous veno-venous hemofiltration on the course of acute pancreatitis. World J Gastroenterol 2005; 11:4815-21.

[84] Chung KK, Juncos LA, Wolf SE, Mann EE, Renz EM, White C et al. Continuous renal replacement therapy improves survival in severely burned military casualties with acute kidney injury. J Trauma 2008; 64:S179-85.

[85] Uchino S, Bellomo R, Goldsmith D, Davenport P, Cole L, Baldwing I, et al. Super high flux hemofiltration: a new technique for cytokine removal. Intensive Care Med 2002;28:651-5.

[86] De Vriese AS, Colardyn FA, Plilippé JJ, Vanholder RC, De Sutter JH, Lameire NH. Cytokine removal during continuous hemofiltration in septic patients. J Am Soc Nephrol 1999;10:846-53.

[87] Reeves JH, Butt WW, Shann F, Layton JE, Stewart A, Waring PM, et al. Continuous plasmafiltration in sepsis syndrome. Plasmafiltration in Sepsis Study Group. Crit Care Med 1999;27:2096-104.

[88] Ratanarat R, Brendolan A, Piccinni P, Dan M, Salvatori G, Ricci Z, et al. Pulse high-volume haemofiltration for treatment of severe sepsis. Effects on hemodynamics and survival. Crit Care 2005;9:R294-302.

[89] Haase M, Silvester W, Uchino S, Goldsmith D, davenport P, Tipping p, et al. A pilot study of high-adsorption hemofiltration in human septic shock. Int J Artif Organs 2007;30:108-17.

[90] John S, Griesbach D, Baumgärtel M, Weihprecht H, Schmieder RE, Geiger H. effects of continuous haemofiltration vs. intermittent haemodialysis on systemic haemodinamics and splachnic regional perfusion in septic shock patients: a prospective, randomized clinical trial. Nephrol Dial Transplant 2001;16:320-7.

[91] Boga M, Islamoglu, Badak I, Cikirikçioglu M, Bakalim T, Yagdi T, et al. The effects of modified hemofiltration on inflammatory mediators and cardiac performance in coronary artery bypass grafting. Perfusion 200;15:143-50.

[92] Rogiers P. Improvement short-term outcomes with early use of isovolemic hemofiltration in patients with septic shock. Nat Clin Pract Nephrol 2006;2:487-9.

[93] Joannes-Boyau O, Rapaport S, Bazin R, Fleureau C, Janvier G. Impact of high volume hemofiltration on hemodynamic disturbance and outcome during septic shock. ASAIO J 2004;50:102-9.

[94] Kielstein JT, Kretschmer U, Ernst T, Hafer C, Bahr MJ, Haller H. Efficacy and cardiovascular tolerability of extended dialysis in critical ill patients: A randomized controlled study. Am J Kidney Dis 2004;43:342-9.

[95] Rokyta R Jr, Matejovic M, Krouzecky A, Opatrny K Jr, Rucicka J, Novac I. Effects of continuous haemofiltration-induced cooling on global haemodynamics, splanchnic oxygen and energy balance in critically ill patients. Nephrol Dial Transplant 2004;19:623-30.

[96] Shapiro NI, Howel MD, talmor D, Lahey D, Buras J, Wolfe S, et al. Implementation and outcomes of the Multiple Urgent Sepsis Therapies (MUST) protocol. Crit care Med 2006;34:1025-32.

[97] VinsonneauC, Camus C, Combes A, Costa de Beauregard MA, Klouche K, Boulain T, et al. On behalf of hemodiafe study Group. Continuos venonenous hemodiafiltration versus intermittent haemodyalisis for acute renal failure in patients with multiple-organ dysfunction syndrome: A muticentre randomised trial. Lancet 2006;368:379-85.

Chapter 19

Induction Agents for Endotracheal Intubation in Severe Sepsis and Septic Shock

Marie Mullen

Additional information is available at the end of the chapter

http://dx.doi.org/10.5772/49948

1. Introduction

The management of severe sepsis and septic shock remains to this day one of the great challenges in medical care. These two disease entities represent significant morbidity and mortality and cross the threshold of multiple medical disciplines. Worldwide it is estimated that one in ten intensive care unit (ICU) patients carry the diagnosis of severe sepsis (1). For the year 2020, in the United States alone, the projected number of severe sepsis cases will approach 1.1 million (2). These disease entities are not only common, but lethal. Severe sepsis carries a reported mortality of 28% (2). Septic shock has recorded mortality rates as high as 60% (3).

Sepsis has a strong association with respiratory failure. From an epidemiologic perspective, sepsis and pneumonia are the leading causes of acute lung injury (ALI) and acute respiratory distress syndrome (ARDS) (4-5). Reported sepsis-related ARDS incidence levels range from 16%-73% in multiple case series (6-9). Pneumonia is consistently documented as the primary inciting infection in the sepsis literature (10-13).

Severe sepsis and septic shock place critically ill patients at risk for respiratory failure and endotracheal intubation. In addition to epidemiologic evidence, there are multiple known complex physiologic variables in sepsis that explain the high potential risk for respiratory failure (14). Sepsis alters the respiratory drive. Early sepsis is particularly associated with an increase respiratory rate and an increase in coinciding energy expenditure. Components of sepsis-related ventilatory failure include a combination of increased respiratory muscle energy requirements with decreased energy availability and impending respiratory muscle fatigue (14).

Additional contributing factors to sepsis-associated respiratory failure include the interaction between the pulmonary and the cardiac system (14). Sepsis decreases pulmonary dynamic compliance, which leads to an increased in pleural pressure variation with each breath. This change in variation can augment right atrial venous return. A volume-resuscitated patient with sepsis will exhibit a significant increase in right atrial filling pressure. This increased return on the right side can translate to left-sided cardiac dysfunction and contribute to pulmonary edema and cardiac dysfunction (14). Other pulmonary-cardiac interactions include decreased left ventricular dysfunction due to pleural pressure changes. These changes effectively increase cardiac afterload. There is also the added phenomenon of intrinsic myocardial depression that is associated with septic shock (15). The preceding mechanisms for respiratory failure are significant. As severe sepsis and septic shock is a highly complex entity, these physiologic variables are a few of many contributory factors.

As demonstrated, severe sepsis and septic shock place a critically ill patient at high risk for respiratory failure. Correction of this impending failure may require endotrachael intubation. The decision to intubate and ventilate these patients presents significant obstacles as well. Severe sepsis and septic shock patients have potential complex multi-organ dysfunction issues that can create clinical care difficulties before, during, and after the intubation procedure. The choice of pharmacologic agent to facilitate endotracheal intubation should reflect these challenges in care.

2. Intubation in severe sepsis and septic shock

Endotrachael intubation for severe sepsis and septic shock presents multiple hurdles. Prior to intubation, critically ill patients with severe sepsis and septic shock are likely hypoxic. The septic patient is at high risk for oxygen desaturation during the procedure. Figure 1 illustrates the oxyhemoglobin curve and associated desaturation risk based on initial starting oxygen saturation (16). The previously described variables such as increased respiratory effort; increased energy expenditure and respiratory muscle fatigue further increase risk of desaturation despite appropriate maneuvers such as pre-oxygenation (16). Figure 2 further illustrates the effect of critical illness and body habitus on time to oxygen desaturation (17).

Critical illness can further decrease time to profound hypoxia beyond these described desaturation curves (16). Additional desaturation risk can ensue in cases of delayed intubation due to a difficult airway situation. Overall, endotrachael intubation in critically ill patients outside the operating environment is associated with high morbidity and complications (18-20).

The change from negative to positive pressure with intubation and mechanical ventilation represents significant changes in patient hemodynamics. One of the most common hemodynamic changes associated with endotracheal intubation is hypotension. Some studies have reported hypotension occurring in up to 25% of emergency intubations (21).

One notable difficulty element is the associated decrease in venous return with intubation. Venous return reduction occurs from several mechanisms (21). Venous return is a function of the difference of systemic pressure subtracted from right atrial pressure. Vasodilation from induction agents and reduction of catecholemine-associated vascular tone reduce left sided pressures and venous return. Positive pressure ventilation abruptly increases right atrial pressure. Decreased systemic pressure and increased right atrial pressure create a reduction in venous return that is difficult for a critically ill patient to compensate. Ongoing increased right atrial pressure contributing to persistent decreased venous return will translate to decreased left ventricular preload (22).

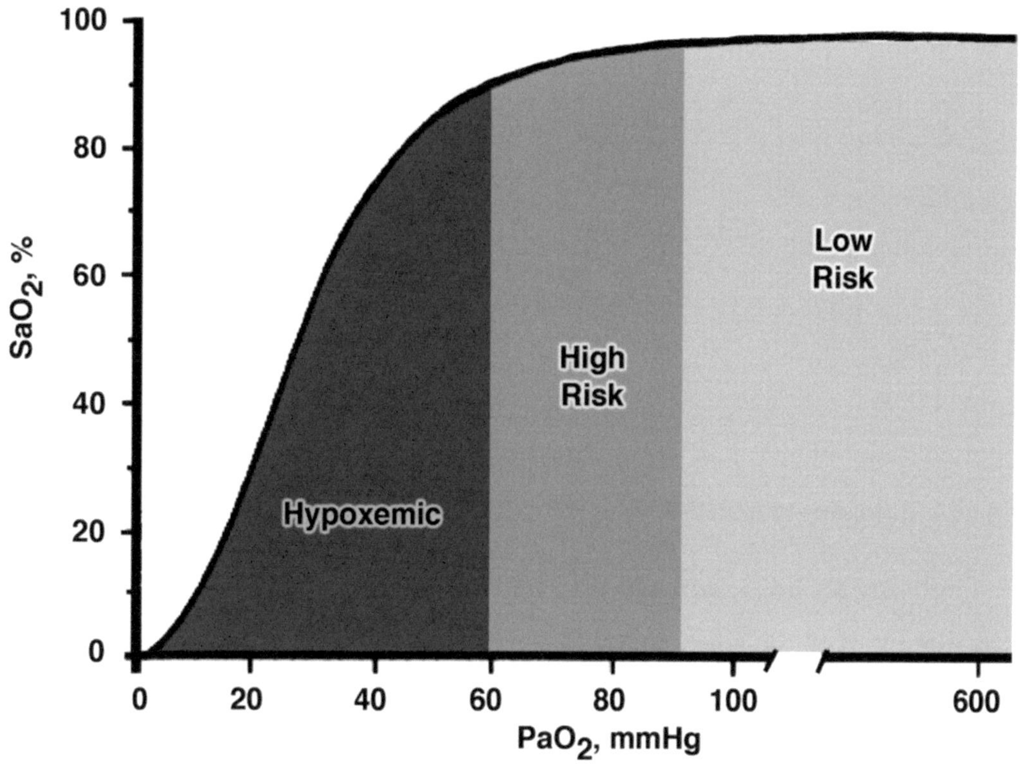

Figure 1. Oxyhemoglobin curve displays risk categories of desaturation (16)

Positive pressure ventilation can further affect left ventricular preload due to the phenomenon of interdependence between the right and left ventricle (22). The increase in thoracic pressure can lead to an increase in pulmonary vascular resistance. This situation results in decreased right ventricular ejection and increasing right ventricular end diastolic volume. Increased right end diastolic volume translates into decreased left end diastolic volume and preload. Mechanical ventilation exerts multiple effects on the cardiopulmonary system that need to be considered when initiating endotracheal intubation. The situation is further complicated in light of the pre-existing cardiopulmonary abnormalities of the sepsis patient (15).

Endotracheal intubation in the severe sepsis and septic shock patient poses many physiologic difficulties. These processes need to be heeded when deciding to intubate and choosing agents to facilitate the procedure.

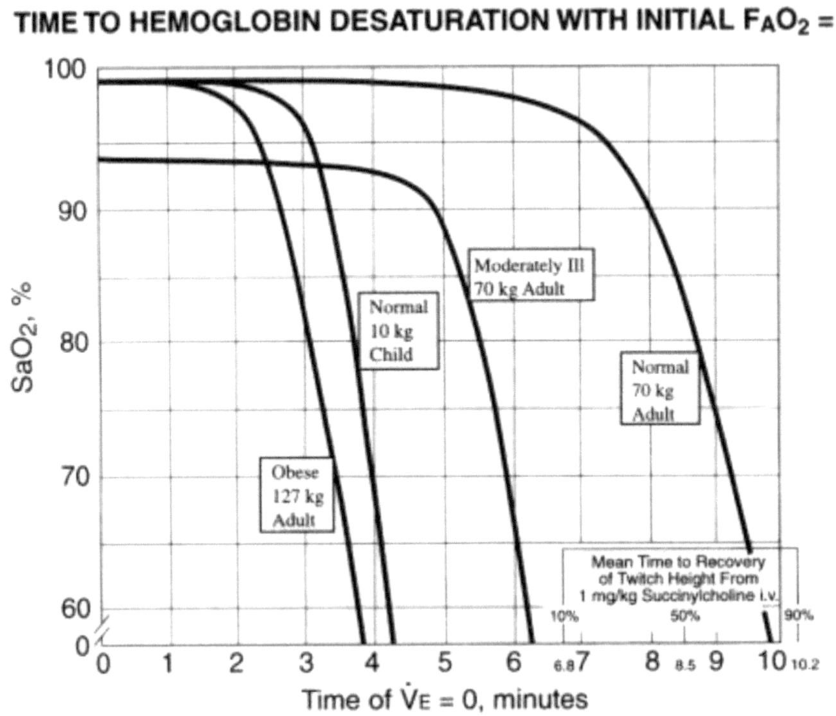

Figure 2. Time to desaturation when apneic with respect to size and medical condition (17)

3. Choosing an induction agent to facilitate intubation

The critically ill severe sepsis and septic shock patient in respiratory failure experiences many physiologic changes. These changes need to be addressed when evaluating the properties of intended induction agents.

As stated, this critically ill population is at high risk for oxygen desaturation. Time of onset for expected effect needs to be considered. An ideal agent would have a short onset of action to prevent undo delay in the procedure. It has been reported that a critically ill patient could theoretically experience serious oxygen desaturation within 23 seconds of apnea (23). This risk of desaturation needs to be evaluated in cases where a paralytic agent in conjunction with an induction agent is the planned intubation strategy.

Septic shock patients are hemodynamically unstable. By definition these patient have fluid-refractory hypotension (24). Induction agents that further contribute to this instability need to be carefully reviewed. The use of induction agents that decrease cardiac output or cause further dilation should be carefully contemplated prior to use. Severe sepsis and septic shock have a documented incidence of myocardial depression (15). Some induction agents may potentiate this cardiac depression as well.

Metabolism of induction agents needs to be examined as well. Severe sepsis and septic shock can exhibit associated organ dysfunction that will potentially affect induction agent metabolism (25). Organ injury that needs to be especially regarded includes renal and hepatic dysfunction.

4. Review of available induction agents

4.1. Etomidate

Etomidate is a non-barbiturate imidazole compound used for induction in endotracheal intubation. The primary mechanism of action is direct action on the gamma amino butyric acid (GABA) receptor (26). As a sedative hypnotic agent, it exhibits many favorable properties that make it a particularly attractive agent to facilitate intubation. Etomidate has a rapid reliable mechanism of action and duration; has minimal affect on many cardiovascular parameters; is neuroprotective and has other favorable attributes as well.

Etomidate is typically dosed at 0.3 mg/kg in adult patients (27). Reported literature dosing for induction is cited as 0.2-0.4 mg/kg (28). It is also recommended to consider a reduction in dosing in the elderly patient due to delayed metabolic clearance (28).

As stated, etomidate has a rapid onset and duration of action with a single bolus dose. In a standard single induction dose, onset to hypnotic effect is 5-15 seconds (28). Duration of action is rapid as well and is dose dependent. Estimated metabolism is 5-14 minutes. Metabolism of the medication is primarily hepatic and the agent is strongly protein bound. Interestingly, hepatic disease and protein metabolism may alter potency of etomidate, but not timing of clinical actions (28).

The strength of etomidate lies in its cardiovascular effects. Etomidate does not significantly impact systolic blood pressure (SBP), mean arterial blood pressure (MAP), central venous pressure (CVP), heart rate, systemic vascular resistance (SVR), cardiac index (CI), stroke volume (SV) in standard bolus dosing (28). The literature in some cases does report a slight decrease in SBP. At high bolus dosing (>0.4mg/kg), one recorded study reports less than a 15% impact on SBP and MAP (29). Etomidate does not adversely alter hemodynamics in the face of valvular or coronary artery disease (28). The literature also reports improvement of coronary blood flow with the use of etomidate without an increase in oxygen consumption (30). Etomidate seems to offer a significant safety profile for hemodynamically compromised patients.

Other advantageous elements of etomidate include its neuroprotective effects. Etomidate is noted to effectively lower intracranial pressure (ICP) (28). Etomidate is able to lower ICP without adversely affecting hemodynamics. In addition, etomidate appears to independently lower cerebral oxygen consumption by several mechanisms (28). The medication also has the ability to lower intraocular pressure. This induction agent again has many attractive properties when considering its use.

Adverse effects of etomidate should be reviewed. Etomidate is linked to myoclonus. Reported rates of this effect can be as high as 30% (28). The literature regarding this agent and seizures remains mixed (28). There have been reports of decreased seizure potential in patients with seizure disorders. Overall, etomidate remains a neuroprotective agent. The induction agent has a moderate risk of nausea and vomiting. This may be a consideration in the non-fasted patient. Etomidate also may have a potential to cause peripheral vascular irritation (28).

The critical care community appropriately expressed concerns about etomidate in regards to its link to critical illness-related corticosteroid insufficiency. Etomidate has a documented ability to inhibit the function of the 11 β-hydroxylase enzyme and subsequently contribute to this phenomenon (31-32). Several retrospective studies or study subsets have even suggested a mortality impact from this suppressive action (33-36).

The literature clearly acknowledges and supports the presence of etomidate-related adrenal insufficiency. The presence of actual mortality remains questionable. Multiple studies retrospective and prospective do not support the presence of increased mortality. Ehrman and Dmello exhibited a lack of mortality in large retrospective cohort studies (37-38).

Prospective studies surrounding the use of etomidate remain encouraging in regards to mortality. Tekwani initially showed no difference in mortality in a prospective observational study of over 100 septic patients receiving etomidate (39). The same author performed a prospective randomized study of etomidate versus midazolam in septic patients, which did not show any increase in length of stay with use (40). A large randomized prospective study comparing etomidate to ketamine in over 400 critically ill patients failed to show a mortality difference between the two agents in regards to administration (41). It should be noted that only 16% of patients in this large cohort carried the diagnosis of sepsis.

Due to the presence of adrenal insufficiency, there is consideration in regards to addition of corticosteroid therapy to patients receiving etomidate. Initial research suggests that in non-shock states this approach may not be effective. A recent prospective study by Payen, et al revealed no significant difference in 28 day mortality, ICU length of stay, ventilator days, or organ failure scales between etomidate treated patients who received moderate dose steroids and those who received a saline control (42). Use of steroids likely should be reserved for septic shock patients with fluid and vasopressor refractory shock (24).

Etomidate remains an attractive induction agent for severe sepsis and septic shock patients. It has a rapid reliable onset and duration of action, which is critical in a highly unstable, hypoxemic patient. The hemodynamic profile is ideal in the setting of hemodynamic instability and potential anticipated clinical decompensation. Vulnerable elderly patients with co-morbidities seem less susceptible to injury with this agent. It has added beneficial effects that do not contribute to potential worsening organ failure.

The issue of adrenal insufficiency continues to give emergency and critical care practitioners pause in regards to use. Based on the most current literature, the corticosteroid insufficiency issue should be acknowledged and respected. At the same time, the current literature does not support an absolute mortality effect. As the intubation procedure under non-operative circumstances can be associated with complications, this reliable medication that preserves hemodynamic reflexes should remain in the induction armamentarium.

4.2. Midazolam

In reviewing available induction agents, midazolam should be included as an option. Midazolam is a member of the benzodiazepine class of medications. As with other benzodiazepines, the medication possesses sedative, hypnotic, amnestic, and anti-anxiolytic properties. The drug specifically is classified as an imidazobenzodiazepine (43). Due its unique structure, midazolam has a significantly rapid onset and short duration of action. These qualities make it an attractive induction medication.

As a benzodiazepine agent, midazolam exerts its influence on the GABA receptor. Midazolam binds to the GABA receptor and potentiates the inhibitory affect of GABA on the receptor (43).

Typical rapid sequence dosing is 0.1-0.3 mg/kg. Onset of action in intravenous dosing is 30-60 seconds. Duration of action is 15-30 minutes (43-45). The lipophilic nature of this drug accounts for its rapid uptake and onset of action. Its rapid metabolism and elimination are subject to several factors.

Midazolam is metabolized through the hepatic system. The cytochrome P450 system is the primary actor in midazolam breakdown. Cytochrome P450-3A4 hydroxylates midazolam to its metabolites, which are ultimately renally excreted (43). This makes midazolam metabolism subject to agents that may interfere with the cytochrome P450 system. Patients taking such agents as ranitidine or macrolide antibiotics may experience a decreased clearance of the medication (43). As elimination is through the renal system, patients with kidney dysfunction may experience a longer sedation period due to slower elimination time (43).

As an induction agent, midazolam has several favorable properties. The rapid action of this medication is a clear advantage. Critically ill patients have a very small respiratory and ventilatory reserve. Rapid action is crucial. The agent has anticonvulsant and muscle relaxant activity. The pharmacology literature has reported that midazolam directly relaxes the muscles of the airway (43). As endotrachael intubation requires optimum conditions, muscle relaxation presents a clear advantage. Midazolam as an agent is also not linked to vomiting and does not have a peripheral vascular irritant effect (45).

Midazolam does have noted cardiovascular effects. Use of midazolam will decrease both systolic and diastolic blood pressure (45). The primary mechanism appears to be vascular dilation and reduction of systemic vascular resistance (SVR) (45). This results in an increase in heart rate as part of the baroreceptor response. Clinicians should expect a lowering of blood pressure and an increase in patient heart rate with the use of this drug. Cardiac index is preserved (45). The degree of blood pressure reduction is not dependent on the presence of cardiac disease, but is more pronounced in cases of volume depletion (45).

The hypotensive effect of midazolam needs to be seriously scrutinized. A case series in the literature revealed at least a 10 percent reduction in systolic blood pressure in patients receiving midazolam for intubation (46). The reduction in blood pressure was doubled for patients age 70 years and older. Reduction in dose still precipitated hypotension in this report (46).

As endotracheal intubation physiologically predisposes a patient to hypotension, midazolam may not be the best induction agent for the severe sepsis and septic shock population. This patient population is often volume depleted and hypotensive prior to the procedure. Midazolam carries the risk of worsening an already tentative hemodynamic situation. Clinician should strongly consider alternative induction agents for this critically ill population.

4.3. Ketamine

Ketamine is a medication with a unique mechanism of action. Due to its many advantageous properties, this agent merits discussion. Structurally, ketamine resembles the hallucinogenic agent phencyclidine (PCP) (47). Ketamine acts as a dissociative agent. The medication essentially dissociates the thalamus from the limbic system. It is different from the previously discussed agents in that it does not interact with GABA receptors. Its primary mechanism of action is its antagonist effect on the excitatory N-methyl-D-aspartate receptor (NMDA) (48). Ketamine also interacts with opioid and muscarinic receptors, which contribute to its unusual qualities and effects (48). These qualities include sedative, hypnotic, analgesic, bronchodilator and cardiac stimulatory effects.

Dosing of ketamine for induction of intubation is typically 1-2 mg/kg (27,49). The sedative effects are rapid and initiate in approximately 30-60 seconds (27,48-49). Primary sedative effects dissipate within 10-15 minutes.

Ketamine is metabolized in the liver and excreted in urine (47). The primary mechanism of breakdown is through the cytochrome P450 system. Of note, decreased renal function does not effect duration of action as active ketamine metabolites are not excreted in the urine (47,51). Limited ketamine use for induction should not be impacted by renal disease. Induction doses of ketamine have not been well studied in severe liver disease. It is thought that a transient induction dose in liver dysfunction should not have a significant clinical impact (51). Certain medications can interfere with ketamine metabolism including diazepam and halothane (47). Prolonged use of ketamine is linked to elevation of liver enzymes (47).

As stated, ketamine has many favorable effects as an induction agent. It has a rapid onset and duration of action. In a potentially difficult, tenuous airway, where timing is critical, this is an important property. Ketamine has the unique ability to increase blood pressure. It is an actual cardiovascular stimulant (47). Ketamine increases heart rate, blood pressure and systemic vascular resistance (SVR) (47). Ketamine acts to increase these parameters through direct central stimulation of the autonomic nervous system and through indirect inhibition of catecholamine uptake (47, 52).

Unlike other agents, ketamine is not linked to hypotension. As the severe sepsis and septic shock patient is at high risk for hemodynamic instability, this stimulatory effect can be valuable. Ketamine has been reported to show a positive inotropic action. This property may be an advantage, as septic patient tend to have myocardial suppression (15). With increased cardiovascular stimulation, comes increased myocardial oxygen demand.

Clinicians will need to balance ketamine use in the setting of coronary artery disease (47). Overall, ketamine increases mean arterial pressure (MAP), SVR, and cardiac index (CI) (47-48,51-52).

Ketamine exhibits other pertinent abilities that merit consideration. Ketamine preserves airway reflexes and thus minimizes aspiration (51). Ketamine is a known bronchodialtor (47,49,51). In a high-risk airway or a patient with respiratory co-morbidities, these properties can give a care provider an additional benefit. In addition, ketamine has direct analgesic action, which may contribute to patient care during an uncomfortable procedure.

Ketamine has neurologic actions, which have generated controversy. Ketamine has both epileptic and anti-epileptic effects. Ketamine has been noted to change EEG patterns to match epileptiform patterns (47). At the same time, evidence of seizure causation is limited and even contradicted in the literature (53-54). Ketamine's impact on intracranial pressure has generated additional controversy. Initial early ketamine literature did report an increase intracranial pressure (47). A more recent literature review challenges these early reports and suggests a possible neuroprotective role for ketamine (55).

Ketamine does have adverse actions that need to be evaluated. Ketamine is associated with increase oral and airway secretions (47). The clinician needs to consider premedication with atropine or glycopyrrolate to counteract this effect. Ketamine does have a small independent risk factor for larnygospasm. The mechanism seems to be linked to airway sensitivity. Ketamine preserves airway reflexes and may cause increase airway responsiveness to secretions (56). Ketamine is connected to a phenomenon known as reemergence. Patients can experience hallucinations, alarming dreams and delirium. As the patient will be intubated, this phenomenon is less significant. It is also attenuated by concomitant benzodiazepines. Ketamine is associated with nausea and vomiting (51).

In review of ketamine, this medication is an option for severe sepsis and septic shock. It is rapidly acting with a short period of duration. Metabolism does not appear to be a significant concern. It preserves airway reflexes in a potentially high-risk situation. Unlike several agents, it does not cause hypotension. It is linked directly to an increase in blood pressure. This is of particular benefit in hypotensive, hemodynamically unstable patients. Ketamine has been shown to specifically improve hemodynamics in a septic shock case history (57). In a large, randomized, blinded study, ketamine and etomidate were both shown to have a comparable safety profile in critically ill patients (41). This particular cohort of over 400 patients included approximately 16% septic individuals. Clinicians do need to balance known adverse effects such as increased secretions and myocardial oxygen demand.

4.4. Propofol

Propofol is a unique induction mediator. It is an alkyl phenol with sedative, amnestic and anesthetic properties (58). Of note, propofol is highly water-insoluble. This necessitates that its commercial preparation dissolve the medication in a lipid emulsion consisting of soybean oil, egg lecithin and glycerol (59). Despite the egg component in the emulsion, current expert consensus does not indicate that an egg allergy prohibits the use of propofol (59).

At the same time, the lipophilic nature of this unusual drug contributes to its rapid onset and offset of activity (60). Propofol aptly crosses the blood brain barrier to exert its sedating effect. Propofol primarily acts on the GABA receptor and potentiates its activity (50). Induction dosing of propofol ranges from 1.5-3 mg/kg (58). Propofol initiates sedative effects within 20-40 seconds on intravenous administration . Duration of action is 5-10 minutes (58, 60-61).

Metabolism of propofol is through hepatic conjugation (60). The medication is renally excreted. It should be noted that chronic renal or hepatic insufficiency do not significantly affect propofol pharmacokinitcs. The use of prolonged propofol use has not been tested in these populations. The metabolism and elimination of propofol has also not been well studied in cases of acute renal or hepatic failure (58, 60).

There are certain populations to consider when adjusting dosing with propofol. Patients greater than 60 years old have a documented decreased clearance of the drug (58,60). This decreased elimination is thought to be secondary to decreased cardiac output and hepatic blood flow. The obese patients can present a challenge when using this medication as well. Propofol has an increased saturation in fatty tissue and a subsequent decrease in plasma clearance. Use of propofol in obese patients should be dosed according to ideal body weight in the obese patient to insure safety (60).

Propofol as an induction medication has attractive attributes. Its rapid onset of action and short duration of action is a definite benefit for the unstable patient who requires intubation. It also does not seem to be affected by chronic renal or hepatic insufficiency. Propofol has a known bronchodilator ability and has been used in patients with chronic obstructive pulmonary disease with success (60). Propofol also has anti-emetic properties as well (62). Such qualities suggest propofol has good potential as an induction drug.

For a patient with neurologic injury, propofol offers neuroprotective effects. Propofol has been shown to either maintain or reduce intracranial pressure in patients with neurologic injury (60). The medication also has been shown to improve cerebral auto-regulation.

Propofol does have certain qualities that limit its use. Propofol significantly reduces blood pressure. Studies have shown that propofol can reduce blood pressure 30% from baseline (58). Propofol exhibits this suppressive effect to a greater degree than other induction agents including certain barbiturates and midazolam (58, 60). The reduction in blood pressure is presumed to be due to a decrease in systemic vascular resistance and cardiac contractility (60). Propofol also reduces heart rate despite the reduction in blood pressure. The medication has been linked to prolonged bradycardia (58). Elderly patients seem to be particularly susceptible to these effects. Research has shown a decrease in cardiac index in elderly surgical patients who received propofol (58). These effects will give the clinician pause when approaching the hemodynamically unstable, volume depleted, or elderly patient. As severe sepsis and septic shock patients can potentially be included in such categories; propofol appears to be a less ideal medication.

Propofol appears to impact the immune system. The lipid emulsion component of propofol has been shown to have some suppressive affect on the immune system (60). Propofol in one study exhibited inhibitory effects on neutraphil function (62). Of note, the effect appears to be more significant in cases of prolonged infusion.

Propofol has additional issues to address. Though transient, propofol does cause pain at the site of injection. If a propofol infusion is used after induction, the phenomenon of propofol infusion syndrome needs to be considered. Propofol infusion syndrome is an often-fatal entity that consists of metabolic acidosis, renal failure, cardiac failure and rhabdomyolysis. It is linked to prolonged propofol infusion at higher doses. The disease also is connected to pressor and steroid use in conjunction with propofol (64). This problem will not affect short-term induction use. The clinician does need to be mindful that initiating a propofol infusion may be detrimental to a sepsis patient who may later require vasopressors or steroids.

In general, the unfavorable hemodynamic profile displayed by propofol does not make it an ideal mediator for intubation in severe sepsis and septic shock patients. The negative effects likely outweigh its rapid action and other positive attributes. This is especially pertinent in the light of the hemodynamic changes induced by endotracheal intubation itself.

4.5. Thiopental and methohexital

Thiopental and methohexital are barbiturate sedative induction agents. Due to their rapid onset of action, these two medications are classified as ultra short acting. As barbiturates, thiopental and methohexital exhibit their effect at the level of the inhibitory GABA receptor (50). Thiopental also may have a secondary mechanism of inhibiting the NMDA receptors (50). These processes lead to the expected effect of sedation.

Typical induction dose for thiopental is 3-5 mg/kg (50,65). Methohexital is usually dosed at 1-2 mg/kg (50,66-67). Both agents have a swift onset of action at 10-30 seconds (50). Thiopental is rapidly metabolized and has a duration of 5-10 minutes (50). Methohexital is metabolized 3-4 times more quickly than thiopental and has a duration of action of 4-7 minutes (50,68). The duration of action is comparable despite the faster metabolism of methohexital. This originates from the fact that actual clinical effect is due to redistribution of the medication in the body. In both agents, redistribution to other tissues is swift (50).

Metabolism of both these barbiturates is hepatic with renal elimination. Due to a balance in clearance and elimination, renal insufficiency does not seem to impact thiopental dosing or duration of action. Of note, phenobarbital is one of the few barbiturates affected by renal dysfunction. Plasma clearance of thiopental also remains unaffected by cirrhosis or decreased hepatic blood flow (65). There are factors that do impact duration of action and dosing. Decreased clearance of thiopental in elderly patients indicates a reduction in dose for expected onset of effect. Some authors recommend a reduction in dose of 25-50% for older individuals. Half-life of thiopental is increased in younger females and obese individuals (65).

As an induction drug, both thiopental and methohexital have a rapid onset and short duration of action. These qualities make these medications potential options for critically ill patients with a need for rapid airway management. Thiopental has significant neuroprotective effects as well. The medication has been shown to decrease intracranial pressure, cerebral oxygen demand , and to decrease the actions of damaging neuro-excitatory transmitters (65). Critically ill patients with brain injury may reap the reward of these beneficial actions.

Thiopental and methohexital do have a marked negative impact on the cardiovascular system. Thiopental has been shown to profoundly lower mean arterial pressure and cardiac output (65). The primary mechanism appears to be vasodilatation. The negative inotropic effect is not entirely defined. There also tends to be a resulting increase in heart rate. Increased heart rate can negatively impact an already tachycardic septic patient or a patient with coronary artery disease. These agents do not appear to offer any benefit to the hemodynamically unstable or volume depleted patient.

There are added negative aspects of barbiturates as induction agents for septic patients. The barbiturates appear to impact immunosuppression. Both thiopental and methohexital were linked to inhibition of granulocyte recruitment and phagocytosis (69). Thiopental has also been linked directly to lymphocyte destruction (70). These agents appear to have a potential negative impact on the immune system response.

Thiopental and methohexital have other concerning attributes. Methohexital has been linked to laryngospasm (68). Both medications have been connected to bronchospasm and are not recommended for patients with asthma (50,65,68,71). Both these agents are contraindicated in cases of porphyria. The medications may increase the activity of γ-aminolevulinic acid synthetase and precipitate an acute episode (50,68).

These agents for multiple reasons do not appear to be ideal induction agents for severe sepsis and septic shock patients. Of note, thiopental is not manufactured in the United States as of 2011.

4.6. Dexmedetomidine

Dexmedetomidine is a newer sedative medication under investigation as an adjunct to intubation. It is currently approved primarily for sedation of critically ill patients in the intensive care environment. As it is a potential intubation facilitator, it will be mentioned in this chapter. It has many potential pitfalls that do not make it ideal for use in severe sepsis and septic shock.

Dexmedetomidine is a centrally acting alpha-2 agonist with sedative, amnestic, and sympatholytic properties. It has the additive effect of preserving airway reflexes (72-74). Due to these properties, it is under evaluation as an adjunct for awake fiberoptic intubation (73).

As an induction agent, dexmedetomidine is not as rapid as the other discussed agents. Use in the intubating environment requires a bolus of 0.5-1 mcg/kg over 10 minutes (73-75). An infusion follows ranging from 0.2-0.7 mcg/kg/hour until the procedure is complete (73, 75). This is not consistent with the rapid acting agents previously discussed. The medication does offers a significant degree of sedation, comfort and airway protection. For the particularly high-risk airway, this drug creates an environment of "cooperative anesthesia" and has been shown to facilitate the awake intubation (73). The medication again is not as short acting as other medications reviewed. Onset of action is in 5-10 minutes and duration of action extends from 60-120 minutes. When time is critical, dexmedetomidine nay not fit the best pharmacologic profile

Dexmedetomidine is metabolized through the hepatic system. Unlike several of the previously described agents, drug clearance is impacted by hepatic failure and low hepatic blood flow. Elimination is through renal and fecal routes (74). In regards to metabolism, elderly patients have been found to be particularly sensitive to dexmedetomidine. Reduction of bolus dosing in this population is encouraged (74).

As an alpha-2 agonist, dexmedetomidine causes a decrease in mean arterial blood pressure and heart rate. Of note, With the initial bolus, a transient increase of mean arterial pressure can occur (50,74). This is felt to be due to a temporary stimulation of peripheral alpha-2 receptors (50,74). Overall, dexmedetomidine reduces MAP, SVR, cardiac index and heart rate. These attributes are dose dependent and have been diminished with dose reduction or elimination of bolus administration. Dexmedetomidine has been linked to sinus arrest during intubation (74). In a hemodynamically, volume depleted, or inotropically challenged patient this side effect profile is not helpful. As severe sepsis and septic shock patients have many of these attributes, dexmedetomidine may not be the best induction option.

Dexmedetomidine does deserve mention, as it is becoming a select option for induction and sedation. Dexmedetomidine preserves airway integrity, ventilatory response and reduces risk of bronchconstriction (74). In a tenuous airway situation, such qualities are clearly favorable.

While not a first line induction choice, dexmedetomidine may have a role in the sedation of sepsis patients under the appropriate circumstances. Dexmedetomidine appears to have anti-inflammatory properties. In one study, the use of dexmedetomidine reduced the serum levels of tumor necrosis factor (TNF), interleukin-1 and interleukin-6 in comparison to midazolam (76). Use of dexmedetomidine as a sedative agent in another case study reduced delirium, ventilator days, and 28-day mortality in comparison to lorazepam (77). While the medication may not be an optimal emergency intubation agent, future avenues in its use as a sedative are intriguing.

4.7. Methoxycarbonyl-etomidate (MOC-etomidate) and carboetomidate

Etomidate as discussed has a very favorable profile in regards to use in severe sepsis and septic shock. The controversy ensues in regard to etomidate's tendency to suppress the adrenal axis (31-32). In the interest of remaining up to date, it is important to mention etomidate analogues that may resolve the adrenal suppression debate.

Methoxycarbonyl-etomidate is an ultra short-acting analogue of etomidate (78). It was designed to maintain the favorable hemodynamic profile of etomidate and avoid the adrenal axis suppression component. Like etomidate, MOC-etomidate does act at the GABA receptor. In recent animal studies, this medication exhibited similar sedative potency and was found to have a half-life of 4 minutes as opposed to 40 minutes for etomidate (78). In initial promising research, the drug did not impact adrenal function. This may be due to its extremely swift onset and metabolism. There was some decreased potency in comparison to etomidate and its ultra rapid action will be a factor in future dosing. Multiple questions remain and this data remains extremely preliminary. It is important for the clinician to be aware of the next generation of agents.

Carboetomidate is another analog designed for a better side effect profile as well. Carboetomidate generation focused specifically on adrenal suppression issues (79). The medication was designed to have a reduced affinity for 11 β–hydroxylase. This particular analog maintained a similar hypnotic effect to etomidate, a stable hemodynamic profile, and had a third less adrenal suppression activity. It also did have a slightly less hypnotic effect in regards to etomidate (79). Carboetomidate remains another future potential agent in the care of critically ill patients. Clearly, ongoing research is required.

5. Conclusions

As reviewed, endotracheal intubation of the critically ill septic patient is one of the most significant challenges an emergency medicine or critical care practitioner will face. The intubation procedure itself is associated with profound physiologic changes. Performing this procedure on a patient with underlying hemodynamic, respiratory, and additional organ compromise can be arduous. Agents to rapidly and safely accomplish this procedure need to be chosen. The caregiver needs to be aware of induction agent side effects, mechanism of action, metabolism, and duration of action. This knowledge is as important as the actual procedural skill. Intubation under adverse circumstances can be worsened with poor choice in induction mediator.

Severe sepsis and septic shock is a particularly special circumstance. Critically ill septic patients are literally a maelstrom of organ failure. Induction mediators can help or hinder an already difficult task. This chapter is designed to facilitate the best choices for this particular patient care scenario.

In review of induction medications, rapid onset with short duration of action, preservation of hemodynamic parameters, and low adverse side effect profile are key components for success. Table 1 summarizes the qualities of the previously discussed agents. For severe sepsis and septic shock, two particular candidates rise to the occasion. Ketamine and etomidate appear to be the best current induction options.

The recommendation of etomidate may elicit some controversy. The adrenal suppression effect of this medication is well described in the literature. At the same time, multiple studies continue to show a paucity in mortality impact. The endocrine suppression is evident. The mortality figures are not. For rapid, reliable induction without hemodynamic compromise in a critical moment, etomidate does serve this purpose. Future agents and analogues may make this controversy obsolete.

Induction agent	Class	Dose (IV)	Onset of Action	Duration of Action	Metabolism	Hemodynamic Effects	Special Consideration
Etomidate	Non-barbiturate Sedative hypnotic	0.3mg/kg	5-15 sec	5-14 min	Hepatic	None or slight decrease in MAP Minimal impact on SVR/ CI/ SV	Preservation of hemodynamic status Neuroprotective Adrenal suppression
Midazolam	Benzodiazepine	0.1-0.3 mg/kg	30-60 sec	15-30 min	Hepatic	Decreased MAP/SVR	Risk of hypotension Affected by renal insufficiency
Ketamine	Dissociative	1-2 mg/kg	30-60 sec	10-15 minutes	Hepatic	Increased MAP/ SVR/ CI	Increased myocardial oxygen consumption Increased secretions
Propofol	Non-barbiturate Sedative hypnotic	1.5-3 mg/kg	20-40 sec	5-10 minutes	Hepatic	Decreased MAP/SVR/ CI	Caution with elderly patients Risk of hypotension
Thiopental	Barbiturate	3-5 mg/kg	10-30 sec	5-10 minutes	Hepatic	Decreased MAP/SVR/ CI	Risk of hypotension Vasodilator Immunosuppression
Methohexital	Barbiturate	1-2 mg/kg	10-30 sec	4-7 minutes	Hepatic	Decreased MAP/SVR/ CI	Risk of hypotension Vasodilator Immunosuppression
Dexmedetomidine	Non-barbiturate Sedative hypnotic	0.5-1 mcg/kg over 10 minutes Drip 0.2-0.7 mcg/kg hour	5-10 minutes	60 -120 minutes	Hepatic	Decreased MAP/ SVR/ CI Reduced heart rate	Risk of hypotension Risk of bradycardia

MAP- Mean arterial pressure, SVR- Systemic vascular resistance, CI- Cardiac index, SV- Stroke volume

Table 1. Summary of Induction Agent Attributes

Ketamine is another agent that appears well suited for induction of the severe sepsis and septic shock patient. Ketamine preserves airway reflexes, increases blood pressure and systemic vascular resistance, and serves as a bronchodilator. In a prospective trial, ketamine and etomidate exhibited a similar safety profile for a wide range of critically ill patients; including patients with sepsis (41). Due to increased myocardial oxygen consumption, ketamine may be a less optimal choice for patients with known coronary artery disease.

All other agents discussed suppress the hemodynamic profile to some degree. Best choice for intubation induction for severe sepsis and septic shock remains etomidate and ketamine. Circumstances may preclude the use of these agents. The practicing clinician is cautioned to review the remaining sedation agents carefully in the context of the clinical picture. In the case that the need arises for another drug choice, the most rapid acting medication with the least duration of action and least adverse side effect profile should be administered. The informed clinician needs to be aware of the side effect profile and prepare accordingly.

Successful intubation in severe sepsis and septic shock patients is a critical skill. Choosing the best medication to accomplish this task is a significant component of the battle. The well-informed practitioner can make all the difference in this challenging situation.

Author details

Marie Mullen
Department of Emergency Medicine, University of Massachusetts, Worcester, MA, USA

6. References

[1] Linde-Zwirble WT, Angus DC. Severe sepsis epidemiology: Sampling, selection, and society. *Crit Care Med* 8 (2004) : 222–226.
[2] Angus DC, Linde-Zwirble WT, Lidicker J, et al. Epidemiology of severe sepsis in the United States: Analysis of incidence, outcome, and associated costs of care. *Crit Care Med* 29 (2001): 1303–1310.
[3] Annane D, Aegerter P, Jars-Guincestre MC, Guidet B. Current epidemiology of septic shock: the CUB-Rea Network. *Am J Respir Crit Care Med* 168 (2003): 165-172.
[4] Piantadosi C, Schwartz D. The Acute Respiratory Distress Syndrome. *Ann Intern Med* 141(2004): 460-470.
[5] Rubenfeld GD, Herridge MS. Epidemiology and outcomes of acute lung injury. *Chest* 131 (2007): 554–562.
[6] Pepe PE, Potkin R, Holtman-Reus D, Hudson L, Carico J. Clinical predictors of the adult respiratory distress syndrome. *Am J Surg* 144 (1982): 124-128.
[7] Montgomery AB, Stager MA, Carrico CJ, Hudson LD. Causes of mortality in patients with the adult respiratory distress syndrome. *Am Rev Respir Dis* 132 (1985): 485–489.
[8] Kaplan R, Sahn S, Petty T: Incidence and Outcome of the Respiratory Distress Syndrome in Gram-Negative Sepsis. *Arch Intern Med* 139.8 (1979): 867-869.

[9] Eggimann P, Harbarth S, Ricou B, Hugonnet S, et al. Acute Respiratory Distress Syndrome after Bacteremic Sepsis Does Not Increase Mortality. *Am J Respir Crit Care Med* 167 (2003): 1210–1214.
[10] Brun-Buisson C, Meshaka P, Pinton P, Vallet B: EPISEPSIS Study Group: EPISEPSIS: a reappraisal of the epidemiology and outcome of severe sepsis in French intensive care units. *Intensive Care Med* 30 (2004): 580-588.
[11] Bernard GR, Vincent JL, Laterre PF, LaRosa SP, et al. Recombinant human protein C Worldwide Evaluation in Severe Sepsis (PROWESS) study group: Efficacy and safety of recombinant human activated protein C for severe sepsis. *N Engl J Med* 344 (2001): 699-709.
[12] Vincent JL, Sakr Y, Sprung CL, Ranieri VM, et al. Sepsis Occurrence in Acutely Ill Patients Investigators: Sepsis in European intensive care units: results of the SOAP Study. *Crit Care Med* 34 (2006): 344-353.
[13] Blanco J, Muriel-Bombín1 A, Sagredo V, Taboada F, et al. Incidence, organ dysfunction and mortality in severe sepsis: a Spanish multicentre study. *Critical Care* 12 (2008): R158.
[14] Madger S. Bench-to-bedside review: Ventilatory abnormalities in sepsis. *Crit Care* 13.1 (2009): 202.
[15] Parker MM, Shelhamer JH, Bacharach SL, et al. Profound but reversible myocardial depression in patients with septic shock. *Ann Intern Med* 100 (1984): 483-490.
[16] Weingart S, Levitan R. Preoxygenation and Prevention of Desaturation During Emergency Airway Management. *Annals of Emergency Medicine* 59.3 (2012): 165–175.
[17] Benumof J, Dagg R, Benumof R. Critical hemoglobin desaturation will occur before return to an unparalyzed state following 1-mg/kg intravenous succinylcholine. *Anesthesiology* 87 (1997): 979–982.
[18] Griesdale D, Bosma T, Kurth T, Isac G, et al. Complications of endotracheal intubation in the critically ill. *Intensive Care Med* 34 (2008): 1835–1842.
[19] Schwartz D, Matthay M, Cohen NH. Death and other complications of emergency airway management in critically ill adults. A prospective investigation of 297 tracheal intubations. *Anesthesiology* 82 (1995): 367–376.
[20] Walz J, Zayaruzny M, Heard S. Airway management in critical illness. *Chest* 131 (2007): 608–620.
[21] Manthous C. Avoiding Circulatory Complications During Endotracheal Intubation and Initiation of Positive Pressure Ventilation. *The Journal of Emergency Medicine* 38.5 (2010): 622–631.
[22] Pinsky M. The hemodynamic consequences of mechanical ventilation: an evolving story. *Intensive Care Medicine* 23 (1997): 493–503.
[23] Farmery A, Roe P. A model to describe the rate of oxyhaemoglobin desaturation during apnoea. *Br J Anaesth* 76 (1996): 284–291.
[24] Dellinger R, Levy M, Carlet J, et al. Surviving Sepsis Campaign: International guidelines for management of severe sepsis and septic shock. *Crit Care Med* 36 (2008): 296–327.
[25] Levy M, Fink M, Marshall J, Abraham E, et al. 2001 SCCM/ESICM/ACCP/ATS/SIS International Sepsis Definitions Conference. *Crit Care Med* 31.4 (2003): 1250-1256.

[26] Yang J, Uchida I: Mechanisms of etomidate potentiation of GABAA receptor-gated currents in cultured postnatal hippocampal neurons. *Neuroscience* 73.1(1996): 69-78.
[27] Walls R: Airway. In Marx J, et al (eds.). Rosen's Emergency Medicine. Philadelphia. Elsevier/Mosby. 2009. 3-22
[28] Bergen J, Smith D. A review of etomidate for rapid sequence intubation in the emergency department. *J Emerg Med* 15 (1997): 221-230.
[29] Criado A, Maseda J, Navarro E. et al. Induction of anaesthesia with etomidate: haemodynamic study of 36 patients. *Br J Anaesthesia* 52 (1980): 803-806.
[30] Kettler D, Sonntag H, Donath U, et al. Hemodynamics, myocardial mechanics, oxygen requirements, and oxygen consumption of the human heart during induction of anaesthesia with etomidate. *Anaesthesist* 23(1974): 116-121.
[31] Jong F, Mallios C, Jansen C, Scheck P. Etomidate Suppresses Adrenocortical Function by Inhibition of 11 ◉-Hydroxylation. *Journal of Clinical Endocrinology and Metabolism* 59.6 (1984): 1143-1147.
[32] Schenarts CL, Burton JH, Riker RR. Adrenocortical dysfunction following etomidate induction in emergency department patients. *Acad Emerg Med* 8.1 (2001): 1–7.
[33] Annane D, Sebille V, Charpentier C et al. Effect of treatment with low doses of hydrocortisone and fludrocortisone on mortality in patients with septic shock. *JAMA* 288.7 (2002): 862–871.
[34] den Brinker M, Joosten KF, Liem O et al. Adrenal insufficiency in meningococcal sepsis: bioavailable cortisol levels and impact of interleukin-6 levels and intubation with etomidate on adrenal function and mortality. *J Clin Endocrinol Metab* 90.9 (2005): 5110–5117.
[35] Malerba G, Romano-Girard F, Cravoisy A, et al. Risk factors of relative adrenocortical deficiency in intensive care patients needing mechanical ventilation. *Intensive Care Med* 31.3 (2005): 388–392.
[36] Sprung CL, Annane D, Keh D et al. Hydrocortisone therapy for patients with septic shock. *N Engl J Med* 358.2 (2008): 111–124.
[37] Ehrman R, Wira C, Lomax A, Hayward A, et al. Etomidate use in severe sepsis and septic shock patients does not contribute to mortality. *Intern Emerg Med* 6 (2011): 253–257.
[38] Dmello D, Taylor S, O'Brien J, Matuschak G. Outcomes of Etomidate in Severe Sepsis and Septic Shock. *Chest* 138.6 (2010): 1327-1332.
[39] Tekwani K, Watts H, Sweis R, Rzechula K, Kulstad E. A Prospective Observational Study of the Effect of Etomidate on Septic Patient Mortality and Length of Stay. *Acad Emerg Med* 16.1 (2009): 11–14.
[40] Tekwani K, Watts H, Sweis R, Rzechula K, Kulstad E. A Comparison of the Effects of Etomidate and Midazolam on Hospital Length of Stay in Patients With Suspected Sepsis: A Prospective, Randomized Study. *Annals of Emergency Medicine* 56 (2010):481–489.
[41] Jabre P, Combes X, Lapostolle F et al. Etomidate versus ketamine for rapid sequence intubation in acutely ill patients: a multicentre randomised controlled trial. *Lancet* 374(2009): 293–300.

[42] Payen, J, Dupuis C, Trouve-Buisson T, Vinclair M, et al. Corticosteroid After Etomidate in Critically Ill Patients. *Crit Care Med* 40.1(2012): 29-35.
[43] Nordt S, Clark R. Midazolam: a review of therapeutic uses and toxicity. *J Emerg Med* 15.3 (1997): 357-365.
[44] Sagarin M, Barton E, Sakles J, Vissers R, et al and On behalf of the National Emergency Airway Registry (NEAR) Investigators. Underdosing of Midazolam in Emergency Endotracheal Intubation. *Academic Emergency Medicine* 10 (2003): 329–338.
[45] Reves J, Fragen R, Vinik H, et al. Midazolam: Pharmacology and uses. *Anesthesiology* 62 (1985): 310-324.
[46] Choi Y, Wong T, Lau C. Midazolam is more likely to cause hypotension than etomidate in emergency department rapid sequence intubation. *Emerg Med J* 21.6 (2004): 700-702.
[47] Reich D, Sivay G. Ketamine: an update on the first twenty-five years of clinical experience. *Canadian Journal of Anesthesia* 36.2 (1989): 186-197.
[48] Hirota K, Lambert D. Ketamine: its mechanism(s) of action and unusual clinical uses. *Br J Anaesth.* 77.4 (1996): 441-444.
[49] Porter K. Ketaminc in prehospital care. *Emerg Med J* 21 (2004): 351-354.
[50] Reves JG, et al. Intravenous anesthetics. In Miller R, et al (eds): Miller's Anesthesia. Philadelphia, Elsevier/Churchill Livingstone. 2009: 719-768.
[51] Taylor, E: Ketamine. In Bissonette B (ed.) Pediatric Anesthesia. Shelton, CT. People's Medical Publishing House. 2011: 376-386.
[52] Hanouz JL, Persehaye E, Zhu L, Lammens S, et al. The inotropic and lusitropic effects of ketamine in isolated human atrial myocardium: the effect of adrenoceptor blockade. *Anesth Analg* 99.6 (2004): 1689-1695.
[53] Corssen G, Little S, Tavakoli M. Ketamine and Epilepsy. *Anesth Analg.* 53.2 (1974): 319-335.
[54] Pruss H, Koltcamp M. Ketamine successfully terminates malignant status epilepticus. *Epilepsy Research* 82 (2008): 219-222.
[55] Himmelseher S, Durieux M. Revising a dogma: ketamine for patients with neurological injury? *Anesth Analg* 101.2 (2005): 524-534.
[56] Green S, Krauss B. Clinical Practice Guideline for Emergency Department Ketamine Dissociative Sedation in Children. *Annals of Emerg Med* 44.5 (2004): 460-471.
[57] Yli-Hankala A, Kirvelä M, Randell T, Lindgren L. Ketamine anaesthesia in a patient with septic shock. *Acta Anaesthesiologica Scandinavica* 36.5 (1992): 483–485.
[58] Sebel P, Lowden J. Propofol: A New Intravenous Anesthetic. *Anesthesiology* 71.2 (1989): 260-277.
[59] Hepner D, Castells M. Anaphylaxis During the Perioperative Period. *Anesth Analg* 97.5 (2003): 1381-1395.
[60] McKeage K, Perry C. Propofol: a review of its use in intensive care sedation of adults. *CNS Drugs* 17.4 (2003): 235-72.
[61] Hopson L, Schwartz R. Pharmacologic Adjuncts to Intubation. In Roberts J, Hedges J (eds): Clinical Procedures in Emergency Medicine. Philadelphia Elsevier/Saunders. 2010: 99-107.

[62] Skues M, Prys-Roberts C. The pharmacology of Propofol. *J Clin. Anesth* 1.5 (1989): 387-400.

[63] Inada T, Taniuchi S, Shingu K, Kobayashi Y, et al. Propofol depressed neutrophil hydrogen peroxide production more than midazolam, whereas adhesion molecule expression was minimally affected by both anesthetics in rats with abdominal sepsis. *Anesth Analg* 92.2 (2001): 437-441.

[64] Vasile B, Rasulo F, Candiani A, Latronico N. Propofol infusion syndrome. *Intensive Care Med 29* (2003): 1417–1425.

[65] Russo H, Bressolle F, Pharmacodynamics and pharmacokinetics of thiopental. *Clin Pharmacokinet* 35.2 (1998): 95-134.

[66] Doze V, Westphal L, White P. Comparison of propofol with methohexital for outpatient Anesthesia. *Anesth Analg* 65.11 (1986): 1189-1195.

[67] Avramov MN, Husain M, White P. The comparative effects of methohexital, propofol, and etomidate for electroconvulsive therapy. *Anesth Analg* 81.3 (1995): 596-602.

[68] Martone C, Nagelhout J, Wolf S. Methohexital: a practical review for outpatient dental anesthesia. *Anesth Prog* 38.6 (1991): 195–199.

[69] Ploppa A, Kiefer R, Nohé B, Haeberle H, et al. Dose-dependent influence of barbiturates but not of propofol on human leukocyte phagocytosis of viable Staphylococcus aureus. *Crit Care Med.* 34.2 (2006): 478-483.

[70] Keel M, Mica L, Stover J, Stocker R, et al. Thiopental-induced apoptosis in lymphocytes is independent of CD95 activation. *Anesthesiology* 103.3 (2005): 576-584.

[71] Hirota K, Ohtomo N, Hashimoto Y, Kudo T, et al. Effects of thiopental on airway calibre in dogs: direct visualization method using a superfine fibreoptic bronchoscope. *Br J Anaesth* 81.2 (1998): 203-207.

[72] Brummett C. Dexmedetomidine: A Clinical Review. *Seminars in Anesthesia, Perioperative Medicine and Pain* 25.2 (2006):41–42.

[73] Unger R, Gallagher C. Dexmedetomidine sedation for awake fiberoptic intubation. *Seminars in Anesthesia, Perioperative Medicine and Pain*, 25.2 (2006): 65-70.

[74] Wagner D, Brummett C. Dexmedetomidine: as safe as safe can be. *Seminars in Anesthesia, Perioperative Medicine and Pain* 25.2 (2006): 73-83.

[75] Lacy CF, et al. (Eds). Lexi-Comp's Drug Information Handbook, 21st ed. Lexi-Comp Inc, Hudson, OH. 2012.

[76] Memiş D, Hekimoğlu S, Vatan I, Yandim T, et al. Effects of midazolam and dexmedetomidine on inflammatory responses and gastric intramucosal pH to sepsis, in critically ill patients. *Br J Anaesth.* 98.4 (2007): 550-552.

[77] Pandharipande P, Sanders R, Girard T, McGrane S. Effect of dexmedetomidine versus lorazepam on outcome in patients with sepsis: an a priori-designed analysis of the MENDS randomized controlled trial. *Crit Care* 14.2 (2010): R38.

[78] Cotten J, Husain S, Forman S, et al. Methoxycarbonyl-etomidate: a novel rapidly metabolized and ultra-short-acting etomidate analogue that does not produce prolonged adrenocortical suppression. *Anesthesiology* 111 (2009): 240–249.

[79] Cotten J, Forman S, Laha J, et al. Carboetomidate: A pyrrole analog of etomidate designed not to suppress adrenocortical function. *Anesthesiology* 112 (2010): 637–644.